W9-AFF-237

Pathology of
the Uterine Cervix,
Vagina, and Vulva

OTHER MONOGRAPHS IN THE SERIES *MAJOR PROBLEMS IN PATHOLOGY*

VIRGINIA A. LIVOLSI, M.D.
Series Editor

Published

Katzenstein: *Katzenstein and Askin's Surgical Pathology of Non-Neoplastic Lung Disease,* 3rd edition

Striker, Striker, and D'Agati: *The Renal Biopsy,* 3rd edition

Fox: *Pathology of the Placenta,* 2nd edition

Isaacs: *Tumors of the Fetus and Newborn*

Foster and Bostwick: *Pathology of the Prostate*

Carter and Patchefsky: *Tumors and Tumor-like Lesions of the Lung*

Helliwell: *Pathology of Bone and Joint Neoplasms*

Neiman and Orazi: *Disorders of the Spleen,* 2nd edition

Owen and Kelly: *Pathology of the Gallbladder, Biliary Tract, and Pancreas*

Virmani, Burke, Farb, and Atkinson: *Cardiovascular Pathology,* 2nd edition

Forthcoming

Leonard: *Diagnostic Molecular Pathology*

Foster and Ross: *Pathology of the Urinary Bladder*

LiVolsi: *Pathology of the Thyroid,* 2nd edition

Tomaszewski: *Renal Neoplasms*

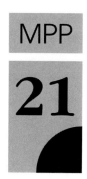

MPP

21

YAO S. FU, M.D.

Senior Pathologist
Chief of Anatomic Pathology
Department of Pathology
Northridge Hospital Medical Center
Northridge, California

Pathology of the Uterine Cervix, Vagina, and Vulva

Volume 21 in the Series
MAJOR PROBLEMS IN PATHOLOGY

second edition

SAUNDERS
An Imprint of Elsevier Science
PHILADELPHIA LONDON NEW YORK ST. LOUIS SYDNEY TORONTO

SAUNDERS
An Imprint of Elsevier Science

The Curtis Center
Independence Square West
Philadelphia, PA 19106

PATHOLOGY OF THE UTERINE CERVIX, VAGINA, AND VULVA   ISBN 0–7216–5756–7
Copyright 2002, 1989, Elsevier Science (USA). All rights reserved.

No part of this publication may be reproduced, stored in a retrieval system, or transmitted in any form or by any means, electronic, mechanical, photocopying, recording, or otherwise, without prior permission of the publishers (Saunders, The Curtis Center, Independence Square West, Philadelphia, PA 19106-3399).

Notice

Pharmacology is an ever-changing field. Standard safety precautions must be followed, but as new research and clinical experience broaden our knowledge, changes in treatment and drug therapy may become necessary or appropriate. Readers are advised to check the most current product information provided by the manufacturer of each drug to be administered to verify the recommended dose, the method and duration of administration, and contraindications. It is the responsibility of the treating physician, relying on experience and knowledge of the patient, to determine dosages and the best treatment for each individual patient. Neither the Publisher nor the editor assumes any liability for any injury and/or damage to persons or property arising from this publication.

The Publisher

First Edition 1989

Library of Congress Cataloging-in-Publication Data

Fu, Yao S.
    Pathology of the uterine cervix, vagina, and vulva / Yao S. Fu—2nd ed.
      p.; cm.—(Major problems in pathology ; v. 21)
    Includes bibliographical references and index.
    ISBN 0–7216–5756–7
    1. Cervix uteri—Diseases.   2. Vagina—Diseases.   3. Vulva—Diseases.   I. Title.   II. Series.
    [DNLM: 1. Cervix Uteri—pathology.   2. Vagina—pathology.   3. Vulva—pathology.   WP
470 F949p 2002]
RG310 .F8 2002
614.1—dc21   2002017020

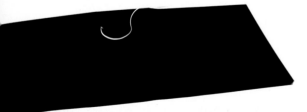

MA/MVY

Printed in the United States of America
Last digit is the print number: 9   8   7   6   5   4   3   2   1

To James W. Reagan, M.D. (1918–1987)
A pioneer in cytopathology and gynecologic pathology,
a great pathologist with immense experience and integrity,
and an inspiring and caring mentor

To my family,
Anne, Karin, Victor, and Eva,
with love

Preface

Since the publication of the first edition in 1989, diagnosis and management of diseases of the female lower genital tract have undergone significant changes. In the current edition, the basic information and the best classic figures from the first edition are retained. New data are added to provide a better understanding of the pathophysiology of the disease processes. Their gross and microscopic diagnostic features, particularly differential diagnosis, are emphasized and complemented by the use of immunohistochemical stains and ultrastructural studies. Illustrations of tumors include not only the typical ones, but also the less common variations. Specialized techniques and pathologic parameters relevant to the prognosis and management of patients are discussed. As with the first edition, the goal of the current edition is to make accurate pathologic evaluations an integral part of clinical decisions.

I am indebted to Diane Voigt and Joyce Masloski for their excellent secretarial assistance and to my colleagues Dr. Warren Allen and Dr. Carl Sohn for their support. I am grateful to Acquisitions Editor Natasha Andjelkovic, Ph.D., and to Senior Project Manager Lee Ann Draud at Elsevier Science for solving problems and producing a fine book.

YAO S. FU, M.D.

Contents

1

HANDLING AND REPORTING OF SPECIMENS FOR PATHOLOGIC EXAMINATION

The anatomic location of the cervix, vagina, and vulva allows diseases of these sites to be detected by direct visual examination, microbiologic cultures, cytologic smears, and tissue biopsies. On the basis of these initial findings, further diagnostic procedures or therapy may be planned. Optimal histologic studies depend on proper processing, embedding, and preparation of tissue samples. Pertinent clinical information provided by the physician further enhances the pathologic interpretation and reduces the possibility of misinterpretation and the resulting potentially grave consequences. In reporting the results, the pathologist should provide an accurate evaluation of the disease process, including factors related to further planning of diagnostic procedures, therapy, and prognosis. In this chapter, proper handling and reporting of specimens from the female lower genital tract are discussed.

TYPES OF SPECIMENS SUBMITTED FROM THE UTERINE CERVIX

Biopsy

Obtaining the Sample

Punch biopsies of the cervix may be taken from clinically apparent abnormalities, such as erosion, ulcer, white epithelium, space-occupying lesions, and otherwise abnormal-appearing epithelium. Biopsy may also be performed under the guidance of colposcopy to confirm an abnormality initially detected by cellular studies. The colposcope, a stereoscopic microscope with an attached illuminating system, enables the gynecologist to visualize the transformation zone and surface abnormalities at a magnification of 6 to 50. Local application of 1% to 2% acetic acid helps to remove excess mucus and secretions, dehydrates the epithelium, and enhances the visualization of the vasculature.

The abnormal squamous epithelium with increased cellularity gives a white and opaque ap-

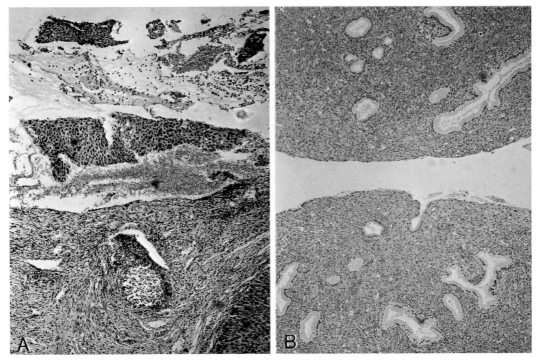

Figure 1–1. *A,* Partially fragmented and denuded dysplastic epithelium resulting from excessive trauma at the time of biopsy. *B,* The endocervical epithelium is completely denuded following dilation and curettage (D&C). (H&E)

pearance, sometimes with an uneven surface and irregular contour. Capillaries in the stromal papillae present as punctate dots and a mosaic pattern characterized by honeycomb-like islands of epithelium demarcated by dilated capillaries. With invasive carcinomas, the abnormal vessels become engorged and tortuous. Colposcopy has also been used to delineate vaginal, vulvar, and penile lesions.

Because most cervices harboring intraepithelial neoplasia have no distinct gross abnormalities, colposcopic examination delineates the abnormal areas for biopsy and determines the extent of disease. When the entire lesion and squamocolumnar junction are visualized, the examination is referred to as satisfactory or adequate. Depending on the size and appearance of the abnormal area, multiple biopsies

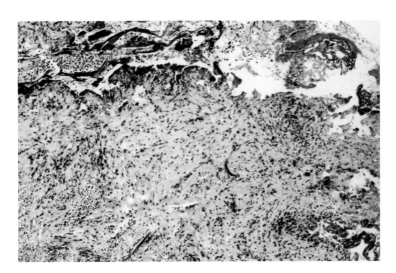

Figure 1–2. Coagulative necrosis and acute inflammatory reactions 3 days after laser therapy. (H&E)

may be necessary to ensure sampling of the most severe focus. Schiller's test is also used to define areas of nonglycogenated epithelium, which in some instances are neoplastic.

Biopsy samples should be obtained with the use of a sharp instrument to avoid distortion and the crushing artifacts. The small square-jawed biopsy instruments such as Kevorkian's or Young's punch require frequent resharpening to obtain optimal samples. When multiple biopsies are taken, the location of each sample should be identified.

For optimal histologic examination of cervical tissues, the physician must understand that instrumentation of the canal, manipulation of the cervix, or trauma in any form may remove the altered surface epithelium. Vaginal scrubs, particularly vigorous ones, should be avoided. Recent biopsy or cytologic studies

not only may dislodge abnormal epithelium but also may result in reparative changes, making the evaluation of the specimen more difficult (Fig. 1–1). Tissue damage following cryosurgery, electrocautery, or laser therapy takes an average of 10 to 12 weeks to heal completely (Fig. 1–2). Under these circumstances, it may be desirable to delay the cervical smear and biopsy. It should be noted that the strong iodine solution (Lugol) used in the Schiller's test to identify abnormal epithelium before cervical biopsy or conization produces significant artifacts (Fig. 1–3). Because of its hyperosmolality, the cells in the upper half or upper third of the epithelium undergo shrinkage and, most critically, loss of chromatinic details (see Fig. 1–3).[2] Mitotic figures become difficult to recognize and therefore accurate grading of dysplasia is hampered. When pos-

Figure 1–3. Artifacts following the use of strong iodine solution. *A,* Sharp demarcation between the affected and unaffected epithelium. *B,* Cellular shrinkage, nuclear hyperchromasia, chromatinic homogenization, and loss of nuclear details in the affected upper half of the epithelium. (H&E)

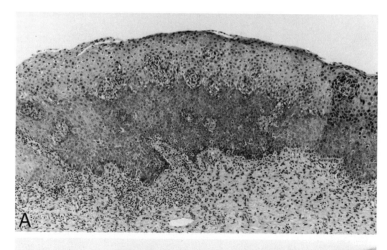
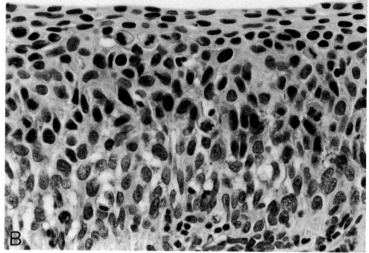

sible, an alternative to the strong iodine solution is recommended.

Orientation of Specimen

Of all the steps involved in specimen processing, none is more crucial than the proper orientation for perpendicular sectioning through the mucosal surface. Tangential and near-horizontal (parallel to the mucosal surface) sections not only are useless for diagnosis but also are a potential source of misinterpretation (Figs. 1–4 and 1–5). Such sections do not allow (1) distinction between a benign epithelial hyperplasia and neoplasia; (2) evaluation of the severity of intraepithelial neoplasia, because of the lack of full-thickness epithelium; (3) separation between intraepithelial and invasive neoplasia (Fig. 1–6); and (4) accurate determination of the depth of stromal invasion. When an invasive carcinoma is sectioned at a 45-degree angle, its depth of invasion is 40% greater than the actual depth in a vertical plane. Once the tissue is embedded incorrectly, multiple deeper cuts occasionally may yield interpretable sections. With small biopsies, this maneuver often proves futile. As a result, re-embedding or another biopsy is ultimately required.

Several methods have been used to orient the colposcopically directed biopsies. A simple method recommended by many colposcopists is to place the tissue on a piece of paper towel or Gelfoam with the mucosal surface upward. The blood, serum, and mucus at the base of the tissue form a coagulum, which helps to adhere the tissue to the paper towel or Gelfoam. The tissue is then immersed into the fixative upside down. After 2 to 3 hours of fixation, the tissue, along with the paper towel or Gelfoam, can be placed in the cassette and processed for paraffin infiltration. At the time of embedding in paraffin, the tissue is separated from the un-

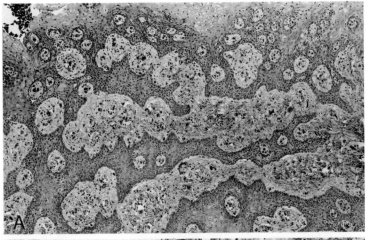
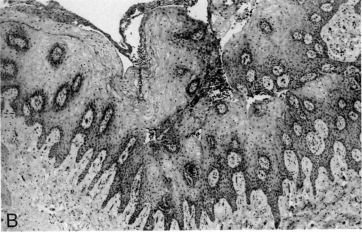

Figure 1–4. *A,* Near-horizontal section through the base of squamous mucosa. *B,* Normal squamous mucosa cut tangentially appears to be thickened and hyperplastic with elongated and pointed rete pegs. (H&E)

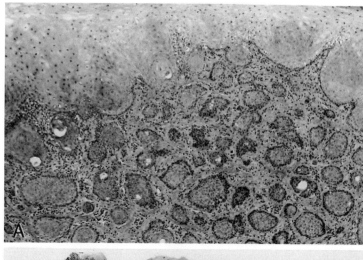

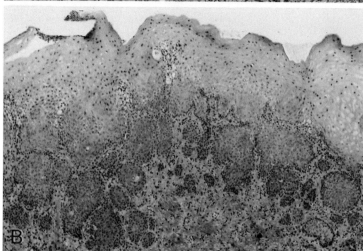

Figure 1–5. *A,* This biopsy from the transformation zone is sectioned tangentially almost parallel to the surface, resulting in many islands of squamous metaplasia in the stroma. *B,* In the deeper cut, the tissue orientation is somewhat improved. (H&E)

derlying paper towel. If Gelfoam is used, the tissue and Gelfoam can be embedded as a unit for sectioning. The histotechnologist should be instructed to embed the tissue in such a manner that sections are cut vertically to the mucosa. If the tissue is larger than 3 to 4 mm, it can be bisected. Multiple levels of sections, usually three or more, are customarily prepared for small biopsies. All tissues received are processed and examined.

If, on the other hand, the specimen is simply dropped into a fixative, the tissue curls up into an amorphous, distorted mass because of a greater degree of shrinkage of the stroma than of the overlying epithelium. Any further attempt to orient this fixed tissue is difficult, if not impossible.

Fixation in Bouin's or Zenker's solution may better preserve nuclear details and provide superior cohesion of the tissue to the paper towel

than does formalin; however, these fixatives may interfere with certain histochemical reactions, such as the Feulgen stain for nuclear DNA. In our experience, buffered formalin provides equally satisfactory results. In examining the histologic sections, the pathologist should recognize the appearance of artifacts and tangentially cut sections and realize that these sections are a potential source of overinterpretation.

Endocervical Curettage (ECC)

Indications

Curettage of the cervical canal is most often performed in conjunction with colposcopy and cervical biopsies in an attempt to determine whether any abnormal epithelium extends beyond the colposcopically visible areas. Under

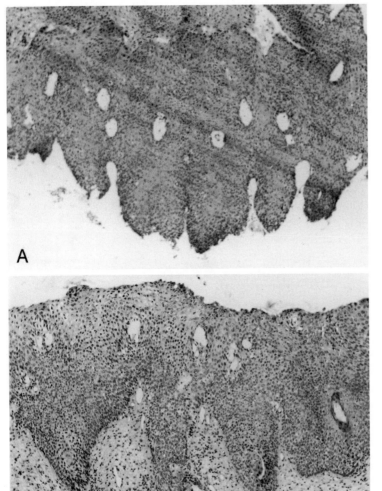

Figure 1-6. *A,* This solid sheet of abnormal squamous epithelium demonstrates long and broad rete pegs. It is impossible to determine whether or not stromal invasion has occurred. The quality of the section also suffers from multiple knife marks. *B,* It is necessary to re-embed the tissue. The diagnosis proves to be a severe squamous dysplasia. (H&E)

these circumstances, the colposcopist is primarily interested in knowing whether or not abnormal epithelium is present in the endocervical curettings.

Whether all women undergoing colposcopic examination should receive endocervical curettage (ECC) remains controversial. Moseley et al.[24] contend that ECC should be performed only for women with satisfactory colposcopy results, because all patients having unsatisfactory results of colposcopy require conization regardless of the findings on ECC.

In the study by Williams et al.,[37] 159 women with cytologic diagnosis of atypical squamous cells of undetermined significance or a low-grade squamous intraepithelial lesion underwent colposcopic examination and ECC. Only 4 (2.5%) had abnormal cells in the endocervi-

cal curettings. The authors suggest that in a woman with a low-grade squamous intraepithelial lesion and satisfactory colposcopic examination the chance of finding abnormal cells in the endocervical curettings is small and this procedure can be avoided. According to the authors' review of the literature, the rate of satisfactory colposcopy for women with cervical intraepithelial neoplasia (CIN) varies from 54% to 95%. Among women with unsatisfactory colposcopic examination, the frequency of finding dysplasia within the ECC is in the range of 25% to 50%.[23,25]

In a survey of more than two thousand women with abnormal cervical smears studied by colposcopy, cervical biopsy, and ECC, Hatch et al.[10] found positive endocervical curettings in 14% of women with satisfactory colposcopy, 52% of women with unsatisfactory colposcopy, and 39% of women without detectable lesions. More important, endocervical curettings contained more severe lesions than did cervical biopsies in 16% of women with unsatisfactory colposcopy and in 31% of those without visible lesions. Several invasive carcinomas were detected only in the endocervical curettings. Because the diagnosis of cervical squamous lesions is improved by ECC, these authors recommend ECC for all women undergoing colposcopy.[10] The treatment modality may be modified for intraepithelial neoplasia based on the findings of endocervical curettings. For example, in women whose endocervical curettings indicated more advanced change than that shown by the cervical biopsy, a diagnostic conization is performed.[10]

Curettings of the endocervix are also submitted as part of a fractional curettage designed to obtain separate specimens from the endocervical canal and the endometrial cavity. The purpose of this procedure usually is to determine the primary site (endocervical or endometrial) of origin and the extent of a glandular neoplasm. For example, in a patient with endometrial carcinoma, involvement of the cervix indicates an International Federation of Gynecology and Obstetrics (FIGO) clinical Stage II disease. Even if fractional curettage is properly performed, starting with the ECC and followed by uterine sounding, cervical dilation, and endometrial curettage, the samples may fail to determine the primary site. In the case of endocervical carcinoma, the endometrial sample is frequently contaminated with the tumor as the curette is being withdrawn from the cervical canal. As a result, both endocervical and endometrial samples may contain tumor tissue.

Method of Preparation

The specimen may be processed as either a cytologic smear or, more commonly, a histologic specimen. For the latter, tissue fragments should first be placed on a suitable substrate before immersion into the fixative because of the minute and fragmented nature of the specimen. This ensures easy handling of the specimen as an aggregate and processing of all fragments for histologic examination. If placed on gauze or immersed directly into the fixative, minute fragments are difficult to retrieve.

Method of Reporting

In reporting the findings of endocervical curettings, three categories may be used[29]:

1. Insufficient for diagnosis: The specimen contains only blood, mucus, or inflammatory exudate. Endocervical cells are absent or extremely few in number.
2. Negative ECC: The specimen has a sufficient number of endocervical cells or glands, but no abnormal or neoplastic epithelium is identified. This negative finding, when accompanied by a complete visualization of the lesion colposcopically, implies that the cervical canal is uninvolved. The sample often contains metaplastic squamous epithelium and sometimes endometrium from the lower uterine segment. In women who have had prior cervical conization or who are postmenopausal, the amount of endocervical tissue in ECC may be scanty.
3. Positive ECC: This diagnosis is made if fragments of abnormal squamous or glandular epithelium are identified. The report indicates the severity and type of abnormality. The sample should be evaluated with caution, because the precise site of origin of the changes and the full extent of the disease usually cannot be fully evaluated. The presence of abnormal epithelium provides sufficient evidence to warrant additional study, such as a loop electrosurgical excision procedure (LEEP) or cervical conization, to rule out more advanced disease existing in the cervical canal that cannot be adequately visualized by colposcopy. In rare instances, unsuspected in situ or invasive squamous cancer or glandular neoplasm may be identified in the endocervical curettings. This indicates the need for additional studies.

It should be noted that in ECC large sheets of condyloma or dysplastic epithelium may appear (Fig. 1–7). This finding by itself, in the absence of stromal invasion, should not be overdiagnosed as invasive carcinoma. It merely indicates that an abnormal epithelium is embedded en face and cut parallel to the mucosal surface.

In positive ECC samples from patients with endometrial carcinoma, the relationship between the cervical tissue and the tumor tissue deserves a clear characterization. In most instances, the specimens contain fragments of tumor without any connection with the cervical tissue. In such cases, the diagnosis should reflect the mere presence of tumor but no evidence of cervical involvement.

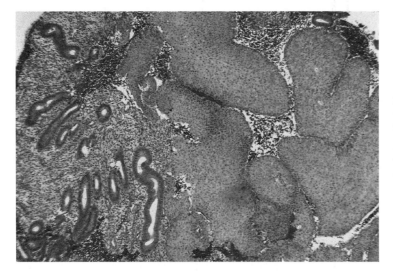

Figure 1–7. Endocervical curettings contain endometrial tissue and large sheets of condylomatous change. The presence of a large sheet of abnormal epithelium alone without stromal invasion should not lead to the diagnosis of invasive squamous carcinoma.

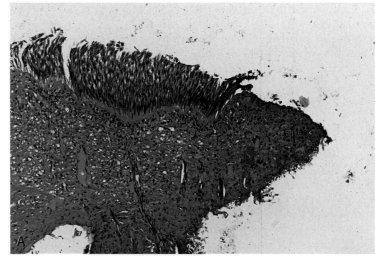

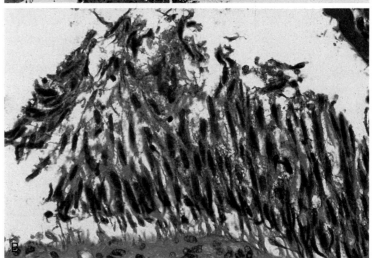

Figure 1–8. Effect on cells by thermal damage. *A* and *B,* Nuclear elongation and chromatin homogenization makes distinguishing between normal and dysplastic cells difficult.

Excisional Biopsy and Cervical Conization

A portion of cervix may be removed by excision, LEEP, cold knife conization (CKC), or laser conization. In recent years, LEEP has become widely used because it is easy to perform, has a high cure rate, and is well tolerated by patients as an office procedure. It has fewer side effects and complications than CKC and is more cost-effective. The removed tissue is suitable for the diagnosis of most cervical lesions.[9] It does have some disadvantages: depending on the experience of the operator, thermal damage, tissue disruption, and poor orientation may cause considerable difficulty in diagnosis and in assessing excision margins.

Thermal effects cause tissue to undergo coagulative necrosis, evaporation, vacuolation, and mucosal elevation, detachment, denuda-tion, and stripping. The affected epithelial cells present with nuclear distortion, elongation, and homogenization of chromatin (Fig. 1–8A and B). In the study by Montz et al.,[22] extensive tissue damage, crush artifact, and distortion precluded assessment of ectocervical margins in 20% and endocervical margins in 44% of specimens (Fig. 1–9A).

In the study of Wright et al.,[38] two zones of thermal effects were described on excision margins: (1) 50-micron–thick carbonization and charring and (2) coagulative necrosis (Fig. 1–9B). The latter damage measured 150–830 (mean 396 ± 28) microns in the LEEP specimen and 130–750 (mean 411 ± 54) microns with laser conization specimens ($P = 0.79$). On the other hand, Parasekevaidis et al.[26] compared the thermal damage in laser conization and LEEP specimens and found a mean depth

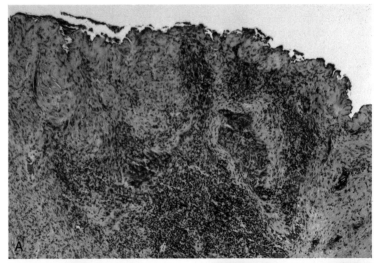

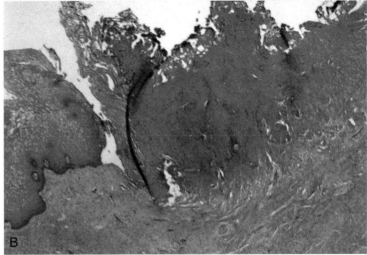

Figure 1–9. Thermal effects. *A*, The crushed cells in the stroma make it difficult to distinguish between normal and dysplastic tissue. *B*, On excision margin, an outer layer of carbonization of the tissue with irregular borders results from evaporation of the tissue. The second layer has the appearance of coagulative necrosis characterized by homogenized eosinophilic tissue.

of 0.49 ± 0.16 mm in the former and 0.22 ± 0.09 mm in the latter (P <0.001). It appears that considerable variation exists depending on the operator.

The tissue damage following LEEP and conization is followed by acute and chronic inflammation with development of foreign body reaction and vascular proliferation (Fig. 1–10). The overlying epithelium is healed by re-epithelialization. Sometimes beneath the re-epithelialized epithelium, entrapped nests of squamous or glandular cells simulate invasive carcinoma, especially because of their active nuclear appearance and irregular configuration (Fig. 1–11). The endocervical cells may demonstrate nuclear irregularity, hyperchromasia, nucleoli, and mitotic figures (Fig. 1–12). As a result of the excision of cervical tissue, ciliated tubal metaplastic glands may appear directly beneath the ectocervical squamous mucosa (Fig. 1–13).

McLaughlin et al.[20] described the effect of local lidocaine injection before LEEP procedure. The needle tract resulted in nests of dysplastic cells in the space, thus simulating vascular lymphatic space invasion (Fig. 1–14). In addition, detached fragments of dysplastic epithelium may be identified in the vascular spaces (Fig. 1–15). The key to recognizing this artifact is the lack of any tissue reaction adjacent to the dysplastic epithelium.

Indications

LEEP and conization have been used for the diagnosis and treatment of squamous and glandular intraepithelial lesions.[17] Some gynecologists advocate conization for all patients with squamous severe dysplasia or carcinoma in situ.[17] Cervical conization is most useful when invasive squamous cancer or adenocarcinoma is suspected on the basis of cellular evidence but no evidence of disease exists either on clinical inspection or at colposcopy. This procedure is also used for the treatment of early invasive cervical carcinoma.[3]

At the completion of conization, additional fragments of tissue may be sampled from the cervical canal through the use of the so-called apical biopsy. Some gynecologists may also perform endometrial curettage. Based on the study by Helmkamp et al.,[11] this procedure is recommended as part of the conization for perimenopausal or postmenopausal women, in patients suspected of having intrauterine abnormalities, and in the presence of abnormal glandular cells in cytologic samples.

Although LEEP is used in the diagnosis and treatment of cervical adenocarcinoma in situ,[5] others propose the use of CKC for this disease. They have shown a larger number of positive margins when LEEP is used as compared to CKC.[1]

In this study by Tseng et al.,[33] loop conization in the case of microinvasive squamous carcinoma of the cervix was found to have a much higher frequency of positive margins (17% versus 0% by CKC [$P = 0.02$]). In addition, the authors experienced difficulty in determining the depth and width of stromal invasion as a result of poor orientation and tissue fragmentation when multiple pieces were submitted to the lab-

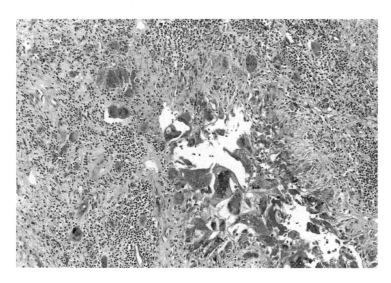

Figure 1–10. On the edge of the cauterized tissue are foreign-body reactions associated with necrosis and histiocytes and lymphocytes.

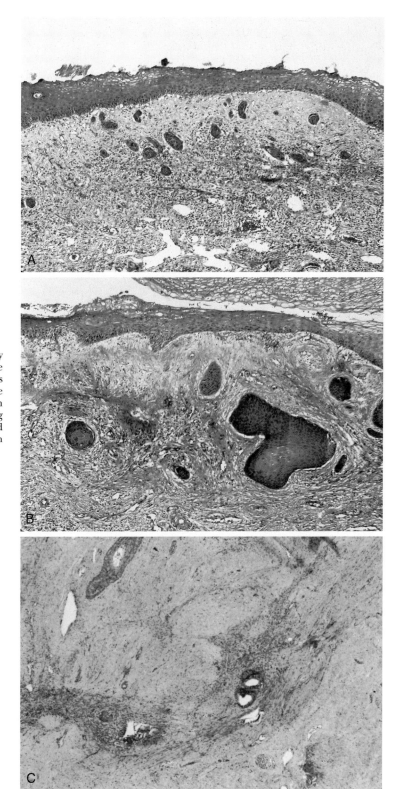

Figure 1–11. Effects of prior surgery such as cryotherapy, LEEP, or cone biopsy. *A* and *B,* Area of previous LEEP is re-epithelialized. Notice the irregular nests of remaining benign epithelial cells in the stroma. *C,* Along the tract of the incision are entrapped endocervical tissue and tissue from the lower uterine segment.

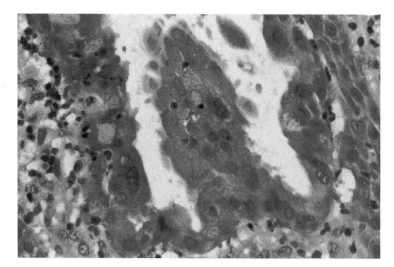

Figure 1–12. Effects of previous surgery. The adjacent endocervical cells reveal reactive atypia with nuclear enlargement, irregularity, and small nucleoli.

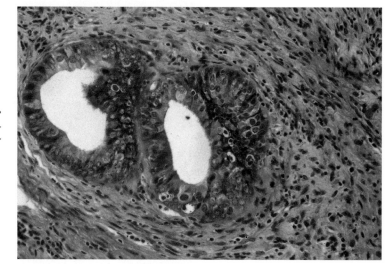

Figure 1–13. Effects of previous LEEP or cone biopsy. Ciliated tubal metaplastic glands appear beneath the re-epithelialized squamous mucosa.

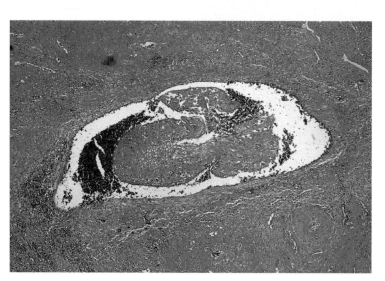

Figure 1–14. Entrapped dysplastic epithelium within the stroma resulting from needle tract. This nest of dysplastic cells is associated with hemorrhage and empty space, simulating vascular lymphatic space invasion.

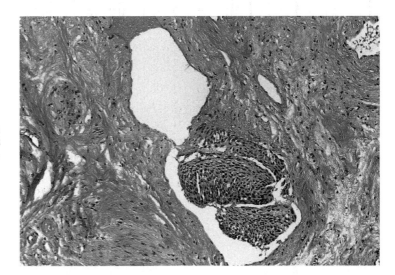

Figure 1–15. Pseudovascular invasion resulting from artifact of entrapment of dysplastic epithelium within a vein.

oratory. This problem does not occur with the use of CKC.[33]

Methods of Sectioning

LEEP specimens usually consist of one fragment each from the anterior lip and posterior lip of the cervix and a third sample from the cervical canal. The excision margins ideally should be inked or oriented by a suture. Without proper orientation, the specimen may be improperly embedded and the diagnostic area may not be visible.

Several different methods are used for processing the conization specimen. A fixed conization specimen makes taking proper vertical sections difficult, because its rigid consistency prevents the cervix from opening. For this reason, it is preferable to receive the specimen unfixed and to use the method advocated by Christopherson.[4] Using a single-edged, sharp razor blade, the cone is opened by cutting through the anterior lip of the cervix in a plane parallel to the long axis of the canal at the site identified as 12 o'clock. The specimen is pinned out flat on a corkboard or paraffin wax by inserting pins through the subepithelial connective tissue. Care should be taken to avoid touching the epithelium or pinning the mucosal surface.

After preliminary fixation of the specimen for a minimum of 2 hours, the entire specimen is serially sectioned into 12 or more segments. Using the suture to identify the 12 o'clock position, the cervix is sampled around the clock. A sharp, single-edged razor blade is used, and all cuts are made perpendicular to the mucosal surface. Each segment is placed in a properly labeled cassette. To avoid sectioning the two apposing sides of a single cut, each successive specimen should be placed in the cassette in a similar manner (Fig. 1–16). Using India ink to mark the opposite surface to be sectioned may further facilitate this process. In addition, the ectocervical and the endocervical mucosa resection margins are marked with ink.

In some laboratories, the conization specimen is divided into four quadrants (12 to 3 o'clock, 3 to 6 o'clock, 6 to 9 o'clock, and 9 to 12 o'clock). This method, although usually adequate for the identification of the lesion in relation to the quadrant involved, makes direct correlations of colposcopic and histologic findings difficult. It should be emphasized that the entire cervical conization specimen must be submitted for histologic examination. Random sampling may cause serious diagnostic errors as a result of inadequate studies.

Holzner[13] has reviewed and illustrated other methods of sectioning the conization specimen, including serial sagittal sections of the cervix at 3 to 5 mm intervals. Each block is then embedded separately and sectioned subserially or serially when necessary. Such a method may not provide an adequate survey of the entire transformation, especially at the 3 or 9 o'clock position.

A more complex method is advocated for assessing the tumor volume. The fixed cone specimen is bisected by a medial sagittal cut. Each piece is then embedded entirely for step sectioning of the cut surfaces. Sections may be col-

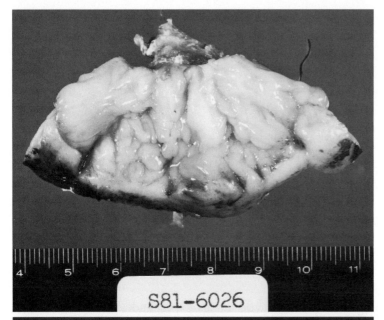

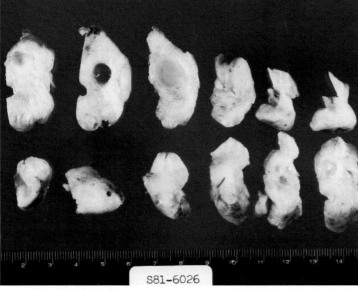

Figure 1–16. A cervical conization specimen is open at the 12 o'clock position, which is marked with a black suture. After adequate fixation, the surgical margins are painted with ink. The entire specimen is sectioned along the long axis of the cervical canal and around the clock. Each segment is placed in the cassette consistently to avoid sectioning of the same cut surface.

lected at intervals of 100 to 200 μm. The overall thickness of the tumor is determined from the thickness and number of sections collected and discarded. When this information is taken into consideration along with the length of tumor along the cervical canal and the depth of invasion, the tumor volume can be estimated. For assessing the volume of microinvasive carcinoma of the cervix, about 60 to 70 sections are prepared from each specimen. This method of sectioning is not performed in most laboratories because of its cost and labor-intensive nature.

Method of Reporting

Reports of the LEEP and conization specimens should specify the type of abnormal epithelium present and its severity, histologic grade, location, extent, and relationship to the surgical margins. A close relationship between the excision margin and residual disease or recurrent squamous dysplasia is well documented. In the case of cervical squamous dysplasia treated by LEEP, residual disease was found in 75% (9 of 12) of women if the excision margin and ECC were both positive, in 3% (1 of 38) of women if both were negative, and in 43% (3 of 7) if either one is positive.[8]

In the study by Parasekevaidis et al.,[27] 782 women with CIN were treated with large LEEP of the transformation zone. The excision margins were reported to be clear in 88.2%, positive in 8.7%, and uncertain due to thermal damage in 3.1%. Among women with incomplete excision followed for at least 2 years, the treatment failure rate was 29.5%. In contrast, when the margins were clear, only 4.9% of women developed recurrent CIN.

In a study with the use of a multiple logistic regression model, the risk factors for the development of recurrent CIN included glandular involvement, the presence of satellite lesions on colposcopic examination, and age over 40 years. In the authors' review of the literature, the treatment failure rate with clear margins on conization ranged from 1.9% to 6%.[27]

In the study by Phelps et al.,[28] hysterectomy was performed within 6 months of conization. The frequency of finding residual dysplasia in the hysterectomy specimens was 23% with negative excision margins on conization and 47% for positive conization margins ($P < 0.01$). Others have presented similar findings.[18] These studies indicate the importance of reporting excision margins on conization specimens. Women who have positive margins with CIN are likely to have persistent CIN. In addition, the possibility of more serious lesions, such as coexisting invasive carcinoma, cannot be excluded.

In dealing with invasive tumors, the type of stromal response, the depth of stromal invasion, and the presence of vascular and lymphatic involvement should be indicated. The location of the change is usually expressed in relation to the squamocolumnar junction and the clock positions. The depth of stromal infiltration of a malignant process is determined by measurement with a calibrated ocular micrometer. The points of measurement from the deepest portion of the tumor to the mucosal surface, to the basement membrane of the squamous epithelium, or to the origin of invasion should also be specified. This information is particularly crucial for microinvasive carcinoma. Evaluation of the surgical margins includes the ectocervical (distal), endocervical (proximal), and deep borders.

Multiple sections may be necessary to evaluate early stromal invasion or to identify multiple cellular elements. Quality control is desirable, and one should discuss the quality of the conization specimens with the responsible physician if possible. A shallow or fragmented cone should be avoided, because these specimens taken with this method are difficult to orient. In addition, the full extent of the disease and lines of resection cannot be adequately studied.

Frozen Sections

In the study by Hoffman et al.,[12] 159 cone specimens were submitted for frozen section diagnosis. Of the 20 specimens reported as negative for CIN, 5 (25%) had CIN I or CIN II on the permanent sections. Among the 36 specimen with frozen section diagnosis of CIN I or CIN II, 19% had no CIN on the permanent sections. Of the 51 specimens diagnosed as having CIN III, permanent sections revealed CIN II in 6%, CIN III in 90%, and microinvasive carcinoma in 4%. Among 12 cases with the frozen section diagnosis of microinvasive carcinoma, permanent sections contained CIN III in 25%, microinvasive carcinoma in 67%, and frankly invasive carcinoma in 8%. All eight specimens with frankly invasive carcinoma were confirmed on the permanent sections. Based on the authors' calculation, the frozen section diagnosis of CIN III has a sensitivity of 74%, a specificity of 91%, a positive predictive value of 88%, and a negative predictive value of 79%.[12]

Intraoperative frozen section of conization specimens should be reserved for special cases, for several reasons. Frozen sectioning of the entire conization specimen is time-consuming. More important, the diagnosis of early invasive carcinoma is more difficult with frozen sections than with permanent sections. In such cases, small foci of questionable invasion may become exhausted during the preparation for frozen sections. Nuclear details and important prognostic features, such as tumor depth and capillary-lymphatic invasion, may be sufficiently altered by frozen artifacts to prevent their recognition on the permanent section. When a discrepancy exists between the frozen section and the permanent section diagnosis, determining which is the correct diagnosis to guide further management of the patient can be very difficult. For these reasons, it is preferable to expedite the conization specimens by reporting the results within 24 hours. This allows the performance of hysterectomy within 48 hours following conization, if necessary.

Total Hysterectomy and Radical Hysterectomy

A total hysterectomy may be performed for various non-neoplastic and neoplastic conditions of the cervix. Hysterectomy specimens are preferably received fresh. The specimen is bisected to expose the entire endometrial cavity and the cervix. Abnormalities seen on gross examination are recorded. The number of sections taken from the cervix depends in part on the disease process. If the hysterectomy is performed primarily for non-neoplastic or benign conditions of the uterus and no gross abnormality is noted in the cervix, sections are taken from the 12, 3, 6, and 9 o'clock positions to include the squamocolumnar junction.

If a total hysterectomy is performed for an intraepithelial neoplasia or early invasive carcinoma of the uterine cervix, the cervix should be amputated from the uterus and submitted for histologic examination in a manner similar to that described for cervical conization specimens. In the presence of residual tumor, the extent of the disease is documented, including any extension into the endometrial cavity and vagina. If the ovaries, uterine tubes, and parametrial tissue are included, suitable samples should be taken for histologic examination.

A radical or modified radical hysterectomy is performed most frequently for an invasive carcinoma of the cervix. The cervix is removed en bloc along with the uterus, soft tissue around the uterine cervix, and upper vagina (Fig. 1–17). The outer excision margin at 12 o'clock and 6 o'clock indicates the clearance between the cervix and fascial tissue that separates the urinary bladder and the rectum, respectively. The excision margins at 3 o'clock and 6 o'clock, representing the right and left parametrial margins, respectively, usually include fibroadipose tissue and possibly lymph nodes.

Histologic sections should include different areas in the tumor and the deepest portion of the tumor in relation to the parametrium and surgical margins. Findings of these sections provide valuable prognostic information and the basis for additional therapy (Fig. 1–18). If the tumor is confined within the deep cervical stroma, the neoplasm is classified as FIGO surgical stage IB. When it extends beyond the deepest portion of cervical stroma and involves parametrial fibroadipose tissue, the tumor is at least FIGO surgical stage IIA.

Pelvic and para-aortic lymphadenectomy is usually performed.

Pelvic Exenteration

This procedure is performed primarily for locally advanced, persistent, or recurrent gynecologic malignancies. In pelvic exenteration, the uterine structures are removed en bloc with the urinary bladder (anterior exenteration), rectum (posterior exenteration), or both (total

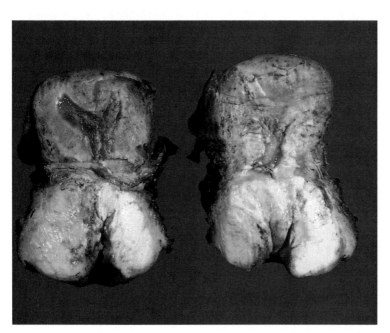

Figure 1–17. Radical hysterectomy for a locally advanced cervical squamous cell carcinoma. Sections of parametrium are critical in the determination of whether this is a FIGO stage IB or IIA tumor.

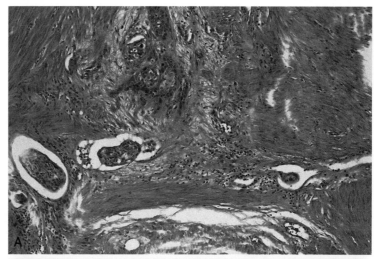

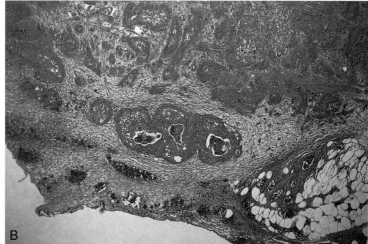

Figure 1–18. Sections of parametrium reveal: *A,* vascular space invasion; *B,* extension into parametrium; and *C,* tumor extension beyond the cervix into the parametrial fat.

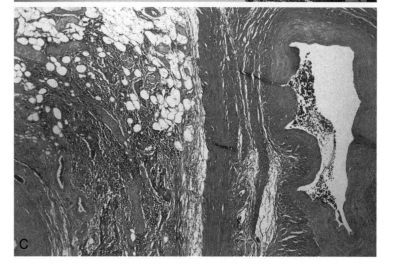

pelvic exenteration). Other structures may be resected as clinically indicated. The pathologist should be aware of the anatomy and the orientation of the specimen. The extent of the disease and the lines of resection should be evaluated. Prior biopsy results, if available, should be compared with the findings in the current specimen, especially in patients who previously have had radiotherapy.

TYPES OF SPECIMENS SUBMITTED FROM THE VAGINA

Biopsies of the vagina are ideally taken under colposcopic examination or after Schiller's staining and may be either punch biopsies or excisional biopsies, depending on the clinical impression and therapeutic plan. Grossly abnormal changes, white epithelium, hyperkeratosis, unstained foci with Schiller's test, and areas showing an abnormal vascular pattern are sampled. As with cervical biopsies, great care should be taken in orienting the samples.

Partial vaginectomy may be performed for in situ neoplasms. For invasive carcinomas, partial or radical vaginectomy may be accompanied by hysterectomy and pelvic lymphadenectomy. The clinician should mark the suspected area or identify it in the pathology laboratory, because vaginal intraepithelial or superficially invasive carcinoma may not be apparent grossly. It tends to be obscured by the mucosal folds or atrophic mucosa. As in the evaluation of cervical neoplasms, the nature and extent of the disease and the relationship of the disease to the lines of resection should be evaluated.

TYPES OF SPECIMENS SUBMITTED FROM THE VULVA

Biopsy

Neoplastic and non-neoplastic diseases of the vulva sometimes coexist or mimic each other in clinical appearance. The liberal use of biopsy is the most effective means of detecting an early neoplastic disease. Colposcopy and/or the application of 1% toluidine blue solution followed by destaining with 3% acetic acid may be helpful in delineating the neoplastic tissue for biopsy. Toluidine blue solution reacts with the nuclear DNA and stains positively in areas with increased cellularity.

Biopsy of the vulva may be obtained by using a Keyes cutaneous punch or a scalpel to remove a circular core of skin. The biopsy should include the underlying subcutaneous tissue. A small shaving biopsy may be difficult to orient and rarely includes the base of the lesion. Morphologic distinction among vulvar dystrophy, epithelial hyperplasia, condyloma, intraepithelial neoplasia, and invasive neoplasm, especially verrucous carcinoma, requires full-thickness skin samples and proper orientation. In a large lesion with a variegated appearance, several samples are required to ensure adequate representation.

Excisional biopsy is generally performed for well-circumscribed lesions (cysts, pigmented lesions, masses, or papules). If possible, an ellipse is removed, which includes the underlying subcutaneous tissue. This procedure is for diagnosis and, in some instances, definitive therapy. The lines of resection should therefore be studied carefully.

Superficial Vulvectomy

Partial or complete excision of the vulvar skin, along with the perineal body or perianal tissue followed by full thickness skin graft, is usually performed to remove large confluent or multicentric foci of squamous carcinoma in situ. Adequate sampling of all grossly abnormal areas is essential to detect early occult invasive carcinomas, which occur in 6% to 8% of vulvectomy specimens removed for vulvar carcinoma in situ. Because vulvar squamous carcinoma in situ is often multifocal, lines of resection must be carefully examined histologically. Parallel sections along the surgical margins are preferred over radial sections; the latter are preferred when the lesion lies in close proximity to the margins. An exact relationship between the lesions and the margin can be established by taking radial sections. A diagram indicating the method of sectioning is always useful for major resection specimens.

Total Vulvectomy

In this procedure, the entire vulva and the underlying tissue up to the deep fascia are removed. It is advocated for the treatment of Paget's disease of the vulva. Because of the thick subcutaneous tissue, proper fixation of the specimen is needed before sections are taken. In 30% of women with Paget's disease of the vulva, an associated invasive carcinoma of the sweat glands or of the Bartholin's gland exists. The extent and depth of the associated invasive carcinoma have bearing on the prognosis and additional therapy, such as radiotherapy or inguinal node dissection.

Radical Vulvectomy

A radical vulvectomy specimen consists of an en bloc resection of the entire vulva and underlying tissue up to the deep fascia as well as dissection of the superficial inguinal and femoral lymph nodes or superficial and deep inguinal and femoral lymph nodes. Lymph nodes are sometimes removed separately through additional incisions. This procedure is performed for invasive carcinoma. In handling such specimens, proper orientation of the specimen is important, as is a clear understanding of the anatomic demarcations, the surgical margins, and the subdivision of the lymph nodes.

After adequate fixation by pinning out the specimen, sections are taken to demonstrate the depth and extent of the disease and the surgical margins. Urethral, vaginal, and rectoanal margins deserve special attention because of the likelihood of incomplete excision in advanced tumors. If the tumor is within 5 mm of these sites, the distance between the two should be measured and documented.

HANDLING OF LYMPH NODES

Lymph nodes removed from different regions of the pelvic and para-aortic chains are usually received in the laboratory with indication of the anatomic site. Each group is submitted separately. In the case of groin node dissection, the node-bearing areas are divided according to anatomic location.

Method of Preparation

Enlarged lymph nodes are isolated. The remainder of the fat pad is sliced serially at 2 to 3 mm intervals. By palpation and inspection of the sliced fat, lymph nodes as small as 2 to 3 mm can be identified. All lymph nodes are submitted in their entirety for histologic examination after proper sectioning and orientation.

In most instances, the lymph node is dissected through the hilum, and the cut surfaces are submitted for histologic sections. This method, as estimated by Wilkinson and Hause,[35] has only a 30% chance of detecting 1 mm metastasis in a 5 mm spherical lymph node. If the 5 mm lymph node is cut at center and two additional sections are embedded as shown in Figure 1–19, the chance of detecting the same metastasis is increased to 83%.[35]

The lymph nodes ideally are cut at 2 mm intervals, and each slice is embedded alternately. At least two histologic sections are prepared: an initial cut and a second cut 1 mm below the ini-

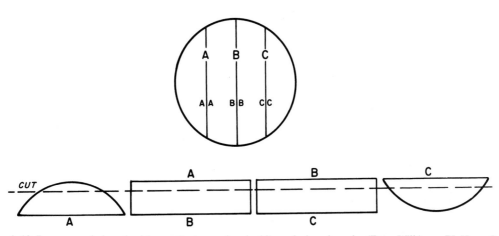

Figure 1–19. Recommended method for sectioning and embedding of a lymph node. (From Wilkinson EJ, Hause L. Probability in lymph node sectioning. Cancer 33:1269, 1974; used by permission.)

tial cut. This method improves the detection of occult metastasis to 100%.[36]

Intraoperative Consultation

In the study by Eltabbakh and Trask,[7] the accuracy of scrape cytology and frozen section of the abdominal lymph nodes removed during surgery for gynecologic malignancies was compared. After the lymph node was bisected, the cut surface was scraped using the edge of a glass slide and the material smeared onto the other slides and fixed immediately in alcohol and stained with a rapid hematoxylin and eosin (H&E) stain. The accuracy of scrape cytology was 95.8% as compared with 87.5% by frozen sections. The average

time needed to perform scrape cytology was 14 minutes as compared with 25 minutes for frozen section diagnosis.

The false-negative results were attributed to sampling, screening, and interpretation errors. False-positive interpretations were due to misinterpretation of lymphocytes, histiocytes, and endothelial cells as neoplastic cells. Cells of benign glandular inclusions may also be overinterpreted as malignant cells. The combination of scrape cytology and frozen section did not improve the accuracy rate in this study. Scrape cytology is appropriate for use by pathologists who are familiar with this method.[7]

Sentinel lymph node sampling for malignant melanoma and breast carcinoma following the injection of blue dye or a radioactive substance to the primary site has become widely accepted.

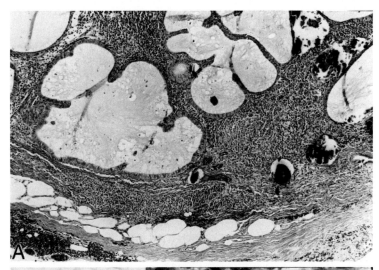

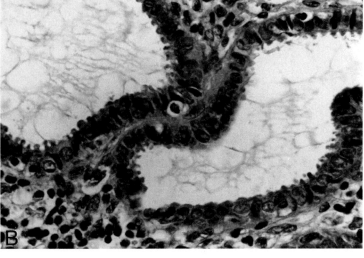

Figure 1–20. Benign glandular inclusions in a pelvic lymph node. *A,* Dilated glands are located underneath the capsule and within the parenchyma. Multiple psammoma bodies are also present. *B,* The lining epithelium resembles that of tubal mucosa and consists of ciliated cells, nonciliated cells, and intercalated cells. (H&E)

These lymph nodes are frequently submitted intraoperatively for immediate interpretation by frozen section or cytology, or both.[19,34] This technique has been used in the staging of vulvar squamous cell carcinoma.

Sentinel Lymph Nodes

In the study by Terada et al.,[32] sentinel lymph nodes were successfully identified in nine women with vulvar squamous cell carcinoma, including one patient who had two separate primaries. In one case, the lymph node was not identified by isosulfan blue dye. It was identified with the use of technetium Tc 99m—labeled sulfur colloid and gamma counter. Of the 15 sentinel lymph nodes, one was found to be positive on the H&E stained slide. Of the 14 remaining lymph nodes, two were found to contain metastasis by immunohistochemical stain for cytokeratin. Of the three positive nodes, therefore, one was detected by H&E stain and two required immunohistochemical stains for cytokeratin. These authors have demonstrated technical feasibility for the detection of sentinel lymph nodes in the femoral inguinal regions.[32]

Kamprath et al.[15] described the use of technetium Tc 99m the day before surgery to identify pelvic and para-aortic lymph nodes in women with cervical cancer. More studies are needed to define the techniques and to determine their accuracy.

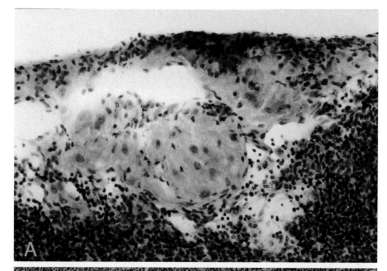

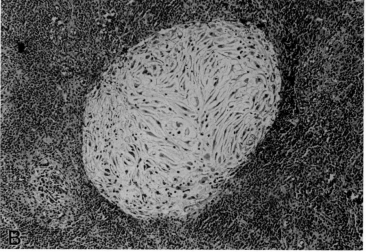

Figure 1–21. Decidual changes in a pelvic lymph node. *A,* Clusters of decidual cells located in the subcapsular sinuses may simulate metastatic carcinoma. The abundant eosinophilic cytoplasm, uniform nuclei, and history of pregnancy strongly suggest the possibility of decidual cells. *B,* Decidual cells can also follow the fibrous septum and extend into the parenchyma. (H&E on frozen section).

Benign Changes in Pelvic and Para-aortic Lymph Nodes

Benign glandular inclusions (endosalpingiosis) of pelvic and para-aortic lymph nodes are found in 5%[30] to 14%[16] of women undergoing lymphadenectomy for gynecologic cancers. The glands are located mainly in the fibrous capsule or peripheral portion of the lymph nodes (Fig. 1–20). Rarely, exuberant proliferation of glands results in replacement of lymphoid follicles.[16] Most of the glands are cystically dilated and lined by a single layer of columnar to cuboidal epithelium, which is often ciliated and resembles tubal epithelium (see Fig. 1–20).[16] Less frequently, the epithelium is proliferative, is pseudostratified, or forms papillary infoldings associated with psammoma bodies. Rarely, epithelial clusters may be found within the sinusoidal spaces.[6,14,16] The uniform nuclear appearance, inconspicuous nucleoli, and lack of mitosis are helpful in distinguishing these inclusions from adenocarcinoma. These glandular inclusions may be associated with squamous metaplasia and endo-salpingiosis of the pelvic peritoneum and omentum.[21,31]

During pregnancy, decidual change may occur in the fibrous septum of the pelvic lymph node with or without associated glandular inclusions (Fig. 1–21). At the time of intraoperative frozen section, these decidual cells containing large nuclei, prominent nucleoli, and abundant eosinophilic cytoplasm may be mistaken for malignant squamous cells, especially without the knowledge of pregnancy. It is important to recognize these benign changes in the lymph nodes to avoid overdiagnosis.

CONCLUSIONS

The foregoing discussion emphasizes the importance of obtaining samples with an optimal technique and the proper handling of the specimens received. Pathologists are in a position to monitor and, if necessary, improve the quality of the sample obtained and to provide accurate interpretation of the changes observed. These can be achieved through a close collaboration with the physicians and an understanding of the clinical settings and disease processes.

REFERENCES

1. Azodi M, Chambers SK, Rutherford TJ, et al. Adenocarcinoma in situ of the cervix: Management and outcome. Gynecol Oncol 73:348, 1999.
2. Benda JA, Lamoreaux J, Johnson DR. Artifact associated with the use of strong iodine solution (Lugol's) in cone biopsies. Am J Surg Pathol 11:367, 1987.
3. Burghardt E, Holzer E. Diagnosis and treatment of microinvasive carcinoma of the cervix uteri. Obstet Gynecol 49:641, 1977.
4. Christopherson WM. Dysplasia, carcinoma in situ and microinvasive carcinoma of the uterine cervix. Hum Pathol 8:489, 1977.
5. Duggan BD, Felix JC, Muderspach LI, et al. Cold-knife conization versus conization by the loop electrosurgical excision procedure: A randomized, prospective study. Am J Obstet Gynecol 180:276, 1999.
6. Ehrmann RL, Federschneider JM, Knapp RC. Distinguishing lymph node metastasis from benign glandular inclusions in low-grade ovarian carcinoma. Am J Obstet Gynecol 136:737, 1980.
7. Eltabbakh GH, Trask CE. Scrape cytology for intraoperative evaluation of lymph nodes in gynecologic cancer. Obstet Gynecol 95:67, 2000.
8. Felix J, Muderspach LI, Duggan B, Roman LD. The significance of positive margins in loop electrosurgical cone biopsies. Obstet Gynecol 84:996, 1994.
9. Ferenczy A, Choukroun D, Arseneau J. Loop electrosurgical excision procedure for squamous intraepithelial lesions of the cervix: Advantages and potential pitfalls. Obstet Gynecol 87:332, 1996.
10. Hatch KD, Shingleton HM, Orr JW, et al. Role of endocervical curettage in colposcopy. Obstet Gynecol 65:403, 1985.
11. Helmkamp BF, Denslow BL, Bonfiglio TA, et al. Cervical conization: When is uterine dilatation and curettage also indicated? Am J Obstet Gynecol 146:893, 1983.
12. Hoffman MS, Collins E, Roberts WS, et al. Cervical conization with frozen section before planned hysterectomy. Obstet Gynecol 82:394, 1993.
13. Holzner JH. Histologic verification of cervical cancer. Curr Top in Pathol 70:67, 1981.
14. Hsu YK, Parmley TH, Rosenshein NB, et al. Neoplastic and non-neoplastic mesothelial proliferations in pelvic lymph nodes. Obstet Gynecol 55:83, 1980.
15. Kamprath S, Possover M, Schneider A. Laparoscopic sentinel lymph node detection in patients with cervical cancer. Am J Obstet Gynecol 183:1648, 2000.
16. Kheir S, Mann WJ, Wilkenson JA. Glandular inclusions in lymph nodes. Am J Surg Pathol 5:353, 1981.
17. Killackey MA, Jones WB, Lewis JL. Diagnostic conization of the cervix: Review of 460 consecutive cases. Obstet Gynecol 67:766, 1986.
18. Lapaquette TK, Dinh TV, Hannigan EV, et al. Management of patients with positive margins after cervical conization. Obstet Gynecol 82:440, 1993.
19. Liberman L. Pathologic analysis of sentinel lymph nodes in breast carcinoma. Cancer 88:971, 2000.
20. McLaughlin CM, Devine P, Muto M, Genest DR. Pseudoinvasion of vascular spaces: Report of an artifact caused by cervical lidocaine injection prior to loop diathermy. Hum Pathol 25:208, 1994.
21. Mills SE. Decidua and squamous metaplasia in abdominopelvic lymph nodes. Int J Gynecol Pathol 2:209, 1983.

22. Montz FJ, Holschneider CH, Thompson LDR. Large-loop excision of the transformation zone: Effect on the pathology interpretation of resection margins. Obstet Gynecol 81:976, 1993.

23. Morrow CP, Townsend, DE. Synopsis of Gynecologic Oncology. 3rd ed. New York, John Wiley & Sons, 1987.

24. Mosely KR, Dinh TV, Hannigan EV, et al. Necessity of endocervical curettage in colposcopy. Am J Obstet Gynecol 154:992, 1986.

25. Oyer R, Hanjani R. Endocervical curettage: Does it contribute to the management of patients with abnormal cervical cytology? Gynecol Oncol 25:204–211, 1986.

26. Parasekevaidis E, Kitchener HC, Malamou-Mitsi V, et al. Thermal tissue damage following laser and large loop conization of the cervix. Obstet Gynecol 84:752, 1994.

27. Parasekevaidis E, Lolis E, Koliopoulos G, et al. Cervical intraepithelial neoplasia outcomes after large loop excision with clear margins. Obstet Gynecol 95:828, 2000.

28. Phelps JY III, Ward JA, Szigeti J II, et al. Cervical cone margins as a predictor for residual dysplasia in post-cone hysterectomy specimens. Obstet Gynecol 84:128, 1994.

29. Richart RM, Fenoglio CM. Principles of diagnosis. In Corscaden's Gynecologic Cancer, 5th ed. Gusberg SB, Frick HC II (eds). Baltimore, Williams & Wilkins, 1978, pp 24–68.

30. Schnurr RC, Delgado G, Chun B. Benign glandular inclusions in para-aortic lymph nodes in women undergoing lymphadenectomies. Am J Obstet Gynecol 130:813, 1978.

31. Shen SC, Malviya V, Bansal M, et al. Benign glandular inclusions in lymph nodes, endosalpingiosis and salpingitis isthmica nodosa in a young girl with clear cell adenocarcinoma of the cervix. Am J Surg Pathol 7:293, 1983.

32. Terada KY, Shimizu DM, Wong JH. Sentinel node dissection and ultrastaging in squamous cell cancer of the vulva. Gynecol Oncol 76:40, 2000.

33. Tseng CJ, Liang CC, Lin CT, et al. A study of diagnostic failure of loop conization in microinvasive carcinoma of the cervix. Gynecol Oncol 73:91, 1999.

34. Weaver DL, Krag DN, Ashikaga TA, et al. Pathologic analysis of sentinel and nonsentinel lymph nodes in breast carcinoma. Cancer 88:1099, 2000.

35. Wilkinson EJ, Hause L. Probability in lymph node sectioning. Cancer 33:1269, 1974.

36. Wilkinson EJ, Hause L, Hoffman RG, et al. Occult axillary lymph node metastasis in invasive breast carcinoma: Characteristics of the primary tumor and significance of the metastasis. In Sommers SC, Rosen PP (eds). Pathology Annual, Vol 17, Part II, Norwalk, Conn., Appleton Century Crofts, 1982, pp 67–91.

37. Williams DL, Dietrich C, McGroom J, et al. Endocervical curettage when colposcopic examination is satisfactory and normal. Obstet Gynecol 95:801, 2000.

38. Wright TC, Richart RM, Ferenczy A, Koulos J. Comparison of specimens removed by CO_2 laser conization and the loop electrosurgical excision procedure. Obstet Gynecol 79:147, 1994.

2

DEVELOPMENT, ANATOMY, AND HISTOLOGY OF THE LOWER FEMALE GENITAL TRACT

The development of the female genital tract is closely influenced by chromosomes XY and XX. In chromosome Y is a gene called testis-developing factor (TDF), which is needed for the development of testis. Without TDF, gonads proceed as ovaries, leading to the development of a female embryo. In addition, the Sertoli cells of fetal testis secrete müllerian-inhibiting substance (MIS), which causes müllerian ducts to regress, a process that is usually completed by day 77. In female embryos, MIS appears in an insignificant amount to allow the development of tubes, the uterus, and part of the vagina. The receptor of MIS is believed to be located in the stromal cells of müllerian ducts.[42]

Both testes are required to produce a sufficient amount of MIS to suppress completely the müllerian ducts. In the presence of a testis and a contralateral streak, ovary, or ovotestis, for example, a fallopian tube, uterus, and vagina are formed on the side with the ovary. Only after the müllerian ducts become well formed do granulosa cells of the ovary begin to secrete MIS.[42]

For development of the müllerian ducts to proceed normally, they need to follow the framework of mesonephric/wolffian ducts, which are located medially. The importance of epithelial and stromal cell interactions during müllerian development has been recognized.[8,42]

Leydig cells in the testis secrete testosterone, which is converted to dihydrotestosterone (DHT) by 5α-reductase in the tissue. The lack of dihydrotestosterone causes undifferentiated external genital tissue to become a vulva. For a detailed and excellent discussion of normal and abnormal sexual development of the female genital system, readers are referred to the work of Robboy et al.[42]

DEVELOPMENT OF THE UTERINE CERVIX AND VAGINA

The uterus is derived from a pair of müllerian (paramesonephric) ducts, which are formed by invagination of coelomic epithelium during the 6th week of gestation. At this time, urogenital sinus and wolffian (mesonephric) ducts are already established. The blind ends of müllerian ducts grow caudally and parallel to the mesonephric ducts. After crossing the mesonephric ducts at the pelvic region, the müllerian ducts lie close to the midline and fuse to form a common lumen (Fig. 2–1A). Simultaneously, a transverse, peritoneal fold is formed in each side, extending from the müllerian duct to the lateral bony pelvis. These folds correspond to the broad ligaments of the uterus. The

fused müllerian duct, called the uterovaginal primordium or uterovaginal canal, reaches to the dorsal wall of the urogenital sinus between the openings of the mesonephric ducts at about the 8th to 9th week.[34] This area where müllerian, mesonephric, and urogenital sinus epithelia meet is called the müllerian, or sinus, tubercle (Fig. 2–1B).

At about the 11th week (60 mm crown-rump length), proliferation of epithelial cells in the region of the müllerian tubercle results in a solid, so-called vaginal, plate (Fig. 2–2A). Subsequent canalization and continued proliferation and elongation of the vaginal plate result in the formation of the vagina. Bulmer[3] and others[52] concluded that vaginal epithelium derived from the urogenital sinus, whereas its musculature and supporting connective tissue derived from the uterovaginal primordium. The paired sinovaginal bulbs grew from the urogenital sinus into the caudal end of the uterovaginal primodium, whereas Forsberg,[18] Forsberg and Kalland,[19] Koff,[26] Cunha,[8] and others favor a dual origin, that is, the epithelium of the upper vagina is of müllerian origin and that of the lower vagina derives from the urogenital sinus. Based on the experimental model, Forsberg[18] and Forsberg and Kalland[19] observed that the upper three-fifths of the vagi-

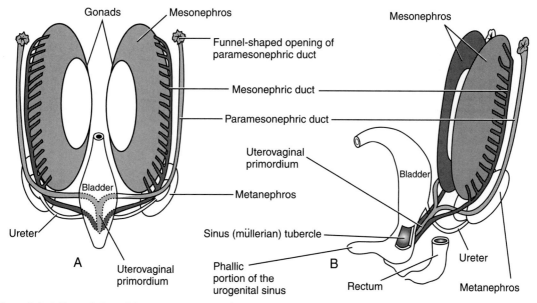

Figure 2–1. *A,* Frontal view of the posterior wall of a 7-week embryo showing the mesonephric and paramesonephric ducts during the indifferent stage of development. *B,* A lateral view of a 9-week fetus showing the müllerian tubercle on the posterior wall of the urogenital sinus. (From Moore KL. The Developing Human: Clinically Oriented Embryology, 3rd ed. Philadelphia, W.B. Saunders, 1982; used by permission.)

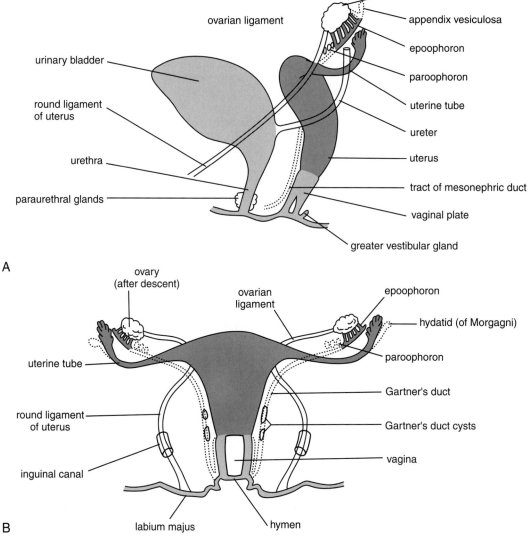

Figure 2–2. *A,* Female genital tract in a 12-week fetus. Note the solid vaginal plate formed in the region of the müllerian tubercle. *B,* Female genital tract in a newborn. (From Moore KL. The Developing Human: Clinically Oriented Embryology, 3rd ed. Philadelphia, W.B. Saunders, 1982; used by permission.)

nal epithelium is of müllerian origin, whereas only the lower two-fifths is derived from the urogenital sinus.

Several findings support that the vagina and cervix are lined by a contiguous layer of columnar epithelium and are surrounded by mesenchyme of müllerian origin.[39–41] Beginning at the 10th to 11th week and continuing into the next several weeks, the vagina lengthens. Simultaneously, squamoid cells grow upward from the lining of the urogenital sinus to replace the müllerian epithelium lining the vagina and ectocervix.[39–41]

As early as the 9th to 10th week, proliferation of the müllerian mesenchyme causes fusiform thickening of the cervix and constriction between the cervix and corpus uteri. By the 20th week, the uterus is a well-developed organ, and the vagina is canalized.[34] From 7 months, the cervical canal starts to form mucosal folds, branches, and clefts, making its distinction from the endometrium possible. Synthesis of acid mucopolysaccharide is evident by 8.5 months.[34] At term, a columnar mucus-secreting epithelium is recognizable. During the late fetal life and continuing to infancy, the size of the cervix is disproportionally large at three to five times the length of the corpus (Fig. 2–2B).

DEVELOPMENT OF THE VULVA

In the 4th week of embryonic life, the hindgut empties into a sac-like structure, the endodermal cloaca. The allantois, arising from the ventral and cranial portions of the cloaca, extends into the umbilical cord. Meanwhile, mesenchymal cells originating in the region of the caudal end of the embryonic sac, the primitive streaks, migrate to the cloacal membrane to form a pair of slightly raised folds, the cloacal folds. They fuse anteriorly to form the genital tubercle. Between the 4th and 7th weeks of development, the cloaca is subdivided into a posterior portion, the primitive anorectum, and an anterior portion, the ventral cloacal remnant. This is achieved by a downward growth of a transverse mesodermal ridge, the urorectal septum. The cloacal folds are similarly separated into genital (urethral) folds anteriorly and anal folds posteriorly.[10]

Before this division is complete, the wolffian (mesonephric) ducts connect to the dorsolateral parts of the ventral cloacal remnants. The part of the ventral cloacal remnant below the ductal openings is the urogenital sinus. The upper part of the ventral cloacal remnant gives rise to the bladder and urethra. The urogenital sinus shortens, and the inner aspect of the urogenital sinus evolves into the vestibule. By the 8th week, the original cloacal membrane is perforated by urogenital and anal openings.[32] The indifferent stage of the external genitalia persists until the 9th week. The decisive stage in the male and female external genitalia occurs approximately from day 60 to day 70.

If the testis is absent or abnormal, the external and internal genital organs will be female oriented. The genital tubercle remains as the clitoris, and the genital folds remain as the labia minora. Further development of the mesenchymal tissue produces the genital swellings or labioscrotal folds, which develop into the labia majora. The Bartholin's glands (major vestibule glands) arise from the endodermal epithelium lining the vestibule in the 3rd month. With canalization of the vagina by the 5th month, the lumen is separated from the urogenital sinus by a thin tissue plate, which is the hymen.

The blood vessels are laid down as elsewhere in the body, and new channels develop from the pre-existing vascular endothelium. The lymphatics originate from veins located in the abdominal wall and migrate caudally, along with ectodermal elements destined to be located in the perineum. The regional lymph nodes within the inguinal ligament and in the femoral triangle remain stationary. As a result, the lymphatic drainage in the vulvar area is first directed caudally, then horizontally, and, finally, cephalad. The nerve fibers arising early in the embryonic life are well developed by 8 to 14 weeks. Later, encapsulated nerve endings are formed.

ANATOMY AND HISTOLOGY OF THE VULVA

Gross Anatomy and Histology

The female external genitalia include the mons pubis, the labia majora, the labia minora, the clitoris, the vestibule, and the Bartholin's glands. These are collectively referred to as the vulva.

The labia majora are longitudinal, bilateral folds of cutaneous fat and the remains of the round ligaments. They are covered by skin and its appendages, including hair follicles, sebaceous glands, sweat glands, and apocrine glands.

These structures are part of the development of secondary sex characteristics. The apocrine glands secrete by detachment of the apical portion of the cytoplasm ("decapitation"), which is rich in secretory granules. The sebaceous glands secrete by loss of the secretory cells along with their accumulated secretion (holocrine). The sweat glands discharge their secretory granules through a pore-like opening of the luminal cell membrane, and the secreting cells remain intact (merocrine).[15] Secretory cells of sweat glands and apocrine glands contain periodic acid–Schiff (PAS) positive, diastase-resistant substance, mostly neutral mucopolysaccharide. Ducts of sebaceous glands and apocrine glands are connected with hair follicles through pilosebaceous unit. In the non–hair-bearing areas, the apocrine glands open directly on the skin in a manner similar to that of sweat glands.

Depending on the anatomic site, the hair follicle may be located 3 to 4 mm below the epidermis. The basal layer of the epidermis is continuous with that of the pilosebaceous unit and hair sheath. Thus, the neoplastic cells derived from squamous cell carcinoma in situ, Paget's disease, and malignant melanoma may involve these structures by direct extension. For this reason, an effective eradication of these neoplasms requires removal of skin to a sufficient depth. In small vulvar biopsies in which the hair follicles are cut tangentially, aggregates of in situ carcinomatous cells may be found isolated in the dermis without any contact with the hair follicles. This feature may simulate an invasive neoplasm.

The labia minora are two skin folds that are in contact with the labia majora laterally, border the vestibule medially, and form the fourchette posteriorly. They join anteriorly to form the prepuce of the clitoris above and the frenulum of the clitoris below. The labia minora consist primarily of vascular connective tissue devoid of adipose tissue. The surface is covered by nonkeratinizing squamous epithelium containing numerous sebaceous glands, but apocrine glands are rare and hair follicles are absent.

The clitoris comprises two corpora cavernosa, vascular erectile tissue, and connective tissue. It is supported by suspensory ligaments. Each corpus is connected to the rami of the pubis and ischium by a crus similar to that of the penis. Although the corpus spongiosum is not represented in the clitoris, the body of the clitoris is capped by a small mass of erectile tissue, the glans clitoris.

The vestibule is an elongated area bordered by the labia minora medially, the frenulum of the clitoris anteriorly, and the fourchette posteriorly. It is covered by stratified squamous epithelium, beneath which are tubular mucus-secreting glands, referred to as minor vestibular glands. Squamous metaplasia may occur in the glands and ducts. In the study by Slone et al.,[49] neuroendocrine cells are demonstrated in the minor vestibular glands. These cells are few in number and evenly distributed throughout the glands in the acini and ducts. In the areas of squamous metaplasia, these cells remain. They express either chromogranin or synaptophysin or both. On average, 1.6 to 1.8 chromogranin/synaptophysin-positive cells occur per gland. The mean number is slightly increased in the presence of moderate or marked chronic inflammation.[49]

The Bartholin's glands are two small round bodies lying deeply in the posterior aspect of the labia majora and normally are not palpable. The ducts, 2.5 cm long, open onto the posterolateral aspect of the vaginal orifice at the junction of the hymenal ring and labia minora. Histologically, the Bartholin's glands consist of lobules of mucus-secreting cells with abundant clear, vacuolated cytoplasm and basally located nuclei. The terminal and secondary ductules are lined by stratified columnar epithelium that increases in thickness as the main duct is approached (Fig. 2–3). The main excretory duct is lined by stratified epithelium having the appearance of transitional epithelium of the urinary tract.[43] At the orifice, it merges with the stratified squamous epithelium of the vagina. This divergent cell population in the Bartholin's glands can give rise to different types of carci-

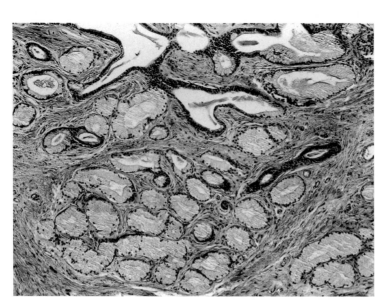

Figure 2–3. Normal Bartholin's gland. Lobules of mucous glands connect to terminal and secondary ductules. (H&E, ×80)

noma. Between the vaginal orifice and the anus is the fibromuscular perineal body.

Lymphatic System

In the subcutaneous tissue of the vulva is an extensive multilayered meshwork of fine lymphatic vessels in the form of minute papillae. The collecting lymphatics of the prepuce and the anterior portion of the labia form a dense network of large lymphatic vessels, called the presymphyseal plexus, in the vicinity of the symphysis pubis. For the most part, they drain to the ipsilateral or contralateral superficial inguinal lymph nodes. Lymphatics draining the lower portion of the labia, the fourchette, and the perineum reach directly to the superficial inguinal nodes, bypassing the presymphyseal plexus (Fig. 2–4).[36] Lymphatics of the perineum or fourchette also anastomose with those of the anus. As a result, a

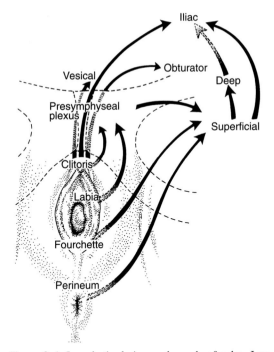

Figure 2–4. Lymphatic drainage channels of vulva. Lymphatics and regional lymph nodes of perineum, fourchette, and labia are located within the subcutaneous tissue of vulva, mons veneris, and femoral triangle. The clitoris, on the other hand, drains to primary lymph node sites within the pelvis. (From Plentl AA, Friedman EA. Lymphatic System of the Female Genitalia. The Morphologic Basis of Oncologic Diagnosis and Therapy. Philadelphia, W.B. Saunders, 1971; used by permission.)

retrograde spread of perineum or fourchette carcinoma may occur in the thigh.

The lymphatics of the glans clitoris differ from the remaining vulva by having dual drainage. From the presymphyseal plexus, lymphatic vessels drain to superficial inguinal nodes and also to the uppermost deep inguinal lymph nodes (Cloquet's or Rosenmüller's) and the external iliac lymph node (see Fig. 2–4). The latter pathway explains metastatic carcinoma to Cloquet's lymph nodes in the absence of superficial inguinal lymph node metastasis.[36]

The collecting lymphatic trunks of the clitoris also reach to the iliac and obturator lymph nodes by passing beneath the symphysis along with the dorsal vein of the clitoris or above the symphysis between the insertions of the rectus muscles. The lymphatics of the Bartholin's glands have access to both the femoral and pelvic lymph nodes.[36]

The superficial inguinal lymph nodes are the primary drainage for most of the external genitalia. They usually number 8 to 12 and lie in the superficial fascia just beneath and parallel to the inguinal ligament. Efferent vessels drain further to the deep inguinal or lower external iliac lymph nodes (see Fig. 2–4).

Deep inguinal lymph nodes are generally secondary, receiving drainage from the superficial inguinal lymph nodes and the presymphyseal plexus. They are located in the inguinal canal medial to the femoral vein. The uppermost lymph nodes (Cloquet's or Rosenmüller's) are the most constant, varying from one to three in number. Their efferent vessels extend to the external iliac nodes.[36]

In summary, the lymphatics of the labia, fourchette, and perineum drain, for the most part, to the superficial and deep inguinal lymph nodes. The clitoris, on the other hand, has direct access to the pelvic lymph nodes through suprapubic and infrapubic trunks.

Blood Vascular Supply

The labia majora and minora are supplied by the superficial branches of the femoral artery (external pudendal artery) and the internal iliac artery (internal pudendal artery).[24] The clitoris, vestibule, and Bartholin's glands are supplied by branches of the internal pudendal artery. The venous return parallels the arterial supply.

Nervous System

The external genitalia and perineum are richly supplied with myelinated and nonmyelinated nerve fibers from the pudendal nerve (S2 to S4), which is responsible for the motor (sympathetic) and sensory functions. Branches of the ilioinguinal nerve (L1) supply the mons pubis and anterior portion of the labia majora, whereas branches of the posterior femoral cutaneous nerve innervate the posterior part of the labia majora.

Free nerve endings are numerous in the vulva. They form a network around the cells in the stratum germinativum. These fibers may terminate as free endings or with small endbulbs. Pacinian corpuscles situated deep in the subcutaneous tissue are related to the sensation of pressure and possibly to alteration of the blood supply.[27]

ANATOMY AND HISTOLOGY OF THE VAGINA

Gross Anatomy

The adult vagina is a collapsed tube that extends from the uterine cervix to the vestibule. Normally, the vagina is directed upward and backward, and its long axis forms an angle of about 90 degrees with that of the uterus. The uterine cervix protrudes into the upper vagina, and the covering epithelium of the cervix is continuous with that of the vagina. The anterior wall of the vagina measures 6 to 7.5 cm in length; the posterior wall measures about 9 cm. The recess between the uterine cervix and the vagina is referred to as the vaginal fornix. The posterior vaginal fornix is somewhat deeper than the anterior or lateral recesses. Only in the posterior vaginal fornix is the vagina covered by peritoneum. The vagina may be somewhat constricted in its upper and lower aspects and slightly dilated in its mid-portion.[24]

The vagina lies anterior to the rectum and is separated by the rectovaginal fascia. It is posterior to the urinary bladder and urethra. The vagina opens in the vestibule formed from the urogenital sinus. The vestibule lies beneath the urethra and between the inner margins of the labia minora. The vagina, urethra, and ducts of the Bartholin's glands open into the vestibule. The size and shape of the vaginal orifice are related to the state of the hymen. When the inner edges of the hymen are in apposition, the vaginal opening resembles a cleft. When stretched, the hymen may persist in the form of a ring-like structure above the readily recognized vaginal orifice.

In the vagina of the nulliparous woman, the mucosa may form longitudinal ridges anteriorly and posteriorly. From these ridges arise multiple secondary ridges, between which are recesses of variable depth. The mucosa may appear to be studded with multiple papillae because of the complex pattern of ridges and recesses. This is more likely to be observed near the vaginal orifice of the virgin than in the multiparous woman.

The hymen is a thin membrane located at the entrance of the vagina into the vestibule. When intact, it is referred to as an imperforate hymen. One or more central openings are commonly found. In the annular hymen is a central opening of moderate size. A central septum, as observed in the septate hymen, results in two or more openings in the membrane. In the cribriform pattern, there are many small openings. After coitus, the persisting membranous remnants are referred to as the carunculae myrtiformes. In the parous woman, only a thin rim of the membrane may persist.

The hymen is covered on both the vaginal and vestibular aspects by stratified squamous epithelium. A central core of vascularized connective tissue, elastic fibers, and a few nerves separates the epithelial coverings.

Lymphatic System

Plentl and Friedman's monograph contains a detailed summary of the lymphatic system of the vagina.[36] Their contribution forms the basis of this review. The complexities of the vaginal lymph vascular system account, in part, for the divergent views expressed in the literature.

The lymphatic system of the vagina begins as a delicate network of small channels involving the mucosa and lamina propria of the entire vagina. Anastomoses exist between a superficial network of lymphatic channels and a deeper system of intercommunicating lymphatics involving the submucosa and muscularis. The lymphatics of the vagina terminate in a perivaginal plexus from which arise collecting trunks related to the lateral aspects of the vagina. The latter represent the efferent lymphatics of the vagina.

Although the vaginal lymphatics contain numerous anastomoses, the lymph drainage tends to follow several more or less constant patterns related to the anatomic aspects of the vagina. The lymphatics of the anterior vaginal wall drain into the lymph nodes of the lateral pelvic wall, whereas the lymph vascular channels of the posterior vaginal wall drain into the deep pelvic, rectal, and aortic lymph nodes (Fig. 2–5). The lymphatics of the vaginal vault and lateral aspects of the urinary bladder anastomose and ultimately empty into the most caudal interiliac lymph nodes. The lymphatic channels of the posterior portion of the upper vagina drain into the most dorsal group of interiliac lymph nodes. The lymphatics within the distal or lower aspect of the vagina converge into the two to four collecting channels, which ultimately form two major trunks. One of these channels drains into the interiliac lymph nodes, which also receive the drainage of the upper vagina. The other trunk drains into the inferior gluteal lymph nodes, which lie near the ischial spine.

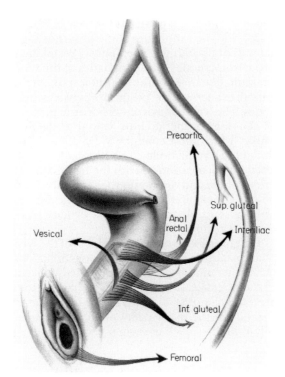

Figure 2–6. Schematic presentation of major lymphatic drainage of vagina. (From Plentl AA, Freidman EA. Lymphatic System of the Female Genitalia: The Morphologic Basis of Oncologic Diagnosis and Therapy. Philadelphia, W.B. Saunders, 1971; used by permission.)

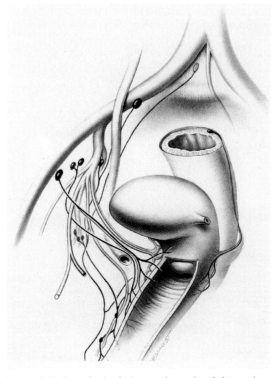

Figure 2–5. Lymphatic drainage channels of the vagina. From the proximal posterior vagina and vaginal vault, the lymphatics terminate in the rectal lymph nodes, whereas from the upper anterior vagina, several trunks terminate in the interiliac lymph nodes. Lateral trunks arise from all portions of the vagina, leading to the pelvic floor, superior gluteal, and, occasionally, the common iliac lymph nodes. From the distal portion of the vagina, the lymphatics terminate in the inferior gluteal lymph nodes. Small intercalate nodes may occur along the collecting trunks arising from the lower vagina. (From Plentl AA, Friedman EA. Lymphatic System of the Female Genitalia: The Morphologic Basis of Oncologic Diagnosis and Therapy. Philadelphia, W.B. Saunders, 1971; used by permission.)

In addition to the major pathways described, there are lymphatic channels throughout the vagina that converge into the lateral collecting trunks related to the vaginal artery. These drain into the superior gluteal lymph nodes and occasionally empty into the iliac lymph nodes.

The small lymphatics related to the posterior vaginal wall form a network that is in continuity with the lymphatics of the anterior rectal wall. Anatomists have extensively discussed this interrelationship between the lymphatics of the genital and gastrointestinal systems.

Initially, it was believed that above the level of the hymen, the lymphatics drained into the pelvic lymph nodes, whereas below the level of the hymen, the drainage flowed into the femoral lymph nodes. More recent evidence indicates that there are intercommunications between the lymphatics in this site. As a result, the femoral lymph nodes may occasionally receive the lymphatic drainage of the lower vagina. Anastomoses also occur between the lymphatics of the vagina and the urinary bladder.

As illustrated in Figure 2–6, the lymphatics of the anterior vaginal wall drain into the lymph nodes of the lateral pelvic wall or vesicle lymph nodes, and the lymphatics of the posterior vaginal wall drain into the deep pelvic, rectal, and aortic lymph nodes. The lymphatics of the vaginal vault, like those of the uterine cervix, drain into the lateral and posterior pelvic lymph nodes. The lymphatics from the central portion of the vagina merge into lateral collecting trunks, which most commonly drain the superior gluteal lymph nodes. The lymphatics of the distal vagina anastomose with the lymphatics of the vestibule and drain into the femoral lymph nodes. The vaginal lymphatics may anastomose with those of the uterine cervix, urinary bladder, and rectum.

The complex nature and variability of the lymphatic channels in the vagina impose limitations on any attempt to present a simplified concept of the drainage of the vaginal lymphatics. However, the pathologist should have a basic understanding of the major pathways that may be involved in the spread of vaginal neoplasms.

Blood Vascular Supply

The blood supply of the vagina derives from the vaginal artery, which arises from the uterine or adjacent internal iliac artery and anastomoses with the uterine, inferior vesicle, and middle rectal arteries. The vaginal artery also anastomoses with the azygos artery over the dorsal aspect of the vagina.[9] The veins of the vagina are collected into the lateral channels, which communicate with the uterine, vesicle, and rectal veins, emptying into a vein opening and then into the internal iliac vein (Fig. 2–7).[24]

Nervous System

A rich nerve supply in the vulva is in sharp contrast to that of the vagina, where only a small number of nerve fibers penetrate the tunica propria and terminate in the epithelium as free endings. No pacinian or Meissner's corpuscles

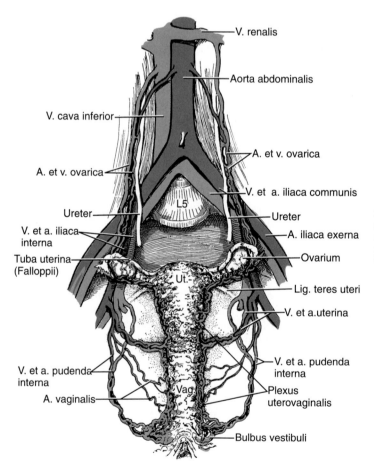

Figure 2–7. Vascular supply to the vagina and uterus. (From Clemente CD [ed]. Gray's Anatomy, 30th American ed. Philadelphia, Lea & Febiger, 1985; used by permission.)

are found in the vaginal muscularis and tunica propria. Nerve fibers are found mainly in vaginal musculature and adventitia.[27] Consequently, sensation of light touch and pain are absent in the vagina of most women, accounting for the fact that infection of the vagina is usually asymptomatic. Only when vaginal discharge reaches the vulva, where nerve endings are numerous, do symptoms such as pruritus (Merkel's and Meissner's endings) and pain (free endings) occur.

Histology

The vagina is covered by stratified squamous epithelium 150 to 200 μm in thickness. The mature stratified squamous epithelium of the vagina can be subdivided into several different layers, which vary in thickness depending on their hormonal stimulation.[35,51] From the base to the surface, the epithelium is divided into deep, intermediate, and superficial zones (Fig. 2–8). The basilar epithelium is also referred to as the stratum cylindricum, or basal cell layer. Above this is the deep spinous layer, or parabasal zone, over which lies the intermediate zone. Above the intermediate zone, a poorly defined intraepithelial layer of Dierks[11] may be identified in some epithelium (see Fig. 2–8). Over the surface is the superficial cell layer.

The basal cell layer is a single layer of columnar cells. The long cell axis is vertically arranged in relation to the surface. The cells have a basophilic cytoplasm and a relatively large oval nucleus. Mitoses may be identified in

the cells. In 3 of 100 cases studied by Nigogosyan et al.,[33] melanocytes were identified in the basal cell layer of the vagina.

The deep spinous layer is poorly demarcated from the overlying cell layers and usually comprises four or five layers of small polygonal cells. Intercellular bridges may be observed. The cells have a basophilic cytoplasm and a relatively large centrally placed round nucleus. Mitoses may be observed in the deep cells of this layer.

The intermediate cell layer varies more in thickness than do the other layers. The cells that make up this layer have prominent intercellular bridges. In sections cut perpendicular to the surface, the long cell axis is parallel to the surface and the cells have a naviculare configuration. The lateral aspects of the cells are thin, and the cytoplasm is more abundant in the mid-portion of the cells. The cytoplasm is basophilic and often divided into a thin, dense ectoplasmic zone and a central clear endoplasm. The nuclei are round, oval, or irregularly shaped, with a finely granular chromatin. A perinuclear clear zone surrounds some nuclei. Nuclear displacement may be associated with accumulated glycogen.

Overlying the intermediate layer, the intraepithelial layer of Dierks may be identified. This layer is not always present, is poorly understood, and may be homologous to an intraepithelial layer observed in the epithelium of rodents during the early stages of cornification. When observed in humans, this is manifested by several layers of flattened cells with intensely acidophilic cytoplasm and small, often pyknotic nuclei.

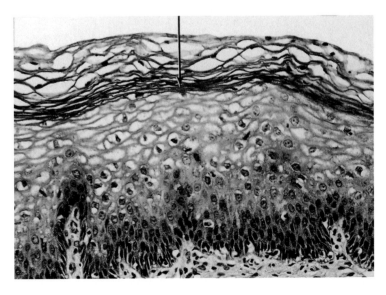

Figure 2–8. Normal vaginal mucosa, including basal cell layer, deep spinous layer, intermediate layer, intraepithelial layer of Dierks (arrow), and superficial layer.

The superficial layer is variable in thickness and comprises cells that are polygonal when viewed from above and flattened when viewed in a section cut perpendicular to the surface. The cytoplasm is acidophilic, and the nuclei are centrally located, small, round, and pyknotic. Granules believed to be composed of keratohyalin may be identified in the cytoplasm.

In the newborn, the vaginal epithelium matures under the influence of the maternal hormones, and the mucosa may resemble that of the adult vagina. Without the stimulation afforded by the maternal hormones, the vaginal epithelium of the infant is reduced in thickness, and little evidence of maturation is apparent before the onset of menstrual cyclic activity. With estrogenic stimulation, the thickness of the vaginal mucosa is increased as a result of cellular maturation. Ovulation and progesterone secretion lead to a diminished maturation and increased cellular desquamation. After conception, the vaginal epithelium resembles that observed during the luteal phase of the cycle.

In the postmenopausal period with cessation of cyclic hormonal stimuli, the vaginal epithelium is reduced in thickness and cellular maturation is diminished. Considerable variation exists in the length of time required for the transition to an atrophic epithelium and in the degree of atrophy that occurs.

Beneath the squamous mucosa lies the lamina propria, which is composed of fibrous connective tissue, a dense network of elastic fibers, and vascular spaces. Within the superficial aspect of the lamina propria, there is sometimes a band-like zone of loose connective tissue containing atypical stromal cells (Figs. 2–9 and 2–10) extending from the cervix[6] to the vagina.[13] These atypical stromal cells have scant cytoplasm and are polygonal to stellate in form. Most are multinucleated or contain hyperchromatic nuclei with multiple lobes (see Figs. 2–9 and 2–10); only a few are mononucleate. Mitoses are not observed. These atypical stromal cells are similar to those seen within the cervix and vaginal fibroepithelial polyps.

Underlying the lamina propria is the muscularis, comprising circularly and longitudinally arranged smooth muscle bundles. Longitudinally arranged bundles are more numerous in the outer aspect of the muscularis. Striate muscle fibers of the bulbocavernosus muscle form a sphincter around the ostium of the vagina. The adventitia is a thin coat of dense connective tissue adjoining the muscularis. The connective tissue of the adventitia merges with the stroma, connecting the vagina to the adjacent structures. Within this layer are many veins, some nerve bundles, and small groups of nerve cells. Remnants of the mesonephric duct are sometimes found in this location.

On scanning electron microscopy, the surface of the superficial cells is roughened, and terminal bars may be identified. A complex network of ridges is evident over the surface of the epithelium.[15]

Intrinsic stimuli are believed to be responsible for the epithelial changes. As a result of extrinsic stimuli, a thick layer of anucleated

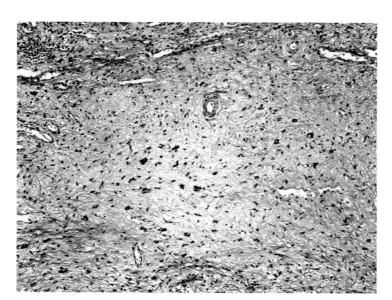

Figure 2–9. Band-like area comprising loose connective tissue and multinucleated cells running the length of the vagina. This tissue may also occur in the cervix. (H&E)

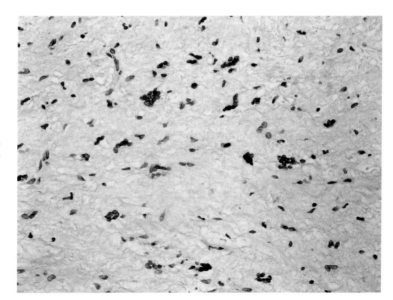

Figure 2–10. Multinucleated cells occurring in the band-like area illustrated in Figure 2–9. (H&E)

squames may cover the surface of the vaginal mucosa. Beneath this, a granular cell layer may develop. In the presence of pronounced hyperkeratosis, the vaginal epithelium resembles the epidermis. Less frequently, parakeratosis may be present over the surface.

ANATOMY AND HISTOLOGY OF THE UTERINE CERVIX

Gross Anatomy

At birth, the uterus is about 3 cm long. During the first 2 years of life, the uterus continues to grow but then reaches a plateau. The size of the uterus remains unchanged between 2 and 9 years of age, at which time the cervix is larger than the corpus. By 13 years of age, the length of the cervix and corpus is about equal owing to substantial growth of the corpus between 9 and 13 years.[53]

The adult cervix is cylindrical in shape. The portion that projects into the vagina is called the ectocervix, or portio vaginalis. The ectocervix, consisting of anterior and posterior lips, contains an external os roughly in the center. In nulliparous women, the cervix is 2.5 to 3.0 cm in length and 2.5 cm. in diameter. The external os is small and circular. In multiparous women, the cervix is larger and has a slit-like horizontal external os. Healed lacerations may be present. The ectocervix is covered by a smooth, opaque, white mucosa contiguous with

that of the vagina. The vaginal mucosa is reflected around the cervix, forming the fornices. On inspection, the anterior lip is shorter and thicker and projects lower than the posterior lip. The posterior fornix is deeper than the anterior fornix because of the slightly downward and backward position of the cervix. The endocervix or cervical canal, bounded by external os and internal os, is a fusiform cavity. The mucoid mucosal surface has a tree-like pattern with a medial longitudinal ridge and multiple oblique folds referred to as plicae palmatae.

During pregnancy, the cervix becomes enlarged as a result of edema and increased vascularity in the stroma. The squamous mucosa is thickened, and endocervical epithelium often extends onto the ectocervix. In postmenopausal women, the cervix is small, and stenosis of the cervical canal may occur.

The anterior wall of the cervix is in close apposition to the urinary bladder. The peritoneum is reflected at the dome of the bladder. Posteriorly, the peritoneum covers most of the supravaginal portion of the cervix, constituting the anterior wall of the rectouterine pouch of Douglas. A higher level of peritoneal reflection on the anterior cervical wall is a useful marker for orienting the hysterectomy specimen.

The uterosacral and cardinal ligaments provide major support for the cervix. The uterosacral ligaments, arising from the presacral fascia between the second and fourth sacral vertebrae and extending medially toward the cervix, vaginal fornix, and rectum, maintain the relationship between the cervix and rectum. The cardinal ligaments of Mackenrodt, arising from the anterior, posterior, and superior margins of the cervix, extending to the lateral pelvic wall and merging with the upper fascia of the pelvic diaphragm, suspend the cervix in the pelvis. The parametrium is a loose connective tissue located between the supravaginal portion of the cervix and urinary bladder. It extends laterally and merges with broad ligaments. The uterine arteries reach to the lateral wall of the cervix in the parametrial tissue, and the ureters run downward and forward within it at a distance of about 2 cm from the cervix. This area corresponds to point A of the radiotherapist for calculating the radiation dosage.

The cervix has several important functions. It acts as a barrier between the sterile endometrial cavity and the bacteria-laden vagina. The alkaline to neutral cervical mucus inhibits vaginal floras, which generally favor an acid environment. The physical, biochemical, and immunologic properties of the cervical mucus are important for sperm transport. The isthmus acts as a sphincter during childbirth.

Lymphatic System

The lymphatics of the cervix derive from a superficial set beneath the cervical mucosa and peritoneum as well as a deep set located within the stroma. The lymphatics beneath the mucosa anastomose to form collecting channels, which are perpendicular to the cervical canal and radiate outward. In the stroma, they become parallel to the canal and form larger, perforating vessels.[36] The second set of lymphatics originates from the fibromuscular stroma and joins the collecting vessels of the mucosa and serosa to form efferent vessels. Lymphatics derived from the isthmus merge freely with the cervical branches. Efferent lymphatic trunks of the cervix and corpus lie side by side in parallel course without anastomosis until they reach the regional lymph nodes.

According to Plentl and Friedman,[36] there are three major trunks: lateral, posterior, and anterior. The lateral trunks further subdivide into upper, middle, and lower branches (Fig. 2–11). The upper branches, consisting of two or three large lymphatics, leave the anterior and lateral wall of the cervix along with the uterine artery and vein. Coursing through the upper edge of the cardinal ligament, they ter-

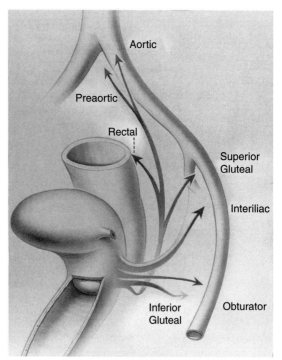

Figure 2–11. Major lymphatic trunks of the cervix. They consist of three lateral sets, which start in the cardinal ligament and reach the pelvic wall in a pattern consistent with their level of origin. The uppermost set follows the uterine artery upward, where it may be interrupted by the parauterine node, and it terminates in the uppermost interiliac nodes. The middle set takes a similar course and reaches the deeper iliac nodes, commonly referred to as obturators. The lowest set of lateral lymphatics immediately sweeps downward toward the posterior pelvic wall and discharges its lymph into all nodes of this area, including inferior and superior gluteal, common iliac, and preaortic nodes. Trunks arising from the posterior cervix follow the uterosacral ligament to drain into the gluteal, common iliac, superior rectal, and preaortic and aortic nodes. The location of these nodes is illustrated in Figure 2–12. (From Plentl AA, Friedman EA. Lymphatic System of the Female Genitalia: The Morphologic Basis of Oncologic Diagnosis and Therapy. Philadelphia, W.B. Saunders, 1971; used by permission.)

minate in the highest interiliac lymph nodes, which are located between the external iliac and hypogastric arteries, also referred to as internal iliac or hypogastric lymph nodes. The middle branches, originating in the middle portions of the cardinal ligament, drain into the external iliac, lower and deeper interiliac, and common iliac lymph nodes. Those located in the deep interiliac group and midway along the medial aspect of the external iliac chain are referred to as obturator lymph nodes. The lower branches, the smallest and least constant, drain into the inferior and superior gluteal, sacral, and subaortic lymph nodes. The posterior trunk reaches to the subaortic as well as the common iliac and para-aortic lymph nodes. The anterior trunk terminates in the interiliac lymph nodes (Figs. 2–11 and 2–12).[36]

Communications between the major trunks are common, and considerable individual variations exist. Lymphatics of the cervix may drain directly into the common iliac or para-aortic lymph nodes, which explains the occurrence of metastasis in the para-aortic lymph nodes without involvement of lymph nodes at the lower levels in patients with cervical cancer.

Blood Vascular Supply

The cervix is supplied mainly by the cervico-vaginal branch of the uterine artery, which enters at the level of isthmus and descends to give off small branches to the cervix (see Fig. 2–7).

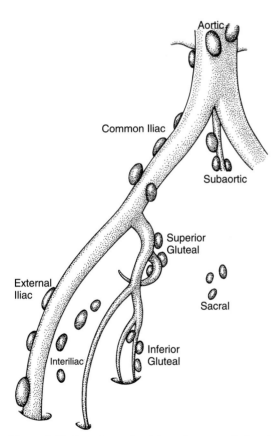

Figure 2–12. Locations of pelvic and para-aortic lymph nodes. (From Plentl AA, Friedman EA. Lymphatic System of the Female Genitalia: The Morphologic Basis of Oncologic Diagnosis and Therapy. Philadelphia, W.B. Saunders, 1971; used by permission.)

The terminal branches anastomose with the azygos vaginal arteries to form a complex network around the cervix. The venous drainage is essentially parallel to that of the arterial system.

Nervous System

The cervix is innervated by the sympathetic and parasympathetic systems derived from the pelvic plexus. The endocervix and the isthmus contain the highest concentration of nerve fibers. Only occasionally do free endings enter the papillae of the native squamous epithelium, which may explain the relative lack of painful sensation in the ectocervix.

Histology, Ultrastructure, Autoradiography, and Immunohistochemistry

Ectocervix

The native squamous epithelium of the cervix is contiguous with and similar to the vaginal epithelium described previously. Under electron-microscopic examination, a progressive upward differentiation from the basal cell layer is evident.[15] The basal cells contain abundant ribosomes and occasional tonofilaments. Other cytoplasmic organelles are few in number. The convoluted nuclei have chromatinic aggregates and occasional nucleoli. The basal plasmalemma is anchored to the basal lamina with hemidesmosomes.

In parabasal cells, squamous differentiation manifests as an increase of tonofilaments, tonofilament-desmosome complexes, and numerous desmosomes at regular intervals. A small amount of glycogen may be present. A high level of proliferative activity is evidenced by the complex nuclear appearance, the presence of nucleoli, and numerous microvillous processes projecting into the intercellular spaces (Fig. 2–13).

In the intermediate cells, squamous differentiation is fully developed. Glycogen, tonofilaments, and desmosomes are more numerous than are parabasal cells (Fig. 2–14). As the superficial cells reach to the upper layers, the nuclei and desmosomes undergo degeneration and eventually become disintegrated. A complex network of microridges can be seen by scanning electron microscopy. These microridges are believed to be important for the horizontal stability of the epithelium.[15]

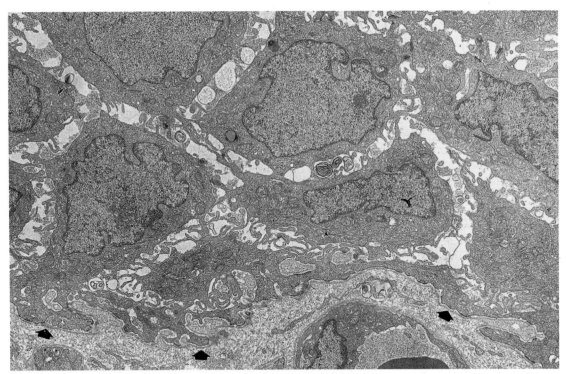

Figure 2–13. Native squamous mucosa of the cervix. The basal and parabasal cells have scanty cytoplasm consisting mainly of ribosomes, mitochondria, and tonofilaments. The lateral cell borders have numerous microvillous processes, which are joined to the neighboring cells by occasional desmosomes. The basal cell membranes contain multiple hemidesmosomes and are ensheathed by a layer of basal lamina (arrows). (×7280)

Autoradiographic studies with the use of tritiated thymidine demonstrate two distinct populations of proliferative cells. More than 90% of these cells are located in the deepest two parabasal layers. Only a few cells in the basal layer undergo DNA synthesis. Intermediate and superficial cells are inactive.[1,45]

Immunohistochemical stains on the ectocervical squamous mucosa demonstrate p53 expression in a few parabasal and basal cells. The basal cells, the parabasal cells, and some of the intermediate squamous cells express p63 diffusely. In contrast, Ki-67–positive cells are limited to the deep parabasal layers. The basal cells are entirely negative for Ki-67, indicating a lack of proliferative activity in the basal cells. Bcl2 is weakly positive in the basal cells and in a few parabasal cells (Fig. 2–15).

These observations confirm that, in the normal ectocervical squamous mucosa, Ki-67–positive cells are confined to the parabasal layers.[21] Bcl2 and p63 expressions are seen in the basal cells and in some parabasal cells. These findings support the theory that p63 is a marker of stem cells, which are responsible for cellular proliferation, renewal, and regeneration in both normal and abnormal conditions.[55,57]

The parabasal cells have a cell cycle generation time of 3 days, compared with 30 days for the basal cells.[1] The overall generation time for the cervical squamous epithelium is estimated at 5.7 days.[38] The differences in the cell cycle kinetics of parabasal and basal cells suggest that basal cells act primarily as reserve cell compartments, which become activated on stimulation. For example, if atrophic squamous mucosa in postmenopausal women is treated with estrogen, the generation time for parabasal cells is reduced to 1.7 days and to 11 days for basal cells.[1] These normal patterns observed through autoradiography and ultrastructure provide a better understanding of the dynamic processes involved in pathologic conditions and especially in neoplasia.

Endocervix

A single layer of tall columnar mucus-secreting cells and a variable number of ciliated cells cover the cervical canal. Cells resembling in-

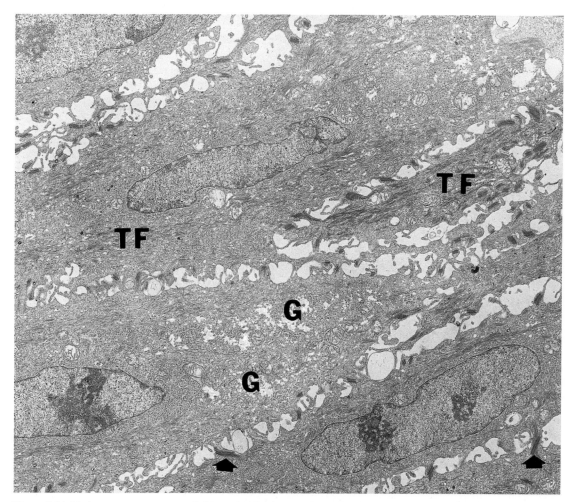

Figure 2–14. Native squamous mucosa of the cervix. The intermediate cells contain abundant glycogen (G), tono-filaments (TF), and regularly spaced desmosomes (arrows). (×7280)

tercalated cells of the endometrium and tubal epithelium are occasionally seen, as are argyrophilic cells located beneath the columnar cells.[20] The endocervical epithelium covers the surface and the underlying clefts, tunnels, and crypts (Fig. 2–16). Although these are often referred to as endocervical glands, they are not true racemose glands. The mucus-secreting cells are 30 to 35 μm in height and 5 to 9 μm in width. The nuclei are oval and basally located. During active secretion, the nuclei are shifted to the middle third of the cell. In postmenopausal women, the endocervical epithelium is low columnar or cuboidal. Dense, inspissated globules are sometimes found in the lumen and appear as basophilic bodies in cervical smears.

Endocervical glands in multiparas and older women often appear in distinct clusters of 20

to 50 oval or round, crowded glands of varying sizes. The lining cells are cuboidal or flattened. Connection of these glands with the main or secondary clefts is demonstrated by serial sections. Fluhmann[16,17] suggests the term *tunnel cluster* for this normal variation (Fig. 2–17). A layer of cuboidal or flattened endocervical cells lines the majority of these cystic glands, and their lumens contain mucinous material (Fig. 2–17). These are referred to as type B cystic tunnel clusters.[16,17]

Type A tunnel clusters consist of branching cystic and tubular glands, which are lined by a layer of tall columnar cells (Fig. 2–18). Both type A and type B tunnel clusters maintain a lobular pattern; the borders of type A, however, are less well defined than are those of type B. By immunohistochemical stain, carcinoembryonic antigen (CEA) was not seen in the cytoplasm of

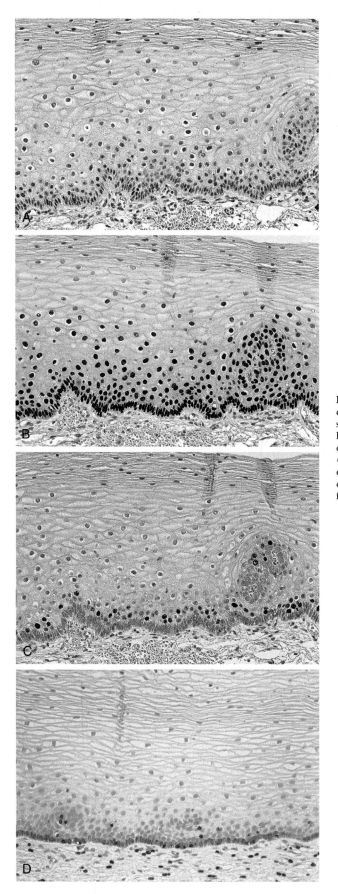

Figure 2–15. Immunohistochemical stains of ecto-cervical squamous mucosa. *A,* Stain for p53 demonstrates rare positive cells in the parabasal and basal layers. *B,* P63 is expressed by basal cells, parabasal cells, and occasional intermediate squamous cells. *C,* Ki-67 is expressed in a few cells in the parabasal cells. Notice the lack of expression in the basal cells. *D,* Bcl2 is expressed in the basal cells and a few parabasal cells. (See color section.)

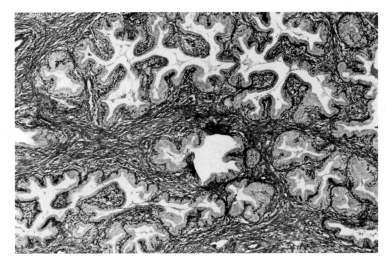

Figure 2–16. Endocervical glands form branching patterns with active secretion. (H&E)

these endocervical cells, but it was evident focally on the luminal borders in 52% of cases.[47] Because of the potential confusion of tunnel clusters with glandular neoplasms, a more detailed discussion of tunnel clusters and hyperplastic changes will be provided in Chapter 8.

The secretory activity reaches a peak at the time of ovulation and subsides subsequently. During active secretion, the cells are tall and form papillary infoldings. The mucous granules are secreted by fusion with the apical cell membrane (merocrine) or by breakdown of the apical cytoplasm (apocrine).[14,15]

Between the endocervix and the lower uterine segment, the glands are often lined by tubal ciliated and nonciliated cells and occasionally by oxyphilic cells. Their nuclei are slightly larger than those of endocervical and endometrial cells. In addition, chromocenters, small nucleoli, and occasionally mitotic figures are present (Fig. 2–19). A more detailed discussion of ciliated tubal metaplastic glands and tunnel clusters is presented in Chapter 8.

Ultrastructurally, a uniform population of mucus-secreting cells and ciliated cells is observed (Fig. 2–20). By autoradiographic technique, cells on the surface are more often labeled by tritiated thymidine than are those in the crypt, but the difference in labeling index is minimal and does not demonstrate a distinct relationship between cells lining the surface and those in the crypt.[22]

The mucus produced by the endocervical cells has different physical and biochemical properties during the menstrual cycle. At the mid-cycle, it is more abundant, watery, and less viscous than at other phases of the cycle. Mucins are composed of macromolecular chains arranged in filaments. Several filaments form a unit, called a micelle. Longitudinal

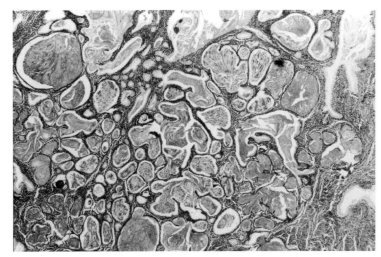

Figure 2–17. Type B tunnel clusters. Closely apposed cystic glands typical of so-called tunnel cluster in postmenopausal women. Most glands are dilated, lined by flattened cells. The lumens are filled with inspissated mucus. (H&E)

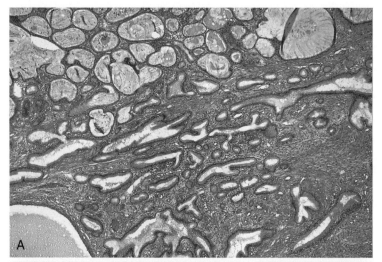

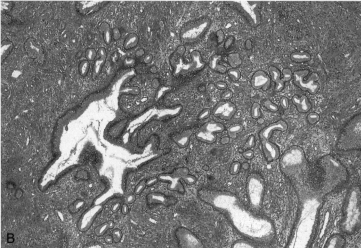

Figure 2–18. Type A tunnel clusters. *A,* Adjacent to the type B cystic glands are clusters of branching type A glands. *B,* These glands are lined by a layer of tall columnar cells and grow in a lobule.

Figure 2–19. High in the cervical canal adjacent to the lower uterine segment, the glands are often lined by ciliated cells and nonciliated tubal cells. The nuclei are slightly larger than endocervical and endometrial cells, contain small nucleoli, and occasionally undergo mitosis. These cells should not be confused with glandular dysplasia or neoplasia. (H&E)

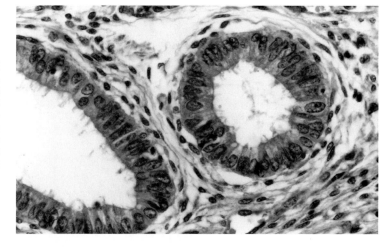

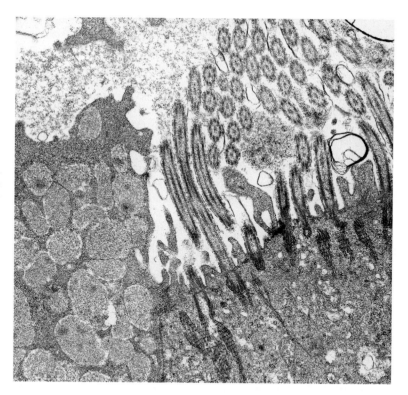

Figure 2–20. Normal endocervical cells. Nonciliated, mucous cells contain vacuoles. Ciliated cells have well-developed ciliary shafts, basal bodies, and rootlets. (×17,500)

chains of micelles form rods of mucus. They become arranged in parallel fashion at or just before ovulation.[2] This arrangement explains the fern or arborizing pattern seen in a smear of mucus and is believed to facilitate upward movement of the sperm through the cervical canal.

In other phases of the cycle, interbranching of the micelles creates a mechanical barrier to sperm transport. Therefore, the property of the cervical mucus plays a role in the passage of sperm. Certain pathologic conditions of the cervix may directly or indirectly affect sperm migration, such as secretion of abnormal mucus, which is toxic to sperm; stenosis or malposition of the cervix; and inadequate secretion of cervical mucus, for example, following cervical conization. Study of the cervical mucus is part of the work-up for women with infertility problems.[2]

Transformation Zone

The squamocolumnar junction may be abrupt or gradual, and its location in relation to the anatomic external os varies, depending on the age, hormonal influence, parity, and shape of the cervix. At the squamocolumnar junction,

the native squamous epithelium may be in direct apposition to the endocervical epithelium, or, more frequently, there is a metaplastic squamous epithelium between the two epithelia. This area between the original and the new squamocolumnar junctions is referred to as the transformation, or transition, zone (T-zone).

When endocervical epithelium extends to the ectocervix, the condition is often referred to as cervical erosion, ectropion, eversion, or ectopy. It has been emphasized that the red, mucoid, eroded appearance of so-called cervical erosion is no more than columnar epithelium overlying the stromal capillary bed and represents a physiologic response to the cervicovaginal conditions.[48] The anterior lip of the cervix is more frequently involved than is the posterior lip; however, both may be involved.

During the late fetal and neonatal life, the columnar epithelium often lies on the ectocervix, a phenomenon attributed to maternal hormonal milieu.[23,30] At approximately 1 year of age, elongation of the upper cervix results in an upward movement of the squamocolumnar junction.[23] Thereafter, until adolescence, the squamocolumnar junction appears, to the naked eye, at or near the external os. However, in a colposcopic study of children between 1 and 13 years of age, 43% of the subjects reveal columnar epithelium on the ectocervix.[29] It is possible that some degree of cervical eversion results from inserting the vaginal speculum for colposcopy.

During adolescence, the appearance of the squamocolumnar junction is variable, depending on hormones, menarche, coitus, and pregnancy. In virginal cervices of adolescents, 28% of the squamocolumnar junctions are situated within the cervical canal, whereas 72% occupy an ectocervical position.[48] After the onset of menarche, 88% of the subjects studied had squamocolumnar junctions located on the ectocervix with varying degrees of squamous metaplasia.[48] This increase in the frequency of cervical eversion after menarche is most likely caused by newly secreted estrogens and progesterones. In sexually active adolescents and adults, the T-zone tends to retract to within the cervical canal.[48]

In the primigravid cervix during the early part of the first trimester, the transformation zone comprises large areas of columnar epithelium without squamous metaplasia. With progression of the pregnancy, metaplastic epithelium increases in area and maturity. Multigravid cervix during pregnancy undergoes similar changes, but its extent is limited.[48] In adult women after the third decade of life, a gradual increase in the maturity of squamous metaplasia takes place. With increasing age, the squamocolumnar junction becomes sharply defined and often recedes within the cervical canal.

Squamous Metaplasia

Squamous metaplasia of the cervix refers to a process by which columnar epithelium is replaced or transformed into a stratified squamous epithelium. This change is observed from the late fetal stage to the eighth decade of life. In most instances, this represents a physiologic response to the hormones and to the exposure of the acid vaginal environment.[48] Other possible causes include trauma, inflammation, chronic irritation owing to a variety of physical and chemical agents, and coitus (exposure to prostaglandin in the semen). Morphologic changes related to squamous metaplasia have been divided into three stages: reserve cell hyperplasia, immature squamous metaplasia, and mature squamous metaplasia.[4,5] A spectrum of these stages often coexists in the same cervix and may involve the surface or the underlying glands, or both.

The earliest change, reserve cell hyperplasia, is characterized by the presence of a single row of primitive, cuboidal cells located between the endocervical cells and the basement membrane (Fig. 2–21). Subsequent proliferation of reserve cells results in two to five layers (Fig. 2–22). They have uniformly round to oval nuclei with finely granular chromatin and occasional chromocenters. The cytoplasm is scant, amphophilic, and sometimes vacuolated. The nucleocytoplasmic ratio is high (Fig. 2–23). The cell borders are poorly defined, giving a syncytial and basaloid appearance. When reserve cells replace the branching endocervical glands, the

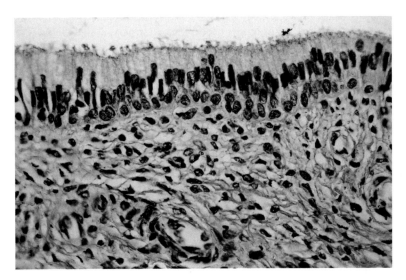

Figure 2–21. Reserve cell hyperplasia. In the earliest stage, a row of polygonal cells appears between the basement membrane and endocervical cells. (H&E)

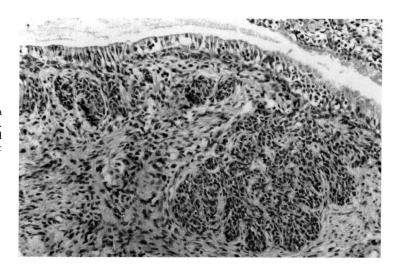

Figure 2–22. Reserve cell hyperplasia occurs in the endocervical glands. The immature reserve cells arranged in a solid pattern superficially mimic a neoplasia. (H&E)

solid growth pattern and immature appearance of the cells may suggest an intraepithelial or even invasive neoplasm. However, the reserve cells have uniform nuclear size and shape and lack mitotic activity.

Multilayered cells resembling parabasal cells of the native squamous epithelium characterize the next stage of development, immature squamous metaplasia. They have slightly more abundant eosinophilic cytoplasm than do the reserve cells, and the cell borders are better defined. The cytoplasm may be vacuolated. Glycogen and intercellular bridges are usually absent. Overlying endocervical cells and a distinct basal cell layer may be seen (Fig. 2–24).

In mature squamous metaplasia, the cells develop into distinct basal, parabasal, and intermediate layers. Cells located in the superficial layers have abundant eosinophilic cytoplasm,

distinct cell borders, and varying amounts of glycogen (Fig. 2–25). The overlying endocervical cells are desquamated. The base of the epithelium is flat without rete pegs. Extension into the underlying glands with complete replacement of pre-existing endocervical cells results in solid nests of squamous cells with smooth, regular borders. A fully developed mature squamous metaplasia is indistinguishable from the native squamous epithelium. The only clue to its metaplastic origin is the presence of underlying glands.

Autoradiographic study of squamous metaplasia demonstrates that most of the labeled cells are located in the deepest two layers. In addition, scattered labeled cells are apparent throughout the epithelium.[45] This pattern is distinctly different from that of native squamous epithelium, in which the labeled cells are

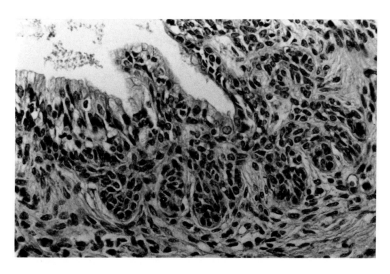

Figure 2–23. The reserve cells have scanty cytoplasm and uniformly round to oval nuclei to resemble basaloid cells. Small chromocenters or nucleoli may be present. Mitotic figures are rarely found. (H&E)

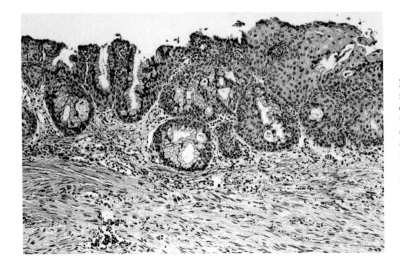

Figure 2–24. Immature squamous metaplasia. Progressive squamous differentiation in the right half of the figure manifests by an increase of eosinophilic cytoplasm and well-defined cell borders. With increasing thickness of the metaplastic cells, the overlying endocervical cells are desquamated. (H&E)

confined to the deepest parabasal layers and occasional basal cells.[1,45]

Histogenesis of Squamous Metaplasia

The origin of reserve cells and squamous metaplasia has been controversial for some time. Meyer,[31] based on his observations of fetal cervices and cervical erosion in adults, proposed a direct ingrowth of basal cells from the immediately adjacent squamous epithelium that undermined and eventually replaced the columnar layer. To explain the occurrence of isolated squamous metaplasia located high in the cervical canal and cervical polyp, he suggested that some of the basal cells became segregated (embryonic tests) during prenatal and postnatal development of the cervix.

Carmichael and Jeaffreson[4,5] initiated the concept of subcolumnar basal cells as reserve depots from which squamous and columnar cells could originate. This concept was based largely on the presence of mucin in the subcolumnar basal and metaplastic squamous cells.[5] Subsequently, other authors supported this hypothesis.[25]

Other authors have proposed that cervical stromal cells give rise to reserve cells. In fetal cervices older than 19 to 20 weeks, Song[50] observed subepithelial stromal cells migrating into the columnar cells. Reid et al.[37] found squamous metaplasia occurring in areas of the cervix that previously had been cauterized up to a depth of 5 mm, which presumably destroyed any pre-existing embryonic rests, native squamous epithelium, or endocervical epithe-

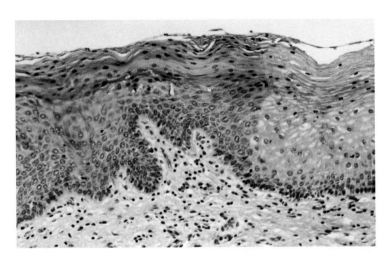

Figure 2–25. Mature squamous metaplasia. The metaplastic cells, although mature, are not fully glycogenated, allowing for distinction from the native squamous mucosa. (H&E)

lium. Mononuclear cells derived from circulating blood started to appear in the acellular area 24 to 48 hours after tissue destruction. They continued to migrate and eventually reached the mucosal surface to form a new epithelium.[37]

Electron-microscopic studies of the earliest stage of squamous metaplasia have demonstrated that reserve cells have a variable appearance. Some are completely undifferentiated, containing mainly a few mitochondria and rough endoplasmic reticula. No tonofilaments or hemidesmosomes are discernible.[28] Others resemble basal cells of the native squamous epithelium. They contain abundant mitochondria and rough endoplasmic reticula, occasional tonofilaments, and hemidesmosomes on the basal plasmalemma (Fig. 2–26). In addition, mucin-like granules and evidence of ciliogenesis are observed in a few reserve cells.[22] These ultrastructural features do not support an origin from undifferentiated embryonic cells or basal cells of the native squamous epithelium. Furthermore, the theory of an ingrowth of basal cells from the adjacent squamous epithelium fails to explain isolated squamous metaplasia occurring within the endocervical epithelium.

Lawrence et al.[28] have described "epithelioid" stromal cells beneath the reserve cells as viewed with electron microscopy. These cells have pinocytic vesicles, hemidesmosome-like structures, and basal lamina. Their appearance, however, is different from that of macrophages or reserve cells. Despite an extensive search, none of these cells contained tonofilaments or came in contact with the reserve cells.[28] The nature of these cells and their relationship to reserve cells remain to be determined.

Organ culture studies of human endocervix maintained up to 24 weeks reveal progressive squamous transformation of endocervical cells.[46] Starting from the fourth week, metaplasia starts from the top of the papillae and ridges and progresses laterally. The endocervical epithelium is replaced by multilayered squamoid

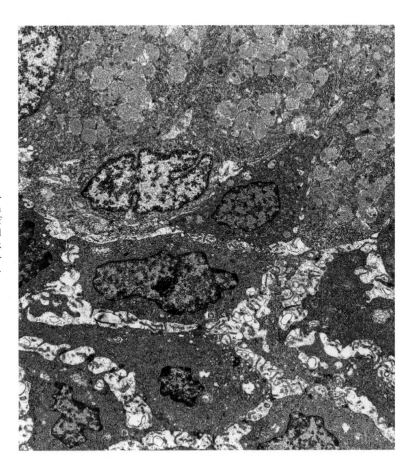

Figure 2–26. Reserve cell hyperplasia. The reserve cells beneath the mucinous cells share many of the features of basal or parabasal cells, such as scanty cytoplasm, lack of glycogen, and numerous microvillous cytoplasmic processes. (×25,000)

cells through progressive loss of mucus-secreting and ciliated cells. In the early stage, mucus-secreting cells, while retaining mucous granules, Golgi complexes, and rough endoplasmic reticulum, gradually increase the amount of tonofilaments and tonofilament-desmosome complexes from 12 to 24 weeks in vitro. A few scattered spindle cells are found in the stroma. Although active proliferation of stromal cells is occasionally found beneath the columnar epithelium, migration of stromal cells into the epithelium is not observed. The changes observed in vitro may be different from those of an in vivo environment, but these studies support direct transformation of endocervical cells into metaplastic squamous cells.[46]

The histogenesis of squamous metaplasia is further elucidated by the study of p63 gene by Yang et al.[55,57] P63 gene is a homologue of p53 tumor suppressor gene.[55] In the immunohistochemical stain of mouse squamous epithelia, p63 is localized entirely to the basal cell layer. Parabasal cells do not express p63. P63 is believed to be the marker of stem cells, which are responsible for epithelial regeneration and proliferation.[56] In this model, the stem cells and basal cells with p63 allow self-renewal and differentiation into transient amplifying cells (TACs). TACs may contain p63 to permit limited proliferation and terminal differentiation.[56]

With the use of immunohistochemical stains, reserve cells are positive for keratin, which indicates an origin from epithelial rather than stromal cells. In the areas of reserve cell hyperplasia and immature squamous metaplasia, occasional cells express p53, whereas p63 is strongly expressed by both reserve cells and immature metaplastic cells (Fig. 2–27). Ki-67 is demonstrated in only a few cells located in the deep layers of the immature squamous metaplasia. CEA is variable and may be positive in the superficial layers of immature squamous metaplasia (see Fig. 2–27E). Bcl2 is strongly expressed in the reserve cells and basal cells in the immature squamous metaplasia (see Fig. 2–27F).

In the endocervix, the endocervical cells are negative for p53 (Fig. 2–28B). Occasional p63-positive cells beneath the endocervical cells appear both on the mucosal surface and in the underlying glands (see Fig. 2–28C). Ki-67 is almost negative, indicating low proliferative activity of the endocervical cells (see Fig. 2–28D). Bcl2 is expressed in some of the cells beneath the endocervical cells in a way that is somewhat

similar to p63 expression (see Fig. 2–28E). It is interesting that in some areas of endocervix, p63-positive cells appear in a discontinuous, isolated fashion, suggesting a localized origin of these stem/basal cells. This pattern of expression also raises the question of potential differentiation of these cells into both squamous and glandular cells.[57] Thus, in the presence of human papillomavirus (HPV) infection, it is not surprising that stem cells affected by HPV can evolve into atypical squamous metaplasia, squamous neoplasia, and glandular neoplasia.[7]

Transitional Cell Metaplasia

A new type of metaplasia, designated as transitional cell type, was described recently. Weir et al.[54] report 63 examples of transitional cell metaplasia of the cervix or vagina from patients 50 to 84 years of age (mean 67.6 years). All but two were postmenopausal. This metaplasia is found incidentally in hysterectomy specimens, endocervical or endometrial curettage, cervical biopsy or conization, and vaginal biopsies. Its location includes ectocervix (14 cases), T-zone (43), vagina (10), and a combination of these(4). This metaplasia has several characteristics. It is hyperplastic with multiple layers of immature cells, usually with a vertical arrangement of the nuclei. The nuclei are oval to elongated and frequently contain longitudinal nuclear grooves. The cell arrangement sometimes becomes horizontal in the superficial layers. The cells have low nuclear cytoplasmic ratios and occasionally perinuclear halos. The mitotic activity is absent or rare (Figs. 2–29 and 2–30). A mild to moderate degree of atypia was seen in only two cases.[54]

The study by Egan et al.[12] includes 31 cases with transitional cell metaplasia of the uterine cervix. In addition, some women had this change in the vaginal mucosa. Their age varied from 30 to 87 years (mean 62 years). Of the women in this study, 81% were postmenopausal and 19% were premenopausal. Six women presented with abnormal cervical smears. All others presented with various benign conditions of the uterus. This represents an essentially incidental finding. Histologically, one can see umbrella-like cell layers on the surface. Similar to the report of Weir et al.,[54] the cells have low nuclear cytoplasmic ratios, and no mitotic activity is seen. One of the distinct features is the presence of nuclear grooves. Chromatin particles are finely gran-

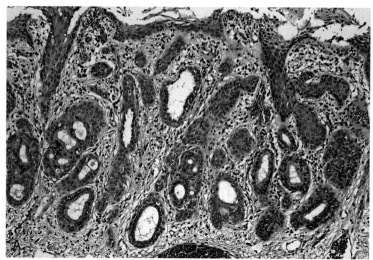

Figure 2–27. *A,* Reserve cell hyperplasia and immature squamous metaplasia. *B* to *F,* Immunochemical stains. *B,* P53 is seen in some of the reserve cells and immature metaplastic squamous cells. *C,* P63 is expressed by reserve cells and immature metaplastic squamous cells. A few cells beneath the endocervical cells are positive, consistent with reserve cells. *D,* Ki67 is positive in only a few metaplastic squamous cells and reserve cells. *E,* CEA is positive in the superficial layers of squamous metaplasia. Endocervical cells are negative for CEA. *F,* Bcl2 is expressed by immature metaplastic squamous cells and reserve cells. (See color section.)

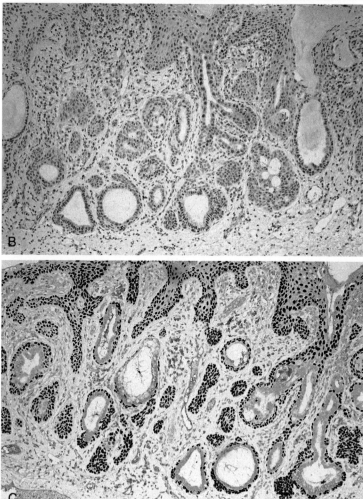

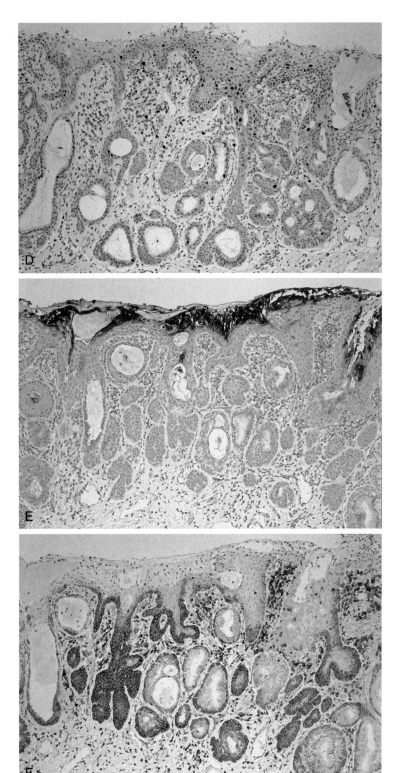

Figure 2–27. *Continued.* D,E,F

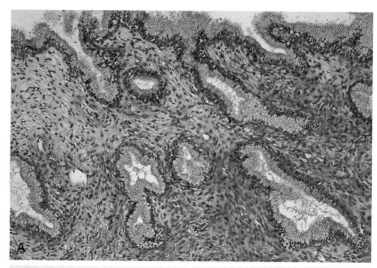

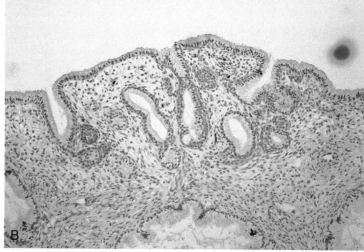

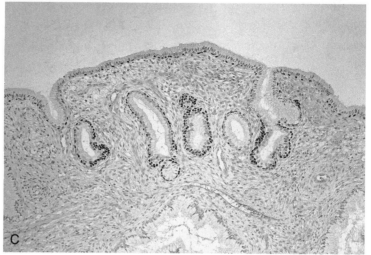

Figure 2–28. *A,* Normal endocervix. *B* to *E,* Immunohistochemical stains. *B,* P53 is negative. *C,* P63-positive cells on the endocervical mucosa appear in a discontinuous fashion, whereas a layer of positive cells is seen in the base of the endocervical glands. *D,* Ki-67 is negative. *E,* Bcl2 is expressed in cells beneath the endocervical cells in a manner similar to that of p63 in *C.* (See color section.)

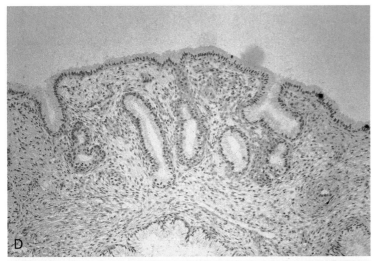

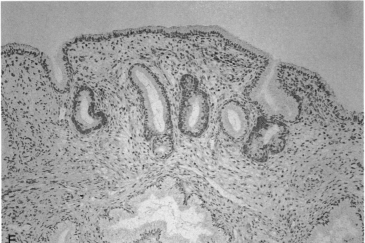

Figure 2–28. *Continued.* D,E

ular. Nucleoli are inconspicuous. No glycogen can be demonstrated by PAS stain. This metaplasia sometimes extends into the underlying endocervical glands. Serotonin and calcitonin may be expressed by immunohistochemical stains.

Transitional cell metaplasia may be confused with dysplastic epithelium; the distinguishing features are summarized in Table 2–1. By immunohistochemical stains, p63 is seen in the entire thickness of transitional cell metaplasia, not unlike its appearance in squamous basal cells (Fig. 2–31A). Ki-67 positive cells are very few in number, indicating a lack of or low proliferative activity (see Fig. 2–31B). As is discussed in Chapter 8, abundant Ki-67 positive cells are scattered within the high-grade dysplastic squamous epithelium.

Stromal Tissue

Between the rete pegs of the squamous epithelium is a network of capillaries that can be visualized by colposcopic examination. The cervical stroma consists largely of fibrous tissue. The smooth muscle, contributing approximately 10% to 15% of the stroma, varies in amount depending on its anatomic location. At the isthmus, the inner longitudinal muscle fibers of the corpus form a spiral pattern and act as a sphincter. About 50% to 60% of the stroma is made up of smooth muscle.[44] The middle half of the endocervix contains terminal fibers of uterine smooth muscle. The lower half of the endocervix and ectocervix is largely devoid of smooth muscle fibers, except around the blood vesssels.[44] Elastic tissue is found only in the wall of the

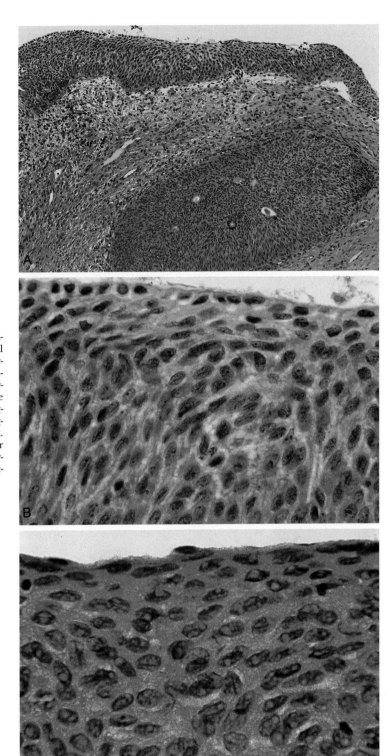

Figure 2–29. Transitional cell metaplasia. *A,* It occurs on the endocervical mucosa and the underlying endocervical glands. *B,* On a higher magnification, they have oval to elongated hyperchromatic nuclei and a moderate amount of cytoplasm. No mitotic figures are evident. *C,* On a higher magnification, nuclear grooves are evident. Some of the cells contain nuclear vacuoles. Occasional nuclei are surrounded by clear halos. (See color section.)

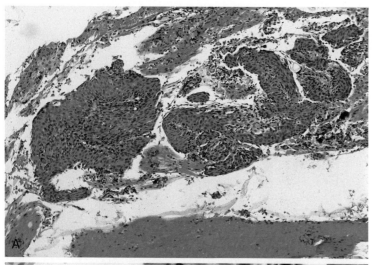

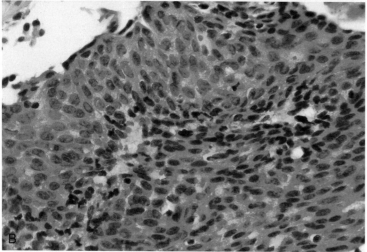

Figure 2–30. Transitional cell metaplasia. *A*, In endocervical curettage, their immature appearance may simulate high-grade dysplasia. *B*, High magnification demonstrates distinct nuclear appearance with nuclear grooves. Notice the lack of mitotic figures.

Table 2–l. Pathologic Characteristics of Transitional Cell Metaplasia and Its Mimickers

	TCM	HGSIL	Atrophy	Immature SM
Thickness	Thick (>10 layers)	Variables (8–12)	Thin (<5 layers)	Variables (5–10)
Maturation	None, streaming	None, disorganized	None	None to some at surface
Mitoses	Rare, normal	Abundant, abnormal	Rare, normal	Present, normal
N/C ratio	Low	High	High	High
Chromatin	Fine	Hyperchromatic	Fine-pyknotic	Coarse-hyperchromatic
Nuclei	Oval spindled, tapered ends, wrinkled	Oval-spindled, irregular	Round-oval, smooth	Oval, smooth
Halos and grooves	Present	Absent	Absent	Absent
Serotonin, calcitonin	Present	Absent	Present	Present

TCM, transitional cell metaplasia; HGSIL, high-grade squamous intraepithelial lesion; SM, squamous metaplasia. (From Weir et al. Am J Surg Pathol 21:510, 1997.)

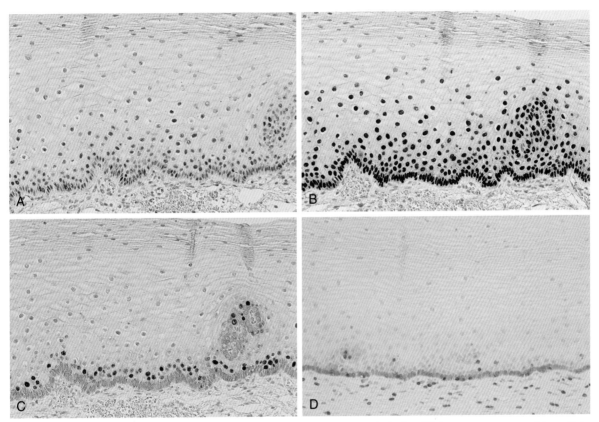

Figure 2–15. Immunohistochemical stains of ectocervical squamous mucosa. *A,* Stain for p53 demonstrates rare positive cells in the parabasal and basal layers. *B,* P63 is expressed by basal cells, parabasal cells, and occasional intermediate squamous cells. *C,* Ki-67 is expressed in a few cells in the parabasal cells. Notice the lack of expression in the basal cells. *D,* Bcl2 is expressed in the basal cells and a few parabasal cells.

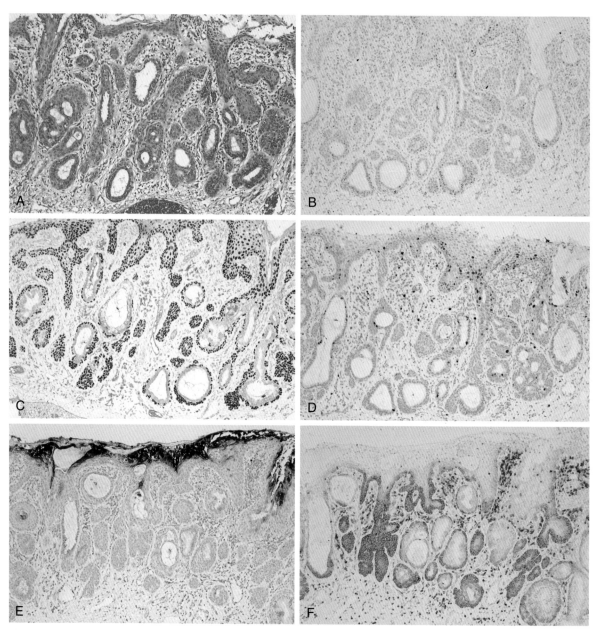

Figure 2–27. *A*, Reserve cell hyperplasia and immature squamous metaplasia. *B* to *F*, Immunochemical stains. *B*, P53 is seen in some of the reserve cells and immature metaplastic squamous cells. *C*, P63 is expressed by reserve cells and immature metaplastic squamous cells. A few cells beneath the endocervical cells are positive, consistent with reserve cells. *D*, Ki67 is positive in only a few metaplastic squamous cells and reserve cells. *E*, CEA is positive in the superficial layers of squamous metaplasia. Endocervical cells are negative for CEA. *F*, Bcl2 is expressed by immature metaplastic squamous cells and reserve cells.

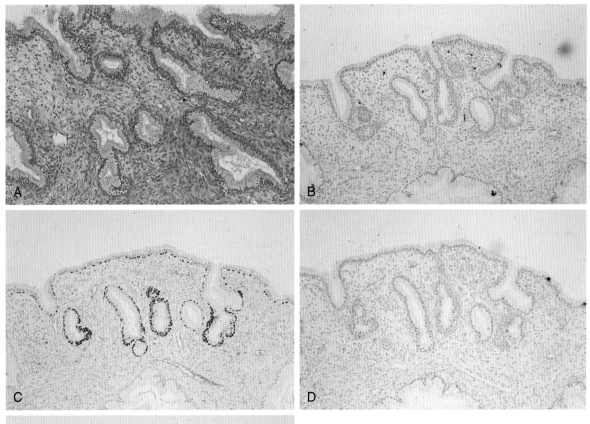

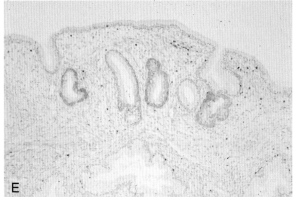

Figure 2–28. *A,* Normal endocervix. *B* to *E,* Immunohisto-chemical stains. *B,* P53 is negative. *C,* P63-positive cells on the endocervical mucosa appear in a discontinuous fashion, whereas a layer of positive cells is seen in the base of the endocervical glands. *D,* Ki-67 is negative. *E,* Bcl2 is expressed in cells beneath the endocervical cells in a manner similar to that of p63 in *C.*

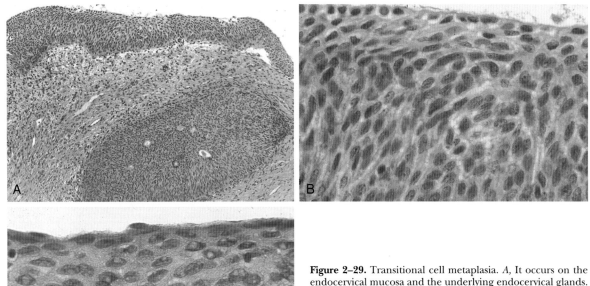

Figure 2–29. Transitional cell metaplasia. *A*, It occurs on the endocervical mucosa and the underlying endocervical glands. *B*, On a higher magnification, they have oval to elongated hyperchromatic nuclei and a moderate amount of cytoplasm. No mitotic figures are evident. *C*, On a higher magnification, nuclear grooves are evident. Some of the cells contain nuclear vacuoles. Occasional nuclei are surrounded by clear halos.

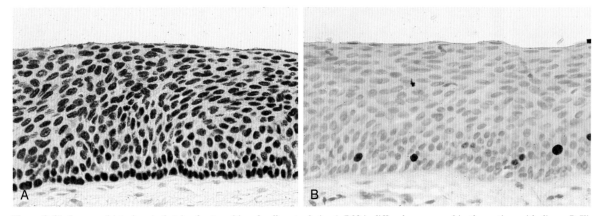

Figure 2–31. Immunohistochemical stains for transitional cell metaplasia. *A*, P63 is diffusely expressed in the entire epithelium. *B*, Ki-67 positive cells are limited to a few cells in the parabasal layers.

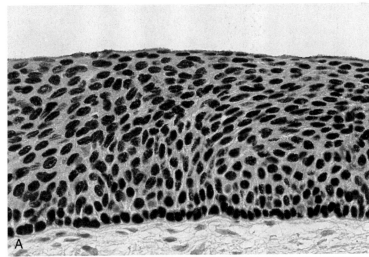

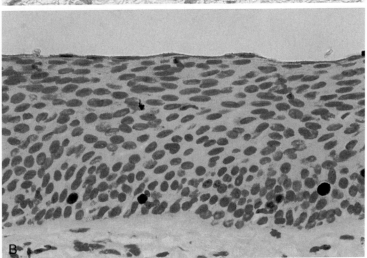

Figure 2–31. Immunohistochemical stains for transitional cell metaplasia. *A,* P63 is diffusely expressed in the entire epithelium. *B,* Ki-67 positive cells are limited to a few cells in the parabasal layers. (See color section.)

blood vessels.[17] Nerve fibers and lymphatics often accompany the blood vessels.

REFERENCES

1. Averette HE, Weinstein GD, Frost P. Autoradiographic analysis of cell proliferation kinetics in human genital tissues. I: Normal cervix and vagina. Am J Obstet Gynecol 108:8, 1970.
2. Blasco L. Clinical approach to the evaluation of sperm-cervical mucous interactions. Fertil Steril 28:1133, 1977.
3. Bulmer O. The development of the human vagina. J Anat 91:490, 1957.
4. Carmichael R, Jeaffreson BL. Basal cells in the epithelium of the human cervical canal. J Pathol Bact 49:63, 1939.
5. Carmichael R, Jeaffreson BL. Squamous metaplasia of the columnar epithelium in the human cervix. J Pathol Bact 52:173, 1941.
6. Clement PB. Multinucleated stromal giant cells of the uterine cervix. Arch Pathol Lab Med 109:200, 1985.
7. Crum CP. Contemporary theories of cervical carcinogenesis: The virus, the host, and the stem cell. Mod Pathol 13:243, 2000.
8. Cunha GR. The dual origin of vaginal epithelium. Am J Anat 132:387, 1975.
9. Curtis AH, Anson BJ, Ashley FL, et al. The blood vessels of the female pelvis in relation to gynecological surgery. Surg Gynecol Obstet 75:421, 1942.
10. Deter RL. Embryology. In: Gardner HL, Kaufman RH (eds). Benign Diseases of the Vulva and Vagina. Boston, G.K. Hall, 1981, p 13.
11. Dierks K. Der normale meusuelle Zyklus der menschlichen Vaginalschleimhaut. Arcj f Gumal 130:46, 1927.
12. Egan AJM, Russell P. Transitional (urothelial) cell metaplasia of the uterine cervix: Morphological assessment of 32 cases. Intl J Gynecol Pathol 16:89, 1997.
13. Elliot GB, Elliot JDA. Superficial stromal reactions of lower genital tract. Arch Pathol 95:100, 1973.
14. Ferenczy A, Richart RM. Scanning electron microscopy of the cervical transformation zone. Am J Obstet Gynecol 115:151, 1973.

15. Ferenczy A, Richard RM. Female Reproductive System: Dynamics of Scan and Transmission Electron Microscopy. New York, John Wiley & Sons, 1974.

16. Fluhmann CF. Focal hyperplasia (tunnel clusters) of the cervix uteri. Obstet Gynecol 17:206, 1961.

17. Fluhmann CF. The Cervix Uteri and Its Diseases. Philadelphia, W.B. Saunders, 1961.

18. Forsberg JG. Cervicovaginal epithelium: Its origin and development. Am J Obstet Gynecol 115:1025, 1973.

19. Forsberg JG, Kalland T. Embryology of the Genital Tract in Humans and in Rodents. In: Herbst AL, Bern HA (eds). Developmental Effects of Diethylstilbestrol (DES) in Pregnancy. New York, Thieme-Stratton, 1981, p 4.

20. Fox H, Kazzaz G, Langley FA. Argyrophil and argentaffin cells in the female genital tract and in ovarian mucinous cysts. J Pathol Bacteriol 88:479, 1964.

21. Geng L, Connolly DC, Isacson C, et al. Atypical immature metaplasia (AIM) of the cervix: Is it related to high-grade squamous intraepithelial lesion (HSIL)? Hum Pathol 30:345, 1999.

22. Gould PR, Barter RA, Papadimetriou JM. An ultrastructural, cytochemical, and autoradiographic study of the mucous membrane of the human cervical canal with reference to subcolumnar basal cells. Am J Pathol 95:1, 1979.

23. Graham CE. Uterine cervical epithelium of fetal and immature human females in relation to estrogenic stimulation. Am J Obstet Gynecol 97:1033, 1967.

24. Gray H. Anatomy of the Human Body, 29th ed. Goss AM (ed). Philadelphia, Lea & Febiger, 1973.

25. Howard L, Erickson CC, Stoddard LD. A study of the incidence and histogenesis of endocervical metaplasia and intraepithelial carcinoma. Cancer 4:1210, 1951.

26. Koff AK. Development of the vagina in the human fetus. Contrib Embryol 24:59, 1933.

27. Krantz KE. Innervation of the human vulva and vagina. A microscopic study. Obstet Gynecol 12:382, 1958.

28. Lawrence ED, Shingleton HM. Early physiologic squamous metaplasia of the cervix: Light and electron microscopic observations. Am J Obstet Gynecol 137:661, 1980.

29. Linhartova A. Extent of columnar epithelium of the ectocervix between the ages of 1 and 13 years. Obstet Gynecol 52:451, 1978.

30. Madile BM. The cervical epithelium from fetal age to adolescence. Obstet Gynecol 47:536, 1976.

31. Meyer R. Die epithelentwicklung der cervix und portio vaginalis und die pseudoerosio gongenita. Arch Gynak 91:579, 1910.

32. Moore KL. The Developing Human: Clinically Oriented Embryology. Philadelphia, W.B. Saunders, 1973, p 212.

33. Nigogosyan G, de la Pava, S, Pickren JW. Melanoblasts in vaginal mucosa. Cancer 17:912, 1964.

34. O'Rahilly R. The embryology and anatomy of the uterus. In: Norris HJ, Hertig AT, Abell MR (eds). The Uterus. Baltimore, Williams & Wilkins, 1973, p 17.

35. Papanicolaou GN, Traut HF, Marchetti AA. The Epithelia of Women's Reproductive Organs: A Correlative Study of Cyclic Changes. New York, The Commonwealth Fund, 1948.

36. Plentl AA, Friedman EA. Lymphatic System of the Female Genital Tract: The Morphologic Basis of Oncologic Diagnosis and Therapy. Philadelphia, W.B. Saunders, 1971.

37. Reid BL, Singer A, Coppleson M. The process of cervical regeneration after electrocauterization. Aust NZ J Obstet Gynecol 7:125, 1967.

38. Richart RM. A radiographic analysis of cellular proliferation in dysplasia and carcinoma in situ of the uterine cervix. Am J Obstet Gynecol 86:925, 1963.

39. Robboy SJ. A hypothetic mechanism of diethylstilbestrol (DES)-induced anomalies in exposed progeny. Human Pathol 14:831, 1983.

40. Robboy SJ, Hill EC, Sandberg ED, et al. Vaginal adenosis in women born prior to the diethylstilbestrol era. Human Pathol 17:488, 1986.

41. Robboy SJ, Taguchi O, Cunha GR. Normal development of the human female reproductive tract and alterations resulting from experimental exposure to diethylstilbestrol. Human Pathol 13:190, 1982.

42. Robboy SJ, Bernhardt PF, Parmley T. Embryology of the Female Genital Tract and Disorders of Abnormal Sexual Development. In: Blaustein's Pathology of the Female Genital Tract, 4th ed. Kurman RJ (ed). New York, Springer-Verlag, 1994, pp 3–29.

43. Rorat E, Ferenczy A, Richart RM. Human Bartholin's gland, duct, and duct cyst. Arch Pathol 99:367, 1975.

44. Rorie DK, Newton M. Histologic and chemical studies of the smooth muscle in the human cervix and uterus. Am J Obstet Gynecol 99:466, 1967.

45. Schellhas HF, Heath G. Cell renewal in the human cervix uteri: A radioautographic study of DNA, RNA, and protein synthesis. Am J Obstet Gynecol 104:617, 1969.

46. Schurch W, McDowell EM, Trump BF. Long-term organ culture of human uterine endocervix. Cancer Res 38:3723, 1978.

47. Segal GH, Hart WR. Cystic endocervical tunnel clusters: A clinicopathologic study of 29 cases of so-called adenomatous hyperplasia. Am J Surg Pathol 14:895, 1990.

48. Singer A. The cervical epithelium during pregnancy and the puerperium. In: Jordon JA, Singer A (eds). The Cervix. London, W.B. Saunders, 1976, p 105.

49. Slone S, Reynolds, Gall S, et al. Localization of chromogranin, synaptophysin, serotonin, and CXCR2 in neuroendocrine cells of the minor vestibular glands: An immunohistochemical study. Int J Gynecol Pathol 18:360, 1999.

50. Song J. The Human Uterus: Morphogenesis and Embryological Basis for Cancer. Springfield, Ill., Charles C Thomas, 1964.

51. Stockard CR, Papanicolaou GN. The existence of a typical oestrous cycle in the guinea pig with a study of its histological and physiologic changes. Am J Anat 22:225, 1917.

52. Ulfelder H, Robboy SJ. The embryologic development of the human vagina. Am J Obstet Gynecol 126:769, 1976.

53. Valdes-Dapena MA. The Development of the Uterus in Late Fetal Life, Infancy and Childhood. In: Norris HJ, Hertig AT, Abell MR (eds). The Uterus. Baltimore, Williams & Wilkins, 1973, p 40.

54. Weir MM, Bell DA, Young RH. Transitional cell metaplasia of the uterine cervix and vagina: An underrecognized lesion that may be confused with high-grade dysplasia. A report of 59 cases. Am J. Surg Path 21:510, 1997.

55. Yang A, Kaghad M, Wang Y, et al. P63, a p53 homolog at 3q27–29, encodes multiple products with transactivating, death-inducing, and dominant-negative activities. Mol Cell 2:305, 1998.

56. Yang A, Schweitzer R, Sun D, et al. P63 is essential for maintaining proliferative capacity of ectoderm involved in limb, craniofacial, and epithelial development. Nature 398:714, 1999.

57. Yang A, Yang YM, Sun D, et al. P63: A p53 homologue that is a differentiation-specific marker in cervical squamous epithelium. Mod Pathol 12:178A, 1999.

3

DEVELOPMENTAL ANOMALIES AND CYSTS OF THE LOWER FEMALE GENITAL TRACT

DEVELOPMENTAL ANOMALIES OF THE VULVA

Developmental anomalies of the vulva are related to sex chromosome abnormalities, hormonal imbalances, target organ insensitivity, developmental defects, and other factors that remain to be clarified. The development of a male-oriented sex organ requires the presence of a testis and its secretory products, including testosterone and müllerian-inhibiting substances. The formation of testis depends on a Y chromosome and one or more X chromosomes. If there is no Y chromosome but two or more X chromosomes, an ovary will be produced.

If the testis is absent or abnormal, the external genitalia will be female-oriented, regardless of the sex chromosomes and the presence or absence of an ovary. Thus, in women with Turner's syndrome and other forms of gonadal dysgenesis, the external genitalia are female oriented, but secondary sexual development does not occur and the müllerian derivatives remain infantile. Other somatic anomalies are common. Rarely, agenesis of müllerian ducts may be associated with gonadal dysgenesis.[20]

57

In true hermaphrodites, the genitalia may be of normal male type or female type, or both. Both the testis and ovary are present. They may be located on opposite sides or coexist in the same gonad as ovotestis. The sex chromosomes are usually of the normal female pattern but, in some cases, are either of male type or of a mosaic form.[80]

In patients with testicular feminizing syndrome, despite the presence of X, Y chromosomes and testes, the phenotype is female. It is believed that the target organs fail to respond to androgens. The vulva appears normal or sometimes hypoplastic. The vagina is short and ends in a blind pouch without a uterus. After puberty, virilization of the vulva with a hypertrophic clitoris may be seen in an incomplete form of the syndrome. The pubic and axillary hair is absent. The testes are often located in the inguinal canal, abdominal cavity, or labia majora. Their removal is recommended because of the increased risk of developing malignant germ cell tumors.[35]

Newborns with congenital adrenal hyperplasia (adrenogenital syndrome) and, less commonly, an excess of exogenous or maternal androgen (such as luteoma of pregnancy) develop hypertrophy of the clitoris. In such cases, labioscrotal fusion is common. Later in life, hypertrophy of the clitoris is most often secondary to androgen-producing ovarian or adrenal tumors.[35]

Hypertrophy of the labia minora may be seen at birth or later in life. The known etiologic factors include filarial infections, congenital lymphedema, and manipulations.[75] Rarely, it is associated with multiple sclerosis. The hypertrophic labia minora protrude in a wing-like manner from the vulva. Resection with a plastic repair is necessary if symptoms occur.

Aplasia of the vulva is presumably due to the developmental failure of the urogenital sinus. A small uterus, tubes, and ovaries were present in the case described by Dunn.[24] Hypoplasia (infantilism) of the vulva when associated with hypoplasia of the remainder of the genital structures is usually secondary to hypopituitary dwarfism or Turner's syndrome.

Persistence of an unperforated cloacal membrane may result in obliteration of the introitus by a thick membrane.[62] The cloacal membrane normally is perforated by the urogenital opening to form the urogenital sinus. Duplication of the vulva is extremely rare and may be partial or total.

In summary, work-up of patients with anomalies of the external genitalia requires appropriate physical examination, hormonal assays, and chromosome karyotyping, including buccal mucosa for sex chromatin.[35]

DEVELOPMENTAL ANOMALIES OF THE VAGINA AND CERVIX

Congenital malformations of the vagina and cervix are generally part of uterine maldevelopment, resulting from abnormal development and fusion of the müllerian ducts.[41] Less commonly, the anomalies are related to the abnormal transitions between urogenital sinus and müllerian epithelium.

The frequency of uterine malformation is estimated to be 1 in 300 women.[8] Most malformations are detected during puberty or adult life because of menstrual disorders, infertility, abortion, premature delivery, abruption, or abnormal fetal position. The cause of cervical malformations in most instances is unknown. Some of the malformations occur in women with trisomy D (46, XX, 13+). In this condition, 45% of women have a double or septate uterus, often coexisting with cleft face.[6] Intrauterine exposure to thalidomide may be associated with uterus didelphys and pseudodidelphys.[8] Vaginal adenosis and gross abnormalities of the cervix, corpus, and uterine tubes have been reported in women exposed to diethylstilbestrol (DES) in utero.

Developmental Defects of the Müllerian Ducts

Agenesis or absence of the uterus and cervix is the result of bilateral agenesis or aplasia of the urogenital primordium or müllerian ducts in the early stage of development. Arrest of the mesonephric duct is accompanied by the absence of the ipsilateral müllerian duct at the comparable level. The kidney is frequently absent on the side without hemi-uterus. The other müllerian duct develops into a uterus unicornis (Fig. 3–1).[8]

Vaginal agenesis is often associated with anomalies of the uterus or urinary tract. The external genitalia may appear normal, but the vagina may exist only as a small indentation or pouch. Complete vaginal agenesis associated with uterine agenesis may be first suspected by a history of amenorrhea or by unsuccessful attempts at first intercourse. Vaginal agenesis oc-

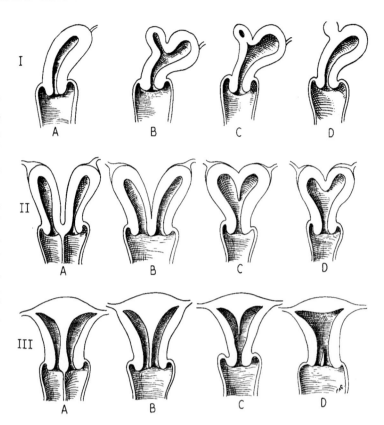

Figure 3–1. Congenital malformations of the uterus. I: Aplasia of one duct. *A,* Uterus unicornis unicollis, dysplasia of one duct. *B,* Asymmetric uterus bicornis with rudimentary horn. *C,* Asymmetric uterus bicornis with partially atretic rudimentary horn. *D,* Asymmetric uterus bicornis with atretic rudimentary horn. II: Defect in the fusion of the müllerian ducts. *A,* Uterus duplex or didelphys with double vagina. *B,* Uterus bicornis duplex. *C,* Uterus bicornis unicollis. *D,* Uterus arcuatus. III: Defect in the resorption of müllerian ducts. *A,* Uterus septus duplex with septate vagina. *B,* Uterus septus duplex. *C,* Uterus subseptus. *D,* Uterus biforis. (Reproduced by permission from Schiller W. The female genitalia. In: Pathology, 2nd ed. Anderson WAD [ed]. St Louis, CV Mosby, 1953.)

curring in the presence of a functional uterus may result in an accumulation of blood that distends the uterus. Atresia of the vagina may exist alone and may result from incomplete canalization of the embryologic primordium.

Abnormal development of the cervical segment of the müllerian ducts results in an absence of cervix (uterus acollis), small cervix (uterus parvicollis), and deformed cervix (cochleate uterus). These anomalies may be associated with changes in the upper vagina.

Defects in the fusion of müllerian ducts may be complete or partial (see Fig. 3–1). In the complete form, a uterus didelphys with a complete duplication of vagina, cervix, and corpus results. More frequently, there is fusion of the vagina (pseudodidelphys) or the lower portion of the uterus. In bicornis uterus, the lower portion of the corpus is joined with the formation of two horns. The cervix may be double (bicollis) (Fig. 3–2) or single (unicollis) (Fig. 3–3). Similarly, the vagina may be single or double. This may be associated with uterus didelphys.

Incomplete resorption of the fused müllerian ducts causes the persistence of a septum, which may be complete (uterus septum), ex-

tending from the corpus to the cervix, or incomplete (uterus subseptum), confined to the corpus or to the external os (uterus biforis) (see Fig. 3–1). In the vagina, the longitudinal septum may be contiguous with that of the uterine corpus or cervix. Incomplete or partial longitudinal vaginal septum is more often encountered and usually occurs without uterine anomalies.

Transverse vaginal septum may also exist in the vagina, most commonly at the junction of the upper and middle thirds of the vagina. When complete and imperforate, there may be symptoms and signs of hydrometrocolpos or hematometrocolpos. Incomplete or perforated vaginal septum unassociated with narrowing of the vagina is less likely to produce significant symptoms.

An imperforate hymen is usually not recognized in young children unless the accumulated vaginal secretion is sufficient to cause protrusion of the hymen. It is more commonly recognized after puberty when the accumulated secretions produce hydrohematocolpos. Because the cervix and uterine body are more resistant to distention, the initial dilation occurs in the vagina, and

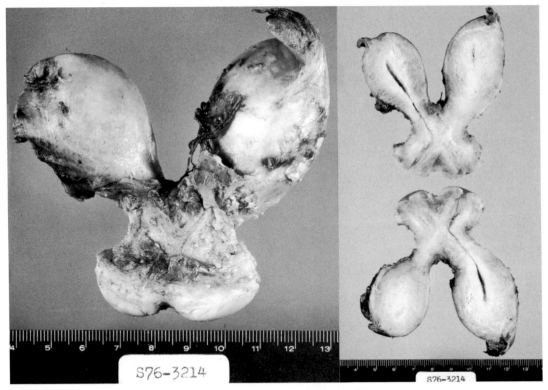

Figure 3–2. Uterus bicornis duplex bicollis.

only with an increasing accumulation of secretion does hydrohematometra or hydrohemato-salpinx occur. This may be associated with cyclic abdominal pain, a palpable abdominal mass, or urinary retention.

Modified cloaca may be formed by the anomalous development of anatomic structures in proximity to the vagina. As a result, the intestine, urinary tract, and vagina may open into a common channel. In some cases, either the rec-

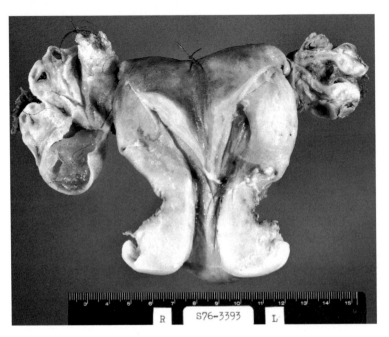

Figure 3–3. Uterus bicornis unicollis and dermoid cyst of right ovary.

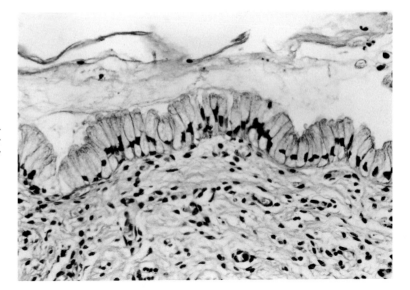

Figure 3–4. Adenosis. Vaginal mucosa replaced by simple columnar epithelium similar to that normally observed in endocervix.

tum or the urethra may open into the vagina. Exstrophy of the urinary bladder may occur.

Vaginal Adenosis

Definition and Frequency

The process currently designated as vaginal adenosis has been recognized for many years. The first description of the entity is credited to Von Preuschen in 1877.[109] In the early literature, similar, if not identical, changes were referred to as vaginal adenomatosis,[11,105] vaginitis adenofibrosa,[59] and endocervicosis. Some authors erroneously considered adenosis to be a malignant process and referred to it as infiltrating diffuse adenoma with malignant change[40] or primary adenocarcinoma of the vagina.[99] In addition, those vaginal cysts, which may be the residuum of a pre-existing adenosis, were initially referred to as diffuse adenosis[70] and later as vaginal adenosis.[71] Adenosis currently is defined as the presence of glandular (columnar) epithelium or its mucinous products occurring in the vagina (Figs. 3–4 to 3–6).[100]

Relatively few studies in the literature provide information on the frequency of vaginal adenosis. Von Preuschen[109] found the process in 4 of 36 vaginal specimens, whereas others were unable to demonstrate adenosis in any of

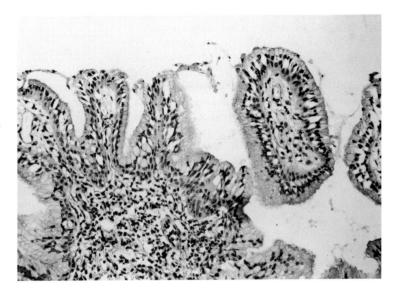

Figure 3–5. Adenosis. Surface of vagina is replaced by mucinous columnar epithelium in papillary projections. This is unusual.

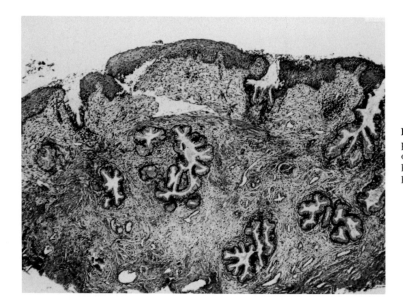

Figure 3–6. Adenosis. Metaplasia replaces most of the surface epithelium once covered by columnar epithelium. Glands are numerous in the lamina propria.

14 vaginal specimens.[78] The first comprehensive study of the vagina was reported by Sandberg et al.[96,97] In this study, none of 13 vaginas of prepubertal females contained adenosis, whereas 9, or 40.8%, of 22 vaginas in postpubertal women were found to have evidence of adenosis. The youngest individual with adenosis in this series was born in 1938—the year in which DES was first synthesized. Thus, none of the cases in this study are related to intrauterine exposure to DES (Fig. 3–7). More recently, Robboy et al.[92] reported 41 women with vaginal adenosis who were born before 1942. They ranged in age from 24 to 88 years (median 44 years). Only 15% were symptomatic. In other women, the vaginal adenosis was found incidentally in the histologic sections of vaginal specimen or clinically as nodule or cyst.

A wide variation exists in the reported frequency of adenosis in the offspring of women treated with DES during pregnancy.[104] Herbst and colleagues[46] observed adenosis in 35% of the cases in their study, whereas in studies by Sherman et al.[103] it was present in more than 90% of the women examined. A number of factors are known to have a bearing on the occurrence rate of adenosis in women with intrauterine exposure to DES.[67] Of these, the most important are the method of case selection, the age at which the patient is examined, the definition of adenosis, the time in pregnancy when DES was first given and the dosage used, and whether the cervicovaginal hood is considered to be of vaginal or cervical origin.

In women exposed to DES in utero, the frequency of vaginal epithelial changes (macroscopic changes identified by colposcopy or iodine staining as well as the microscopic changes of adenosis) was found to be related to the method of case selection.[67] Vaginal epithelial changes were identified in 34% of the women identified on the basis of record review, in 59% of the documented walk-ins, and in 65% of the documented physician referrals. As the result of multiple biopsies, most women with vaginal epithelial changes were ultimately proved to have vaginal adenosis.[85] The frequency of 34%[85] observed in women identified on the basis of record review is believed to be a reasonable estimate of the occurrence of adenosis in the offspring of women given DES in pregnancy.

Location

The currently accepted definition of adenosis is restricted to those processes having columnar epithelium or its mucinous products occurring in the vagina.[100] It does not provide for the recognized involutionary changes associated with adenosis, even though the latter are currently not known to be related to any other process originating in the vagina. Comparable changes are reported to involve the vagina and the vulva as well as the inner aspect of the hymen[64] and may be associated with imperforate hymen.[2] As with the controversy about the origin of the cervicovaginal hood, it is difficult to determine whether columnar epithelium in-

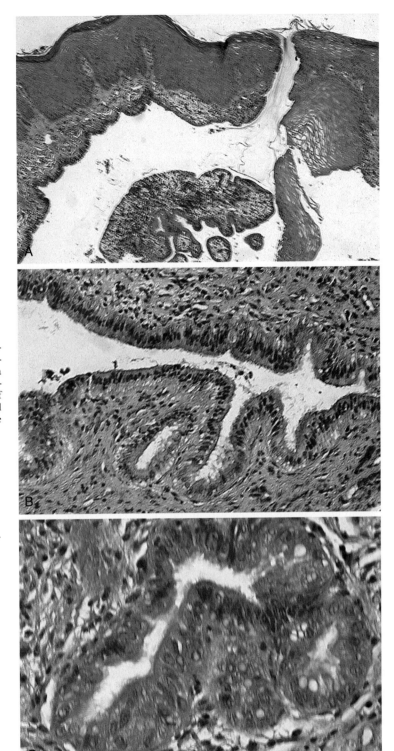

Figure 3–7. Vaginal adenosis in a 54-year-old woman without DES exposure. *A,* The overlying vaginal mucosa is hyperkeratotic. The vaginal adenosis is predominantly cystic. *B,* Some of the glands are lined by endocervical mucinous cells. *C,* Other glands are lined by ciliated tubal epithelium.

volving this structure warrants the designation of vaginal adenosis. Adenosis involved the anterior vaginal wall in 81% of cases and was confined to this site in 56% of cases.[64] The posterior and lateral vaginal walls were less frequently involved. In women identified on the basis of record review, vaginal epithelial changes were identified in the upper one third of the vagina in 23%, in the middle third in 9%, and in the lower third in 2% of cases.[85] Adenosis is most likely to be found in the upper one third of the anterior vaginal wall.

Pathology

On gross or colposcopic examination, adenosis may appear as red, velvety epithelium, which may be arranged in grape-like clusters[105] or as white areas with or without punctation or characterized by mosaicism.[15] The gross or colposcopic appearance depends on the age of the patient and the involutionary stage of the adenosis.

Early in the evolutionary process, columnar epithelium may involve the surface epithelium alone (see Fig. 3–4).[67] When confined to this location, the epithelium may have a papillary growth pattern (see Fig. 3–5). This is reported to occur in less than 10% of cases.[100] The columnar epithelium may involve the surface and be contiguous with columnar epithelium-lining glands occurring in the lamina propria or may be identified only in glands confined to the lamina propria (see Fig. 3–6). The latter is more common and is related to the age of the patient and the site studied within the vagina.[2] Columnar epithelum-lined glands were ob-

served in the lamina propria of 40% of the samples from the upper one third of the vagina, in 62% of the samples from the middle third of the vagina, and in 100% of the samples obtained from the lower third of the vagina.[85]

The columnar epithelium associated with adenosis may resemble the epithelium of the endocervix, endometrium, or uterine tube (Figs. 3–4 to 3–8) or may be represented in the form of mucinous droplets. Mucin-containing cells are reported to occur in 62%[56] to 85% of cases.[85] Cells of the tubuloendometrial type are reported to occur in 21% of cases.[85] Mucinous droplets were observed in 43% of cases.[85]

The distribution of the various types of columnar epithelium is related to the duration of the adenosis and the site of involvement within the vagina. When confined to the surface, the epithelium is usually of the mucinous type and only rarely is of the tubuloendometrial type. Glands present in the lamina propria may be lined with mucinous epithelium or tubuloendometrial cells. The latter were observed in 40% of the cases studied by Robboy et al.[85] The frequency of this cell type is also related to the site of involvement in the vagina. Tubuloendometrial cells were present in 20% of the specimens from the upper one third of the vagina, in 31% of the changes in the middle third of the vagina, and in 100% of the changes in the lower third of the vagina. This cell type is also observed more frequently in adenosis of the anterior wall than of the posterior or lateral vaginal wall.

Droplets of mucin without identifiable columnar cells are commonly observed within metaplastic epithelium. The latter may repre-

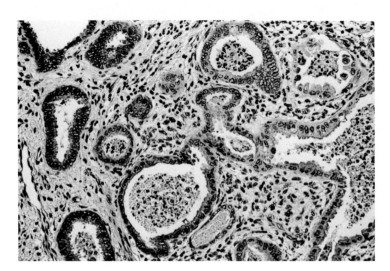

Figure 3–8. Adenosis involving lamina propria. The lining epithelium is tubuloendometrial type and does not resemble the endocervical epithelium more commonly found.

sent reserve cell hyperplasia, immature squamous metaplasia, or a metaplastic squamous epithelium (Figs. 3–6 and 3–9) whose maturity approaches or is equivalent to that of the normal native stratified squamous epithelium of the vagina. The amount and maturity of the metaplastic epithelium increases with the duration of the adenosis. Hyperkeratosis may occur over the surface of the mature metaplastic epithelium.

Often associated with the epithelial changes of adenosis is an infiltration of lymphocytes or plasma cells in the adjacent stroma. Less frequently, neutrophils are seen. The infiltrate is usually more pronounced in the vicinity of the glands lying within the lamina propria, and it may be observed beneath columnar epithelium covering the surface of the vagina.

Adenosis involving the surface of the vagina is reflected in appropriately obtained cellular samples. In samples collected by scraping the four quadrants of the vagina, changes in the surface epithelium are readily detected,[63] and the evidence obtained correlates with the findings of an experienced colposcopist.[9]

Columnar epithelium of the mucinous type may exist alone or in combination with metaplasia.[39] The latter may reflect reserve cell hyperplasia, immature squamous metaplasia, or mature squamous metaplasia. Droplets of mucin may be evident in metaplastic cells. In adenosis of long duration, only metaplasia may be evident. This may be associated with evidence of hyperkeratosis.[9,32,64] Microglandular hyperplasia may coexist with adenosis.[82]

Merchant and Gale[60] reported a 36-year-old DES-exposed daughter, who presented with mild squamous dysplasia of the cervix and extensive vaginal adenosis. In the latter, endocervical cells, ciliated tuboendometrial cells, and metaplastic intestinal cells—including goblet cells, Paneth cells, and argentaffin cells—were present. Pillai et al.[68] reported a 29-year-old woman from India, who presented with a 3×4 cm polypoid, red growth in the posterior fornix and constriction in the upper third of the vagina. Biopsy of the growth showed endocervical glands. This is an example of vaginal adenosis without DES exposure.

The development of vaginal adenosis and clear cell adenocarcinoma following topical (fluorouracil [5-FU]) treatment for cervical or vaginal condyloma and dysplasia has also been reported. They are discussed in the section on the morphogenesis of adenosis.

Natural Evolution

Considerable knowledge has accumulated regarding the natural history of vaginal adenosis. In newborns exposed to DES in utero, a mucinous type of columnar epithelium may occur on the vaginal surface.[50] In other respects, however, the changes are unlike those observed in the adult. Some stimulus occurring at the time of puberty may cause the "ripening" of the process. Adenosis is rarely observed in the prepubertal patient and is more commonly detected after puberty. Although the difficulties inherent in examining females in the immedi-

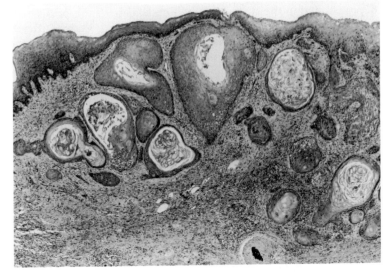

Figure 3–9. Adenosis. As the result of involution, the surface epithelium and the pre-existing glands of the lamina propria are replaced by metaplastic squamous epithelium. (H&E, ×38) (From Ng ABP, Reagan JW, Nadji M, Greening S. Natural history of vaginal adenosis in women exposed to diethylstilbestrol in utero. J Reprod Med 18:7, 1977; used by permission.)

ate postpubertal period may have some bearing on the frequency of the change at this time in life, some evidence suggests that a latent period is involved.

Changes are initially observed in the surface epithelium and are later observed in the lamina propria. In both the surface epithelium and the epithelium lining the glands in the lamina propria, involution occurs in a high percentage of women (see Figs. 3–6 and 3–9). This entails the development of squamous metaplasia, which ultimately becomes as mature as the native stratified squamous epithelium of the vagina (see Fig. 3–9). The metaplastic epithelium replacing the glands in the lamina propria may ultimately disappear, although the mechanism responsible for this is unknown. The change may persist for many years in a small number of cases.

The overall mean age at detection of adenosis was 20.9 ± 4.1 years based on cellular evidence and 20.4 ± 3.4 years based on histopathologic evidence.[113] Burke et al.[25] reported the mean age at first detection to be 21.3 years. Columnar epithelium alone was evident in the surface epithelium at a mean age of 19.9 ± 4 years. Columnar epithelium with immature squamous metaplasia was first detected at a mean age of 20.5 ± 3.9 years. Squamous metaplasia alone was first detected at a mean age of 22.7 ± 4.1 years. Associated hyperkeratosis was evident at a mean age of 23.6 ± 3.8 years. In women with prior evidence of adenosis, conversion to a mature squamous epithelium was observed at a mean age of 24.2 ± 6.9 years. In studies by Zerner et al.,[113] biopsies documented an involution of the changes in the lamina propria that paralleled the regression demonstrated in the surface epithelium by cellular findings.

After 6 years follow-up of 953 women having prior evidence of adenosis demonstrated by cellular samples, only 5% of the women had persisting columnar epithelium.[32] Because biopsies were used only rarely in this study, the disappearance of the change cannot be attributed to inadvertent removal at the time of biopsy.[15,32] Burke et al.[15] have documented the spontaneous involution of adenosis by direct visualization under colposcopy and by biopsy. Of women with vaginal columnar epithelium followed for more than 3 years, all had replacement by white epithelium, which usually reflects the presence of squamous metaplasia in the surface epithelium. It is of particular interest that involution occurred earlier in the vagina than in the cervicovaginal collar. Whether there is an increased risk for the development of squamous dysplasia in vaginal squamous metaplasia is discussed in Chapter 7.

Morphogenesis

Adenosis has been produced in experimental animals exposed to stilbestrol in utero and in newborn mice treated with stilbestrol.[27,58,69] Adenosis confirmed by directed biopsies was identified in three of eight offspring of rhesus monkeys treated with DES during pregnancy.[42] Comparable changes were not observed in control animals. Changes compatible with adenosis have been observed in mice treated with estradiol-17 and stilbestrol during the neonatal period[20] and in mice treated with estrogen during the perinatal period.[69] When pregnant mice were treated with varying daily doses of DES during the period of major organogenesis, a dose-related increase in the abnormalities of the genital tracts in the offspring occurred. Excess vaginal cornification was a common finding in mice exposed in utero to DES. The unstated number of mice developing adenosis apparently were exposed to a lower dose of stilbestrol.

In humans, vaginal adenosis is indistinguishable histologically in women with or without DES exposure.[88,92] According to Robboy et al.,[87,89,92,93] the mesenchyme of the müllerian ducts plays an important role in the differentiation of the müllerian epithelium. In the DES-exposed progeny, the cervical mesenchyme apparently spreads into the vagina. This mesenchyme hinders the upward growth of urogenital sinus epithelium and results in the persistence of müllerian epithelium in the vagina. After puberty, the müllerian epithelium in the upper vagina is induced by the residual cervical stroma to develop into mucinous cells. In the lower vagina, where cervical stroma is absent, the native vaginal mesenchyme influences the müllerian epithelium to become tuboendometrial cells. When cervical and vaginal stromas are mixed, both types of epithelium occur. In nonexposed women, the vaginal adenosis is attributed to an imperfect replacement of müllerian epithelium, leaving behind some müllerian rests. Incomplete separation of the mesenchyme in the cervix and uterine corpus in DES-exposed females is believed to be the cause of gross deformities in the uterine cavity (e.g., T-shape) and cervix (e.g., ridges and hypoplastic fornices).

Dungar and Wilkinson[23] reported 8 women, aged 26 to 45 years, who received 5-FU topical treatment for cervical HPV infection or CIN 1. This treatment lasted 2 to 17 weeks and consisted of 3 to 10 applications. Five women also had undergone prior laser ablation. Adenosis was found in the upper third of the vagina with replacement of squamous mucosa by columnar epithelium, typically on the surface of the vagina, consisting of a layer of low cuboidal or mucus-secreting cells. Ciliated tuboendometrial epithelium was found in one case, and nonglycogenated squamous metaplasia occurred in some cases. Extension into the stroma, when present, was less than 2 mm in all cases. Marked acute and chronic inflammation was present. It is speculated that 5-FU treatment caused dysfunction of the inner stromal tissue or that 5-FU interferes with epithelial cell receptor for normal stromal induction to result in adenosis.

Bornstein et al.[12] reported on a 40-year-old woman who initially had received 5% 5-FU topical treatment for vaginal condyloma. This was followed by laser ablation for persistent vaginal condyloma. A year later, she developed vaginal adenosis consisting of tuboendometrial epithelium and squamous metaplasia.

Goodman et al.[36] reported on a 44-year-old woman with urethral and bladder condyloma who received intraurethral 5-FU cream in 1979. In 1983, she required laser ablation for vulvar and perianal condylomas. Vaginal condyloma in this patient was treated in 1986 with one full applicator of 5% 5-FU. Mucosal sloughing de-

veloped a week later and lasted about 3 months. Eight months later, a red papillary lesion appeared in the vaginal fornices that had previously been denuded by 5-FU. Biopsy showed papillary adenosis. This patient had no DES exposure history. Forty months after the vaginal 5-FU treatment, she was found to have an abnormal Pap smear, mild cervical dysplasia, residual vaginal adenosis, and clear cell carcinoma of the vagina. In the vaginal adenosis, ciliated tuboendometrial glands were found adjacent to the clear cell adenocarcinoma, which included 0.4 cm in situ carcinoma and 1.5 cm superficially invasive carcinoma less than 2 mm in depth. Except for atypical adenosis, no residual tumor was found in the hysterectomy and vaginectomy specimens.[36]

Atypical Variants of Adenosis

Atypical variants of adenosis have been described in the literature.[3,31,85,90,91] Robboy et al.[85] refer to five examples, Antonioli et al.[3] described two cases, and Fu et al.[31] evaluated three examples of glandular atypicality. In atypical adenosis, the glands are irregular and the epithelium is usually of the tuboloendometrial type without ciliation. The epithelium is of the simple pseudostratified or columnar type. Both cellular and nuclear enlargement may be apparent. The nuclei are sometimes varied in size and shape and have a hyperchromatic, finely granular chromatin. Small nucleoli and infrequent mitoses may exist (Figs. 3–10 and 3–11).

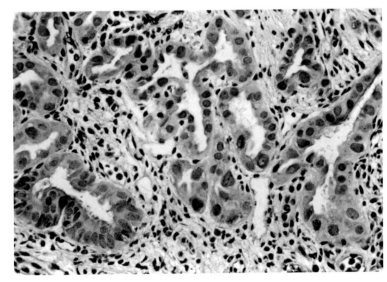

Figure 3–10. Atypical adenosis. Tuboloendometrial-type glands are in close proximity to other glands. Pseudostratification, some hyperchromasia, and rare macronucleoli are present.

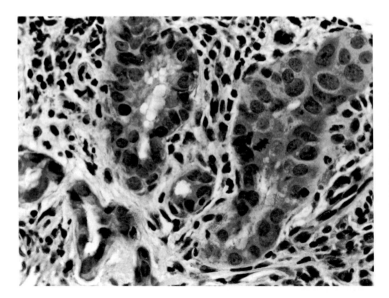

Figure 3–11. Atypical adenosis. The tubuloendometrial-type glands are pseudostratified, and the nuclei are enlarged and hyperchromatic. Macronucleoli are present in some cells. A single normal metaphase is present. Despite severe nuclear atypia, these glands are separated by fibrous stroma without evidence of invasion. This is the same case as shown in Figure 3–10.

Hobnail cells with enlarged nuclei bulging into the glandular lumens are sometimes present. The DNA ploidy pattern was polyploid in two cases and appeared to have an early aneuploid pattern in a third case.[31]

In subserial sectioning of 17 vaginal and 3 cervical clear cell adenocarcinomas, mucinous glands were generally found above the tumor, whereas tuboendometrial glands tended to surround or be located at the inferior border of the tumor.[90] In 60% of cervical and 75% of vaginal clear cell adenocarcinomas, atypical adenosis of the tuboendometrial type has been identified. This may be the forerunner of clear cell cancer.[91] Adenosis may rarely be associated with a non–clear cell type of adenocarcinoma. Ray and Ireland[77] reported a mucin-positive adenocarcinoma coexisting with vaginal adenosis. The patient was a 38-year-old woman with no history of DES exposure. The issue of squamous neoplasia in DES-exposed women[29,72,74,81,86,92] is discussed in Chapter 7.

Prasad et al.[74] reported on a 34-year-old woman who presented with a 3-cm fungating mass just inside the hymenal ring located at 11 o'clock. A small cell carcinoma was found in continuity with adjacent benign and atypical adenosis consisting of tuboendometrial cells. Neuroendocrine differentiation in small cell carcinoma was confirmed by neurosecretory granules with the use of electron microscopy and expression of chromogranin, bombesin, serotonin, and pancreatic polypeptides by immunohistochemistry stains.

Microglandular Hyperplasia of Vaginal Adenosis

Microglandular hyperplasia was initially described in the uterine cervices of women receiving oral contraceptives. More recently, the change has been observed in the vaginas or cervices of women receiving oral contraceptives who have pre-existing vaginal adenosis associated with prenatal exposure to DES.

In eight cases reported by Robboy and Welch,[82] the women, ranging in age from 17 to 25 years, were asymptomatic. The lesions were discovered on routine examination. In five cases, there was involvement of both the cervix and vagina, and in three cases, the lesions were confined to the vagina. The vaginal involvement was widespread in four cases, limited to the upper one third in two cases, related to the middle third in one case, and related to the lower third in another case. The lesions resembled multiple cauliflower-like nodularities, were flat and granular, or presented as a discrete polyp.

The lesion is composed of glandular acini, which vary in size, are closely related, and are arranged in a honeycomb or reticular pattern (Fig. 3–12). The lining epithelium is of low columnar or cuboidal epithelium and has indistinct cell boundaries. The cytoplasm is homogeneous and amphophilic and, in some cells, contains mucin. The nuclei are small, are uniform in size and shape, and have a finely granular chromatin. Often, little or no de-

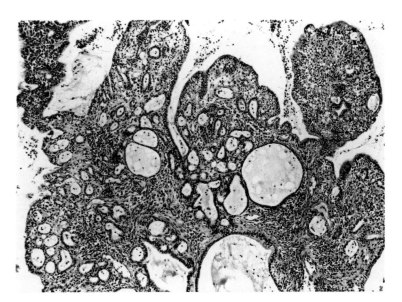

Figure 3–12. Microglandular hyperplasia of vagina in a woman with adenosis who is receiving oral contraceptives. Note the reticular pattern and lack of hyperchromasia.

tectable stroma exists between the glands, and, when present, the stroma is often edematous and infiltrated by neutrophils and lymphocytes. Metaplastic squamous epithelium can occur in the glands. In seven of eight cases,[82] adenosis was also present. Microglandular hyperplasia is benign and may be removed with biopsy, or it may involve following cessation of oral contraceptive use. It is important not to confuse microglandular hyperplasia with clear cell carcinoma.

Gross Abnormalities of the Cervix

In cervical ectropion (erosion), the ectocervix is partially or completely covered by columnar mucinous epithelium, which is often associated with squamous metaplasia. Occasionally, tubo-endometrial epithelium may coexist with mucinous epithelium. Regression of cervical ectropion occurs in most women over time.[4]

Gross structural abnormalities in the form of ridges, pseudopolyps, and hypoplasia of the cervix occur in 22% to 58% of women with a history of DES exposure in utero.[45,98] Ridges exist in several forms. Most frequently, a circular or transverse depression divides the ectocervix into two parts. The inner portion is lined by columnar epithelium and the outer zone by native or metaplastic squamous epithelium. This condition is also referred to as concentric ridge,[43] vaginal hood,[72] or pericervical collar.

Protrusion of the anterior cervical lip with a jagged, irregular or smooth, round mound caused by an excessive amount of stroma is called cock's comb cervix[72] or anterior cervical protuberance.[98] The surface is covered by squamous or columnar epithelium.

Pseudopolyp is a localized, broad-based excrescence arising from the wall of the endocervix near the external os and varying in size from 5 mm to several centimeters.[98] It lacks the stalk commonly found in an ordinary cervical polyp. The surface is invariably covered by endocervical epithelium and the underlying stroma is highly vascular. Some pseudopolyps are associated with ridges.[43] Profuse bleeding often follows disruption of the tissue; therefore, biopsy of pseudopolyp is contraindicated.

Although the abnormalities of the uterus (T-shaped cavity, small cavity, and constriction) and uterine tube may contribute to the increase of infertility and pregnancy wastage in DES-exposed women,[7,53] the effects of cervical abnormalities in this regard are uncertain.

CYSTS OF THE VULVA

Cysts of the vulva are relatively common, most of them being epidermal cysts or cysts of the Bartholin's glands. Other cysts are derived from embryonic remnants or congenital anomalies or arise secondary to infection of the urethral or paraurethral glands. Because mesonephric (wolffian) and paramesonephric (müllerian) ducts meet and terminate at the müllerian tubercle in the dorsal wall of the urogenital sinus, cysts derived from these remnants can occur in the vulvar region.

Mucinous Cysts

Mucinous cysts typically occur in the labium minus and vestibule as asymptomatic, subcutaneous, and unilateral nodules. They range in size from a few millimeters to 3 cm.[83] The cysts are lined by a single layer of tall columnar mucus-producing cells. Ciliated cells, reserve cell hyperplasia, and squamous metaplasia are common associated findings (Fig. 3–13). Smooth muscle is absent in the subepithelial stroma. The uncertain histogenetic origin of these cysts is reflected by multiple designations, such as urogenital sinus remnant, mucous cyst of the vulvar vestibule,[30] and paramesonephric or müllerian mucinous cysts.[38,49]

A close resemblance of the mucinous and ciliated cells to those present in the endocervix, endometrium, and fallopian tube suggests a paramesonephric origin.[38,49] Robboy et al.,[83] on the other hand, have demonstrated that the cells seen in mucinous cysts are identical to those of the Bartholin's gland cysts. They believe that the mucinous cysts are derived from endodermal remnants of the urogenital sinus and pathogenetically resemble mucoid cysts of the urethra and mucinous carcinoma of the urinary bladder.[83] Inflammation and obstruction of the neck of a gland leads to cystic formation. Excision,

the treatment of choice, is both diagnostic and therapeutic.

Epidermal Cysts

Epidermal cysts are usually multiple and less than 1 cm in diameter. They are located mainly on the labia majora and around the clitoris. They may follow inflammation and obstruction of the pilosebaceous follicle or implantation of squamous epithelium through episiotomy repair or may arise spontaneously. The cysts are lined by squamous epithelium and contain keratinous material and cellular debris. Sebaceous cells are occasionally found in the lining epithelium. Rarely, pilomatrixoma or calcifying epithelioma of Malherbe can occur on the vulva.[35,80]

Dermoid Cysts

Dermoid cysts are lined by epidermis and its appendages, including hair follicles, sebaceous glands, and sweat glands. These rare cysts are found along the perineal raphe.

Pilonidal Sinuses and Cysts

These occur mainly in the sacrococcygeal region but have been reported in the clitoris and elsewhere on the vulva.[76] Chronic granulomatous inflammation and sometimes abscess for-

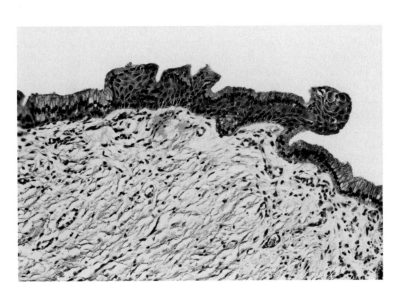

Figure 3–13. Mucinous cyst of vulva lined by tall columnar mucinous cells and metaplastic squamous cells.

mation develop as a reaction to hairs that are inverted or implanted by trauma.

Cysts of the Canal of Nuck

These result from herniation of the peritoneal sac through the inguinal canal to the insertion of the round ligament in the labium majus. It corresponds to the hydrocele in the male. Because of communication with the peritoneal cavity, local excision is often followed by recurrence. The lining mesothelial cells may be highly reactive and may be confused with malignant mesothelioma. Clinically, varicocele of the vulva may be confused with this condition.[35]

Cysts of Urethral or Paraurethral Origin

Small cysts may be found in the distal urethra or urethral orifice following inflammation or occlusion of periurethral glands and Skene's ducts.

Cysts of the Bartholin's Glands

Cyst formation of the Bartholin's glands results from blockage of the major excretory duct or one or more of the larger ducts while the distal glandular cells continue to produce mucin. Most cysts are unilateral and unilocular, involving the main excretory duct. Less fre-quently, they are bilateral and multiloculated. Ductal obstruction may be secondary to infection or may be caused by atresia of the duct, inspissated mucus near the ductal orifice, or mechanical trauma.[35] Bacterial culture of the cystic content is sterile in most cases,[55] supporting the fact that factors other than infection can cause Bartholin's gland cysts.[35]

The lining of the cyst varies. It may be normal transitional epithelium of the excretory duct, stratified squamous epithelium, cuboidal mucinous epithelium, or compressed atrophic epithelium (Fig. 3–14). The lining epithelium may be completely absent. The glandular elements may be intact or atrophic. The extent of the histologic change depends on the cystic pressure and the severity and duration of disease.

The preferred treatment for Bartholin's abscess and cyst is marsupialization. If a concomitant neoplastic disease is suspected, excision is preferred, especially in women older than 40 years. In such cases, the need for a thorough histologic study of the surrounding tissue is apparent.

Subpubic Cartilaginous Cysts

Alguacil-Garcia and Littman[1] reported two cases of subpubic cartilaginous cyst involving two postmenopausal women. In one woman, the cyst was located in the left labium majus, was 2 cm in size, and was associated with groin pain and paresthesias of the thigh. In the sec-

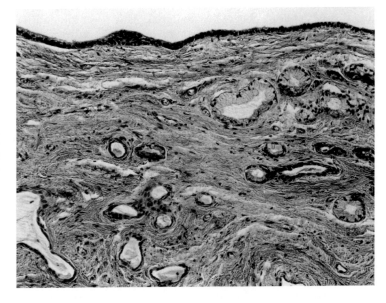

Figure 3–14. Bartholin's gland cyst. The cyst is lined in part by cuboidal mucinous cells and transitional epithelium. The adjacent Bartholin's gland has undergone atrophy and fibrosis.

ond woman, a 4 to 5 cm cystic subpubic mass extended into the urethra and vagina. Grossly, the cysts had dense, fibrous walls. They contained yellow-tan cheesy material. Histologically, the fibrous capsule consisted of irregular layers of degenerated fibrocartilaginous tissue. Secondary to degeneration, abundant mucinous material and acellular debris were produced. The authors suggested an origin from the symphysis pubis. The ligament and bursa-like tissue may have undergone degeneration to cause a cystic mass. However, no radiologic evidence showed that this mass was connected to the pubic bone.

CYSTS OF THE VAGINA

Although some authors have found that more than 50% of vaginal cysts are traumatic inclusion of vaginal stratified squamous epithelium,[21] others have reported müllerian cysts to be the most common type of vaginal cysts. In either case, squamous inclusion cysts and müllerian cysts constitute 60% to 80% of vaginal cysts. Epidermal inclusion cysts occur most often in the anterior or posterior walls and less frequently in the lateral wall.[21] They are usually asymptomatic and are detected in the childbearing years.

Patients with vaginal inclusion cysts ranged from 20 to 35 years of age. Most patients had undergone prior surgical procedures involving the vagina. The cysts were small, averaging 1.6 cm in diameter, were located in the upper part of the lamina propria, and, on transection, contained thick, yellow, cheese-like material. The cysts were lined with stratified squamous epithelium. Rupture of the cysts was associated with an infiltration of lymphocytes, plasma cells, and giant cells of a foreign-body type.

Approximately 35% to 44% of the vaginal cysts were of müllerian type and were detected in women aged 20 to 66 years (mean 36.1 years).[21,73] They were usually located in the anterior or anterolateral aspects of the vagina and, less frequently, in the lateral or posterior vaginal wall. They ranged from 1.4 to 7 cm in diameter[52,73] and some contained mucin.

The lining epithelium was composed of columnar or cuboidal mucus-secreting cells or an epithelium resembling that normally observed in endometrium or uterine tube. Squamous metaplasia was occasionally observed. In less than half of the cases, clusters of small glands were found in the adjacent connective tissue. These were lined by epithelium similar to that observed in the adjacent cyst. When present, the surface epithelium was of a stratified squamous type. It is difficult to determine how many of these cysts may have originated in adenosis.

Cysts believed to be of mesonephric origin are rare. These measure up to 2 cm in greatest diameter and are incidental findings in the lateral vaginal wall. The cysts are lined by a simple columnar or cuboidal epithelium that does not show mucin with the mucicarmine or Alcian blue stains.

Cysts lined by urothelium are rare. They are usually small, measuring 1 to 3 cm in diameter. They are typically suburethral in location but may occur elsewhere in the vagina. The lining epithelium resembles that of the paraurethral glands or Skene's ducts.

CYSTS OF THE CERVIX

Mesonephric Remnants, Cysts, and Hyperplasia

Because of a close embryonic relationship between the müllerian and mesonephric ducts, remnants of the mesonephric duct are found in relation to the uterine tube, ovary, broad ligament, lateral wall of the uterus, and vagina. In the adult cervix, the reported frequency varies from 0.4% to 22%.[47] Typically, mesonephric remnants consist of a main branching duct, the ampulla, and clusters of small tubular glands, usually located 3 to 6 mm beneath the surface of the endocervix (Fig. 3–15). In some samples, only tubular glands are present. The lining epithelium is made up of a layer of cuboidal to low columnar, nonciliated cells. The cells are taller in the ampulla. The cytoplasm is amphophilic or eosinophilic and does not react with PAS or mucicarmine stain. The amorphous material in the lumen may stain with PAS or mucicarmine stain.

Most of the mesonephric remnants are readily recognized in a conization or hysterectomy specimen. It should be emphasized that varying degrees of hyperplasia, nuclear atypia, and mitoses (up to 2 per 10 high-power fields) occur in 40% of cases seen in consultation.

Hyperplasia of the mesonephric remnants is rare. When it does occur, however, considerable diagnostic difficulty is encountered. In one study,[26] 71% of the referring pathologists had seriously considered the possibility of adeno-

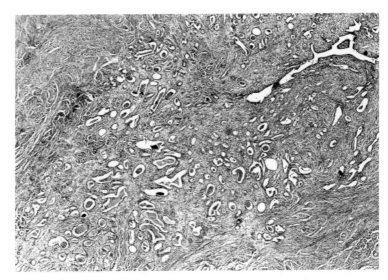

Figure 3–15. Remnants of mesonephric ducts consist of clusters of tubular glands and branching ducts with eosinophilic secretion in the lumen.

carcinoma. In another report, 45% of lobular hyperplasias and 36% of diffuse hyperplasias were considered to be malignant by the referring pathologist.[101] The hyperplasias of the mesonephric remnants are divided into lobular type (Fig. 3–16), diffuse type (Fig. 3–17), and ductal variant (Fig. 3–18). The ductal hyperplasia involves the large mesonephric ducts forming papillary projections (see Fig. 3–18). In contrast, lobular and diffuse mesonephric hyperplasias are characterized by proliferation of small tubular glands, which are lined by one to two layers of cuboidal cells with mild nuclear atypia and rare mitotic figures (see Figs. 3–16B and 3–17B). The mitotic activity is rare, less than 1 mitotic figure per 10 high-power fields in one study,[101] and up to 3 mitotic figures per 10 high-power fields in the other.[26] In the majority of cases, the tubular glands contain eosinophilic, homogeneous material, which is PAS positive. In the background are usually larger and more dilated ducts.

The ratio of lobular type to diffuse type is about 4 to 1.[26,101] In lobular hyperplasia, the lobular architecture is maintained, whereas in the diffuse type, there is extensive diffuse proliferation. In both types, the proliferating glands extend deeply into the stroma and, in most cases, close to the excision margin of the cervical conization. The dimension of lobular hyperplasia was 4.0 to 22.0 mm, and diffuse hyperplasia was 13.0 to 25.0 mm.[26] The mean size was 11.8 mm in lobular hyperplasia and that of diffuse type was 15.7 mm.[101] The mean age of women with lobular hyperplasia was 35 years, as compared with 46 years for women with the

diffuse type.[101] In the great majority of cases, mesonephric hyperplasia is an incidental finding in the cervical conization or hysterectomy specimens.

Ferry and Scully[26] described a case in which the tubular glands were lined by several layers of pseudostratified columnar cells thought to be endometrioid metaplasia or epididymal differentiation.[101] Another unusual pattern is the retiform pattern of intercommunicating, angulated tubular glands to simulate rete testes and rete ovary.[101]

In extremely florid lesions, tubular glands are diffuse and situated deeply in the stroma. This change was designated atypical mesonephric hyperplasia.[102]

Mesonephric hyperplasia can be distinguished from well-differentiated adenocarcinoma by the uniformity of the tubular structures, the lack of apoptotic bodies,[10] and the surrounding normal fibromuscular stroma, rather than the desmoplastic stroma. Most of the "mesonephric carcinomas" reported in the early literature are clear cell carcinomas using the current classification.[44]

In the case of mesonephric adenocarcinoma, confluent, back-to-back glands are lined by tumor cells with nuclear stratification, nuclear atypia, and increased mitotic activity. The possibility of minimal deviation adenocarcinoma (MDA) is often entered into the differential diagnosis. In this tumor, the neoplastic glands are much more irregular in configuration and more complex. Nuclear atypia is evident at least focally. Most of the MDAs have the appearance of the endocervical mucinous type; rarely have

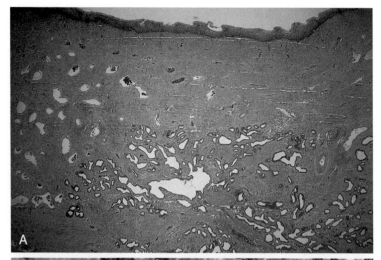

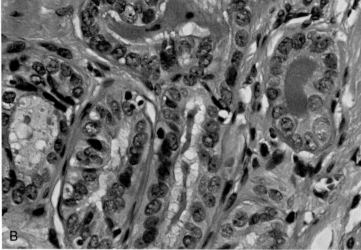

Figure 3–16. Lobular hyperplasia of mesonephric remnants. *A,* On the low-power view, proliferation of cystic ducts and small glands in a lobular pattern are seen. *B,* Small acini are lined by a layer of columnar to cuboidal cells. They demonstrate minor nuclear atypia and small nucleoli. In the glandular space, eosinophilic material is present.

endometrioid and mesonephric cell types been reported.[111] A more detailed discussion on mesonephric carcinoma is found in Chapter 8.

Cysts of the mesonephric duct may occur in the introital area of the vulva and are lined by nonciliated columnar or cuboidal epithelium. In contrast to the mucinous cysts of the vulva, mucin and glycogen production is absent. Furthermore, a layer of smooth muscle is often present beneath the epithelium.

ECTOPIC TISSUES

Ectopic Salivary Gland

Marwah and Berman[57] described ectopic salivary tissue in the left labium majus of a 38-year-

old woman. This solid mass, measuring 4 × 2 × 1 cm, was found during a routine gynecologic examination. Histologically, lobules of a combination of serous and mucinous glands are mixed with ciliated respiratory epithelium and an island of mature hyaline cartilage. In the absence of any other tissue elements, the authors favor a diagnosis of developmental anomaly, choristoma, rather than teratoma.[57]

Benign and Malignant Changes of Supernumerary Breast Tissue

In humans, a pair of bud-like thickenings appears along the ventrolateral body surface from the axillary to the inguinal region during the 6th week of embryonic development. Rudi-

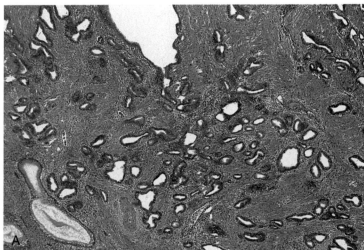

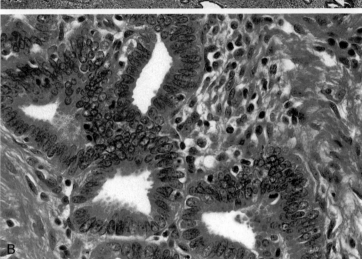

Figure 3–17. Diffuse hyperplasia of mesonephric remnants. *A,* Diffuse proliferation of small to slightly dilated glands is evident. *B,* Some of the glandular cells demonstrate nuclear stratification and rare mitotic figures.

ments of future mammary glands develop at regular intervals along the ectodermal ridges, or so-called milk lines. Normally, only the pectoral pair remains. Persistence of mammary tissue elsewhere along the milk line gives rise to supernumerary breast tissue, the nipples, or both. This occurs in 1% to 6% of women, especially in the axilla.[33]

Supernumerary breast tissue is rare in the vulva (Fig. 3–19). Garcia et al.[33] found only 17 cases reported in the literature up to 1978. In 50% of the cases, the lesion was detected by enlargement or lactational changes during a pregnancy (Fig. 3–20) or the postpartum period. In other cases, the size of the vulvar breast tissue was found to enlarge or fluctuate in relation to the menstrual cycle. All but one of the lesions were located in the labia majora. About one

third of the cases were bilateral. Histologic study of the excised vulvar tissue shows normal mammary tissue. Lactational changes were seen in association with pregnancy.

A variety of benign and malignant changes occur in the supernumerary breast tissue of the vulva, including fibrocystic disease (Fig. 3–21),[79] fibroadenoma,[14,28] intraductal papilloma (see Fig. 3–21),[79] and carcinoma.[48]

The histologic appearance of vulvar supernumerary intraductal papilloma is similar to that of the breast or hidradenoma of the vulva. Intraductal papillomas are generally larger, are less well circumscribed, and have more prominent stromal fibrosis compared with hidradenomas.[59] Lacking the histologic evidence of accompanying mammary tissue, vulvar lesions resembling fibroadenomas and intraductal

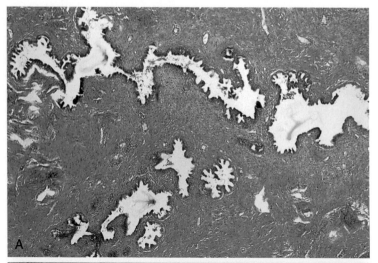

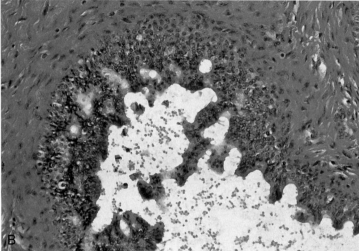

Figure 3–18. Hyperplasia or mesonephric ducts. *A*, These dilated ducts demonstrate papillar proliferation of the lining cells. *B*, Proliferating ductal cells form papillary projections and cribriform spaces.

Figure 3–19. Lobules of supernumerary breast tissue in the vulva. (Courtesy of Robert R. Rickert, M.D., Livingston, New Jersey.)

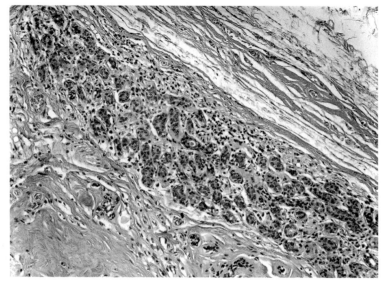

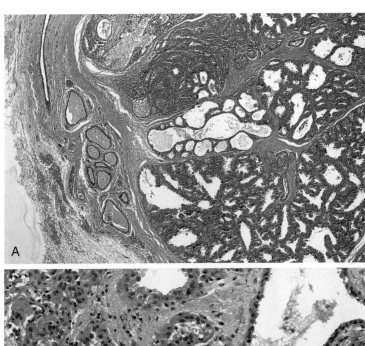

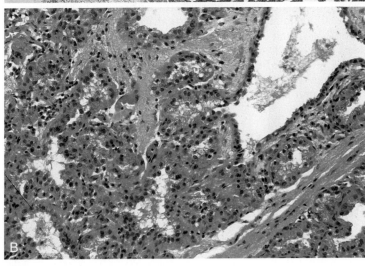

Figure 3–20. Lactational change of vulvar supramammary breast tissue. *A,* Lobules of hyperplastic breast tissue and dilated ducts containing eosinophilic secretions. *B,* Abundant vacuolated cytoplasm in the glandular cells and secretions in the glandular lumens.

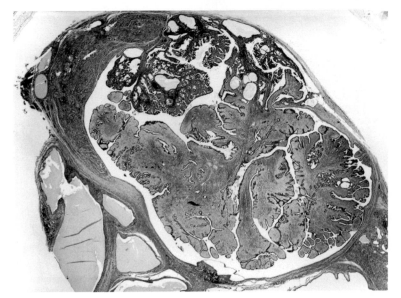

Figure 3–21. Intraductal papilloma and fibrocystic change in supernumerary breast tissue of the vulva. (From Rickert RR: Intraductal papilloma arising in supernumerary vulvar breast tissue. Obstet Gynecol 55:84S, 1980. Reprinted with permission from The American College of Obstetricians and Gynecologists.)

papillomas of the breast are most likely hidradenomas of the sweat glands.[14,79]

Tbakhi et al.[106] reported an unusual case of a 20-year-old woman who developed bilateral vulvar cysts at the age of 15 years. She was found to have two masses in the left labium, each measuring 3.0 to 4.0 cm in size. On the right side were three nodules measuring 1.0 to 2.0 cm. These were excised and had the histologic appearance of benign phyllodes tumor, consisting of leaf-like benign ducts and mildly cellular fibrous stroma without increase of mitotic activity or nuclear atypia. Adjacent to the tumor were lobules of breast tissue. Eight months after the initial excision, two 1.0 cm nodules were found in the left labium majus. These were excised, and phyllodes tumor was confirmed histologically. The fibrous stroma had a moderate cellularity. The mitotic activity was 3 mitotic figures in 50 high-power fields. The authors concluded that the newest lesion represented recurrent benign phyllodes tumor. Cystosarcoma phyllodes rarely arises from the vulvar mammary tissue (Fig. 3–22).

Irwin et al.[48] reported that a 64-year-old woman presented with a 2.7-cm firm, indurated nodule in the left lateral mons pubis deep in the subcutaneous fat tissue. This mass had the histologic appearance of infiltrating mammary carcinoma, consisting of tumor cells arranged in glands and single files. The tumor cells express estrogen and progesterone receptor proteins. One of 14 ipsilateral inguinal and femoral lymph nodes contained metastasis. Although no benign mammary tissue or intraductal carcinoma was identified adjacent to the invasive carcinoma, the authors favor an origin from the supernumerary mammary tissue based on the histologic appearance and positive estrogen and progesterone receptor proteins. After the surgery, the patient received chemotherapy with Cytoxan, methotrexate, and 5-FU, as well as pelvic irradiation and tamoxifen therapy. The follow-up period is brief.

Of the eight women with vulvar mammary carcinoma reviewed by Irwin et al.,[48] four died of disease in from 1 month to 27 months. Three women were alive 1 to 3 years after radical vul-

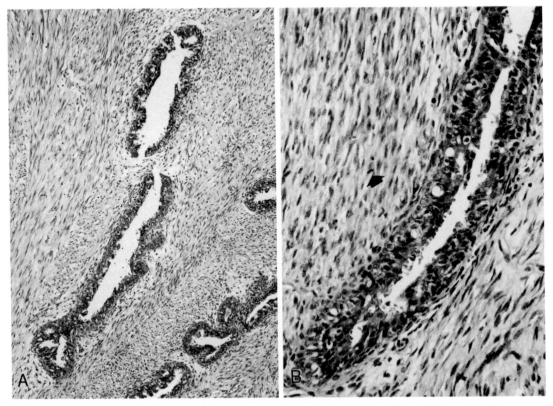

Figure 3–22. Cystosarcoma phyllodes arising in supernumerary breast tissue of the vulva. *A,* Hyperplastic ducts are surrounded by fibrosarcomatous stroma. *B,* Nuclear atypia and occasional mitotic figures (arrow) are evident. (Courtesy of Dr. Denise Hidgehi, Chicago, Illinois.)

vectomy. No follow-up information was available on the eighth patient. The optimal treatment for vulvar breast carcinoma remains controversial.

In terms of the origin of supernumerary mammary tissue of the vulva, van der Putte[107] contends that this tissue is not derived from the mammary ridges or milk lines. He has identified mammary-like glands (MLGs) located in the vulva and, less frequently, in the perineum and anal orifice. MLGs are found deep in the dermis and subcutaneous fat tissue. They are particularly common in the vulva in the areas of the sulcus interlabialis between the labia majorus and minorus.

According to van der Putte,[107] MLGs have a wide range of configuration, from simple, dilated to slightly tortuous tubular glands. They sometimes form outpouchings and acini in a lobular pattern. Secretory cells and myoepithelial cells line these glands. Cytoplasmic snouts sometimes are evident. These glandular cells also express estrogen and progesterone receptor proteins. Van der Putte believes that MLGs are intermediate between eccrine sweat gland and mammary tissue.[107] This view does not explain typical lactational changes seen in the vulvar mammary tissue during pregnancy.

Endometriosis

Vulvar Endometriosis

Vulvar endometriosis most frequently follows accidental implantation of viable endometrium at the time of surgery or vaginal delivery, especially following an episiotomy (Fig. 3–23). Superficial endometriosis appears as a red or purple mass, whereas the deeper implant tends to be blue. Cyclic enlargement in relation to the menstrual cycle is characteristic of this lesion.[34]

Vaginal Endometriosis

Endometriosis of the vagina is uncommon. It is believed to develop from shed endometrial tissue, which implants in an area denuded of its epithelium as a result of trauma. Endometriosis occurring solely in the vagina in the absence of pelvic endometriosis (primary endometriosis) is unusual. Gardner[34] observed 6 cases over a period of time in which 68 cases of cervical endometriosis were observed. Williams[110] described a case of vaginal endometriosis following mucosal chemical burns. Endometriosis is reported to be rare following vaginal plastic procedures and seldom develops after delivery.[34,35]

Vaginal endometriosis is reported to be more common in women with pelvic endometriosis. Nodules may be palpated in the posterior vaginal fornix. With associated hemorrhage, the etiology of the induration is evident. March and Israel[56] reported two cases of rectovaginal endometriosis (primary endometriosis) without evident disease elsewhere in the pelvis. The involvement resulted in the formation of retroperitoneal masses in these women. The histopathologic changes are similar to those associated with endometriosis occurring elsewhere.

Judson et al.[51] reported on a 42-year-old

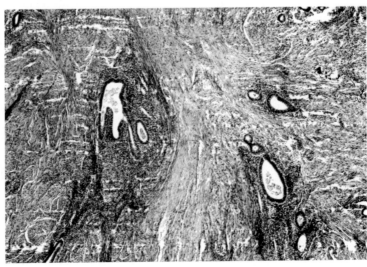

Figure 3–23. Endometriosis in episiotomy scar. Endometrial glands and stroma surrounded by scar tissue.

woman who had undergone a total abdominal hysterectomy for leiomyomas of the uterus. She subsequently developed endometriosis of the sigmoid colon. Two years after the hysterectomy, in June 1994, a 6.0 × 7.0 cm mass was found that involved the vagina and left pelvis. In October 1996, a 6.0 × 3.0 cm mass was excised from the vaginal cuff, and the diagnosis of adenosarcoma arising in endometriosis was made. The adenosarcoma consisted of endometrioid and endocervical mucinous cells. The stromal tissue demonstrates hypercellularity and low mitotic activity up to 3 mitotic figures per 10 high-power fields. There was also liposarcoma consisting of atypical lipoblasts. A recurrent adenosarcoma was removed from this patient's vagina in October 1997. She underwent external radiation therapy and brachyradiotherapy.

This case illustrates the difficulty of arriving at a correct diagnosis of adenosarcoma. Malignant degeneration of endometriosis most frequently results in the development of adenocarcinoma. However, the possibility of adenosarcoma should be kept in mind when the patient complains of persistent symptoms and masses related to endometriosis.

Cervical Endometriosis

Endometriosis of the cervix is divided into superficial (primary) and deep (secondary) types. The former is closely related to prior trauma, surgical procedures (biopsy, curettage, conization, cautery), abortion, and vaginal delivery (Fig. 3–24A). During pregnancy, decidual reaction may occur in the stroma (Fig. 3–24B). It may appear as reddish discoloration or as a nodule. Deep endometriosis involves the outer third of the cervical wall and sometimes extends to the rectovaginal septum or serosal surface.

Although the diagnosis of endometriosis is straightforward, Baker et al.[6] reported a series of 20 cases in which the possibility of endocervical glandular dysplasia or adenocarcinoma in situ was considered in 50% of cases. It is common to find mitotic figures and nuclear stratification in the endometrial cells. The glands sometimes appear hyperplastic with overcrowding and

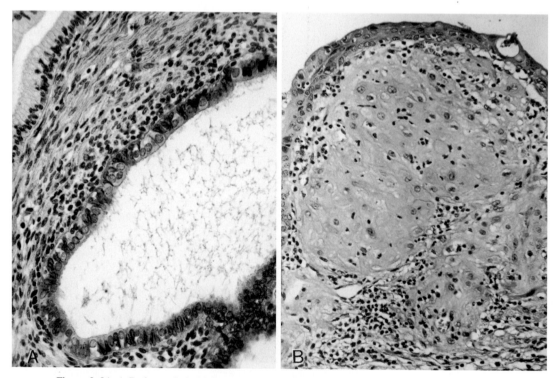

Figure 3–24. *A,* Endometriosis of the cervix. *B,* Decidual change in the stroma during pregnancy.

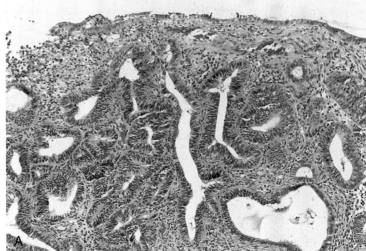

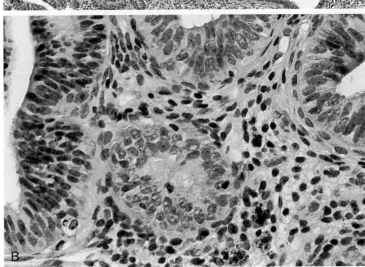

Figure 3–25. Cervical endometriosis. *A,* The endometrial glands are overcrowded and form branching and budding patterns. *B.* The glands are lined by two to three layers of tall columnar cells with rare mitotic figures, but no nuclear atypia is seen.

a back-to-back arrangement. However, nuclear atypia in most cases is absent or minimal (Fig. 3–25). A moderate degree of nuclear atypia was found focally in two cases (10%). Secretory change, ciliated cells, and hobnail cell metaplasia may occur. Stromal edema, hemorrhage, fibrosis, and inflammation sometimes result in distorted glands that simulate invasive adenocarcinoma. In such cases, endometrial stroma is difficult to recognize, further hindering a correct diagnosis. Other less common secondary changes include smooth muscle hyperplasia and perineural space invasion. Serial sections are recommended for these difficult cases.

Clement and Young[18] described a variant of endometriosis consisting predominantly or entirely of endocervical mucinous-type glands,

which they termed *endocervicosis.* They describe six cases of such lesions involving the posterior wall of urinary bladder in women 31 to 44 years of age. In this lesion, the endocervical-type glands are lined by cells with mild nuclear atypia. The surrounding stroma undergoes fibrosis, chronic inflammation, and sometimes smooth muscle hypertrophy. Endocervicosis can occur in the cervix following low cervical cesarean section.

A rare stromal variant of cervical endometriosis, which is made up entirely of endometrial stroma (Fig. 3–26), was reported by Clement et al.[19] The age range of six women was 29 to 64 (mean 43) years. Their presentations included abnormal vaginal bleeding in three women and abdominal swelling owing

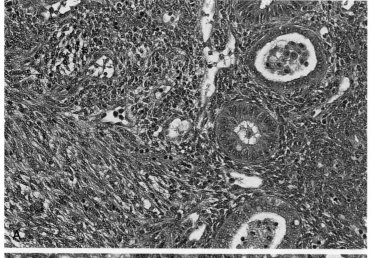
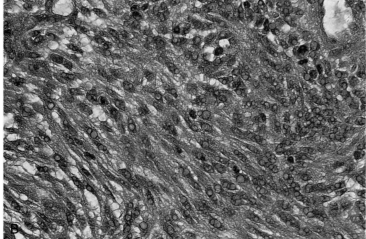

Figure 3–26. *A,* Cervical endometriosis with abundant endometrial stromal tissue. *B,* Sheets of uniform elongated endometrial stromal cells with rare mitotic figures. However, no nuclear atypia is seen.

to ovarian clear cell adenocarcinoma in another woman. The remaining two women were asymptomatic. A red polypoid nodule was visible in four women. Immediately beneath the mucosa were sheets of endometrial stromal cells and spiral arterioles. Hemorrhage was common in the form of blood-filled sinusoid spaces or permeating the stromal cells, which is suggestive of Kaposi's sarcoma. Mitotic activity and nuclear atypia were absent or minimal. This lesion can be distinguished from endometrial stromal sarcoma and other sarcomas by findings of increased mitotic activity, nuclear atypia, and clinical evidence of a mass for sarcoma. Rarely, adenocarcinomas have been reported to arise in the cervical endometriosis.[13,16]

Glial Polyp or Glioma

This lesion occurs more often in the cervix than in the endometrium. Most women present with a polypoid mass and usually have a history of abortion, which occurred a few months to more than 2 years before the diagnosis.[37] It is postulated that fetal brain tissue is mechanically implanted in the cervix or endometrium at the time of curettage.[65] This interpretation is supported by the presence of additional hyaline cartilage, bone, squamous epithelium, and decidual tissue.[37] Histologically, one or more foci of mature glial tissue are covered by endocervical epithelium (Fig. 3–27). Rarely, neurons may be present. The surrounding stroma is often infiltrated by plasma cells and lymphocytes. Recurrence following local excision may occur,

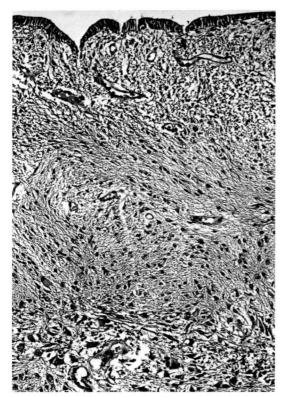

Figure 3–27. Glial polyp of the cervix. Mature glial tissue beneath the endocervical epithelium. Gemistocytic cells with abundant cytoplasm are present in the lower portion of the figure.

but malignant transformation has not been reported.[94]

Young et al.[112] reported on a 15-year-old girl who presented with intractable vaginal bleeding and a polyp protruding from the cervical os. In the hysterectomy specimen, a soft, polypoid, 10×3 cm mass filled the endometrial cavity and invaded the myometrium. The glial cells were mature, were well differentiated, and lacked mitoses. Based on the lack of coital history and recent pregnancy and a large mass invading into the myometrium, the lesion is considered to be a low-grade astrocytoma, possibly derived from germ cell or mesodermal origin. This unusual case seems to be different from other reported cases of glial polyp.

Ectopic Skin and Adnexae and Prostate

Ectodermal elements, such as epidermis, hair follicles, and sebaceous glands, have been described in the cervix.[17,22,25] Whether these are

derived by metaplasia or are ectopic misplaced tissue remains uncertain. Mature hyaline cartilage has also been reported to occur in the cervix,[95] as has Walthard's cell rest.[61,108]

Larraza-Hernandez[54] reported a 38-year-old woman who had a prior cervical biopsy for low-grade squamous dysplasia and condyloma. In the electrocauterized excision specimen, no residual dysplasia was seen. However, clusters of benign prostatic glands were found in the endocervix. These glands showed papillary infoldings, cribriform spaces, and nuclear stratification. The cells expressed prostatic-specific antigen (PSA). The differential diagnosis included microglandular hyperplasia of the endocervix, mesonephric remnants, and cervical adenocarcinoma in situ.

Nucci et al.[66] subsequently reported four cases of ectopic prostatic tissue in the uterine cervix. In three young women, the prostatic tissue was found incidentally in cervix removed for high-grade squamous dysplasia through loop excisions and cone biopsy. In the fourth case, a 77-year-old woman presented with postmenopausal bleeding and was found to have a cervical mass clinically suspicious for fibroid. In all the cases, the prostatic tissue demonstrated papillary proliferation and cribriform glands closely resembling benign glandular hyperplasia of the prostate. These glands were lined by two cell types. Squamous metaplasia occurred in focal areas. These columnar cells demonstrated strong immunoreactivity for PSA and prostatic acid phosphatase. A basal cell layer was also confirmed by expression of high molecular weight cytokeratin. The prostatic tissue was usually identified from beneath the cervical mucosa to deeply (as much as 7.0 mm) into the stroma.

The differential diagnosis considered included endocervical glandular hyperplasia. However, no lobular architecture was seen in the prostatic tissue. Papillary formation, a prominent feature of ectopic prostatic tissue, is not a common finding in lobular endocervical hyperplasia.

Nucci et al.[66] raised three possibilities to explain the development of prostatic tissue in the cervix. One is monodermal teratoma. This event is thought to be unlikely because of the rarity of teratoma in the cervix. The second possibility is metaplasia of the endocervical glands. The third explanation is a malformation derived from the periurethral Skene's glands. During the fetal development, the uterus and urogenital sinus epithelium are quite close to each other. A misplaced Skene's gland into the cervix may induce the development into prostatic tissue, especially with testosterone stimulation. The authors favor the theories of metaplasia or maldevelopment.[66]

REFERENCES

1. Alguacil-Garcia A, Littman CD. Subpubic cartilaginous cyst: Report of two cases. Am J Surg Pathol, 20:975, 1996.

2. Amortegui AJ, Kanbour AI, Silverstein A. Diffuse vaginal adenosis associated with imperforate hymen. Obstet Gynecol 53:760, 1979.

3. Antonioli D, Burke L. Vaginal adenosis: Analysis of 325 biopsy specimens from 100 patients. Am J Clin Pathol 64:625, 1975.

4. Antonioli DA, Rosen S, Burke L, et al. Glandular dysplasia in diethylstilbestrol-associated vaginal adenosis. Am J Clin Pathol 71:715, 1979.

5. Antonioli DA, Burke L, Friedman EA. Natural history of diethylstilbestrol-associated genital tract lesions: Cervical ectopy and cervico-vaginal hood. Am J Obstet Gynecol 137:847, 1980.

6. Baker PM, Clement PB, Bell DA, Young RH. Superficial endometriosis in the uterine cervix: A report of 20 cases of a process that may be confused with endocervical glandular dysplasia or adenocarcinoma in situ. Int J Gynecol Pathol 18:198, 1999.

7. Barnes AB, Colton T, Gundersen JH, et al. Fertility and outcome of pregnancy in women exposed in utero to diethylstilbestrol: Preliminary findings from the DESAD project. N Engl J Med 302:609, 1980.

8. Benirschke K. Congenital anomalies of the uterus with emphasis on genetic causes. In: Hertig AT, Norris HJ, Abell MR (eds). The Uterus. Baltimore, Williams & Wilkins, 1973, p 68.

9. Bibbo M, Gill WR, Azizi F, et al. Follow-up study of male and female offspring of DES-exposed mothers. Obstet Gynecol 49:1, 1977.

10. Biscotti CV, Hart WR. Apoptotic bodies. A consistent morphologic feature of endocervical adenocarcinoma in situ. Am J Surg Pathol 22:434, 1998.

11. Bonney V, Glendining B. Adenomatosis vaginae: A hitherto undescribed condition. Proc Soc Med 4:18, 1911.

12. Bornstein J, Sova Y, Atad J, et al. Development of vaginal adenosis following combined 5-fluorouracil and carbon dioxide laser treatments for diffuse vaginal condylomatosis. Obstet Gynecol 81:896, 1993.

13. Brooks JJ, Wheeler JE. Malignancy arising in extragonadal endometriosis. A case report and summary of the world literature. Cancer 40:3065, 1977.

14. Burger RA, Marcuse PM. Fibroadenoma of the vulva. Am J Clin Pathol 24:9965, 1954.

15. Burke L, Antonioli D, Friedman EA. Evolution of diethylstilbestrol associated genital tract lesions. Obstet Gynecol 57:79, 1981.

16. Chang SH, Maddox WA. Adenocarcinoma arising within cervical endometriosis and invading the adjacent vagina. Am J Obstet Gynecol 110:1015, 1971.

17. Chiarelli SM, Onnis GL. Pilosebaceous structures in the uterine cervix: Case report. Clin Exp Obstet Gynecol 8:15, 1981.

18. Clement PB, Young RH. Endocervicosis of the urinary bladder: A report of six cases of a benign müllerian lesion that may mimic adenocarcinoma. Am J Surg Pathol 16:533, 1992.

19. Clement PB, Young RH, Scully RE. Stromal endometriosis of the uterine cervix. A variant of endometriosis that may simulate a sarcoma. Am J Surg Pathol 14:449, 1990.

20. De Leon FD, Hersh JH, Sanfilippo JS, et al. Gonadal and müllerian duct agenesis in a girl with 46,X,i(Xq). Obstet Gynecol 63:81S, 1984.

21. Deppisch LM. Cysts of the vagina. Classification and clinical correlations. Obstet Gynecol 45:632, 1975.

22. Dougherty CM, Moore WR, Cotten N. Histologic diagnosis and clinical significance of benign lesions of the nonpregnant cervix. Ann NY Acad Sci 97:683, 1962.

23. Dungar CF, Wilkinson EJ. Vaginal columnar cell metaplasia. An acquired adenosis associated with topical 5-fluorouracil therapy. J Reprod Med 40:361, 1995.

24. Dunn JM. Congenital absence of the external genitalia. J Reprod Med 4:57, 1970.

25. Ehrmann RL. Sebaceous metaplasia of the human cervix. Am J Obstet Gynecol 105:1284, 1969.

26. Ferry JA, Scully RE. Mesonephric remnants, hyperplasia and neoplasia in the uterine cervix. A study of 49 cases. Am J Surg Pathol 14:1100, 1990.

27. Forsberg JG. The development of atypical epithelium in the mouse uterine cervix and vaginal fornix after neonatal oestradiol treatment. Br J Exp Pathol 50:187, 1969.

28. Foushee JHS, Pruitt AB Jr. Vulvar fibroadenoma from aberrant breast tissue. Obstet Gynecol 29:819, 1967.

29. Fowler WC Jr, Edelman DA. In utero exposure to DES. Obstet Gynecol 51:459, 1978.

30. Friedrich EG Jr, Wilkinson EJ. Mucous cyst of the vulvar vestibule. Obstet Gynecol 42:407, 1973.

31. Fu YS, Reagan JW, Richart RM, et al. Nuclear DNA and histologic studies of genital lesions in diethylstilbestrol-exposed progeny. II: Intraepithelial glandular abnormalities. Am J Clin Pathol 72:515, 1979.

32. Fu YS, Reagan JW, Richart RM. Cytologic diagnosis of diethylstilbestrol-related genital tract changes and evaluation of squamous cell neoplasia. In: Herbst AL, Bern HA (eds). Development Effects of Diethylstilbestrol (DES) in Pregnancy. New York, Thieme-Stratton, 1981, p 46.

33. Garcia JJ, Verkauf BS, Hochberg CJ, et al. Aberrant breast tissue in the vulva: A case report and review of the literature. Obstet Gynecol 52:225, 1978.

34. Gardner HL. Cervical and vaginal endometriosis. Clin Obstet Gynecol 9:90, 1966.

35. Gardner HL, Kaufman RH. Benign Diseases of the Vulva and Vagina, 2nd ed. Boston, G. K. Hall, 1981.

36. Goodman A, Zukerberg LR, Nikrui N, Scully RE. Vaginal adenosis and clear cell carcinoma after 5-fluorouracil treatment for condyloma. Cancer 68:1628, 1991.

37. Gronroos M, Meurman L, Kahra K. Proliferating glia and other heterotopic tissues in the uterus: Fetal homografts? Obstet Gynecol 61:261, 1983.

38. Hart WR. Paramesonephric mucinous cyst of the vulva. Am J Obstet Gynecol 107:1079, 1970.

39. Hart WR, Zaharov I, Kaplan BJ, et al. Cytologic findings in stilbestrol-exposed females with emphasis on detection of vaginal adenosis. Acta Cytol 20:7, 1976.

40. Haultain JWN. Note on a case of adenoma of the

vagina under observation for 15 years. Tr Edinb Obst Soc 36:160, 1910.

41. Hendrickson MR, Kempson RL. Congenital uterine abnormalities. In: Surgical Pathology of the Uterine Corpus. Philadelphia, W.B. Saunders, 1980, p 17.

42. Hendrix AG, Benirschke K, Thompson RS, et al. The effects of prenatal diethylstilbestrol (DES) exposure on the genitalia of pubertal macaca mulatta. J Reprod Med 22:233, 1979.

43. Herbst AL, Kurman RJ, Scully RE. Vaginal and cervical abnormalities after exposure to stilbestrol in utero. Obstet Gynecol 40:287, 1972.

44. Herbst AL, Norusis MJ, Rosenow PJ, et al. An analysis of 346 cases of clear cell adenocarcinoma of the vagina and cervix with emphasis on recurrence and survival. Gynecol Oncol 7:111, 1979.

45. Herbst AL, Poskanzer DC, Robboy SJ, et al. Prenatal exposure to stilbestrol: A prospective comparison of exposed female offspring with unexposed controls. N Engl J Med 292:334, 1975.

46. Herbst AL, Robboy SJ, Scully RE, et al. Clear cell adenocarcinoma of the vagina and cervix in young females: An analysis of 170 Registry cases. Am J Obstet Gynecol 119:713, 1974.

47. Huffman JW. Mesonephric remnants in the cervix. Am J Obstet Gynecol 56:23, 1948.

48. Irwin WP, Cathro HP, Crosh WW, et al. Primary breast carcinoma of the vulva: A case report and literature review. Gynecol Oncol 73:155, 1999.

49. Janovski NA. Dysontogenetic cyst of the vulva: Report of a case, with reference to etiologic classification of vulvar cyst. Obstet Gynecol 20:227, 1962.

50. Johnson LD, Driscoll SG, Hertig AT, et al. Vaginal adenosis in stillborns and neonates exposed to diethylstilbestrol and steroidal estrogens and progestins. Obstet Gynecol 53:45, 1979.

51. Judson PL, Temple AM, Fowler WC, et al. Vaginal adenosarcoma arising from endometriosis. Gynecol Oncol 76:123, 2000.

52. Junaid TA, Thomas SM. Cysts of the vulva and vagina: A comparative study. Int J Gynecol Obstet 19:239, 1981.

53. Kaufman RH, Adam E, Binder GL, et al. Upper genital tract changes and pregnancy outcome in offspring exposed in utero to diethylstilbestrol. Am J Obstet Gynecol 137:299, 1980.

54. Larraza-Hernandez O, Molberg KH, Lindberg G, Albores-Saavedra J. Ectopic prostatic tissue in the uterus cervi. Int J Gynecol Pathol 16:291, 1997.

55. Lee YH, Rankin LM, Alpert S, et al. Microbiological investigation of Bartholin's gland abscesses and cysts. Am J Obstet Gynecol 129:150, 1977.

56. March CM, Israel R. Rectovaginal endometriosis: An isolated enigma. Am J Obstet Gynecol 125:274, 1974.

57. Marwah S, Berman ML. Ectopic salivary gland in the vulva (choristoma): Report of a case and review of the literature. Obstet Gynecol 56:389, 1980.

58. McLachlan JA, Newbold RR, Bullock BC. Long-term effects on the female mouse genital tract associated with prenatal exposure to diethylstilbestrol. Cancer Res 40:3988, 1980.

59. Meeker JH, Neubecker RD, Helwig EB. Hidradenoma papilliferum. Am J Clin Pathol 37:182, 1962.

60. Merchant WJ, Gale J. Intestinal metaplasia in stilboestrol-induced vaginal adenosis. Histopathology 23:373, 1993.

61. Munsick RA, Janovski NA. Walthard cell rest of the cervix uteri. Am J Obstet Gynecol 82:909, 1961.

62. Nesbitt REL, Abdul Karim RW. Persistent urogenital membrane sinus as a clinical entity. JAMA 205:141, 1968.

63. Ng ABP, Reagan JW, Hawliczek S, et al. Cellular detection of vaginal adenosis. Obstet Gynecol 46:323, 1975.

64. Ng ABP, Reagan JW, Nadji M, et al. Natural history of vaginal adenosis in women exposed to diethylstilbestrol in utero. J Reprod Med 18:1, 1977.

65. Niven PAR, Stansfeld AG. "Glioma" of the uterus: A fetal homograft. Am J Obstet Gynecol 115:534, 1973.

66. Nucci MR, Ferry JA, Young RH. Ectopic prostatic tissue in the uterine cervix. Am J Surg Pathol 24:1224, 2000.

67. O'Brien PC, Noller KL, Robboy SJ, et al. Vaginal epithelial changes in young women enrolled in the National Cooperative Diethylstilbestrol Adenosis (DESAD) Project. Obstet Gynecol 53:300, 1979.

68. Pillai NV, Thye KE, Kumar P. Vaginal adenosis without exposure to diethylstilbestrol: A case report. Asia-Oceania J Obstet Gynecol 17:27, 1991.

69. Plapinger L, Bern HA. Adenosis-like lesions and other cervicovaginal abnormalities in mice treated perinatally with estrogen. J Natl Cancer Inst 63:507, 1979.

70. Plaut A. Diffuse adenosis of vagina: A very rare disease. Am J Pathol 3:581, 1927.

71. Plaut A, Dreyfuss ML. Adenosis of vagina and its relation to primary adenocarcinoma of vagina. Surg Gynecol Obstet 71:756, 1940.

72. Pomerance W. Post-stilbestrol secondary syndrome. Obstet Gynecol 42:12, 1973.

73. Pradhan S, Tobon H. Vaginal cysts: A clinicopathological study of 41 cases. Int J Gynecol Pathol 5:35, 1986.

74. Prasad CJ, Ray JA, Kessler S. Primary small cell carcinoma of the vagina arising in a background of atypical adenosis. Cancer 70:2484, 1992.

75. Radman HM. Hypertrophy of the labia minora. Obstet Gynecol 48:78S, 1976.

76. Radman HM, Bhagavan BS. Pilonidal disease of the female genitals. Am J Obstet Gynecol 114:271, 1972.

77. Ray J, Ireland K. Non–clear-cell adenocarcinoma arising in vaginal adenosis. Arch Pathol Lab Med 109:781, 1985.

78. Ricci JV, Lisa JR, Thom CH Jr, et al. The vagina in reconstructive surgery: A histological study of its structural components. Am J Surg 77:547, 1949.

79. Rickert RR. Intraductal papilloma arising in supernumerary vulvar breast tissue. Obstet Gynecol 55:84S, 1980.

80. Ridley CM. The Vulva. London, W.B. Saunders, 1975.

81. Robboy SJ, Prat J, Welch WR, et al. Squamous cell neoplasia controversy in the female exposed to diethylstilbestrol. Human Path 8:483, 1977.

82. Robboy SJ, Welch WR. Microglandular hyperplasia in vaginal adenosis associated with oral contraceptives and prenatal diethylstilbestrol exposure. Obstet Gynecol 49:430, 1977.

83. Robboy SJ, Ross JS, Prat J, et al. Urogenital sinus origin of mucinous and ciliated cysts of the vulva. Obstet Gynecol 51:347, 1978.

84. Robboy SJ, Keh PC, Nickerson RJ, et al. Squamous cell dysplasia and carcinoma in situ of the cervix and vagina after prenatal exposure to diethylstilbestrol. Obstet Gynecol 51:528, 1978.

85. Robboy SJ, Kaufman RH, Prat J, et al. Pathologic findings in young women enrolled in the National Cooperative Diethylstilbestrol Adenosis (DESAD) Project. Obstet Gynecol 53:309, 1979.

86. Robboy SJ. Risk of cancer, dysplasia for DES daughters found "very low." Med News JAMA 241:1555, 1979.

87. Robboy SJ. A hypothetical mechanism of diethylstilbestrol(DES)-induced anomalies in exposed progeny. Human Pathol 14:831, 1983.

88. Robboy SJ, Hill EC, Sandberg EC, et al. Vaginal adenosis in women born prior to the diethylstilbestrol era. Human Pathol 17:488, 1986.

89. Robboy SJ, Taguchi O, Cunha GR. Normal development of the human female reproductive tract and alterations resulting from experimental exposure to diethylstilbestrol. Human Pathol 13:190, 1982.

90. Robboy SJ, Welch WR, Young RH, et al. Topographic relation of cervical ectropion and vaginal adenosis to clear cell adenocarcinoma. Obstet Gynecol 60:546, 1982.

91. Robboy SJ, Young RH, Welch WR, et al. Atypical vaginal adenosis and cervical ectropion: Association with clear cell adenocarcinoma in diethylstilbestrol-exposed offspring. Cancer 54:869, 1984.

92. Robboy SJ, Prade M, Cunha G. Vagina. In: Sternberg SS (ed). Histology for Pathologists. New York, Raven Press, p 881.

93. Robboy SJ, Bernhardt PF, Parmley T. Embryonoly of the female genital tract and disorders of abnormal sexual development. In: Blaustein's Pathology of the Female Genital Tract, 4th ed. RJ Kurman (ed). New York, Springer-Verlag, 1994, pp 3–29.

94. Roca AN, Guajardo M, Estrada WJ. Glial polyp of the cervix and endometrium. Am J Clin Pathol 73:718, 1980.

95. Roth E, Taylor HB. Heterotopic cartilage in the uterus. Obstet Gynecol 27:838, 1966.

96. Sandberg EC, Danielson RW, Cauwet RW, et al. Adenosis vaginae. Am J Obstet Gynecol 93:209, 1965.

97. Sandberg EC. The incidence and distribution of occult vaginal adenosis. Am J Obstet Gynecol 101:322, 1968.

98. Sandberg EC. Benign cervical and vaginal changes associated with exposure to stilbestrol in utero. Am J Obstet Gynecol 125:777, 1976.

99. Scannell RC. Primary adenocarcinoma of the vagina. Am J Obstet Gynecol 38:331, 1939.

100. Scully RE, Robboy SJ, Welch WR. Pathology and pathogenesis of diethylstilbestrol related disorders of the female genital tract. In: Herbst AL (ed). Intrauterine Exposure to Diethylstilbestrol in the Human. Chicago, American College of Obstetrics and Gynecology, 1978, p 8.

101. Seidman JD, Tavassoli FA. Mesonephric hyperplasia of the uterine cervix: A clinicopathologic study of 51 cases. Int J Gynecol Pathol 14:293, 1995.

102. Shah KH, Kurman RJ, Scully RE, et al. Atypical hyperplasia of mesonephric remnants in the cervix. Lab Invest 42:149, 1980.

103. Sherman AI, Goldrath M, Berlin A, et al. Cervical-vaginal adenosis after in utero exposure to synthetic estrogens. Obstet Gynecol 44:531, 1974.

104. Smith OW. Diethylstilbestrol in the prevention and treatment of complications of pregnancy. Am J Obstet Gynecol 56:821, 1948.

105. Stabler F. Adenomatosis vaginae. J Obstet Gynaecol Br Comm 68:857, 1961.

106. Tbakhi A, Cowan DF, Kuman D, Kyle D. Recurring phyllodes tumor in aberrant breast tissue of the vulva. Am J Surg Pathol 17:946, 1993

107. Van der Putte SCJ. Mammary-like glands of the vulva and their disorders. Int J Gynecol Pathol 13:150, 1994.

108. Villet WT, Marcus PB. Walthard cell rests in the cervix. Gynecol Oncol 5:385, 1977.

109. Von Preuschen F. Uber cystenbildung in der vagina. Archiv F Path Anat U Phys (Virchow) 70:111, 1877.

110. Williams GA. Post-surgical and post-traumatic tumors of the vulva and vagina. Clin Obstet Gynecol 8:309, 1965.

111. Young RH, Scully RE. Minimal-deviation endometrioid adenocarcinoma of the uterine cervix. A report of 5 cases of a distinctive neoplasm that may be misinterpreted as benign. Am J Surg Pathol 17:660, 1993.

112. Young RH, Kleinman GM, Scully RE. Glioma of the uterus. Am J Surg Pathol 5:695, 1981.

113. Zerner J, Fu YS, Taxiarchis LN, et al. A clinicopathologic study of cervix and vagina in DES-exposed progeny. Diagn Gynecol Obstet 2:245, 1980.

4

INFECTIOUS AND INFLAMMATORY DISEASES OF THE LOWER FEMALE GENITAL TRACT

Infectious diseases of the female genital tract can be divided into two major categories on the basis of transmission: venereal and nonvenereal. The venereal diseases, acquired by various forms of sexual contact, are highly contagious with frequent concurrent involvement in both sexes. In addition to the five classic venereal diseases (i.e., syphilis, gonorrhea, chancroid, lymphogranuloma venereum, and granuloma inguinale), genital infections caused by herpes simplex virus type II, papillomavirus, molluscum contagiosum, *Trichomonas vaginalis, Chlamydia trachomatis,* mycoplasma, and *Gardnerella vaginalis* also fulfill the criteria for venereal diseases.[72,92,93,192]

The majority of nonvenereal infectious diseases are related to alterations of the normal vaginal environment and flora.[59,61] In women of reproductive age, the vagina maintains an acidic pH through the production of lactic acid by acidogenic bacilli, which metabolize the glycogen present in the intermediate squamous cells. This acidic environment helps to maintain a balanced host of organisms. Instrumentation, surgery, trauma, immunosuppression, hormonal imbalances, and metabolic disorders are some of the factors known to predispose the vagina to the development of nonvenereal bacterial and candidal vulvovaginitis.[59,61] Extrapelvic systemic infectious diseases may spread through vascular and lymphatic channels to involve the lower female genital tract. Rarely, nonvenereal diseases such as candidiasis, tuberculosis, and amebiasis may be contracted through sexual contact. Finally, the cause of some inflammatory conditions remains unknown.

Proper specimen collection and submission for identification of causative agents are essential for diagnosis and optimal treatment results. Because some infectious agents may be carcinogenic, the possibility exists that infectious and neoplastic diseases coexist.

CLASSIC SEXUALLY TRANSMITTED DISEASES

Syphilis

Syphilis is a major venereal disease in the United States. Although only about 20,000 cases of primary syphilis are reported annually, the actual number of cases is estimated to be 100,000,[60] of which about 20% affect women. For secondary syphilis, the male and female ratio is 1:1.3.[167] Syphilis is caused by the spirochete *Treponema pallidum* and, if untreated, goes through three clinical stages.

The primary lesion, a hard chancre, appears about 3 weeks after inoculation as a round, hard, painless ulcer. Most often, it is solitary and about 1 cm in diameter, but occasionally two or three ulcers may be present. In females, the chancre is most often located on the fourchette or the labia and less frequently occurs around the clitoris or urethral meatus or in the vagina or cervix. Inguinal lymphadenopathy is usually present. Histologically, the ulcer is covered by fibrinous exudate containing spirochetes and neutrophils (Figs. 4–1 and 4–2). In the ulcer bed, endarteritis and plasmacytic infiltration are prominent (see Fig. 4–1). An untreated chancre resolves spontaneously in 3 to 9 weeks after its first appearance.[119] Because of the painless nature and spontaneous healing of the chancre, it often goes unrecognized.

Secondary syphilis may become evident about 6 weeks after the appearance of the chancre.[119] Slightly raised confluent excrescences of so-called condylomata lata appear on the vulva and the adjacent perineum. Histologically, there is a heavy plasmacytic infiltration with prominent endarteritis. The adjacent epidermis is acanthotic. Macular or papular lesions, which ultimately undergo ulceration, may occur in the vagina. These lesions contain large numbers of spirochetes and may resemble chancres; however, capillary proliferation is more marked, and multinucleated giant cells may be present. The secondary lesions involute spontaneously.

Tertiary syphilis rarely involves the lower genital tract. When it occurs, granulomatous inflammation destroys the vulva and the surrounding tissue in the form of ulcers or tumor masses. Tubercles of epithelioid cells and Lang-

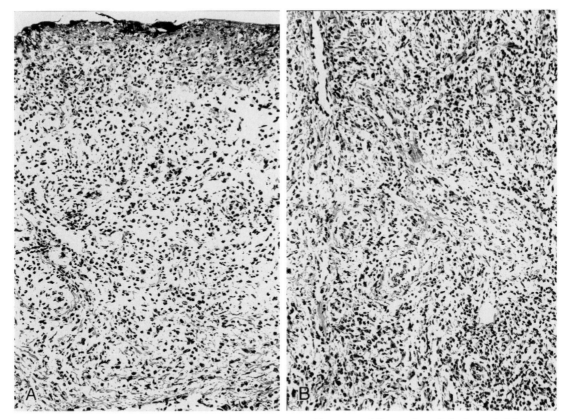

Figure 4–1. Primary syphilitic chancre. *A,* The ulcer bed is covered by neutrophilic exudate. *B,* In the underlying granulation tissue, dense plasmacytic infiltrations, vascular proliferation, and endarteritis are present. (H&E; both, ×200)

hans-type giant cells mix with lymphocytes and plasma cells.

The optimal method for identifying the syphilitic chancre is darkfield examination of the exudate. *T. pallidum* can be identified by its morphology and characteristic movement. The exudate can also be studied with the fluorescent antitreponemal antibodies. The Warthin-Starry silver impregnation stain is useful in the study of primary and secondary lesions (see Fig. 4–2).

Figure 4–2. Primary syphilitic chancre. Warthin-Starry stain demonstrates numerous spirochetes in the ulcer bed and the granulation tissue.

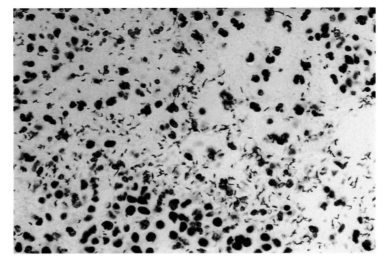

Four weeks after the onset of the chancre, most patients have positive serologic tests for syphilis. If negative, such tests should be repeated weekly for 4 weeks. In patients with primary or secondary syphilis, the positive serologic tests become nonreactive within 12 to 24 months after appropriate therapy. No serologic or morphologic test is available that distinguishes syphilis from yaws, which is caused by *T. pertenue*.

By electron microscopic study, the *T. pallidum* organism has a diameter of 171 nm, with axial filaments of 24 to 27 nm in diameter.[190] The organisms are found in the cytoplasm and nucleus of squamous cells and in a variety of cells, including fibroblasts, neutrophils, macrophages, plasma cells, and endothelial cells of small capillaries and lymphatic channels.[8,190] Their presence in the interstitial tissue may be related to the phenomenon of latency and resistance to treatment.[190]

Gonorrhea

In adults, gonorrhea initially involves the urethra, Skene's ducts, paraurethral glands, or Bartholin's glands. Ascending infection to the endocervix, uterus, fallopian tubes, and peritoneum may follow, especially in untreated cases. Gonorrhea often develops at the time of the menstrual period when the hormonal changes seem to favor its occurrence. The endocervix, with its complex and deeply seated glands, is the favorite site for carriers of gonorrhea (Fig. 4–3). Abscesses of the Bartholin's glands and involvement of the rectum and pharynx occur in some instances. The vagina and vulva are more likely to be involved in prepubertal females because of the susceptibility of atrophic stratified squamous epithelium to the organism, which is diplococcus *Neisseria gonorrhoeae*.

The incubation period varies from 1 to 14 days, averaging 2 to 7 days. Symptoms and signs are absent or minimal in about 50% of cases in females. Electron microscopic studies suggest that the organisms first attach to the transitional or columnar cells by hair-like filaments, the pili, and invade the mucosa by passing through the intercellular spaces.[141] The capsular antigen and toxins of the organisms incite a severe neutrophilic response, producing a purulent discharge from the urethral meatus and vagina.

Cultures are the most reliable method for establishing the diagnosis of gonorrhea. Sam-

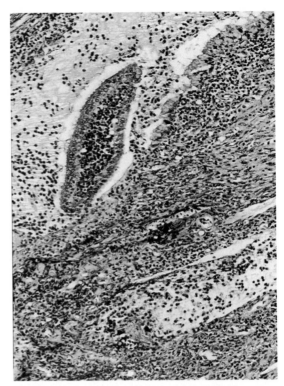

Figure 4–3. Acute cervicitis in association with gonorrhea. The endocervical glands and the adjacent stroma are heavily infiltrated by neutrophils and lymphocytes, and necrosis of the lining of the epithelium is evident.

pling for culture should include specimens from the pharynx and rectum, in addition to those from the genital areas. Immunoassays have been used in detection. Direct smears may be helpful in recognizing acute disease. In gram-stained preparations, the gonococci appear as gram-negative diplococci occurring within leukocytes. The detection rate is 65%.[6] However, *N. catarrhalis* may mimic *N. gonorrhoeae* in stained smears. In chronic cases, the organisms are more difficult to detect in smears and, when identified, may be extracellular. The absence of identifiable diplococci in smears does not rule out the presence of chronic disease. It should be noted that concurrent trichomonas infection is common. Candida is less commonly identified.

Granuloma Inguinale

Granuloma inguinale, a chronic, progressive granulomatous disease involving the skin and subcutaneous tissue of the genital, inguinal, and anal areas, is caused by *Calymmatobacterium granulomatis.* It is a gram-negative encapsulated bacillus and antigenically related to *Klebsiella* and other members of the Enterobacteriaceae. Electron microscopic study suggests that the organisms may be phage modified. This disease is rarely seen in the United States.

In females, the lesions are most commonly found on the labia or in the fourchette and, less commonly, in the vagina and cervix. The initial lesion appears as an eroded papule, which becomes superficially ulcerated, with bright granulation tissue in the ulcer base (Fig. 4–4).[78] Inguinal lesions usually involve the subcutaneous tissue and only occasionally the lymph nodes; genital distortion, mutilation, and elephantiasis may occur with time.

Histologically, the affected dermis is infiltrated by a dense, mixed cellular infiltrate consisting predominantly of mononuclear cells and occasional neutrophils (Fig. 4–5A). Pseudoepitheliomatous hyperplasia of the adjacent skin is often prominent and may be misinterpreted as invasive squamous carcinoma. Rarely, granuloma inguinale coexists with squamous carcinoma.

The diagnosis is based on the finding of Donovan bodies in the biopsy or smears of the ulcer. Donovan bodies are large histiocytes containing numerous organisms in the cytoplasm, which are best demonstrated with Wright's or Giemsa stain (Fig. 4–5B). Culture of the organism is difficult because it requires chick embryo tissue or special media.

Lymphogranuloma Venereum

Lymphogranuloma venereum is caused by *Chlamydia trachomatis.*[162,164] Immunofluorescent typing has identified types LI, LII, and LIII and serotypes of *C. trachomatis* as the specific agent for lymphogranuloma venereum. Like bacteria, the organisms contain a cell wall and both RNA and DNA and are sensitive to antibiotics, but, like viruses, they are obligate intracellular parasites.[60] The organisms have an affinity for deep structures, especially the lymphatics. The disease is most prevalent in tropical and subtropical climates. Fewer than 100 cases are reported annually in the United States.[167]

The initial lesion appears as a single papule or vesicle located in the vicinity of the posterior fourchette. Painless superficial ulcers or inguinal lymphadenitis follows.[174] Proctocolitis and edema of the perianal skin are common. The inflammatory reaction and scarring lead to anorectal stricture. In severe cases, the inguinal lymph nodes form matted buboes. Progressive destruction of the vulva results in fenestrations and tunneling of the vulvar skin. Carcinoma of the vulva or rectum has also been reported.

Histologic changes include intense chronic inflammatory infiltrates beneath the ulcerated skin. Necrotic foci, appearing as fissure-type ulcers, are sometimes bordered by palisaded epithelioid cells and multinucleated giant cells (Fig. 4–6A and B).[174] Lymphangiectasia, dermal

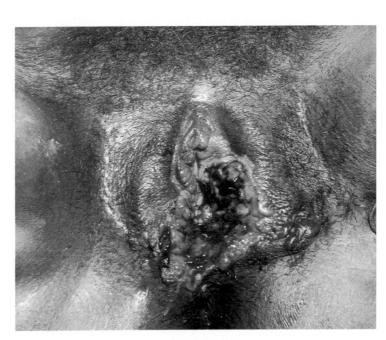

Figure 4–4. Granuloma inguinale. Ulcerated, granular lesion involves the labia minora and fourchette.

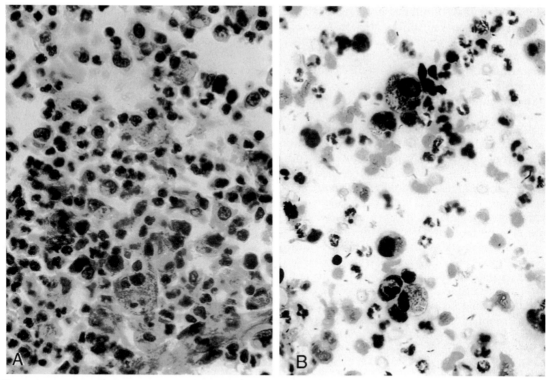

Figure 4–5. Granuloma inguinale. *A,* Large, mononuclear cells with abundant foamy or granular cytoplasm are mixed with lymphocytes, histiocytes, and occasionally neutrophils. *B,* Imprint of the lesion confirms the presence of bacilli in the histiocytes and the Donovan bodies. (*A,* H&E, ×600; *B,* Giemsa's stain, ×600)

fibrosis, and active or healed vasculitis are prominent in some cases (see Fig. 4–6A). The epidermis adjacent to the ulcer demonstrates pseudoepitheliomatous hyperplasia (Fig. 4–6C).

The involved inguinal lymph nodes reveal suppurative necrosis, which coalesces to form stellate abscesses. They are surrounded by palisaded epithelioid cells and occasional multinucleated giant cells (Fig. 4–6D). The adjacent lymphoid tissue sometimes contains atypical lymphocytes. A direct immunofluorescent technique or an indirect peroxidase-antiperoxidase method using antiserum against *C. trachomatis* may be used to confirm the diagnosis.[2] The histologic changes closely resemble cat-scratch disease; however, bacilli are present in cat-scratch disease, which can be demonstrated by Dieterle's stain.[106]

The Frei skin test has been abandoned because of its high false-negative and false-positive results.[72] A complement fixation titer of 1:32 or greater usually indicates active disease.[72] A negative complement fixation test should be repeated in 1 to 3 weeks for suspected cases.

Chancroid

Chancroid is caused by *Haemophilus ducreyi,* a short, plump, gram-negative coccobacillus. In the United States, 5001 cases were reported in 1988, affecting mostly males. About 60% of these cases were reported in New York City.[167] Within 4 to 7 days after exposure, chancroid first appears as a papule on the vulva, usually the fourchette and labia minora, and occasionally on the urethra, vagina, or cervix. It then ulcerates, causing pain and secondary infections. Involvement of the inguinal lymph nodes occurs in 50% of cases. Chancroid is often confused with herpes genitalis. The ulcers of chancroid tend to be larger, deeper, and fewer in number than those of herpes genitalis.

The histologic change is nonspecific chronic inflammation. Occasionally, bacilli can be demonstrated in smears prepared from the ulcer or in the histologic sample of the vulva or lymph node.

Gram stain of smears from the ulcer or lymph nodes for organisms has a variable sensitivity and specificity. Gram-negative bacilli are

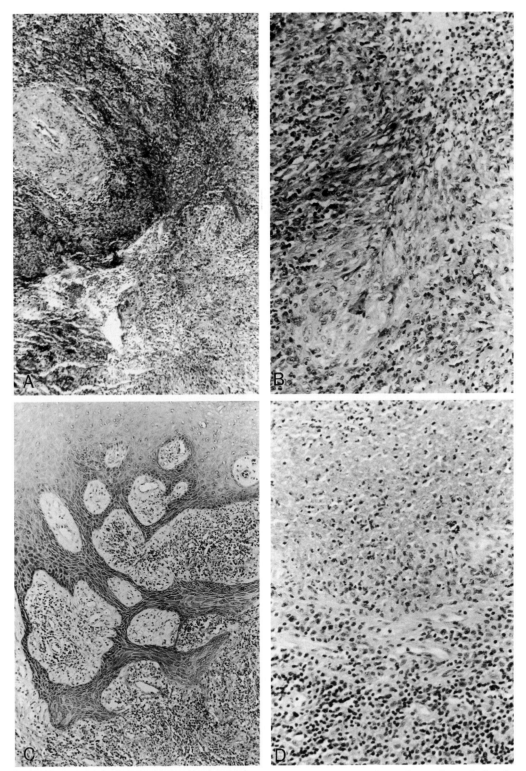

Figure 4–6. Lymphogranuloma venereum. *A,* Deep fissure-type ulcer contains necrotic exudate and granulation tissue. A vasculitis with marked thickening and fibrosis is shown in the left upper corner of the figure. *B,* Part of the ulcer is lined by palisaded epithelioid cells and multinucleated giant cells. *C,* Pseudoepitheliomatous hyperplasia adjacent to the ulcerated squamous epithelium is common. *D,* The involved inguinal lymph node undergoes necrosis. Adjacent to the necrosis, early granulomatous reaction and atypical lymphocytes are present.

arranged in chains or "schools of fish." Owing to secondary infection, the presence of gram-negative bacilli may represent false-positive results. Thus, the specificity is less than 50%. A skin test is available but takes 2 to 3 weeks to become positive after exposure. For isolation of the organism, two media, chocolate agar and rabbit blood with vancomycin, are recommended.[12] Van Dyck and Piot recommend incubation at 33 to 34°C in a 5% to 10% CO_2 and water-saturated condition for 3 to 4 days. Monoclonal immunofluorescence assay has a sensitivity comparable to that of culture but only 60% of culture's specificity.[202]

VENEREAL AND NONVENEREAL VIRAL INFECTIONS

Herpes Genitalis

The herpes simplex virus (HSV) was first isolated from the female genital tract in 1946.[171] Antigenic and biologic differences were subsequently identified between HSV types I and II.[98,135,136] Most genital infections are related to HSV type II, whereas HSV type I more frequently affects the oral cavity and eye.[135] Evidence suggests that 85% to 90% of the genital infections are caused by HSV type II, and the remainder are related to HSV type I.[98,155]

Prevalence

It is estimated that 700,000 new cases of genital herpes and 20 million attacks of recurrent genital herpes occur in the United States annually. The prevalence is related to the age distribution, the nature of the population under study, and the method used to establish the disease. The highest frequency is observed in women in low socioeconomic groups.[154] The lowest prevalence is observed in more affluent women seen in private practice. The reported frequency varies from 0.1% to 6.9%.[72] The disease is sexually transmitted. In one study, 80% of the women exposed to men with clinical evidence of disease excreted the virus or developed antibodies to herpesvirus type II.[155] Herpes genitalis is the most common cause of vulvar ulcers.[72]

Clinical Findings

Symptoms may develop within 3 to 7 days after exposure.[72] A prodrome of paresthesia may appear 12 to 48 hours before the appearance of vesicles, which rupture to cause superficial ulcers. In primary infections, the changes are painful, widespread, and usually midline or bilateral and may involve the vulva, perianal skin, cervix, and vagina. Early in the disease, vesicles last 10 to 12 days and the ulcers persist for 1 to 2 weeks (Fig. 4–7).[167] The ulcers may coalesce and then heal spontaneously. Rarely, disseminated disease follows the primary infection.

With recurrent infection, the lesions are less conspicuous, milder, and usually unilateral, and they may be overlooked. The ulceration observed is similar to that associated with primary infection. The entire course lasts about 10 days. The reactivation of HSV in sacral dorsal root ganglia is believed to be the source of reinfection following stress, menstruation, or external stimuli, such as trauma or overexposure to sunlight.[72]

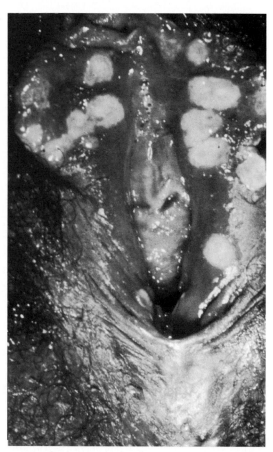

Figure 4–7. Herpes genitalis. Multiple superficial ulcers on the labia minora.

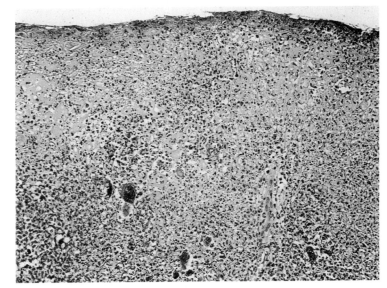

Figure 4–8. Herpes genitalis. Ulcer base demonstrates necrotic tissue, acute inflammatory response, and several multinucleated giant cells.

Pathologic Findings

Our knowledge of the histopathologic changes associated with genital involvement is based on a relatively small sample, because biopsy is not commonly used to establish the diagnosis.[98,211] The changes in primary and secondary disease are similar. Vesicle formation is inconspicuous in samples obtained from the vagina and is seldom as well developed as in lesions arising in the skin. In the vaginal mucosa, the vesicular phase is of limited duration and, when observed, is poorly defined. This is associated with evidence of acantholysis and an infiltration of leukocytes. Ulceration is more common. The surface of the ulcer often lies above the level of the uninvolved mucosa. The ulcer base is covered with fibrin, necrotic debris, and degenerate or necrotic leukocytes. Plasma cells and lymphocytes occur in the underlying stroma (Fig. 4–8). Varying degrees of pseudoepitheliomatous hyperplasia may occur at the margins of the ulcer.

Cells containing viral inclusions are more likely to be observed at the margins of the ulcer or deep in the ulcer base (see Fig. 4–8), but they may be inconspicuous in some lesions. The cells containing inclusions may be mononucleate or multinucleate (Fig. 4–9). Their cytoplasm is altered by degeneration. The enlarged

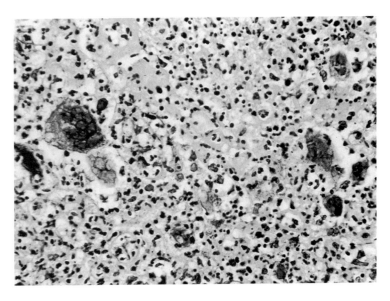

Figure 4–9. Herpes genitalis. Mononucleate and multinucleated giant cells containing organisms are present deep in the wall of the ulcer. Large, discrete inclusions are uncommon.

nuclei contain numerous small viral particles. Such cells have a condensation of chromatin beneath the nuclear membrane. Other cells contain large acidophilic intranuclear inclusions surrounded by clear zones.[72,137,139,211]

The cellular changes associated with herpes genitalis are evident in smears prepared from scrapings of the clinical lesions.[139] These changes are more conspicuous in the nucleus and may be observed in mononucleate or multinucleate cells. It may be difficult to determine the parentage of the affected cells. On the basis of current knowledge, most of the altered cells originate in stratified squamous epithelium.

The cells may be isolated or arranged in aggregates. The amount of cytoplasm is limited in amount in many cells. Less frequently, the amount of cytoplasm is comparable to that observed in mature squamous cells. A diffuse vacuolization of the cytoplasm is evident in some cells, whereas only isolated vacuoles are present in other cells. Considerable variation exists in the intensity of the cytoplasmic staining. In most cells, the cytoplasmic staining is cyanophilic or indeterminate; an eosinophilic cytoplasm is less frequently observed. The cytoplasmic boundaries are poorly defined, and, in some cells, the cytoplasm is fragmented (Fig. 4–10).

In part, the nuclear changes are related to the stage of the infection. Early in the evolution of the infection, the nucleus is relatively large and is characterized by a poorly stained chromatin, throughout which there are minute cyanophilic particles and small vacuoles (see Fig. 4–10). Margination of the chromatin is variable. Somewhat later, the nucleus has a "ground-glass" appearance, with the formation of a chromatic membrane owing to margination of the chromatin (Fig. 4–11A). This characteristic change has been attributed to an increased number of minute viral particles and DNA synthesized by the virus. This is the most common change observed in the disease, accounting for two thirds of the altered cells. Ultimately, the viral particles are concentrated in a well-defined eosinophilic intranuclear mass of variable configuration. It is usually centrally located, in the nuclei of multinucleate cells, and represents the type A inclusion (Fig. 4–11B). A clear zone often surrounds this inclusion. Some investigators maintain that this is an artifact resulting from shrinkage, because it is not observed in living cells. Margination of the chromatinic material also occurs in this cell type.

In association with the cells containing viral inclusions, the cellular sample often contains aggregates of neutrophils and cellular detritus resulting from the destruction of the host tissues. Evidence of epithelial regeneration or a reparative process is observed in a significant number of the samples evaluated.

Diagnosis

Diagnosis may be based on clinical examination alone, with the use of cellular studies, or by culture. Positive cultures were close to 100%

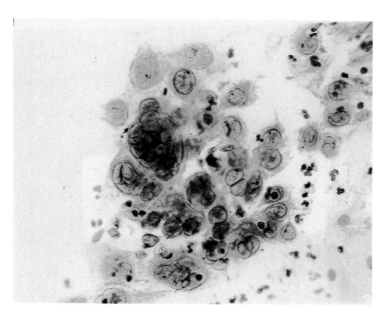

Figure 4–10. A vaginal scraping of herpes genitalis showing early changes. Cells demonstrate margination of the chromatin, small vacuoles, and minute inclusions. Multinucleated giant cells are also present. (Papanicolaou's stain, ×500)

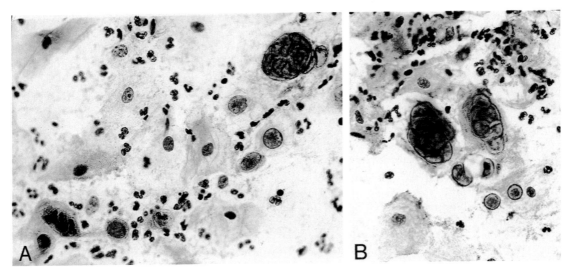

Figure 4–11. Vaginal scrapings of herpes simplex. *A*, The "ground glass" nucleus is characterized by homogeneous, opaque, basophilic material surrounded by a rim of chromatin. *B*, Multinucleated cells with large, discrete inclusions are present. Similar inclusions occur in mononucleated cells. These findings are seen only rarely. (Papanicolaou's stain; *A* and *B*, ×520)

when taken during the vesicle stage, 89% during the pustular stage, and 33% or less from ulcers.[167] Positive culture from the cervix was reported in 88% of women with primary infection and in 12% to 20% of those with recurrent disease.[167] In these cases, the cervix was erythematous and eroded. Detection of HSV antigen or nucleic acid hybridization is reported to have a sensitivity of 80%. Antibody titers are of value in determining whether the infection is primary or secondary.

Smears taken from the base of lesions to examine for viral inclusions have a sensitivity of 67% during the vesicle stage, 75% during the pustular stage, and 50% at the ulcer stage.[211] The smears can be stained with Wright's or Giemsa stain or using the Papanicolaou method and are useful when culture is not possible, for example, when genital ulcers are discovered shortly before childbirth.

Biopsy is seldom necessary to confirm the diagnosis. Diagnostic features are most commonly seen at the edge of the ulcer, where biopsy should be taken, and multiple sections may be necessary to detect the characteristic changes. Most ulcers heal spontaneously in 2 to 3 weeks; however, secondary infection delays the healing process.

Complications

Acute HSV infection occurring during pregnancy has been related to abortion, premature

delivery, and the development of neonatal herpetic infection.[139] The latter may come about by transplacental passage of the virus, by contamination of the newborn during childbirth, or by means of an ascending infection.[136] In the presence of active infection at the time of delivery, Nahmias et al.[136] calculated that during vaginal delivery the infant had a 60% chance of developing a herpetic infection. A similar risk exists when cesarean section is done, after the membranes have been ruptured for more than 6 hours. In subsequent studies, the risk of neonatal infection through vaginal delivery is estimated to be 33% to 50%, in neonates of women with first-episode genital herpes with asymptomatic shedding or lesions, as confirmed by viral cultures.[23,132] The risk is only about 3% when newborns are exposed to women who previously had genital herpes or who have antibodies against the same type of virus isolated by cultures.[23] The risk of neonatal transmission is higher when maternal disease is in the cervix rather than in other genital sites.[132] The oncogenic potential of the virus[96] is questionable and is discussed in Chapters 6 and 8 on cervical and vulvar squamous neoplasia.

Condyloma Acuminatum

Condyloma acuminatum is caused by the papillomavirus, a subgroup of the papovaviruses (papilloma, polyoma, and vacuolating agent plus virus). Human papillomaviruses (HPV) are distinguished not by serotype but rather by genotypes using molecular hybridization techniques.[22,110] A new type of HPV is accepted if its DNA genome has less than 50% homology with the genomes of established HPV types. More than 100 types of HPV have been identified from both genital and nongenital areas. More than 20 types were cloned from the female genital tract.[22,51,73,110,185,217] HPV consists of a naked icosahedral capsid with 72 capsomers. The genome is composed of circular, supercoiled, double-stranded DNA with a molecular weight of about 5×10^6 daltons and 8000 base pairs.[216] HPV genomes consist of three regions: the long controlling (upstream regulatory) region; the early region; and the late region, which codes for viral capsid protein.[165] The function of these genes, and especially their role in cervical carcinogenesis, is discussed in Chapter 8.

HPVs are divided into low- and high-risk types. Low-risk types include HPV types 6, 11, 42, 43, and 44. High-risk groups are HPV types 16, 18, 31, 33, 35, 39, 45, 51, 52, 56, 58, and others. Low-risk HPV types are found in condyloma acuminatum, low-grade squamous dysplasia, and low-grade intraepithelial lesions. The high-risk types are associated with both low- and high-grade intraepithelial lesions and invasive squamous and glandular neoplasms.[8,51,65,110,175,185,217]

In the current World Health Organization (WHO) classification for tumors of the female genital tract, condyloma acuminatum is considered to be a benign neoplasm, whereas flat condyloma is part of the mild dysplasia or low-grade intraepithelial lesions. Flat condyloma and dysplastic change are discussed in the section on intraepithelial neoplasia of individual sites.

The majority of condylomata acuminata are caused by HPV type 6, and about 25% of genital warts are associated with HPV type 11. HPV types 6 and 11 are grouped together in most studies.

Epidemiology

In a population-based study conducted in Rochester, Minnesota, the average annual incidence rate of clinically evident condyloma acuminatum in both sexes rose slowly from 1950 to 1970 and then more rapidly after 1970.[31] The incidence rates in women in creased from 39 per 100,000 between 1965 and 1969 to 109 per 100,000 between 1970 and 1974, and to 126 per 100,000 between 1975 and 1978, representing a 3.2-fold increase in a 10-year period. Females were affected 1.7 times more often than males. A similar trend was also reported by others.[5] The warts occur in the following areas: vulva (66%), vagina (37%), perineum (29%), anus (23%), cervix (8%), and urethra (4%).[31]

Clinical Findings

Condyloma acuminatum is a disease of young women, but children and postmenopausal women occasionally are affected.[187,209] In the vulvar region, the vestibule and the labial folds are affected most commonly. Involvement of the perianal skin, mons pubis, and urethra is less common. Perianal warts may extend into the anus and rectum.

The incubation period, based on the followup studies of penile and vulvar warts, is estimated to be a few weeks to as long as 6 months.[4,142] Initially, the disease appears as a small, warty growth that spreads locally as multiple seedlings. With growth and coalescence, a cauliflower-like, lobulated mass is formed (Fig. 4–12). Extension to the fourchette and lower vagina just inside the hymenal ring is common. In the UCLA series, 53% of patients with vulvar condyloma had additional gross lesions in the vagina (16%) or the cervix (21%), or both (16%).[5] Purola and Savia[152] found evidence of condylomatous changes in the vaginal and cervical smears of most women with vulvar condylomas. Vaginal discharge, secondary infection, and bleeding are common.

When flat and acuminate condylomas are combined, about 80% of vaginal and vulvar condylomas are exophytic (Fig. 4–13). By contrast, the majority of cervical HPV-related changes are flat or inverted, and sometimes are exophytic (Fig. 4–14).[129] These differences in growth pattern suggest that different HPV types preferentially affect a particular anatomic site or epithelium.[156]

In addition to exophytic growth, condylomas may appear as white, thickened epithelium (Fig. 4–15). Rarely, the entire vaginal mucosa is covered by numerous miliary seedlings of so-called condylomatous colpitis (Fig. 4–16). Many genital warts in males and females may have gone undetected without the use of acetic acid, a magnifying lens, or a colposcope.[79]

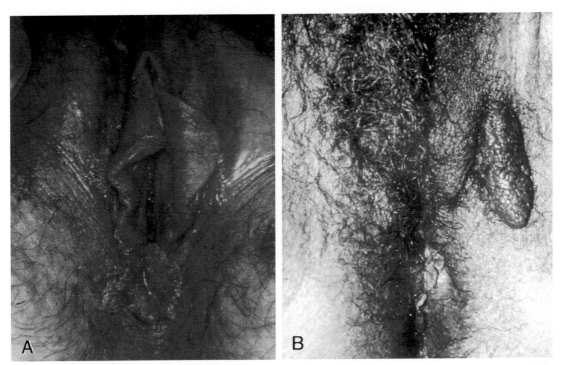

Figure 4–12. *A,* Slightly raised, exophytic condyloma involves the fourchette. *B,* The left labial condyloma has a nodular and pigmented appearance.

Pathologic Findings

Condylomata acuminata produces papillary, exophytic, and acanthotic lesions with elongation and thickening of the rete pegs (Fig. 4–17). Hyperpigmentation of basal layer sometimes occurs (see Fig. 4–17). The surface may be pointed or blunt and is often covered by parakeratosis and hyperkeratosis (see Figs. 4–17 and 4–18). Keratohyaline granules and, rarely, nuclear inclusions are present. A delicate, central fibrovascular core arising from the underlying dermis supports the papillary frond. Surface parakeratosis and hyperkeratosis, although commonly seen, are usually limited in extent. Between the rete pegs, the anastomos-

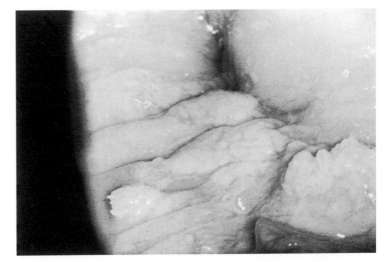

Figure 4–13. Exophytic condyloma as seen by colposcopy reveals finger-like projections and raised white epithelium with mosaic pattern. (Courtesy of Duane Townsend, M.D., Salt Lake City, Utah.)

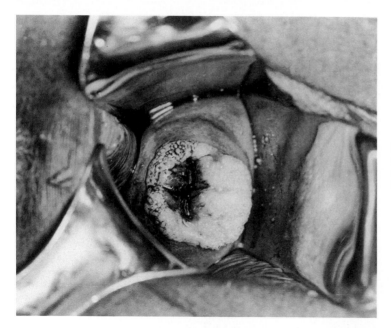

Figure 4–14. Exophytic condyloma involving the entire circumference of the cervix has a granular, cauliflower-like appearance.

Figure 4–15. Flat condyloma of the vagina. (Courtesy of Duane Townsend, M.D., Salt Lake City, Utah.)

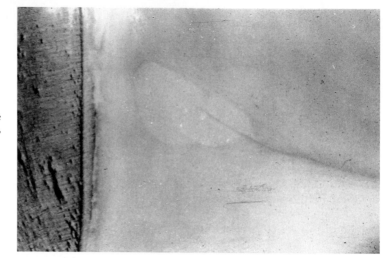

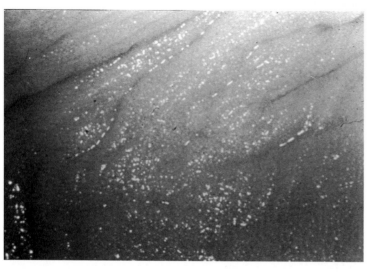

Figure 4–16. Condylomatous vaginitis as visualized under the colposcope with numerous miliary seedings. (From Roy M, et al. Condylomata acuminata: Recent developments. Colposcopist, Summer 1981 issue, by permission of the American Society for Colposcopy and Cervical Pathology.)

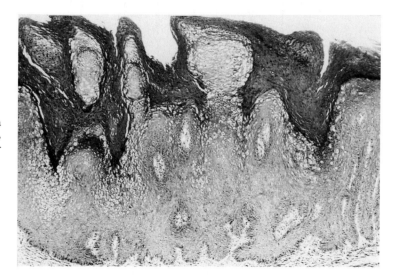

Figure 4–17. Exophytic condyloma with hyperkeratosis, parakeratosis, and koilocytosis. Melanocytes are increased in the basal layer.

ing, dilated capillaries extend to three to four layers beneath the superficial squamous cells, causing the punctation and mosaic patterns seen on colposcopy.

The hallmark of HPV infection is koilocytosis. Koilocytes, which have a perinuclear clear halo, are found in the intermediate and superficial layers of condyloma. The cell borders are accentuated by eosinophilic material. In addition, the nuclei have a wrinkled, popcorn-like appearance (see Fig. 4–19A). Binucleation, multinucleation, hyperchromasia, and pyknosis are sometimes seen (see Fig. 4–19B, C). Nuclear atypism is mild. In the basal and parabasal layers, the cellular polarity and maturation processes are maintained. The basal cells retain

a distinct palisaded arrangement. There is cellular proliferation in the parabasal layers with occasional mitotic figures. Abnormal mitotic figures are absent in condyloma but are seen in intraepithelial neoplasia[18,37,39]

By in situ hybridization, capsid proteins and a specific type of HPV DNA can be visualized by immunohistochemical stains with the use of radioactive or biotin-labeled probes.[64,209] Positive nuclei are generally located in the superficial and intermediate cell layers. Oriel and Almeida[143] demonstrated the viral particles in human genital warts by electron microscopy. These particles, similar to those found in common skin warts, have a 45 to 55 nm diameter (Figs. 4–20 and 4–21) and are found mainly in

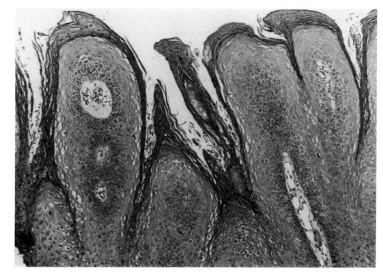

Figure 4–18. Exophytic condyloma of the vulva with long, papillary fronds supported by vascular cores. The surface typically has a pointed appearance, but tangential cuts through the stalk often result in a blunt, smooth surface.

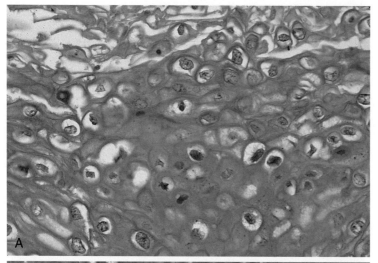

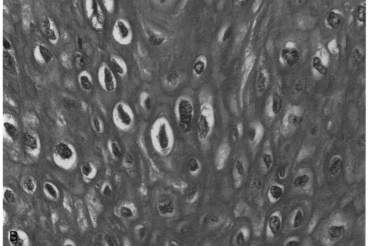

Figure 4–19. *A,* Koilocytes are characterized by enlarged, irregular hyperchromatic nuclei surrounded by perinuclear halos. Cell borders are thickened and distinct. *B,* Some nuclei are binucleated. *C,* In cervical smears, koilocytes also reveal similar characters. The nuclei are enlarged (compared with normal intermediate squamous cells in the background), hyperchromatic, and irregular in shape. Perinuclear halos and thickened cell borders are evident.

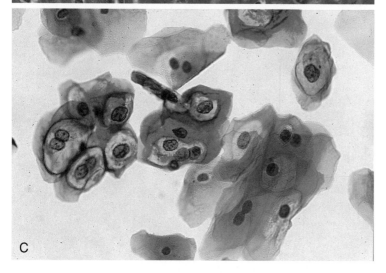

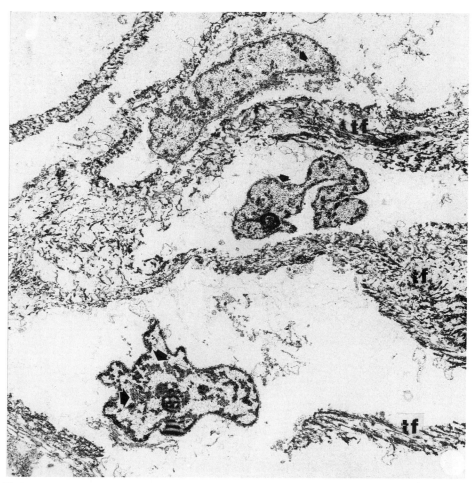

Figure 4–20. Accumulations of fluid and vacuoles are evident in the perinuclear regions of koilocytes. Tonofilaments (tf) form coarse bundles and accumulate near the cell borders, attributing to the eosinophilic cytoplasm and well-defined cell boundaries. The convoluted nuclei contain irregular chromatinic aggregates. Viral particles disperse throughout the nucleus (small arrowheads) or form crystalline aggregates (large arrowheads). (×7800)

the nuclei of superficial and intermediate squamous cells, either dispersed diffusely in the nuclei or arranged in a crystalline pattern[9,30,50]

The koilocytes are characterized by accumulations of fluid and glycogen, cellular debris, and vacuoles around the nucleus. The tonofilaments form coarse bundles and tend to aggregate near the periphery of cytoplasm and cell membranes (see Figs. 4–20 and 4–21); thus, the cell borders appear more accentuated than the normal squamous cells. The desmosomes are poorly preserved (see Fig. 4–21). The nuclei have an angulated or lobulated configuration, an uneven chromatinic material on the nuclear membrane, and coarse chromatin clumps (see Fig. 4–20). These features account for the hyperchromasia and wrinkled appearance seen by light microscopy.[27]

Natural History

Condylomatous growth may regress spontaneously, persist for many years, or become neoplastic.[110,142] In common skin warts, the rate of spontaneous regression in adults is in the range of 30% over a period of 3 to 6 months. Oriel[142] reported that most untreated condyloma acuminatum regressed spontaneously in 3 to 5 years. Regression may be related to the immune response of the patient.

Several factors are known to enhance the growth of condyloma, including pregnancy, altered immune status, oral contraceptives, and poor personal hygiene.[149] During pregnancy, condylomas tend to increase in size and number, and some regress after childbirth, presumably with the return of normal immunity.[72]

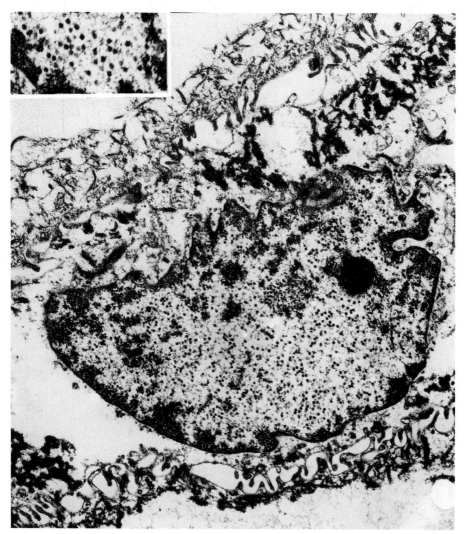

Figure 4–21. The nucleus of this koilocyte contains numerous electron-dense, spherical viral particles (inset). Tonofilaments accumulate near the cell borders. The desmosomes have been disintegrated, a sign of degeneration. (×26,000; inset ×52,000)

Condyloma may reappear in the next pregnancy. Patients who receive immunosuppressive therapy are at increased risk of developing genital warts and squamous neoplasia.[35,83] Among renal transplant patients, the rate of genital warts is estimated to be nine times greater than that of the general population and 17 times greater than that of matched immunocompetent controls. The risk of cervical neoplasia is 16 times greater than that of the general population and nine times greater than that of matched controls.[83]

It is unknown how often vulvar condylomas undergo malignant transformation. As many as 26% of women with vulvar carcinoma in situ have pre-existing or concomitant condylomas.[63]

Occasional reports have documented the development of in situ and invasive squamous carcinoma within the condyloma.[20,107,144]

The infectivity of maternal genital warts to newborns remains to be determined. During a follow-up period of 7 to 42 months, none of 28 infants born to mothers with genital warts had clinical evidence of laryngeal papilloma.[32]

Effects of Podophyllin

Since the report of Sullivan and King,[188] topical application of podophyllin has been used in the treatment of skin and genital warts. It is important to recognize the nuclear alterations induced by podophyllin to ensure that they are not confused with squamous dysplasia or squamous carcinoma in situ.[34,54]

In podophyllin-treated condyloma, the squamous cells undergo degeneration characterized by swelling and vacuolation of the cytoplasm. The nuclei become enlarged, hyperchromatic, or pyknotic (Fig. 4–22 A and B). The nucleoli increase in number and size. Cells of the parabasal and basal layers demonstrate disintegration of chromatinic membranes. The number of cells in the mitotic cycle is increased. The chromosome particles are dispersed in the form of numerous small granules scattered within the nucleoplasm, suggesting an aborted mitosis (Fig. 4–22C). Some nuclei have chromosomes arranged in two or three aggregates. These cells, called "podophyllin cells," resemble colchicine-treated skin with an arrest of mitosis in the metaphase (see Fig. 4–22C).[105] In the dermis, edema and lymphocytic infiltration are present.

The effects of podophyllin usually disappear within 2 weeks of withdrawal of the treatment.[34] It is believed that podophyllin has a direct cytotoxic effect, with profound disturbance of cell metabolism. This eventually leads to necrosis of the condylomatous tissue.[188]

Podophyllin acts by arresting mitosis in metaphase and is not recognized as a carcinogenic agent. Rare examples of neoplasia observed in condylomas following podophyllin treatment most likely represent neoplasia that has failed to be eradicated by the podophyllin treatment.[80] Podophyllin causes local irritation and can be absorbed through the skin. It is not recommended for treating cervical and vaginal condylomas. Its use in pregnant women is best avoided, especially for treatment of large condylomas.

Salicylic acid and trichloroacetic acid are also used in the treatment of skin warts. They act by keratolysis of superficial squamous cells.

Squamous Papillomatosis

Squamous papillae of the vulvar vestibule are thought to be normal variations of pelvic anatomy.[60] In most instances, these papillae have a symmetrical distribution and occur in asymptomatic women. Growdon et al.[79] found similar changes in symptomatic women with pruritus, dyspareunia, pain, or burning. The lesions are located in the vulvar vestibule, especially near the inner aspect of the labia minora, navicular fossa, and hymen. Numerous small, 1 to 2 mm, slightly raised, polypoid nodules cover the affected area. Several longer papillae that have the appearance of a teardrop or rod are scattered over the area (Fig. 4–23). Other investigators have also referred to this lesion as microcondyloma.

Colposcopic examination reveals vascular cores in the papillae and punctation of the surrounding epithelium. Local application of acetic acid enhances the lesion by whitening the abnormal area.[79] Four of six male partners available for examination also demonstrated similar papillary changes on the penile skin, distal shaft, or glans. All were asymptomatic.[79]

Histologically, the papillary fronds are isolated and supported individually by coarse fibrovascular stalks with congestion and mild chronic inflammation. The overlying squamous epithelium is mildly hyperplastic (Fig. 4–24). Koilocytosis may be absent or seen at the base of the stalk (Fig. 4–25). In condyloma acuminatum, proliferating epithelium forms the bulk of the lesion. Koilocytosis is prominent. The fibrovascular cores are often compressed and limited in amount.

Studies by in situ hybridization have confirmed the presence of HPV DNA in some lesions.[168] In the study by Welch et al.,[205] 1% (3 of 295) of women who visited the genitourinary medicine clinic and underwent colposcopic examination of the vulva had vestibular papillomatosis. Of women with vestibular papillomatosis, 9 of 18 (50%) were symptomatic and 13 (72%) had a history of genital warts; 94% of vulvar biopsies had features of HPV effects. HPV 16 DNA was detected by in situ hybridization or PCR in 7 of 18 women (39%). The lesion in 9 (75%) regressed during a mean follow-up period of 9 months. Ten (56%) women had cervical condyloma or dysplasia. Of these, 5 required laser treatment. These authors conclude that this entity is commonly associated with HPV 16 infection.[205]

De Deus et al.[43] studied HPV DNA in normal controls, women with vestibular condyloma, and women with papillomatosis. The normal controls included 25 women who had no abnormal clinical, cytologic, or colposcopic findings in the cervix or vagina. Vulvar biopsies were taken from women with condyloma acuminatum, papillomatosis, and from normal controls. HPV DNA was detected by dot blot in 50% (12 of 24) of vestibular condylomas, 4% (1 of 25) of papillomatosis, and none of normal samples. By PCR, 100% (6 of 6) of condylomas and 7% (1 of 15) of papillomatosis had detectable HPV DNA. About one third of women with papillo-

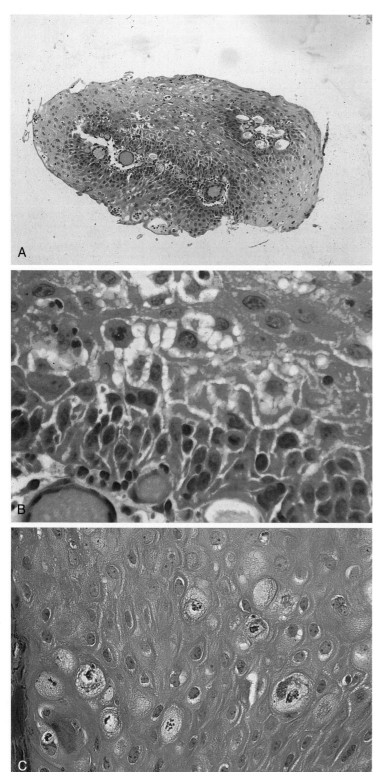

Figure 4–22. Podophyllin-treated condyloma. *A,* Spongiosus and infiltration of inflammatory cells. *B,* Scattered mitotic figures in the parabasal layers. *C,* Multiple podophyllin cells with arrested mitoses and dispersed chromosomes.

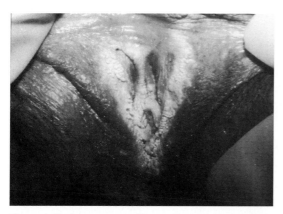

Figure 4–23. Squamous papillomatosis. After topical application of trichloroacetic acid, the affected areas appear white, with multiple papillary and teardrop-like projections on the labia minora and vestibules. Unaffected mucosa retains the normal color. (Courtesy of Dr. William Growdon, Los Angeles, California.)

matosis had focal koilocytosis located at the base of the papillae.[43]

Bergeron et al.,[17] on the other hand, found papillomatosis not associated with HPV. They pointed out that glycogenated squamous cells can be misinterpreted as koilocytes. These conflicting results suggest squamous papillomatosis in many women represents variation in vulvar anatomy. However, some of these women also have HPV infection.

Molluscum Contagiosum

This infection, caused by pox DNA virus, usually occurs on the hands, forearms, and face in children. After puberty, it is typically found on or near the genitalia.[206] A 25% increase in the incidence of molluscum contagiosum in females was reported in England and Wales from 1971 to 1973.[207] The incubation period appears to be from 14 to 30 days.[158] The age of the patients in one study varied from 17 to 26 years, with a mean age of 20.6 years. The lesions are usually asymptomatic, firm, pearly papules measuring 5 to 8 mm in diameter and having an umbilicated center.[206]

The histologic features of molluscum contagiosum are distinctive. Well-defined masses of hyperplastic epidermal cells extend into the dermis (Fig. 4–26). Cells in the stratum granulosum and stratum corneum contain large, homogeneous intracytoplasmic inclusions (molluscum bodies; see Fig. 4–26). These inclusions are eosinophilic when they first appear in the

parabasal cells and become basophilic and "brick-shaped" as the cells reach to the surface. The finding of molluscum bodies in histologic or cellular samples is diagnostic for molluscum contagiosum.

Cytomegalovirus

In the lower female genital tract, cytomegalovirus most often affects the endocervical glands, producing characteristic intranuclear and cytoplasmic viral inclusions.[44] Lymphoid infiltrates with germinal centers are often present in the stroma. The patients may be asymptomatic, or the cytomegalovirus may be associated with erosions and vaginal discharge. The cervix may be the focus of primary infection or a part of the systemic infection, which is usually secondary to immunosuppression.

Although evidence of cytomegalovirus infection is rarely found in pathologic specimens, its occurrence is high in pregnant women younger than 20 years of age (11.4% manifested

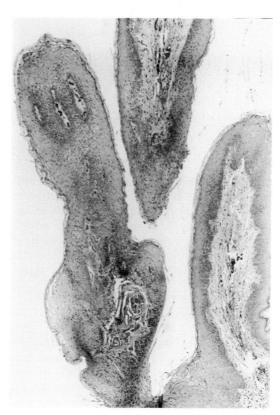

Figure 4–24. Squamous papillomatosis. Papillary fronds are isolated and covered by parakeratotic, slightly hyperplastic, mature squamous epithelium.

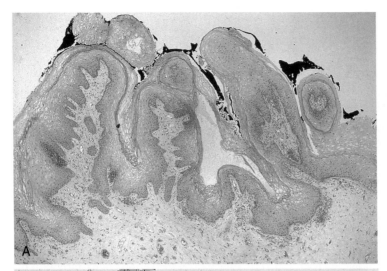

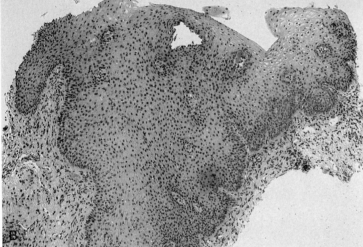

Figure 4–25. Squamous papillomatosis. *A*, Multiple papillary fronds are covered by thickened, hyperplastic, glycogenated squamous epithelium. *B*, At the base of stalk are koilocytes with nuclear hyperchromasia and increased cellularity as compared with the adjacent normal squamous cells.

megaloviruria). Of infants born to these mothers, 10% had congenital infection, with serologic evidence or virus isolation from urine and placenta.[138] Except for a lower birth weight, they had no clinical abnormalities at birth or at subsequent follow-up (12 months).[138] A classic multiple system disorder is rare.

Other Viral Infections

Variolar lesions may involve the vulva and vagina as part of the generalized disease. Vaccinia lesions affect the vulva primarily by accidental inoculation from the vaccination site elsewhere in the patient or on another person.[109] The clinical features depend on the immune status. The histologic changes include dermal inflammation as well as degeneration and vacuolation of the epidermal cells, some of which contain granular cytoplasmic inclusions. The diagnosis can be confirmed by electron microscopy, culture of the virus, or a rising antibody titer.

Varicella (chickenpox) and measles (myxovirus) of the vulva are usually part of a systemic viral infection. Herpes zoster rarely may occur in the anogenital area, with symptoms of motor disturbance of the sacral plexus.[66] Cat-scratch disease of the vulva associated with groin lymphadenopathy may occur. The cutaneous or mucosal lesion may be inconspicuous. The lymph nodes undergo necrosis, and palisading epithelioid cells are evident at the borders of necrosis. Using a modified Dieterle's stain, rod-shaped bacilli can be demonstrated in 66% of lymph nodes affected by cat-scratch disease.[106] Genital ulcers rarely may be asso-

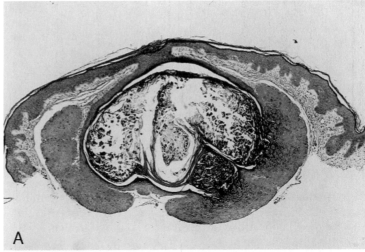

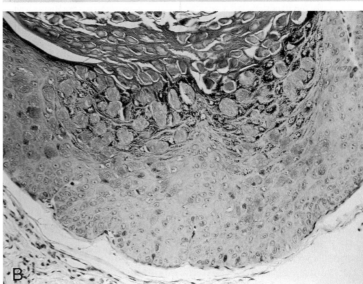

Figure 4–26. Molluscum contagiosum. *A*, Affected epithelium appears hyperplastic and extends downward into the dermis. *B*, Molluscum bodies consist of homogeneous intracytoplasmic inclusions.

ciated with infectious mononucleosis[24] or Epstein-Barr virus infection.[148]

OTHER VENEREAL DISEASES

Trichomoniasis

Causative Organism

Donne initially recognized the organism responsible for trichomoniasis in 1836.[47] Hoehne,[88] in 1916, related the presence of trichomonads to definitive clinical changes. The causative organism was isolated in pure culture by Trussell and Plass.[199] *Trichomonas vaginalis* is a flagellate, often oval or fusiform in shape, measuring 10 to 20 μm in length and 5 to 10 μm in width.[198,199] Although the shape is variable, depending in part on the environment, small organisms tend to be more regular in shape than are large organisms. Four flagellae one to three times the length of the organism arise from the anterior aspect of the protozoa. A small body, the *blepharoplast*, is located at the site of origin of the flagellae. An undulating membrane extends a variable distance from the blepharoplast, often to a site about one half the length of the organism. Also arising from the blepharoplast is the axostyle. The oval nucleus lies in proximity to the blepharoplast and contains chromatin granules and a karyosome. The cytoplasm is finely granular and contains scattered larger aggregates.

Prevalence

Trichomoniasis is a disease of the reproductive years. Although the causative organism may be demonstrated in postmenopausal woman, the prevalence of the disease is related to the population studied. Of 1000 private, nonpregnant patients, only 15.1% had trichomoniasis, whereas in prostitutes the prevalence is as high as 90%.[72]

Clinical Findings

As described by Gardner and Kaufman,[72] *T. vaginalis* may occur in asymptomatic women or may be associated with acute and, more often, chronic disease. Trichomonads may be observed in asymptomatic women with a vaginal pH of 3.8 to 4.2 and having vaginal flora containing numerous lactobacilli. The organisms are few in number, and the patients have no demonstrable evidence of disease. In chronic trichomoniasis, no gross changes in the vulva or vagina are apparent. However, the vaginal secretions have an abnormal volume, odor, and consistency, and the pH is altered.

In acute infection, an abnormal vaginal discharge is associated with gross manifestations of the disease. Erythema is the only finding in two thirds of the patients,[72] whereas in the remaining patients erythema is associated with other changes, including ecchymoses, petechiae, and occasionally pseudomembrane formation. Colpitis macularis (strawberry spots) is considered to be the specific clinical evidence of trichomoniasis. It is seen by naked eye in 1.7% of women with this infection. With the use of colposcopy, this sign increases to 42% of women.

Pathologic Findings

In histopathologic sections, trichomonads cannot be identified within the epithelium.[72] In the acute stages of the disease, necrotic debris and inflammatory cells may occur on the surface of the vaginal epithelium. In the presence of a pseudomembrane, the exudate covering the epithelium is more conspicuous. Acanthosis of the stratified squamous epithelium may be present, together with varying degrees of edema. The latter may produce swelling of the squamous cells with perinuclear halo and spongiosus (Fig. 4–27). With extensive edema, there may be separation of the epithelial cells and the formation of small vesicles. Within the underlying stroma, edema, enlargement of vascular spaces, and an infiltrate of inflammatory cells may occur (see Fig. 4–27). With edema of the stromal papillae, thinning of the overlying epithelium and ulceration may occur. Vascular congestion may explain the erythema observed on clinical examination, and the petechiae are related to localized extravasations of erythrocytes. The stroma, and in some instances the epithelium, are infiltrated by lymphocytes, plasma cells, and fewer neutrophils. Swollen vaginal papillae are the result of localized collections of inflammatory cells. Ulceration may be prominent.

In chronic trichomoniasis, the histopathologic changes are less pronounced. Acanthosis,

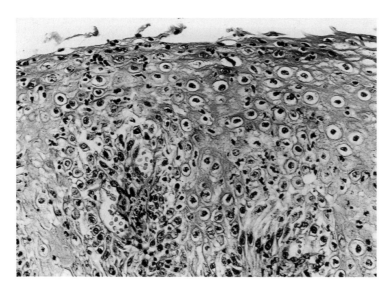

Figure 4–27. Acute trichomoniasis. The vaginal squamous mucosa is spongiotic and diffusely permeated by neutrophils. Most of the squamous cells contain perinuclear clear vacuoles. In contrast to koilocytes, these cells do not have densely eosinophilic cytoplasm and accentuated cell borders. The dermal papillae are enlarged and congested.

spongiosus, edema, and vascular congestion may be observed. The inflammatory infiltrate predominantly comprises lymphocytes and plasma cells. In asymptomatic women with demonstrable trichomonads, there are no significant changes in the vaginal mucosa.

Diagnosis

The wet-mount preparation of vaginal secretions is generally considered to be the optimal practical method for detecting trichomonads.[195] The accuracy of detection is 94%.[6] Actively motile trichomonads may be readily detected. Round organisms are less motile and often encountered in patients who have recently performed a douche or in women who are asymptomatic.[72] If this test is negative, culture of the vaginal swab into modified Diamon's medium is read at 1, 2, 5, and 7 days. Other methods, such as direct fluorescent antibody and acridine orange staining, are less sensitive than is culture.[195]

The classic morphologic features of trichomonads are less apparent in stained preparations. Gram stain, Giemsa stain, iron hematoxylin, acridine orange, and the Papanicolaou staining technique have been used with varying results. With the Papanicolaou technique, the organisms appear as small oval, pear-shaped, or round forms with an indeterminate or slightly eosinophilic cytoplasmic staining reaction (Figs. 4–28 and 4–29). In some forms, an eccentric, pale-staining nucleus may be identified, whereas in others a centrosome may be identified.

Minute eosinophilic cytoplasmic granules may be identified in some stained organisms (see Fig. 4–31). Flagellae are not readily identified in most instances. In stained preparations of the vaginal secretions, which contain a large number of leukocytes in aggregates, trichomonads may be confused with cellular debris, lysed parabasal cells, and small masses of mucus.[72]

Chlamydia Trachomatis Infections

Infections relating to *Chlamydia trachomatis* are believed to be the most prevalent and among the most damaging of the sexually transmitted diseases currently observed in the United States.[183] It is estimated that 3 to 4 million Americans are affected annually. Men, women, and infants may be infected.[183] The disease is associated with serious consequences in women—especially inflammatory disease, infertility, and ectopic pregnancy.

Causative Organism

Chlamydiae are unusual organisms whose characteristics have been established in the last 2 decades. Although classified as bacteria, they have properties shared by both viruses and bacteria. Like viruses, they grow only intracellularly. Unlike viruses, they contain both DNA and RNA, divide by binary fission, and have cell walls similar to those observed in gram-negative bacteria. The genome measures 6.6×10^8 daltons. The infection begins with the entry of 300

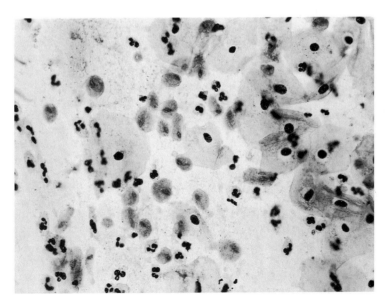

Figure 4–28. Trichomonads observed in a vaginal scraping. Poorly stained pear-shaped organisms can be seen, many of which contain a nucleus and eosinophilic granules in the cytoplasm. Flagellae are seldom seen in such preparations (Papanicolaou's stain, ×450)

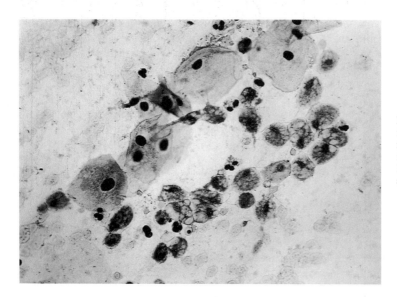

Figure 4–29. Trichomonads observed in a vaginal scraping. Many round forms with vacuolated cytoplasm are not viable. Some squamous cells have perinuclear halo. (Papanicolaou's stain, ×450)

nm elementary bodies into the cell by endocytosis. Inside the cytoplasm, the elementary body is surrounded by a membrane, which is produced by the host cell and later modified by the organisms. In a few hours, the elementary body loses the cell wall to become metabolically inactive, noninfectious reticulate bodies that multiply by binary fission. This process takes place in the form of an inclusion body. Reticulate bodies gain cell wall to become infective elementary bodies. Each inclusion, containing 100 to 1000 elementary bodies, ruptures by lysis or exocytosis.[162,164]

Clinical Findings

C. trachomatis is believed to be responsible for about 50% of reported cases of urethritis unrelated to the gonococcus in men. It is also thought to be responsible for 50% of the cases of acute epididymitis encountered each year in the United States. Although many chlamydial infections in women are asymptomatic, C. trachomatis may cause acute mucopurulent cervicitis,[25] acute pelvic inflammatory disease,[195] or infections of both the mother and the infant during pregnancy and after delivery. The affected cervix appears edematous and congested and is covered by purulent material. The organism is also believed to play a role in the urethral syndrome and in perihepatitis, or Fitz-Hugh–Curtis syndrome.

Infections during pregnancy have been associated with postpartum endometritis, and, in some studies, increases in perinatal mortality

are noted. Infants born to infected mothers may acquire the infection by contact with infected secretions in the cervix or vagina at birth. These newborns are at high risk for developing inclusion conjunctivitis and pneumonia. Another possible complication is otitis media.[86]

Pathologic Findings

The organisms preferentially affect columnar cells. Chlamydial cervicitis is characterized by the presence of a severe inflammatory response in the stroma. The inflammatory infiltrates are typically mixed and consist of lymphocytes, plasma cells, histiocytes, and neutrophils.[40] Lymphoid hyperplasia may be prominent, and the epithelium may be ulcerated. Reactive atypia with nuclear enlargement, hyperchromasia, and prominent nucleoli may be seen in the native squamous, metaplastic, and columnar cells (Fig. 4–30). The stroma undergoes fibrosis. IgG, IgM, and IgA antibodies are produced in response to chlamydial infection. In routine histologic sections and Papanicolaou-stained smears, cytoplasmic vacuoles and questionable inclusion bodies may be seen in the endocervical cells and metaplastic squamous cells; however, it is impossible to positively identify the infectious agents, and these samples are of little diagnostic value.[56] Using a heterologous antisera to *Chlamydia* by immunoperoxidase technique, 7 of 102 cervical biopsies were positive.[40] Antigen-positive cells were limited to the columnar and immature metaplastic cells.

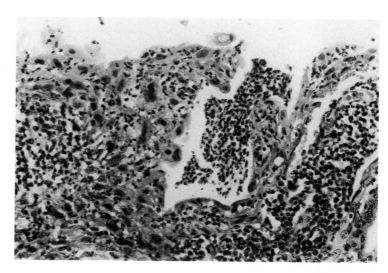

Figure 4–30. This cervical biopsy was taken from a woman with positive culture for *Chlamydia trachomatis*. Metaplastic squamous cells lining the endocervical gland demonstrate nuclear enlargement, irregularity, hyperchromasia, and binucleation. Numerous neutrophils and plasma cells are present in the endocervical gland and stroma. After treatment for Chlamydia, the cervical smears returned to normal.

The sensitivity of this method is not clear, owing to the lack of culture confirmation.

Diagnosis

Methods for diagnosis include tissue culture, immunofluorescent techniques, antigen detection tests, enzyme immunoassay, and serology.[48,49,86,118] Preservation of the specimen in special transport media is crucial for positive results. Culture is probably the most widely accepted method for diagnosis, but it is difficult and expensive. An immunofluorescent technique using commercially available fluorescein-labeled monoclonal antibody resulted in a sensitivity rate of 90% and a specificity rate of 99.6%, compared with those of culture.[86] Training and skills are required to search for elementary bodies under high-power immunofluorescent microscope. Enzyme immunoassay is more objective and is commonly used in laboratories.

Mycoplasma

Three different species of the genus Mycoplasmataceae have been demonstrated in the female genital tract: *Mycoplasma hominis, M. fermentans,* and *Ureaplasma urealyticum.*[122] Although some reports indicate that the organisms are more common in women with vaginitis,[15,41,132] their clinical significance is still controversial.[58] Some authors believe that the organisms are saprophytic in the vagina and are not associated with

distinctive changes[122]; others maintain that the organisms are responsible for clinical infection.[58] In view of the high prevalence of mycoplasma in the genital tract, isolating the organisms by culture is said to be of little value in individual cases.[41,72] The organism is also identified in urethritis.[41]

NONVENEREAL INFECTIONS

Vaginal flora, vaginal epithelial cells, and sex hormones maintain the normal environment or ecology of the vagina. Lactobacilli inhibit other organisms by several mechanisms. They metabolize the glycogen in the intermediate squamous cells to produce lactic acid to keep an acidic pH. Antimicrobial effect is also achieved by producing hydrogen peroxide. Many conditions are known to change the vaginal flora, thereby causing vulvovaginitis, such as antibiotic therapy, immunosuppression, hormonal changes and therapy, irradiation, surgery, and other iatrogenic manipulations.[121]

The isolation or identification of an organism from the vagina of a patient with a vaginal discharge or inflammation does not necessarily imply that the discharge is related to the organism in question.[133] A variety of organisms can be identified in the vaginas of women with vaginal discharge, and many of these organisms are also present in those without recognizable disease. In other cases, the clinical signs and symptoms of vaginal inflammation are secondary to disease of the vulva or upper genital tract.

Some of the organisms that are implicated do not produce distinctive changes, and sometimes more than one organism can be identified in the presence of vaginal inflammation.

Both clinical and laboratory findings are important in investigating the patient with vaginitis. Biopsy is less frequently used. The gynecologist usually examines wet-mount preparations of vaginal discharge. A sample of the vaginal secretion is mixed with physiologic saline solution and examined under the microscope. The identification of fungi is facilitated by mixing the vaginal secretion with 10% to 20% potassium hydroxide (KOH). Samples of the vaginal secretion may also be examined in stained preparations, and cultures are used as well.

Bacterial Vaginosis, Nonspecific Vaginitis, *Haemophilus* Vaginitis, *Gardnerella* Vaginitis

Bacterial vaginosis is characterized by polymicrobial condition symbiosis of a variety of anaerobic and aerobic bacterial flora. These organisms multiply after the disappearance of normal predominant vaginal lactobacilli.

Causative Organism

Gardner and Dukes[70] were first to point out that the changes of "nonspecific vaginitis" were usually related to the presence of an organism initially classified as *Haemophilus vaginalis*. They and others[180] described the clinical and laboratory findings and concluded that, in most cases, the changes were related to the presence of *Haemophilus* vaginitis. With the use of consistent criteria, this disease has been better defined. Lapage[112] suggested that the organism that was initially designated as *H. vaginalis* might belong to the genus Corynebacterium. In 1963, Zinnemann and Turner[215] recommended that the organism be classified as *Corynebacterium vaginale*, and in 1980, the designation *Gardnerella vaginalis* was proposed.[76] The organism is a small, nonmotile gram-negative bacillus with round ends measuring 0.3 to 0.6 microns in width and 1 to 2 microns in length.

The organism is thought to be sexually transmitted.[68,72] Gardner[68] concluded that this form of vaginitis is the most common of the sexually transmitted diseases associated with clinical manifestations. The organism can be isolated from most male partners of infected women, although it is only rarely identified as causing clinically evident disease in the male. The organism has been recovered in 77%[46] to 91%[69] of husbands of infected women. When the male consort is untreated, reinfection in the female usually occurs. This form of vaginitis is frequently associated with other sexually transmitted diseases[11] and is observed with considerable frequency in the sexually promiscuous woman[69] and in 52% of patients with other venereal diseases.[95]

Clinical Findings

The clinical signs and symptoms are usually mild and are often overlooked.[36] Bacterial vaginosis is found in one third of women attending sexually transmitted disease clinics and primary care facilities. The clinical findings are well described by Gardner[68] and Gardner and Dukes.[70] There is considerable variation in the amount of the vaginal discharge, which is gray or white and, less frequently, yellow or green (Fig. 4–31). The discharge is more likely to be adherent to the vaginal wall and is less likely to accumulate in the posterior vaginal fornix. The

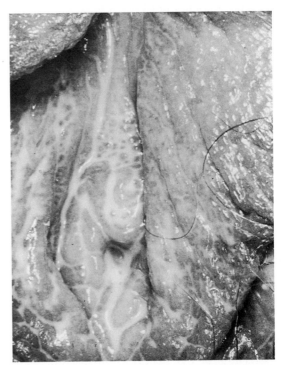

Figure 4–31. Characteristic appearance of exudate in a woman with *Haemophilus vaginalis* vaginitis. (Reproduced with permission from Gardner HL, Kaufman RH. Benign Diseases of the Vulva and Vagina, 2nd ed. Chicago, Copyright © by Year Book Medical Publishers, 1981, p 282)

malodorous secretion is seldom frothy and has a pH of 5.0 to 5.5, only infrequently having a pH of less than 5.0. Erythema and edema of the vagina is only rarely observed, and this may be unrelated to the presence of the organism.

A review by Thompson et al.[194] listed potential complications, including intra-abdominal infections, amniotic fluid infection and premature labor, maternal infection during labor and postpartum, and postcesarean endometritis. They recommend screening of pregnant women for bacterial vaginosis by finding clue cells rather than by culture.

Diagnosis

The diagnosis of bacterial vaginosis is based on the following findings of vaginal discharge: (1) a nonviscous homogeneous consistency, (2) an elevated pH of greater than 4.5, (3) a fishy amine odor after alkalinization with 10% KOH, (4) the presence of clue cells in 10% to 20% or more of epithelial cells, and (5) normal vaginal flora *Lactobacillus* replaced by *G. vaginalis,* anaerobe species, and *Mycoplasma hominis.* At least three of the first four items should be present.[28]

According to Creddia et al.,[35] only clue cells and odor are specific for bacterial vaginosis. On the other hand, Thompson et al.[194] found odor, clue cells, and the presence of Mobiluncus to be specific for bacterial vaginosis. The presence of clue cells on wet mount of vaginal secretion had a sensitivity of 98.2% and a specificity of 94.3%. Under 400 power magnification, the clue cells can be identified by indistinct borders with adherent bacteria.

In wet mounts, the bacilli occur in clumps and in an isolated state. They are often attached to the edges of the squamous cells. Other epithelial cells are covered by organisms, which are evenly dispersed over the surface of the cell. Some epithelial cells are only barely discernible because of the dense accumulation of the organisms, whereas other cells are only partially involved. These characteristic cells are referred to as clue cells (Fig. 4–32).[72,116,126] When clue cells are observed in cellular samples, *G. vaginalis* is identified by culture in more than 87% of cases.[116] Other organisms, such as diphtheroids and cocci, may also adhere to the surface of epithelial cells. These are designated as false clue cells (Fig. 4–33). Elsewhere in wet-mount preparations, neutrophils are infrequent unless there is coexisting infection by other bacteria, and lactobacilli are seldom observed. Although the morphology of the organism is better defined in gram-stained preparations, *G. vaginalis* can be identified in the Papanicolaou-stained sample. Although the epithelial cells have adherent organisms, they are otherwise unaltered. Air-dried vaginal wet mounts can be rehydrated later for more detailed study as needed.[113]

Tissue examination is of no value in identifying the process. The organism acts as a surface parasite, does not invade the vaginal wall, and is not readily detected in the vaginal epithelium. An inflammatory reaction is seldom observed in the underlying stroma.

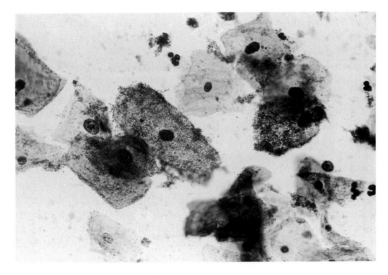

Figure 4–32. "Clue cells" in *Haemophilus vaginalis* vaginitis. Some cells are stippled. These are clue cells typical of *H. vaginalis.* (Papanicolaou's stain, ×400)

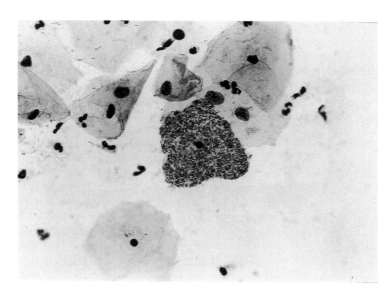

Figure 4–33. Distinctly bacillary organisms cover the surface of one cell. This is a "false clue" cell. (Papanicolaou's stain, ×1080)

Bacterial Vulvovaginitis

Streptococci are commonly observed in the normal vagina. Alpha and gamma types often occur in the presence of *T. vaginalis* but are seldom pathogens in the vagina. Beta streptococci, which are responsible for significant changes in other tissues, are usually unrelated to vaginal infections. According to Gardner and Kaufman,[72] *Streptococcus pyogenes* is the only member of this group that has been implicated in vaginitis. Infections attributed to *S. pyogenes* are rare and are reported to occur in women with low levels of estrogen. The erythematous vagina is associated with a seropurulent-type discharge. The histopathologic changes are not distinctive.

Few infections of the vagina are related to staphylococcus.[111] *Escherichia coli* is a normal inhabitant of the intestinal tract and might be readily introduced into the vagina, but the organism is seldom responsible for vaginitis. On the other hand, Strate et al.[186] reported a xanthomatous pseudotumor of the vagina caused by mucoid *E. coli*. Rod-shaped bacilli were demonstrated in the cytoplasm of foamy histiocytes by Dieterle's silver stain (Fig. 4–34).

Borrelia vincentii and *Fusobacterium plautivincenti* are the organisms associated with fusospirochetosis. This disease is observed in debilitated persons and may result from autoinoculation. Primary and secondary forms of the disease are described. *Bacillus fusiformis* is a long gram-negative rod that may be either curved or straight. *B. vincentii*, which is most

commonly observed with severe disease, is a spirochete 4 to 15 μ in length with 2 to 20 coils. The organisms are observed in lesions characterized by ulceration and edema.[125]

Nonpathogenic corynebacteria, referred to as diphtheroids, are normally found in the vagina. The only proven pathogenic corynebacteria are *C. diphtheriae* (a Klebs-Löffler bacillus related to diphtheritic vaginitis); *C. tenuis,* which causes trichomycosis; and *C. minutissimum,* which is responsible for vulvar erythrasma.[72]

Erythrasma was originally thought to be a fungal infection but is now recognized to be caused by *C. minutissimum* or other related diphtheroid species. This organism is found on normal skin; most often affected are warm, semi-moist areas such as toe clefts and flexural areas, including the groin and intergluteal and genitocrural folds. Diabetes is believed to be a predisposing factor.

The lesion has a brownish-red, finely scaling appearance and is well defined without an active edge. The diagnosis is made by bacterial culture or by the finding of chains of bacilli in smears or biopsies stained by Gram stain. Anaerobes can be readily recovered from the vagina; however, when isolated, they are not clearly related to any distinct clinical entity.

Leptothrix and Leptotrichia are large filamentous bacteria. They are thin, nonbranching, segmented forms (Fig. 4–35). The organisms live symbiotically with known pathogens in the vagina. Gardner and Kaufman[72] stated that the organisms are not known to be responsible for vaginitis.

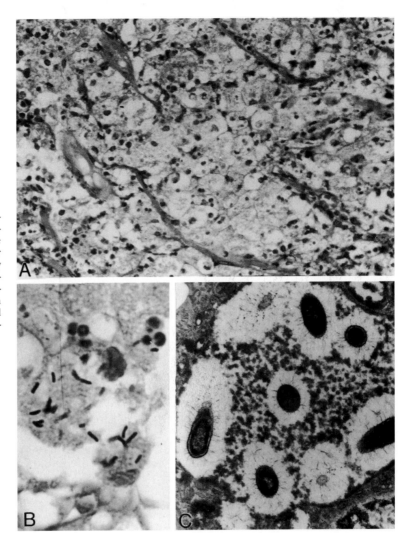

Figure 4–34. *A,* Vaginal xanthomatous pseudotumor caused by mucoid *Escherichia coli.* Bacilli are demonstrated by Dieterle's silver stain (*B*) and electron microscopy (*C*). (*A,* H&E, ×150; *B,* Dieterle silver stain, ×1000; *C,* ×20,500; reproduced with permission from the American Journal of Clinical Pathology, Volume 79, pp 637—643, 1983.)

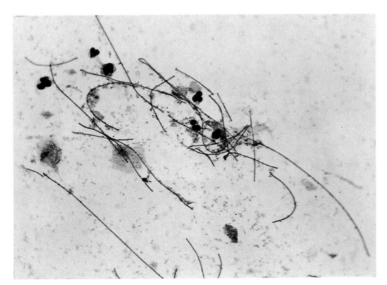

Figure 4–35. Leptothrix observed in vaginal scrapings. Characteristic long, thin, thread-like organisms, which may be beaded. (Papanicolaou's stain, ×560)

Atrophic Vaginitis

As a result of the loss of estrogenic stimulation, a reduction in the thickness of the vaginal mucosa occurs. There is considerable variation in the age at which this takes place and in the degree of atrophy that results. The designation of atrophic vaginitis may be applied to all cases involving atrophy or may be restricted to those in which atrophy is associated with gross tissue changes.[72]

The vaginal folds and rugae disappear, and the mucosa becomes pale. Petechiae or ecchymosis may occur. Adhesions may develop after trauma or, less frequently, without this history. Shrinkage of the tissues leads to varying degrees of stenosis, which first becomes evident in the fornices and ultimately involves the entire vagina. Discharge is variable in amount, and the pH diminishes, usually ranging from 5.5 to 7.0.[72]

As a result of atrophy, the rete pegs are less prominent and the epithelium is reduced in thickness. The nonglycogenated epithelium may become denuded, and ulceration may occur. Minute ulcers and foci of granulation tissue may be present. The underlying stroma may be infiltrated by lymphocytes and plasma cells. Vascular sclerosis may also occur. In the presence of secondary vaginal infection, an acute inflammatory reaction may be observed.

In vaginal scrapings, cells resembling those normally observed in the intermediate or parabasal cell layers are found. The latter should be designated as atrophic cells. These cells are often associated with leukocytes.

Vaginitis Emphysematosa

Vaginitis emphysematosa is a self-limited disease characterized by the presence of multiple discrete, gas-filled cavities within the lamina propria of the vagina. Although many theories have been advanced to explain the process, recent work suggests a relationship between vaginitis emphysematosa and the presence of _T. vaginalis_ and, less often, _G. vaginalis_. More recently, Josey and Campbell[94] suggested impaired immunity as a potential predisposing condition, such as that from alcoholic cirrhosis, corticosteroid therapy, and postoperative wound infection.

The lesion is usually an incidental finding, although it may occur in the presence of vaginal discharge, bloody discharge after inter-course, or genital pruritus. Some women are aware of a "popping" sound resulting from the rupture of the gas-containing cavities.[71] A relationship between the presence of _T. vaginalis_ and vaginitis emphysematosa was observed in 7 of 10 women with vaginitis emphysematosa.[71] The remaining 3 women had _G. vaginalis_. Eradication of the trichomoniasis is reported to be associated with involution of the lesion. In support of this relationship is the production of gas by the subcutaneous inoculation of _T. vaginalis_ in germ-free guinea pigs.

Vaginitis emphysematosa is most pronounced in the upper two thirds of the vagina, and the uterine cervix may be simultaneously involved. The tense cavities may bulge above the level of the vaginal mucosa, or, when smaller, the localized collection of cavities may be appreciated as indurated areas on palpation. Crepitation is not observed.

On histopathologic examination, numerous discrete cavities occur in the lamina propria (Fig. 4–36A). These measure up to 1.5 cm in greatest dimension. There is usually no discernible lining epithelium. Multinucleated giant cells may be found within the cavities and at their periphery (see Fig. 4–36B). Less frequently, stratified squamous or simple columnar epithelium may line the cavities.[71] Fibrosis, histiocytes, or an infiltration of leukocytes may also be found in the cavities.

Desquamative Inflammatory Vaginitis

Desquamative inflammatory vaginitis is a rare form of vaginitis.[67] It resembles the atrophic vaginitis of postmenopausal women, but it also affects premenopausal women with normal ovarian function. It differs from atrophic vaginitis by failing to improve with estrogen therapy. The change is uncommon, being observed in only 8 of more than 3000 women with vaginal infection. Gray and Barnes[75] first described the clinical and microscopic features in 1965, although similar changes were observed in a previously published case classified as exudative vaginitis.[165] Possible causes include local tissue defect, infection, and the use of strong chemical vaginal douches. Microbial cultures have isolated a wide range of gram-positive and gram-negative organisms, especially group B streptococci in 44% of cases.[176] Some cases are associated with lichen planus of the oral and genital regions.

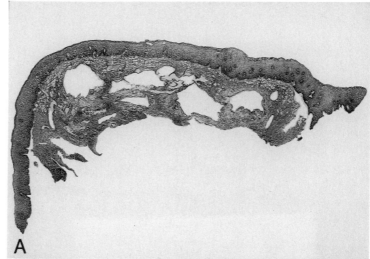

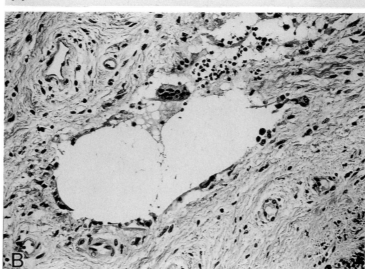

Figure 4–36. Vaginitis emphysematosa. *A,* Multiple gas-filled spaces in lamina propria of vagina. *B,* High-power view of gas-filled space. Note lack of lining epithelium and giant cells.

In one series of 51 women, the mean age was 41.8 (21 to 66) years. The clinical presentation is characterized by diffuse vaginitis, epithelial cell desquamation, profuse and purulent vaginal discharge, and dyspareunia.[176] The mucosa of the upper vagina is acutely inflamed. The margins of the lesion are usually well delineated and may have a serpiginous configuration. Trauma of the epithelium leads to bleeding. The epithelium may be covered by a gray pseudomembrane.[72,165] Vaginal synechiae and stenosis also occur.[141] Vulvar symptoms and signs are relatively minor. Focal ecchymoses may be seen in the vulva, vagina, or cervix, especially in postmenopausal women.[176]

On histopathologic examination, the epithelium is atrophic and thin and sometimes ulcerated.[72] Within the epithelium, there is edema and a dense cellular infiltrate comprising neutrophils, monocytes, plasma cells, and histiocytes (Fig. 4–37A). Hyperkeratosis and parakeratosis may develop. The underlying stroma shows acute and chronic inflammation, congestion, focal hemorrhage, and exudate (see Figs. 4–37B and C). Those associated with lichen planus, liquefied basal cells, and a band-like lymphocytic infiltration are evident.[141] The disease persists for many years and is usually refractory to antimicrobial, estrogen, and corticosteroid treatment.[141] Sobel reported clinical improvement with 2% clindamycin suppositories in more than 95% of patients, although relapse occurred in 30% of cases.[176]

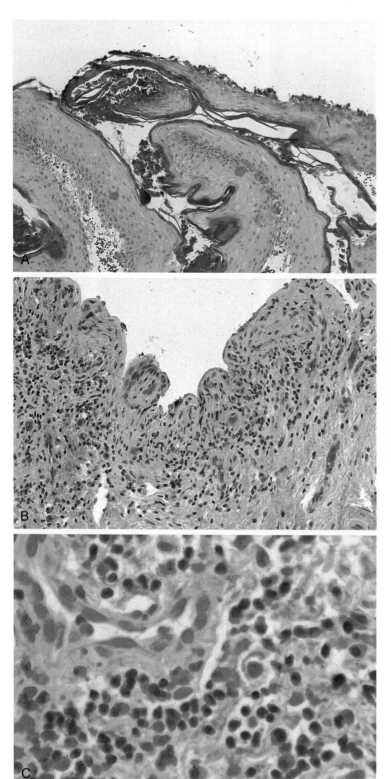

Figure 4–37. Desquamative vaginitis. *A,* Detached desquamated squamous epithelium with focal necrosis and inflammatory reaction. *B,* The superficial stroma demonstrates chronic inflammatory reaction and mild vascular proliferation. *C,* The inflammatory infiltrates consist of lymphocytes, plasma cells, and occasional histiocytes in the perivascular region.

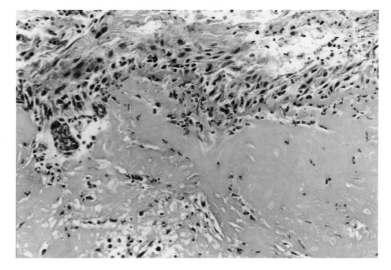

Figure 4–38. Ligneous vulvovaginitis. The mucosa is often denuded or covered by regenerating epithelium. Beneath the mucosa, the deposited material is densely eosinophilic and homogeneous.

Ligneous Vulvovaginitis

Ligneous conjunctivitis is a rare, recurrent, chronic granulomatous inflammation with a wood-like consistency.[179] Some patients may have similar lesions in the nasopharynx, vagina, and vulva. We have seen such a case with multiple yellow 1 to 2 cm nodules removed from the eyelids and vagina.

Histologically, the vaginal lesion is covered by denuded squamous mucosa with areas of regeneration and pseudoepitheliomatous hyperplasia (see Fig. 4–43). The stroma contains deposits of densely eosinophilic, hyalinized, amyloid-like material (Fig. 4–38). At the periphery, occasionally there are lymphocytes, plasma cells, and multinucleated giant cells as well as ingrowth of fibroblasts and capillaries (Fig. 4–39). Special stains for amyloid are negative. A reddish staining reaction with trichrome stain suggests that the material is fibrin.

Tuberculosis

The frequency of tuberculosis varies considerably throughout the world. The disease is often related to socioeconomic conditions and geographic areas.[140,212]

A report based on specimens collected in Madrid, Spain, over a span of 30 years noted 1436 cases of genital tuberculosis.[140] There has been a marked reduction in the frequency of the disease in the last 2 decades, and tubercu-

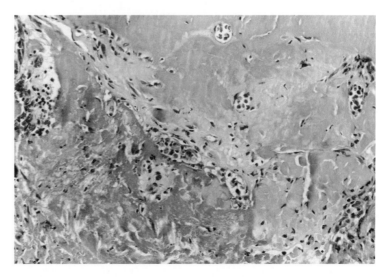

Figure 4–39. Ligneous vulvovaginitis. The amyloid-like material is infiltrated by a small number of lymphocytes, plasma cells, and multinucleated giant cells. Ingrowth of fibroblasts and capillaries is also seen.

losis occurred most commonly in women aged 25 to 35 years. Involvement of the fallopian tubes was observed in 100% of the cases. Vulvovaginal disease was observed in 0.7% of the women, all of whom had coexisting cervical disease. Involvement of the lower genital tract is usually secondary to downward spread from the upper genital tract or pelvis and is less likely to be a result of hematogenous spread from the lung or kidney. Primary tuberculosis of the vulva may be contracted from infected sputum or semen (tuberculous infection of the epididymis or kidney).

The lesion presents as an indurated nodule, an ulcer, or, frequently, as a mass. If limited to the Bartholin's gland involvement is usually unilateral. Involvement of the regional lymph nodes may lead to necrosis, scarring, and lymphedema of the vulva. Histologic changes are characterized by caseating granulomatous inflammation (Fig. 4–40). Identification of acid-fast organisms in the culture, smear, or histologic sample is diagnostic. A negative tuberculin skin test renders the diagnosis unlikely.

Leprosy

Leprosy, caused by *Mycobacterium leprae,* may involve the vulva. In one study, 13% of the patients with leprosy had vulvar involvement.[74] In the female genital tract, the ovary is most frequently affected, followed by the cervix, uterus, and uterine tubes.[19]

Actinomycosis

Actinomycosis of the female genital tract, reported initially in women using an intrauterine pessary, was subsequently linked to the use of intrauterine contraceptive devices (IUDs). Gupta[81] has written a detailed review on this subject.

This organism is a gram-positive, anaerobic bacterium normally found in the oropharynx and intestinal tract. When such an organism has been detected in cervicovaginal smears, 97.2% of the women have been users of various types of IUDs. The remaining women have had foreign bodies in the cervix or vagina.[147] In one study, the detection rate during the first year of IUD use was 5.7%, but it increased to 20% and higher after 2 years.[102] Overall, it was found in this study that 12.6% of IUD users have actinomyces colonies in their cervicovaginal smears.[102] However, other investigators have found a much lower frequency of less than 1%.[147] This divergence may be explained by the population under study and the morphologic criteria for identifying the organism.

In the presence of IUDs, the local environment has apparently been changed to favor an opportunistic infection of actinomyces in the endocervix and endometrium. Additional synergistic action of other anaerobic bacteria and ascending infection may result in pelvic inflammatory disease, tubo-ovarian abscess, or pelvic abscess. About 50% of tubo-ovarian abscesses occur unilaterally.

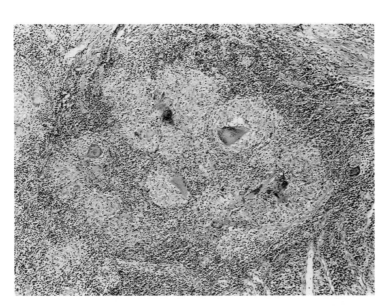

Figure 4–40. Tuberculous granuloma from wall of vagina in a woman with a similar change in the endometrium.

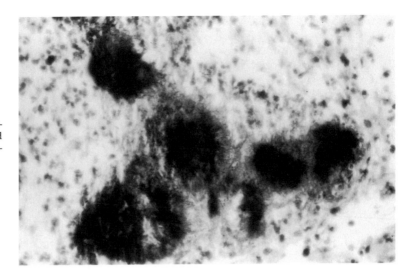

Figure 4–41. Colonies of actinomyces with basophilic center and radiating filaments in the periphery.

In the cervicovaginal smears and tissue sections, the organisms appear as fluffy, basophilic colonies with characteristic parallel, radiating filaments at the periphery (Fig. 4–41). They branch at acute angles, sometimes have a beaded appearance, and are surrounded by neutrophils. Other types of bacterial colonies often coexist with actinomyces. In such cases, the organisms should be verified by Gram, periodic acid–Schiff (PAS), or methenamine silver stain. The clinical significance of identifying actinomyces organisms in the cervicovaginal smears has been controversial. Some investigators have failed to correlate the presence of actinomyces colonies with the symptom or infection[147]; others recommend removal of the IUD and/or institution of antibiotic therapy.[102]

Amebiasis

Amebiasis of the female genital tract usually involves the cervix and upper vagina; rarely is the vulva affected. Multiple irregular ulcerations are covered by necrotic tissue or granulation tissue. The causative organism, *Entamoeba histolytica,* may be identified in the smear or biopsy (Fig. 4–42).[120,200] Cultures are of limited value.

Schistosomiasis (Bilharziasis)

Schistosomiasis is more prevalent in tropical or subtropical climates than in North America. Genital involvement is common in endemic areas[213,214] and is usually caused by *Schistosoma*

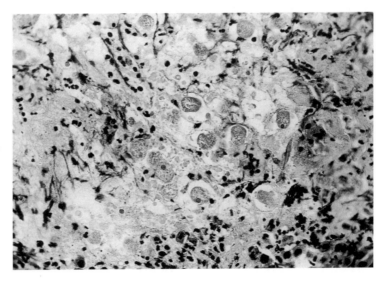

Figure 4–42. Amebiasis of the cervix. The necrotic tissue contains the trophozoites of *Entamoeba histolytica,* which have a small, round nucleus; vacuolated cytoplasm; and phagocytosed red blood cells.

haematobia. Cervical, vulvar, or vaginal lesions may be observed. The lesions are ulcerative or nodular and may present as papillomatous growths. The nature and severity of tissue reactions to the ova are variable. The surface epithelium may be denuded, atrophic, or hyperplastic. Well-preserved or calcified ova may be identified in the stroma. In other instances, venules contain the adult worms. Fibrosis, multinucleated giant cells, and an inflammatory exudate may be observed in the connective tissue. The diagnosis is made by identifying ova or worms in the secretions.

FUNGAL INFECTIONS

In a study by Horowitz et al.,[89] *Candida albicans* (65%) and *C. tropicalis* (23%) were most frequently isolated from patients with mycotic vulvovaginitis. Dermatophytes (3%), *C. humicola* (2%), and *Torulopsis (Candida) glabrata* are less common.

Candidiasis

Candidiasis of the genital tract has been recognized under varied terminology, including vaginal moniliasis; candidal, mycotic, or yeast vulvovaginitis; vaginal thrush; and candidiasis.[72]

Causative Organism

The responsible organism belongs to the genus *Candida.* It is found in humans and animals and is pathogenic only in the presence of a favorable environment and a susceptible host. In an analysis of 100 consecutive cases of vaginal candidiasis, *C. albicans* was found in 67%, *C. tropicalis* in 28%, *C. stellatoidea* in 3%, *C. pseudotropicalis* in 1%, and *C. krusei* in 1% of patients.[72] These fungi are commonly recovered from the intestinal tract, oral cavity, and vagina of normal women.

Clinical Findings

It is currently believed that many factors are important for the development of clinical disease. A variety of host factors have been identified. Diabetes mellitus and pregnancy are important predisposing factors. In pregnancy, this is attributed to the increased glycogen content of the epithelium, the glycosuria occasionally observed in pregnancy, and reduced glucose tolerance leading to elevated levels of blood sugar.[72] Clinical manifestations may be more pronounced before menstruation. Some controversy surrounds the use of oral contraceptives as a predisposing factor. Gardner and Kaufman[72] conclude that this may be associated with a minor increase in the incidence of symptomatic disease and that successful therapy is more difficult when the patient is using oral contraceptives. Antibiotics and corticosteroid administration are believed to be important predisposing factors, as are diabetes mellitus and debilitation. Other factors are also implicated.

Candidiasis is primarily a disease of the childbearing years. Because the organism cannot be demonstrated within the affected tissues, many of the symptoms and signs are believed to be an allergic reaction to the *Candida* or its endotoxins.[72] Rarely, candidiasis presents as a cutaneous infection of the vulva, especially in infants and in diabetics. In this form of candidiasis, the keratinized superficial layers of the epidermis are infected.

Common symptoms include pruritus, edema, dysuria, dyspareunia, and, less commonly, leukorrhea. The inner aspect of the labia and the vestibule are most often involved in the infection, and the disease may extend to the genitocrural folds. Erythema is appreciated in 20% of the cases,[72] and thrush patches are variable in their appearance and occurrence. From 10%[181] to 15%[72] of patients have thrush patches, which are loosely adherent and white or, less frequently, yellow. Some patients have few patches, but in other cases, they are more numerous. Occasionally, a pseudomembrane covers the vaginal mucosa. The amount of vaginal exudate may vary.

Diagnosis

Biopsy is occasionally used in establishing the diagnosis of candidiasis. *Candida* organisms with spores and pseudohyphae are found in the epidermal surface and keratin debris; they rarely invade the vaginal epithelium and can be identified only on the surface of the mucosa.[72,181] Within the mucosa, there is acanthosis, spongiosus, and hyperemia of the lamina propria. In the upper levels of the lamina propria is an infiltrate of lymphocytes, plasma cells, and fewer neutrophils. The infiltrate may focally involve the stratified squamous mucosa. Over the surface of the mucosa may be degenerate squamous cells, neutrophils, and sometimes spores or pseudohyphae of *Candida*. In chronic states, the histopathologic changes are less pronounced.[72]

The diagnosis of candidiasis is not based solely on the identification of the causative organism. *Candida* must be demonstrated in the presence of clinical findings compatible with the disease process.

A rapid identification of *Candida* is facilitated by the use of 10% to 20% potassium hydroxide. When mixed with a sample of the vaginal discharge, neutrophils and erythrocytes disappear; the epithelial cells become transparent; and *Candida*, as well as other filamentous organisms, becomes more apparent. In addition to wet mounts, stained preparations may be used. *Candida* may be grown in culture, although differentiation of the species requires the use of sugar fermentation. Phase contrast may also be used.

Specific identification is not possible by means of cellular examination, although the observed findings may permit a presumptive diagnosis. *Candida* reproduces by budding, which results in the formation of pseudomycelia. Budding yeast cells may be identified. In stained smears, perinuclear halos may be observed in the epithelial cells, along with degenerated leukocytes. It should be noted that vulvovaginal candidiasis may coexist with other infections, especially gonorrhea. However, trichomoniasis rarely coexists with candidiasis.[158]

Torulopsis Glabrata Vaginitis

Smith, Taubert, and Martin[172] reported that *Torulopsis glabrata* was the only fungus identified in vaginal cultures of 6 (9.7%) of 62 pregnant women thought to have vulvovaginal mycosis. Timonen, Salo, and Haapoja[196] isolated the organism from the vaginas of 70 women, only 21 of whom had evidence of vaginal inflammation. According to Kearns and Gray,[101] only 7% of vulvovaginal mycoses are related to this fungus. Gardner and Kaufman[72] regard the fungus as a weak pathogen associated with mild vulvovaginitis associated with vaginal discharge, sometimes accompanied by mild edema.

Whereas specific identification of the fungus depends on culture, the cellular sample obtained in the presence of *T. glabrata* may contain encapsulated or budding yeast cells (Fig. 4–43). These cells may also be associated with Saccharomyces or Cryptococcus. Mycelia of *T. glabrata* are seldom observed in the cellular sample.

Dermal Mycosis

Superficial dermatophytic mycosis involves only the skin and the appendages. The pathogenicity of the organisms is weak and elicits only minor chronic inflammation. Therefore patients are usually asymptomatic. Tinea cruris is found occasionally on the vulva. Tinea versicolor

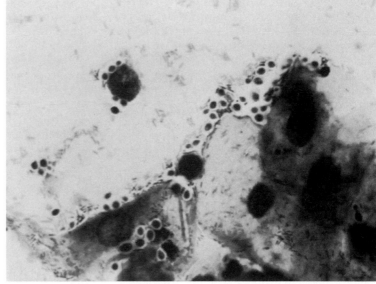

Figure 4–43. Spores in *Torulopsis glabrata.* (Papanicolaou's stain, ×1000; courtesy of Marluce Bibbo, M.D., Thomas Jefferson University, Philadelphia, Pennsylvania.)

(pityriasis versicolor) and tinea circinata are rarely reported on the vulva. Tineas are caused by a variety of organisms. The exact identification of the causative fungi is not clinically important, but the disease should be differentiated from candidiasis and erythrasma.[59]

Tinea cruris of the vulva usually involves the upper inner thighs, perineum, and buttocks. The well-defined and usually symmetrical lesion has an erythematous, slightly raised, vesiculated appearance.[59,72] A positive diagnosis can be made by finding hyphae on a scraping from the edge of the lesion. In PAS-stained biopsy, fungal hyphae can be seen in the stratum corneum.

Rare deep mycoses, such as actinomycosis, phycomycosis, chromomycosis, blastomycosis, sporotrichosis, and coccidioidomycosis, have been reported in the vulva.[26,59,72,158]

OTHER INFECTIOUS AND INFLAMMATORY DISEASES

Acute and Chronic Cervicitis

Many of the infectious diseases, both venereal and nonvenereal, that occur in the vulva and vagina can also involve the cervix. The cervix may appear edematous, congested, ulcerated, or eroded. During acute cervicitis, the epithelium undergoes degeneration and necrosis with neutrophilic infiltration in the stroma. The infection may become chronic. The associated epithelial changes include regeneration, hyperplasia, and squamous metaplasia. The causative agents in many cases of chronic cervicitis are difficult to determine. Most cases of mild chronic cervicitis represent physiologic or reactive changes to local trauma or irritation. A highly reactive epithelium may simulate neoplasia. Similarly, exuberant lymphoid hyperplasia in the stroma can be confused with malignant lymphoma.

Bartholinitis and Bartholin's Gland Abscess

Infection of the Bartholin's gland is caused by a variety of organisms, including gonococcus, E. coli, streptococcus, staphylococcus, T. vaginalis, anaerobic and aerobic vaginal flora, and mycoplasma. Depending on the organisms, both the acinar and ductal elements may become affected.[114] The involved ducts become swollen and edematous, and the drainage is blocked. The secretion rapidly becomes infected, and acute bartholinitis and abscess may develop. Bacterial culture and smears of 34 Bartholin's gland abscesses show that 10 (29.4%) were sterile and that the remaining 24 (70.6%) contained organisms, including gram-negative rods (E. coli and Proteus mirabilis) in 8 cases (23.5%), gonococci in 4 cases (11.8%), and various anaerobic and aerobic vaginal flora in 12 cases (35.3%).[115] In one case, M. hominis was isolated.[115] Rarely, in patients with diabetes and ketoacidosis, Bartholin's gland abscess may be the source of a serious necrotizing fasciitis (progressive synergistic bacterial gangrene).[159]

In chronic bartholinitis, infiltrates of lymphocytes, plasma cells, and histiocytes may be localized or diffuse. The mucinous acinar cells are sometimes atrophic. The ductal epithelium undergoes hyperplasia or squamous metaplasia. The periductal fibrosis may further compromise the lumen, leading to stenosis and cyst formation.

Synergistic Bacterial Gangrene and Necrotizing Fasciitis

Brewer and Meleney,[21] in 1926, described two cases of progressive gangrenous necrosis of the abdominal wall following surgery for a perforated appendix. Staphylococcus aureus and microaerophilic streptococcus were isolated respectively from the center and periphery of necrosis. It was concluded that the gangrene resulted from synergistic actions of these organisms.[21] Wilson,[208] in 1952, applied the term necrotizing fasciitis to 22 patients who presented with extensive necrosis of fascial and subcutaneous tissue with gas formation, involving the abdominal wall, extremities, and groin region. These two conditions are generally regarded as variants of the same disease process.[159] Bacterial cultures usually yield mixed organisms, including staphylococci, aerobic and anaerobic streptococci, bacteroides, and gram-negative aerobic bacilli.

Necrotizing fasciitis of the genital area has been reported following hysterectomy, cesarean section, laparoscopy, episiotomy, and abscess of the Bartholin's gland.[130,159,178,189] Although diabetes mellitus, obesity, hypertension, peripheral vascular disease, chronic illness, and immunosuppression are known predisposing factors, some patients who acquire necrotizing fasciitis are apparently healthy. Typical presentations include edema and erythema of the skin, cellulitis, local anesthesia, and occasionally crepitus. In the early stage of the disease, diagnosis can be difficult because intact skin covers the damaged fascial tissue. An incisional biopsy of the suspected area for frozen section diagnosis is essential.

In a series of 29 women aged 28 to 74 years (median 59 years) with necrotizing fasciitis of the vulva, 20 women were diabetic or obese and 15 had hypertension or peripheral vascular disease. Cultures of the wound yielded more than one organism in 79% of cases. The most commonly isolated organisms, in order of frequency, are Peptostreptococcus (14 patients), *Bacteroides fragilis* (12), *E. coli* (8), beta-hemolytic streptococci (8), Enterococcus (7 cases), and others. Many of the initial lesions were thought to be minor cellulites of the vulva. The importance of immediate diagnosis and radical surgical débridement is reflected by low survival rates of patients whose disease was not treated promptly. Eleven of 15 women who underwent operation more than 48 hours after presentation died.[184]

According to Stamenkovic and Lew,[182] the histologic criteria for necrotizing fasciitis include necrosis of superficial fascia and neutrophilic infiltration of the deep dermis and fascia (Fig. 4–44). Fibrinous thrombi and vasculitis of arteries and veins are often present (Fig. 4–45A and B). Bacterial organisms may be found in the necrotic tissue. In these cases, a correct diagnosis by frozen section led to an immediate radical resection of necrotic tissue, intense antibiotic therapy, and improved survival rates. Patients whose lesions did not meet the histologic criteria for necrotizing fasciitis had abscesses, and they survived. The mortality rate of patients with necrotizing fasciitis has remained high, ranging from 50% to 80%.[159,161]

Vulvar Vestibulitis Syndrome

Vulvar vestibulitis syndrome refers to a group of symptoms and findings confined to the vulvar vestibule, including: (1) severe pain on touch, (2) tenderness to pressure, and (3) erythema of varying degrees.[123] It affects women between 20 and 40 years of age. Other terms used include *hyperesthesia of the vulva, infection of the minor vestibular gland,*[210] and *focal vulvitis.*[146] The causes are usually multifactorial, including clinical or subclinical HPV infection, chronic candidal infection, recurrent bacterial vaginosis, altered vaginal pH, and local irritations, including those caused by iatrogenic agents.

Grossly, the vestibule appears erythematous, especially surrounding the openings of minor vestibular glands. Histologic examination of the excised vulvar vestibule reveals epithelial hyperplasia (Fig. 4–46A), nonspecific chronic inflammation with infiltrations of lymphocytes, plasma cells, and occasionally histiocytes (see Fig. 4–46B) This response is usually mild to moderate, tends to involve the periglandular and perivascular spaces, and spares the glandular tissue. The minor vestibular glands and ducts usually demonstrate squamous metaplasia and chronic inflammation (see Fig. 4–46C and D). Axe et al.[7] report the presence of ade-

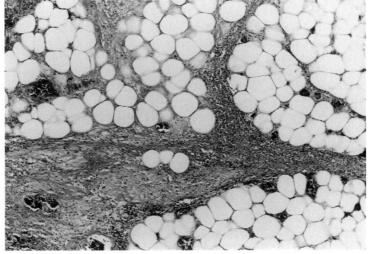

Figure 4–44. Necrotizing fasciitis. Fat necrosis and diffuse neutrophilic infiltrations in the fascia.

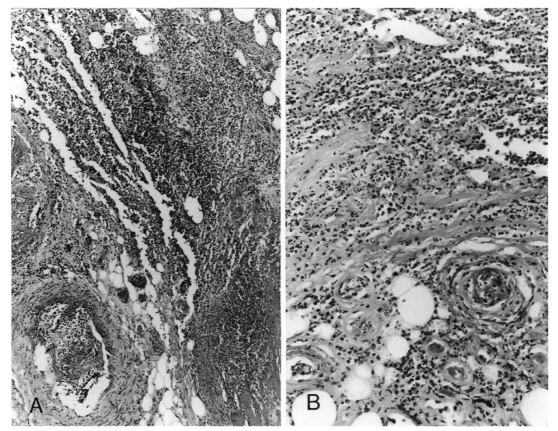

Figure 4–45. Necrotizing fasciitis. *A,* Large areas of necrosis and abscess formation. A vein in the left lower corner contains thrombi. *B,* Vasculitis of arterioles with fibrinoid necrosis and mural thrombi (right lower field).

noma of minor vestibular glands in 12 of 64 (19%) patients. The results of studies of infectious agents have been negative. In one study, 25% of the specimens revealed koilocytosis.[153] Immunologic study of the inflammatory cells suggests a T cell–mediated disease.[153]

In a case-control study, HPV DNA was amplified by PCR using liquid hybridization capture assay of the Digene SHARP signal system. Cells were collected from the opening of the Bartholin's glands with swabs. HPV DNA was found in 29.6% of cases and in 23.9% of controls with a relative risk of 1.4. The prevalence of HPV increased with severity of pain and decreased with increasing duration of pain. The prevalence was 37.5%, 29.6%, and 22.0% for pain duration of 3 to 6 months, 7 to 12 months, and 13 to 24 months, respectively. The *P* value, however, was not significant at 0.1. The authors concluded that because the relative risk did not reach 2.0, HPV was not related to vulvar vestibulitis.[134]

In the study by Prayson et al.,[150] 36 women from 19 to 53 (mean 31) years of age under-

went surgical excision of the vestibule. All had symptoms of vaginal dyspareunia and pain in the vestibular region. All had chronic inflammation, 31% mild, 58% moderate, and 11% severe, in the squamous mucosa and lamina propria. Epithelial changes included spongiosis in 89% of cases, hyperkeratosis and parakeratosis in 78%, hypergranulosis in 3%, and mucosal ulcer in 6%.[150]

Chadha et al.[29] reported 12 women (22 to 51 years; mean 28) who complained of dyspareunia and burning and painful sensation at introitus. Two women were positive for *Candida* in swab, and 1 had *Chlamydia* cervicitis. In punch biopsies, the most common histologic changes included dermal inflammatory infiltrates (100%), epithelial hyperplasia (83%), inflammatory infiltrates of epithelium and periglandular tissue (66%), hyperkeratosis and parakeratosis (50%), squamous metaplasia of vestibular glands (33%), hypergranulosis (16%), mild squamous dysplasia (16%), and spongiosis and koilocytosis (8% each). In the biopsies

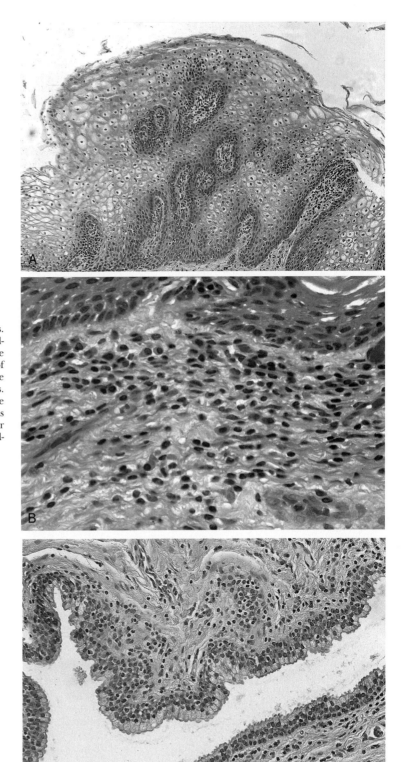

Figure 4–46. Vulvar vestibulitis. *A,* Thickening and hyperplasia of vulvar squamous mucosa. *B,* Moderate chronic inflammation consisting of lymphocytes and plasma cells. There is also proliferation of capillaries. *C,* Mild chronic inflammation in the periglandular tissue. *D,* Squamous metaplasia of the ducts of minor vestibular glands associated with moderate chronic inflammation.

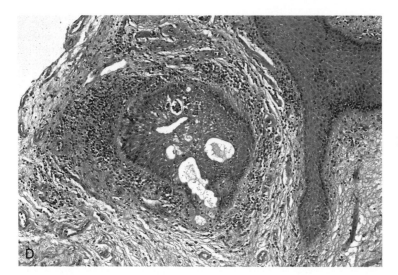

Figure 4–46. *Continued*

of 12 age-matched controls without symptoms and signs of vestibulitis, none of the aforementioned changes were present.[29]

The inflammatory cell infiltrates in the dermis were lymphocytes, plasma cells, mast cells, and monocytes. The severity of inflammation was mild in 5, moderate in 1, and severe in 6. Most lymphocytes are T cells. Plasma cells were positive for IgG in 75% of cases and positive for IgM and IgA in 50% of cases. HPV DNA 6, 11, 16, and 18 by in situ hybridization was negative.[29]

Treatment includes symptomatic relief. Vestibulectomy is reported to be helpful in most patients.[123]

Behçet's Syndrome

Behçet described the triad of genital and oral ulcers and uveitis in 1937.[13] Since then, additional clinical features have been recognized, including skin rash resembling erythema nodosum and erythema multiforme, arthritis, thrombophlebitis, ulcerative colitis, and central nervous system (CNS) disturbances. The International Study Group for Behçet's Disease recommends a new set of criteria that includes recurrent oral ulceration and any two of the following changes: (1) recurrent genital ulceration, (2) typical eye lesions, (3) typical skin lesions, and (4) a positive pathergy test.

The cause of this disease remains unclear. Viral origin and immune deficiency have been suggested. The genital ulcers typically occur on the vulva and rarely in the vagina and cervix. In males, scrotal ulcers are most common. They are painful, sometimes deep ulcerations ranging in size from a few millimeters to 1 cm or greater. The histologic changes are those of a nonspecific chronic inflammation with lymphoplasmacytic and histiocytic infiltrations and vascular changes. The latter are usually in the form of perivascular lymphocytic infiltration. Leukocytoclastic vasculitis occasionally occurs.[33] In severe cases, inflammation and necrosis involve skeletal muscle. Fibrosis, scarring, and destruction of the vulva may follow healing of the ulcers. Children with Behçet's syndrome tend to present initially with oral ulcers, and their disease seems to be milder than that in adults.[104]

The diagnosis of Behçet's syndrome is made by ruling out other ulcerative diseases of the vulva, especially herpes genitalis, syphilis, Crohn's disease, and Stevens-Johnson syndrome (erythema multiforme).

Vulvitis Granulomatosa and Crohn's Disease of the Vulva

Vulvitis granulomatosa is characterized by diffuse enlargement of the labia due to dermal edema, chronic noncaseating granulomatous reaction, and fibrosis. Lymphangiectasia is prominent in some cases. A similar disease can occur in the lip. Some patients with vulvitis granulomatosa proved to have Crohn's disease.[79]

Cutaneous manifestations of Crohn's disease are relatively common. It is estimated that 50% of patients with Crohn's disease have perineal or vulvar lesions in the form of ulcers, abscesses, and fistulae.[72] In severe cases, fenestration and scarring occur on the labia. These manifestations are usually associated with intestinal symptoms or with known Crohn's disease,[45,97] and, rarely, they may precede the intestinal disease.[72] In such cases, the differential diagnosis from other granulomatous inflammations of the vulva, such as hidradenitis suppurativa, actinomycosis, tuberculosis, and granulomatous venereal diseases, becomes important. A correct diagnosis is further hindered because only 50% of the cutaneous lesions of the perineum and vulva demonstrate characteristic noncaseating granulomatous inflammation.

Guerrieri et al.[79] identified 31 cases of Crohn's disease with vulvar involvement. Of these, 20 women had known Crohn's disease, including four who initially presented with vulvar granulomatosa. Eleven patients did not have known Crohn's disease, but eight had simultaneous vulvar/intestinal or extravulvar/perigenital lesions, which is part of Crohn's disease. Crohn's disease is located predominantly in the colon, rectum, and anus. Only 8 of 30 patients had involvement of ileum. A case has been reported in which squamous carcinoma in situ developed in the vulva following Crohn's disease.[151]

Malakoplakia

Malakoplakia is most frequently observed in relation to the urinary tract; less commonly, it involves the kidneys, testes, prostate, epididymis, colon, broad ligament, and inguinal areas. Its location may also be retroperitoneal.[173]

Several cases involving the cervix, vagina, and the Bartholin's glands have been reported.[53,103,145,204] Van der Walt et al.[201] described a firm, partially necrotic, ulcerated, nodular lesion measuring 2×6 cm that was located in the anterior vaginal wall and fornix. In another case, there was involvement of the lateral vaginal wall by three small yellow nodules. The disease was manifested by multiple yellow nodules of the vaginal mucosa, which mimicked leukoplakia in the case described by Lin et al.[117] Paquin et al.[145] described two cases involving Bartholin's gland, which presented with 3.8 and 5 cm cysts containing purulent exudate. Wahl[204] reported two cases involving the cervix: One woman presented with vaginal bleeding and a fungating mass occupying the posterior lip of the cervix; the other woman presented with vaginal discharge and a cervix that was "beefy red and bled easily."

Histopathologic examination reveals numerous histiocytes within the stroma, sometimes associated with plasma cells and neutrophils (Fig. 4–47). The cytoplasm of the histiocytes is vacuolated and poorly stained and, in some instances, contains Michaelis-Gutmann bodies (see Fig. 4–47). The bodies are round, basophilic, and concentrically laminated and measure up to 20 μ in diameter.[173] Other histiocytes contain granules of varying size that stain positive with PAS reagent. The Michaelis-Gutmann bodies have a positive staining reaction for iron with the Perls' Prussian blue method and contain

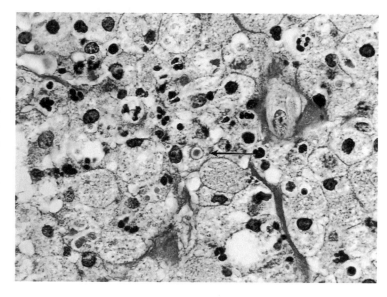

Figure 4–47. Malakoplakia of the cervix. There are numerous large histiocytes, a few inflammatory cells, and a single structure identified by the arrow, which has the features of a Michaelis-Gutmann body. (H&E, ×800; from Falcon-Escobedo R, et al. Acta Cytol 30:281, 1986; used by permission)

calcium as documented by the von Kossa technique. The PAS and Alcian blue stains reveal that the bodies contain neutral mucopolysaccharides. In two of the three reported cases,[117,173] coliform organisms were associated with the lesion. *E. coli* has been implicated in malakoplakia developing in other sites.

Tampon-Related Ulceration

Vaginal ulceration is uncommon. It may be the result of herpes simplex, syphilis, lymphogranuloma venereum, or granuloma inguinale. Vaginal ulceration may also be due to longstanding use of diaphragms and pessaries, medicated silicone rings, detergents, perfumed soaps, foreign bodies inserted into the vagina, or coital lacerations.

Ulceration associated with the use of vaginal tampons has been reported.[62] Of 14 cases in which ulceration was attributed to the use of tampons, seven involved the anterior vaginal fornix, six involved the right lateral vaginal wall or fornix, one involved the cervix, and one was located in the upper posterior vagina. The ulcers were observed in patients at a mean age of 23.8 years, with a range of 15 to 32 years.[10,91] Although microulceration may occur,[91] the ulcers evident on clinical inspection are often sharply demarcated with a red granular base.

Histopathologic examination reveals a separation of the superficial and intermediate layers of the epithelium, and in some cases a cleft occurs between the basal cell layer and the overlying squamous epithelium. The epithelium is lost in the ulcer base, which is infiltrated by neutrophils, lymphocytes, and plasma cells. In four of 10 cases, birefractile fibers were observed in the tissue (Fig. 4–48).[91] Granulation tissue was present in the ulcer base, and dilated vascular channels occurred in the adjacent stroma.

Colposcopic examination showed alterations in the vaginal mucosa associated with tampon usage,[62] including drying, disruption of the epithelial layers, and microulceration. This is believed to be related to altered fluid transfer resulting in impairment of the intercellular bridges and loss of cell cohesion.[62] The colposcopically observed changes, including microulceration, are reversible when the use of tampons is discontinued. Tampons containing superabsorbent materials are said to be more likely to produce transient alterations than are conventional tampons.

Toxic Shock Syndrome

Toxic shock syndrome (TSS) was first described in 1978.[203] A similar, if not identical, syndrome was reported in 1980.[170] This often life-threatening syndrome is usually observed in menstruating women.[128] It is characterized by a brief prodromal illness associated with fever, vomiting, diarrhea, headache, conjunctivitis, ir-

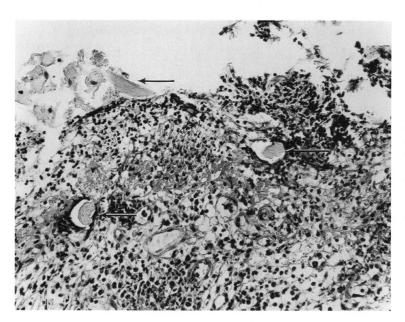

Figure 4–48. Base of tampon ulcer with transected fibers. When they are few in number, polarization may aid recognition. (From Jimerson SD, Becker JD. Obstet Gynecol 56:97, 1980; reprinted with permission from the American College of Obstetricians and Gynecologists.)

ritability, sore throat, myalgia, abdominal tenderness, and rash.[197] Hypotension, shock, respiratory distress, intravascular coagulation, thrombocytopenia, and renal failure may develop. During convalescence, desquamation and peeling of the skin may occur.[128] A simplified definition of TSS includes fever of greater than 102°F, diffuse macular erythema, hypotension, desquamation, involvement of three or more organ systems, and lack of another cause.[157]

Although a similar syndrome has been reported in males,[197] a majority of the currently documented cases occur in females, and many of these women are tampon users.[55] TSS is the result of *S. aureus* infection.[16] More than 90% of menstrually related cases are caused by *S. aureus* strains that produce TSS toxin-1 (TSST-1). Some nonmenstrual TSS is associated with staphylococcal enterotoxins, especially enterotoxins B and C.[157]

Although all types and brands of tampons were linked to TSS, users of "superabsorbent" tampons were particularly at risk. Following removal by the tampon manufacturers of certain chemical substances that enhance absorbency, the number of cases of menstrually related TSS has dramatically decreased since 1980.[157] Of the 179 cases of TSS detected in 1986 and 1987 in five states and one county, 85% involved girls and women, and the remaining 15% involved boys and men. Among the 152 females, TSS occurred during menstruation in 55%, 10% were users of barrier contraception, and 7% were postpartum cases. The other cases, including in both females and males, were caused by *S. aureus* infection from a wide range of body sites. Young women aged 15 to 19 years were at higher risk than were older women, and white females were at greater risk than were nonwhites. The incidence of menstrual TSS in 1991 was estimated at 1 to 3 per 100,000, and the fatality rate was about 2%.[157]

Although little information is available regarding the histopathologic changes, the observed findings suggest that it is toxin mediated.[1,42,193] One case included blister formation, subepidermal and marked interstitial edema, and widespread vasculitis, sometimes associated with platelet thrombi. Within the upper vagina, multiple elevated areas of brown discoloration occurred (Fig. 4–49). The epithelium was partially denuded and focally ulcerated (Fig. 4–50). Subacute vasculitis and perivasculitis were observed in the vagina and elsewhere.[1]

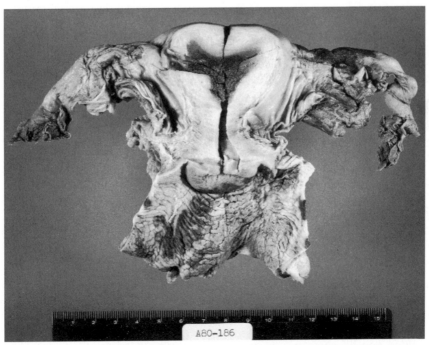

Figure 4–49. Toxic shock syndrome. Multiple areas of brownish discoloration caused by mucosal ulcerations are found in the vagina and cervix. Hemorrhage is noted in the uterus and fallopian tubes. (Courtesy of F.W. Abdul-Karim, M.D., Cleveland, Ohio.)

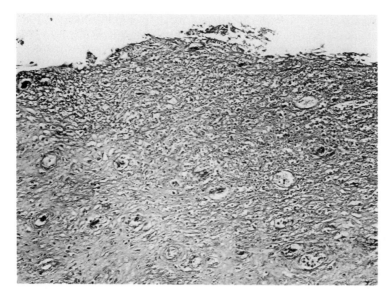

Figure 4–50. Toxic shock syndrome. Mucosal ulcers of the cervix and vagina with neutrophilic and fibrinous exudates. Some of the capillaries contain fibrin thrombi. (H&E, ×50; from Abdul-Karim FW, Lederman MM, Carter R, et al. Human Pathol 12:16, 1981; used by permission)

Potassium Permanganate Burns

It was believed at one time that the insertion of potassium permanganate tablets into the vagina would induce abortion. This misconception by the public allegedly originated on the east coast of the United States and spread westward. The practice resulted in severe vaginal changes. In 1945, McDonough[127] reported 65 cases from Boston, and in 1961 Hill and Thomas[87] described 83 cases from San Francisco.

The vaginal changes are well described by Gardner and Kaufman.[72] Many patients presented with an initial complaint of painless vaginal bleeding, which sometimes was severe enough to require transfusion. The changes were usually present in the upper third of the vagina. The cervix and vulva were less frequently involved. Multiple well-defined, deep ulcers were observed. Active arterial blood was sometimes observed coming from the ulcer base. The adjacent mucosa and ulcer base were covered with a dark brown or black eschar. The sequelae included necrosis in the posterior vaginal fornix with perforation into the cul-de-sac, vesicovaginal fistulas, and scar formation.

Foreign Bodies

Foreign bodies may be found in the vagina in childhood. The objects most often found include wax crayons, pencils, safety pins, hairpins, wads of paper, marbles, twigs, chewing gum, erasers, dried beans, and soap.[72] Sand box vaginitis has been described by Taylor.[191] Henderson and Scott[84] described 11 cases of toilet-tissue vaginitis. The response depends in part on what the foreign body is. Profuse malodorous vaginal discharge may result. Laceration, puncture, and bleeding occur with sharp objects.

Insertion of foreign bodies is less likely to produce significant trauma in the adult parous woman compared with the virgin.[72] Lacerations may result from the breakage of glass objects. Vaginal pessaries left in place for long periods of time may result in laceration.

Giant Cell Arteritis and Necrotizing Arteritis

Giant cell arteritis of small to medium-size arteries has been reported to occur in the ovary, fallopian tube, uterus, and cervix.[14] It typically involves postmenopausal women who may present with fatigue, anemia, fever, weight loss, or abdominal mass. Of the 11 patients reported in the literature, 6 had temporal arteritis, polymyalgia, or rheumatica.[14] In other patients, giant cell arteritis is localized to the female genital tract and associated with ovarian cysts, uterine leiomyomas, or endometrial carcinoma. Schneider[169] reported a case of giant cell arteritis of the cervix following radiotherapy for squamous cell carcinoma.

Histologically, the findings include fibrinoid necrosis of the endothelium and surrounding tissue, mural thrombi, and transmural granulomatous reaction with multinucleated giant cells. The latter involves the medial layer predominantly (Fig. 4–51). Occlusion of the lumen and fibrosis of the vessel wall may follow.

When giant cell arteritis is detected in the female genital tract, involvement of other body sites should be ruled out.[14] Women with symptoms or systemic disease usually require treatment.[14] In a review of the literature, Marrogi et al.[124] found that 11 of 17 women with giant cell arteritis of the female genital tract had symptoms and signs suggestive of systemic vasculitis.[124] Some patients are known to use antihypertensive, antibiotic, or antihistamine drugs.

Francke et al.[57] reported 11 cases of necrotizing arteritis of the polyarteritis-nodosa type involving the cervix. The arteritis was found in women 37 to 74 years of age, the majority of whom presented with menorrhagia, metrorrhagia, or postmenopausal bleeding. Necrotizing arteritis was an incidental finding in cervical biopsy and endometrial curettage for cervical dysplasia or endometrial carcinoma. It was limited to the cervix and isthmus in six women, and additional lesions were found in the uterine corpus or ovary in the remaining five women.

Fibrinous necrosis of the subintimal and medial layers were associated histologically with chronic inflammatory cells, eosinophils, and rare neutrophils in the muscular layer and adventitial layers (Fig. 4–52).

By immunohistochemical stains, 30% to 40% of inflammatory cells are macrophages found mainly in the vicinity of fibrinoid necrosis, 50% to 60% are T lymphocytes, and 0% to 10% are B lymphocytes.[57] Abu-Farsakh et al.[2] also found abundant T lymphocytes and histiocytes but very few B lymphocytes to suggest cell-mediated immune response.[2] Deposits of IgM were found in six specimens, but IgA was entirely negative. In view of the deposits of immune complexes, the authors raised the question of hypersensitivity reactions to drugs, such as antihypertensive agents, hormones, antibiotics, and analgesics.[57]

In a review of the literature, 90% to 100% of women with necrotizing arteritis had involvement of the cervix, and 5% to 10% had multifocal disease in the genital tract.[2,57] However, none had systemic vasculitis. The prognosis was favorable.

Necrotizing Granulomas and Changes Secondary to Prior Surgery

Necrotizing, palisading granulomas resembling rheumatoid nodules have been reported in the uterine cervix,[52] ovary,[85] uterus, and fallopian tube.[160] Although the cause is unknown, all patients had prior surgery to the affected area. Of the three cases involving the cervix, the surgery, including cervical biopsy, fractional curettage, and dilatation and curettage, was performed 3 weeks to 2 years before the diagnosis. One, in addition, had external radiation and intrauterine tandem and ovoids.

Histologically, the granulomas are well defined, round to oval in shape, and deep in the cervical stroma. A large central fibrinoid necrosis is surrounded by palisading epithelioid cells,

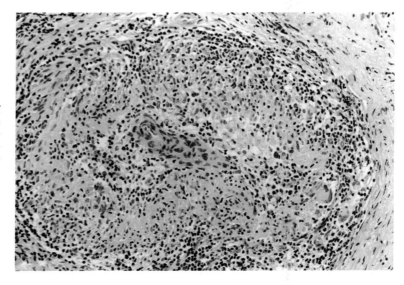

Figure 4–51. Giant cell arteritis of the cervix associated with recent conization. The media layer is involved by a granulomatous reaction. The lumen is almost completely occluded.

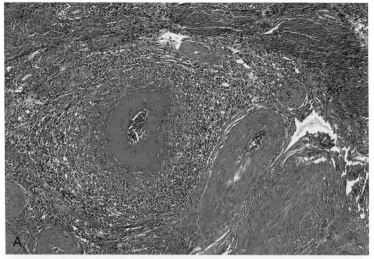

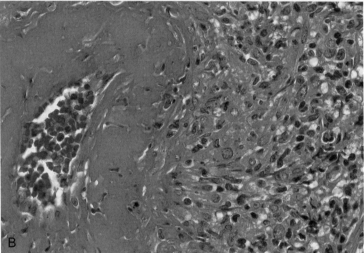

Figure 4–52. Necrotizing vasculitis. *A,* The artery undergoes fibrinoid necrosis of the vessel wall. There is heavy infiltration of inflammatory cells in the perivascular space. *B,* A higher magnification showing fibrinoid necrosis of the vessel wall and infiltrates of lymphocytes, plasma cells, and histiocytes.

Figure 4–53. Necrotizing granuloma of the cervix associated with recent conization. The central fibrinoid necrosis is surrounded by palisading epithelioid cells and multinucleated giant cells. The outer zone contains lymphocytes and fibrous tissue.

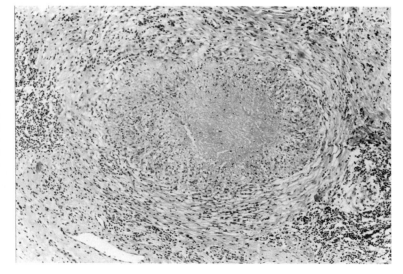

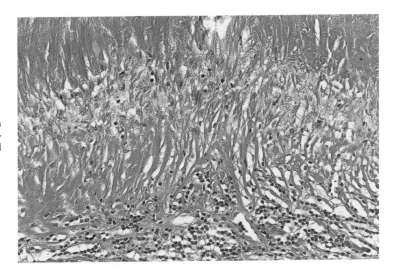

Figure 4–54. Palisading granuloma consisting of necrosis, elongated epithelioid cells, and lymphocytes and plasma cells.

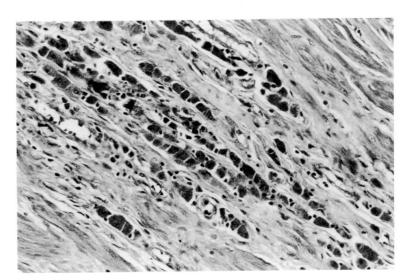

Figure 4–55. Granular cell reaction in the cervix following cesarean section. Granular cells are arranged cords.

occasional Langhans' giant cells, and an outer rim of lymphocytes and plasma cells (Figs. 4–53 and 4–54). Special stains fail to reveal acid-fast and fungal organisms. Clinical surveys rule out the possibility of tuberculosis, sarcoidosis, rheumatoid arthritis, and syphilis. Some authors[52] attribute these granulomas to prior surgery.

Other cervical changes related to prior cervical biopsy, cervical conization, cesarean section, or radiotherapy include localized accumulations of granular cells in the deep stroma of the cervix, which resemble those of granular cell tumor (Fig. 4–55). Sometimes, the cells have the appearance of foamy xanthomatous cells. Both granular and foamy cells react strongly with PAS stain. On the trichrome stain, however, the granular cytoplasm lacks the brilliantly reddish character typically seen in a granular cell tumor. This difference in staining reactions helps to differentiate reactive from neoplastic granular cells.

REFERENCES

1. Abdul-Karim FW, Lederman MM, Carter JB, et al. Toxic shock syndrome: Clinicopathologic findings in a fatal case. Human Pathol 12:16, 1981.
2. Abu-Farsakh H, Mody D, Brown RW, Truong LD. Isolated vasculitis involving the female genital tract: Clinicopathologic spectrum and phenotyping of inflammatory cells. Mod Pathol 7:610, 1994.
3. Alacoque B, Cloppet H, Dumontel C, et al. Histological immunofluorescent, and ultrastructural features of lymphogranuloma venereum: A case report. Br J Vener Dis 60:390, 1984.

4. Almicide JD, Oriel JD, Stannard LM. Characterization of the virus found in human genital warts. Microbiology 1:225, 1969.

5. Anders KH, Hall TL, Fu YS. Epidemiologic and histopathologic studies of female genital warts. In: Fenoglio CM, Wolff MW, Rilke F (eds). Progress in Surgical Pathology, vol 6. Philadelphia, Field and Wood, 1986, pp 33–47.

6. Andrews H, Acheson N, Huengsberg M, Radcliffe KW. The role of microscopy in the diagnosis of sexually transmitted infections in women. Genitourin Med 70:118, 1994.

7. Axe S, Parmley T, Woodruff JD, et al. Adenomas in minor vestibular glands. Obstet Gynecol 68:16, 1986.

8. Azar HA, Pham TD, Kurban AK. An electron microscopic study of syphilitic chancre. Arch Pathol 90:143, 1970.

9. Barrera-Ora JG, Smith KO, Melnick JL. Quantitation of papovavirus in human warts. J Natl Cancer Inst 29:583, 1962.

10. Barrett KF, Bledsoe S, Greer BE, et al. Tampon-induced vaginal or cervical ulceration. Am J Obstet Gynecol 127:332, 1977.

11. Bartlett JG, Onderdork AB, Drude E, et al. Quantitative bacteriology of the vaginal flora. J Infect Dis 136:271, 1977.

12. Becker TM, Larsen SA. Chancroid: Not just another tropical disease. Diagn Med 7:32, 1984.

13. Behçet H. Ober rezidivierende, aphthose, durch ein Virus Verursachte Geschwüre am Mund, am Auge und an den Genitalien. Dermatol Monatschr 105:1152, 1937.

14. Bell DA, Mondschein M, Scully RE. Giant cell arteritis of the female genital tract: A report of three cases. Am J Surg Pathol 10:696, 1986.

15. Bercovici B, Persky S, Rozansky R, et al. Mycoplasma (pleuropneumonia-like organisms) in vaginitis. Am J Obstet Gynecol 84:687, 1962.

16. Bergdoll MS, Crass B, Reiser RF, et al. A new staphylococcal enterotoxin, Enterotoxin F, associated with toxic-shock syndrome *Staphylococcus aureus* isolates. Lancet 1:1017, 1981.

17. Bergeron C, Ferenczy A, Richart RM, Guralnick M. Micropapillomatosis labialis appears unrelated to human papillomavirus. Obstet Gynecol 76:281, 1990.

18. Bergeron C, Ferenczy A, Shah KV, et al. Multicentric human papillomavirus infections of the female genital tract: Correlation of viral types with abnormal mitotic figures, colposcopic presentation, and location. Obstet Gynecol 69:736, 1987.

19. Bonar BE, Robson AS. Gynecologic aspects of leprosy. Obstet Gynecol 9:33, 1957.

20. Boxer RJ, Skinner DG. Condylomata acuminata and squamous cell carcinoma. Urology 9:72, 1977.

21. Brewer GE, Meleney FL. Progressive gangrenous infection of the skin and subcutaneous tissues, following operation for acute perforated appendicitis. Ann Surg 84:438, 1926.

22. Broker TR, Botchan M. Papillomaviruses: Retrospectives and prospectives. In: Botchan M, Grodzicker T, Sharp P (eds). Cancer Cells 4: DNA Tumor Viruses. Cold Spring Harbor, New York, Cold Spring Harbor Press, 1986, pp 17–36.

23. Brown ZA, Benedetti J, Ashley R, et al. Neonatal herpes simplex virus infection in relation to asymptomatic maternal infection at the time of labor. N Engl J Med 324:1247, 1991.

24. Brown ZA, Stenchever MA. Genital ulceration and in-

fectious mononucleosis: Report of a case. Am J Obstet Gynecol 127:673, 1977.

25. Brunham RC, Paavonen J, Stevens CE, et al. Mucopurulent cervicitis—the ignored counterpart in women of urethritis in men. N Engl J Med, 311:1, 1984.

26. Bylund DJ, Manfro JJ, Marsh WL Jr. Coccidioidomycosis of the female genital tract. Arch Pathol Lab Med 110:232, 1986.

27. Casas-Cordero M, Morin C, Roy M, et al. Origin of koilocyte in condylomata of the human cervix: Ultrastructural study. Acta Cytol 25:383, 1981.

28. Catlin BW. Gardnerella vaginalis: Characteristics, clinical considerations, and controversies. Clin Microbiol Rev 5:213, 1992.

29. Chadha S, Gianotten WL, Drogendijk AC, et al. Histopathologic features of vulvar vestibulitis. Int J Gynecol Pathol 17:7, 1998.

30. Chapman GB, Drusin LM, Todd JE. Fine structure of the human wart. Am J Pathol 42:619, 1963.

31. Chuang TY, Perry HO, Kurland LT, et al. Condyloma acuminatum in Rochester, Minn., 1950–1978. I: Epidemiology and clinical features. Arch Dermatol 120:469, 1984.

32. Chuang TY, Perry HO, Kurland LT, et al. Condyloma acuminatum in Rochester, Minn., 1950–1978. II: Anaplasias and unfavorable outcomes. Arch Dermatol 120:476, 1984.

33. Chun SI, Su WPD, Lee S. Histopathologic study of cutaneous lesions in Behçet's syndrome. J Dermatol 17:333, 1990.

34. Connors RC, Ackerman AB. Histologic pseudomalignancies of the skin. Arch Dermatol 112:1767, 1976.

35. Creddia T, Cappa F, Cilfi R, et al. Prevalence of nonspecific vaginitis and correlation with isolation of *Gardnerella vaginalis* in Italian outpatients. Euro J Epidemiol 5:529, 1989.

36. Criswell B, Ladwig CL, Gardner HL, et al. *Haemophilus vaginalis:* Vaginitis by inoculation from culture. Obstet Gynecol 33:195, 1969.

37. Crum CP, Fu YS, Levine RU, et al. Intraepithelial squamous lesions of the vulva: Biologic and histologic criteria for the distinction of condylomas from vulvar intraepithelial neoplasia. Am J Obstet Gynecol 144:77, 1982.

38. Crum CP, Ikenberg H, Richart RM, et al. Human papillomavirus type 16 and early cervical neoplasia. N Engl J Med 310:3812, 1984.

39. Crum CP, Liskow A, Petras P, et al. Vulvar intraepithelial neoplasia (severe atypia and carcinoma in situ). Cancer 54:1429, 1984.

40. Crum CP, Mitao M, Winkler B, et al. Localizing chlamydial infection in cervical biopsies with the immunoperoxidase technique. Int J Gynecol Pathol 3:191, 1984.

41. Csonka GW, Williams REO, Corse J. T-strain mycoplasma in nongonococcal urethritis. Lancet 1:1292, 1966.

42. Davis JP, Chesney PJ, Vergeront JM. Toxic-shock syndrome—epidemiology, pathogenesis, clinical findings and management. In: Medical Microbiology. London, Academic Press, 1984, pp 1–38.

43. De Deus JM, Focchi J, Stavale JN, De Lima GR. Histologic and biomolecular aspects of papillomatosis of the vulvar vestibule in relation to human papillomavirus. Obstet Gynecol 86:758, 1995.

44. Deppisch L. Cytomegalovirus inclusion body endo-

cervicitis: Significance of CMV inclusions in endocervical biopsies. Mt Sinai J Med 48:418, 1981.

45. Devroede G, Schlaeder G, Sanchez G, et al. Crohn's disease of the vulva. Am J Clin Pathol 63:348, 1975.

46. Doll W. Vorkommen von "Haemophilus vaginalis" bei unspezifischer vaginitis? Zentralbl Bakteriol 171:372, 1958.

47. Donne A. Animalcules observes dans les metieres purulentes et al produit des secretions des organes genitaux de l'homme et de la femme. Compt Rend Acad Sci (D) Paris 3:383, 1836.

48. Dorman SA, Danos LM, Caron BL, et al. Detection of *Chlamydia trachomatis* in Papanicolaou-stained cervical smears by an indirect immunoperoxidase method. Acta Cytol 29:665, 1985.

49. Dorman SA, Danos LM, Wilson DJ, et al. The detection of Chlamydia cervicitis by Papanicolaou staining and culture. Am J Clin Pathol 79:421, 1983.

50. Dunn AEG, Ogilvie MM. Intranuclear virus particles in human genital wart tissue: Observations of the ultrastructure of the epidermal layer. J Ultrastruct Res 22:282, 1968.

51. Durst M, Gissmann L, Ikenberg H, et al. A new type of papillomavirus DNA from a cervical carcinoma and its prevalence in cancer biopsies from different geographic regions. Proc Natl Acad Sci USA 80:3812, 1983.

52. Evans CS, Klein HZ, Goldman RL, et al. Necrobiotic granulomas of the uterine cervix. A probable postoperative reaction. Am J Surg Pathol 8:841, 1984.

53. Falcon-Escobedo R, Mora-Tiscareno A, Pueblitz-Peredo S. Malacoplakia of the uterine cervix: Histologic, cytologic and ultrastructural study of a case. Acta Cytol 30:281, 1986.

54. Fitzgerald DM, Hamit HF. The variable significance of condylomata acuminata. Ann Surg 179:328, 1974.

55. Follow-up on toxic-shock syndrome. United States Morbidity Mortality Weekly Report 29:297, 1980.

56. Forster GE, Cookey I, Munday PE, et al. Investigation into the value of Papanicolaou-stained cervical smears for the diagnosis of chlamydial cervical infections. J Clin Pathol 38:399, 1985.

57. Francke M, Mihaescu A, Chaubert P. Isolated necrotizing arteritis of the female genital tract: A clinicopathologic and immunohistochemical study of 11 cases. Int J Gynecol Pathol 17:193, 1998.

58. Friberg J. Genital mycoplasma infections. Am J Obstet Gynecol 132:573, 1978.

59. Friedrich EG Jr. Vulvar Disease. Philadelphia, W.B. Saunders, 1976.

60. Friedrich EG Jr. The vulvar vestibule. J Reprod Med 28:773, 1983.

61. Friedrich EG Jr. Vaginitis. Am J Obstet Gynecol 152:247, 1985.

62. Friedrich EG Jr, Siegesmund KA. Tampon-associated vaginal ulcerations. Obstet Gynecol 55:149, 1980.

63. Friedrich EG Jr, Wilkinson EF, Fu YS. Carcinoma in situ of the vulva: A continuing challenge. Am J Obstet Gynecol 136:830, 1980.

64. Fu YS, Braun L, Shah KV et al. Histologic, nuclear DNA, and human papillomavirus studies of cervical condylomas. Cancer 52:1705, 1983.

65. Fu YS, Sherman ME. The uterine cervix. Silverberg SG, DeLillis RA, Frable WJ (eds). In: Principles and Practice of Surgical Pathology and Cytopathology. Churchill Livingstone, New York, 1997, pp 2343–2409.

66. Fugelso PD. Herpes zoster affecting urination and defaecation. Br J Dermatol 89:285, 1973.

67. Gardner HL. Desquamative inflammatory vaginitis: A newly defined entity. Am J Obstet Gynecol 102:1102, 1968.

68. Gardner HL. Haemophilus vaginalis vaginitis after twenty-five years. Am J Obstet Gynecol 137:385, 1980.

69. Gardner HL, Dampeer TK, Dukes CD. The prevalence of vaginitis: A study in incidence. Am J Obstet Gynecol 73:1080, 1957.

70. Gardner HL, Dukes CD. Haemophilus vaginalis vaginitis. Ann NY Acad Sci 83:280, 1959.

71. Gardner HL, Feret P. Etiology of vaginitis emphysematosa. Am J Obstet Gynecol 88:680, 1964.

72. Gardner HL, Kaufman RH. Benign Diseases of the Vulva and Vagina, 2nd ed. Boston, Massachusetts, GK Hall, 1981.

73. Gissmann L, Wolnik L, Ikenberg H, et al. Human papillomavirus type 6 and 11 DNA sequences in genital and laryngeal papillomas and in some cervical cancers. Proc Natl Acad Sci USA 80:560, 1983.

74. Grabstold H, Swan L. Genito-urinary lesions in leprosy with special reference to the problems of atrophy of the testis. JAMA 149:1287, 1952.

75. Gray LA, Barnes ML. Vaginitis in women, diagnosis and treatment. Am J Obstet Gynecol 92:125, 1965.

76. Greenwood JR, Pickett MJ. Transfer of *Haemophilus vaginalis* (Gardner and Dukes) to a new genus, Gardnerella: *G. vaginalis* (Gardner and Dukes). Int J Syst Bacteriol 30:170, 1980.

77. Growdon WA, Fu YS, Lebherz TB, et al. Pruritic vulvar squamous papillomatosis—evidence for human papillomavirus etiology. Obstet Gynecol 66:564, 1985.

78. Growdon WA, Lebherz TB, Moore JG, et al. Granuloma inguinale in a white teenager—a diagnosis easily forgotten, poorly pursued. West J Med 143:105, 1985.

79. Guerrieri C, Ohlsson E, Ryden G, Westermark P. Vulvitis granulomatosa: A cryptogenic chronic inflammatory hypertrophy of vulvar labia related to cheilitis granulomatosa and Crohn's disease. Int J Gynecol Pathol 14:352, 1995.

80. Gueson ET, Lin CT, Emich JP. Dysplasia following podophyllin treatment of vulvar condylomata acuminata. J Reprod Med 6:159, 1971.

81. Gupta PK. Intrauterine contraceptive devices: Vaginal cytology, pathologic changes and clinical implications. Acta Cytol 26:571, 1982.

82. Gupta PK, Lee EF, Erozan YS, et al. Cytologic investigations in chlamydia infection. Acta Cytol 23:315, 1979.

83. Halpert R, Fruchter RG, Sedlis A, et al. Human papillomavirus and lower genital neoplasia in renal transplant patients. Obstet Gynecol 68:251, 1986.

84. Henderson PA, Scott RB. Foreign body vaginitis caused by toilet tissue. Am J Dis Child 111:529, 1966.

85. Herbold DR, Frable WJ, Kraus FT. Isolated noninfectious granulomas of the ovary. Int J Gynecol Pathol 2:380, 1984.

86. Hermann JE, Howard LV, Armstrong A, et al. Immunoassays for detection of *Neisseria gonorrhoeae* and *Chlamydia trachomatis* in samples from a single specimen (Abstract). International Society for Sexually Transmitted Diseases Research 5:76, 1983.

87. Hill EC, Thomas JM. Potassium permanganate ulcers of the vagina. Obstet Gynecol 18:747, 1961.

88. Hoehne O. *Trichomonas vaginalis* also Haufiger Erreger einer Typischen Colpitis Purulenta. Zentralbl Gynaekol 40:4, 1916.

89. Horowitz BJ, Edelstein SW, Lippman L. *Candida tropicalis* vulvovaginitis. Obstet Gynecol 66:229, 1985.

sponse to an unusual bacterium (mucoid *Escherichia coli*). Am J Clin Pathol 79:637, 1983.

187. Stumpf PG. Increasing occurrence of condylomata acuminata in premenarchal children. Obstet Gynecol 56:262, 1980.

188. Sullivan M, King LS. Effects of resin of podophyllin on normal skin, condylomata acuminata and verruca vulgaris. Arch Dermatol Syphilol 56:30, 1947.

189. Sutton GP, Smirz LR, Clark DH, et al. Group B streptococcal necrotizing fasciitis arising from an episiotomy. Obstet Gynecol 66:733, 1985.

190. Sykes JA, Miller JN, Kalan AF. *Treponema pallidum* within cells of a primary chancre from a human female. Br J Vener Dis 50:40, 1974.

191. Taylor ES. Essentials of Gynecology, 3rd ed. Philadelphia, Lea & Febiger, 1965.

192. Teokharov BA. Non-gonococcal infections of the female genitalia. Br J Vener Dis 45:334, 1969.

193. Thomas D, Withington PS. Toxic shock syndrome: A review of literature. Ann Coll Surg Engl 67:156, 1985.

194. Thomason JL, Gelbart SM, Scaglione NJ, et al. Vaginitis in reproductive-age women. Curr Opin in Obstet Gynecol 2:656, 1990.

195. Thompson SE, Washington AE. Epidemiology of sexually transmitted *Chlamydia trachomatis* infections. Epidemiol Rev 5:96, 1985.

196. Timonen S, Salo OP, Haapoja H. Vaginal mycoses. Acta Obstet Gynecol 45:232, 1966.

197. Toxic-shock syndrome: United States Morbidity Mortality Weekly Report 2–9:229, 1980.

198. Trussell RE. *Trichomonas vaginalis* and trichomoniasis. Springfield, Ill., Charles C Thomas, 1947.

199. Trussell RE, Plass ED. The pathogenicity and physiology of a pure culture of *Trichomonas vaginalis*. Am J Obstet Gynecol 40:883, 1940.

200. Van Coeverden de Groot HC. Amoebic vaginitis. S Afr Med J 37:246, 1963.

201. Van der Walt JJ, Marcus PB, DeWet JJ, et al. Malakoplakia of the vagina: First case report. S Afr Med J 47:1342, 1973.

202. Van Dyck E, Piot P. Laboratory techniques in the investigation of chancroid, lymphogranuloma venereum and donovanosis. Genitourin Med 68:130, 1992.

203. Wager GP. Toxic shock syndrome: A review. Am J Obstet Gynecol 146:93, 1983.

204. Wahl RW. Malacoplakia of the uterine cervix: Report of two cases. Acta Cytol 26:691, 1981.

205. Welch JM, Nayagam M, Parry G, et al. What is vestibular papillomatosis? A study of its prevalence, aetiology and natural history. Brit J Obstet Gynaecol 100:939, 1993.

206. Wilkin JK. Molluscum contagiosum venereum in a women's outpatient clinic: A venereally transmitted disease. Am J Obstet Gynecol 128:531, 1977.

207. Willcox RR. Importance of the so-called "other" sexually transmitted diseases. Br J Vener Dis 51:221, 1975.

208. Wilson B. Necrotizing fasciitis. Am J Surg 18:416, 1952.

209. Woodruff JD, Braun L, Cavalier R, et al. Immunologic identification of papilloma virus antigen in condylomatous tissue from the female genital tract. Obstet Gynecol 56:727, 1980.

210. Woodruff JD, Parmley TH. Infection of the minor vestibular gland. Obstet Gynecol 62:609, 1983.

211. Yen SSC, Reagan JW, Rosenthal MS. Herpes simplex infection in female genital tract. Obstet Gynecol 25:479, 1965.

212. Yllinen O. Genital Tuberculosis in Women: Clinical Experiences with 348 Proved Cases. Helsinki, Mercatorin Kirjapaino, 1960.

213. Youssef AF, Fayad MM, Shafeek MA. The diagnosis of genital bilharziasis by vaginal cytology. Am J Obstet Gynecol 83:710, 1962.

214. Youssef AF, Fayad MM, Shafeek MA. Bilharziasis of the cervix uteri. J Obstet Gynecol Br Comm 77:847, 1970.

215. Zinnemann K, Turner GC. The taxonomic position of "Haemophilus vaginalis" (*Corynebacterium vaginale*). J Pathol Bacteriol 85:213, 1963.

216. zur Hausen H, Gissmann L. Papillomaviruses. In: Klein G (ed). Viral Oncology. New York, Raven Press, 1980, p 433.

217. zur Hausen H. Viruses in human cancers. Science 254:1167, 1991.

5

DERMATOLOGIC DISEASES OF THE VULVA

Dermatologic disorders of the vulvar skin and mucosa can be divided into two large groups.

The first group includes specific, well-recognized dermatologic entities, which are similar to those occurring in the extragenital sites. After this group of dermatoses and infectious vulvitis are excluded, the second group includes a large number of other dermatoses and dermatitis affecting predominantly the vulvar region, including the perineum and perianal area. A major component of these diseases is the category of vulvar dystrophy, the classification of which has undergone several changes in the last 2 decades.

In the classification scheme of the International Society of Gynecological Pathologists, which was subsequently adopted by the International Society for the Study of Vulvar Diseases[39] and the World Health Organization (WHO),[46] vulvar dystrophies and other dermatoses are grouped under vulvar non-neoplastic epithelial disorders (NNED). NNED is listed under "Tumor-like Lesions and Non-neoplastic Disorders" in the WHO classification.[46] In this chapter, discussion begins with specific dermatoses, followed by vulvar non-neoplastic epithelial disorders and other dermatologic diseases.

The clinical and pathologic features of dermatologic diseases are modified by the unique environment of the vulva. The skin of the vulva differs notably from the remaining body surface by its moist, friction-prone, and bacteria-rich environment. This local condition predisposes the vulva to the development of certain dermatologic disorders. The clinical and pathologic manifestations of dermatoses may differ from those occurring elsewhere in the body because of the local factors. Clinical information can be useful in assessing vulvar skin

143

lesions. Some authors have strongly urged the use of dermatologic terminology for vulvar disorders.[26]

SPECIFIC DERMATOSES

Contact Dermatitis

Contact dermatitis of the vulva and vagina is an inflammatory response of the squamous epithelium to a variety of physical and chemical substances, causing either irritation or allergy. Most often, the suspect agents are used for hygienic or therapeutic purposes, such as deodorant spray, douche material, vaginal contraceptives, podophyllin, gentian violet, and 5-fluorouracil (5-FU) cream. Less frequently, the dermatitis is caused by contact with synthetic fibers, detergents, and corrosive chemicals such as concentrated acid and potassium permanganate (abortifacients).[11,17]

The extent of the skin changes depends on the nature, concentration, and duration of exposure to the causative agents as well as the allergic response of the patient. They vary from erythema and edema to vesiculation. In severe cases, bullae and ulcers develop. Histologically, intracellular and intercellular edema (spongiosis) of the squamous epithelium, dilated blood vessels, and edema of the dermis are conspicuous. Inflammatory infiltrations are usually present. Eosinophils may or may not be prominent. Although the histologic changes are not specific, the clinical history and the distribution of the lesions usually help in identifying the causative agent.

Seborrheic Dermatitis

Seborrheic dermatitis usually affects areas with a high concentration of sebaceous glands, such as the scalp, midportion of the face, and presternal and interscapular regions. The folds of the genital area, including the vulva and pubic and perianal areas, are particularly susceptible in obese women. The vulvar eruptions are yellowish-red and are covered by greasy scales. Because of the moisture and friction at these sites, the lesions are likely to have an eczematoid appearance.[17]

The histologic changes are nonspecific, and the diagnosis is made by finding the lesions elsewhere and by ruling out infectious agents, and especially fungal organisms. In the epidermis, acanthosis with elongation and clubbing of the rete pegs occurs. Spongiosis and parakeratosis are often observed and conspicuous. Usually a mild chronic inflammation exists in the dermis.

Psoriasis

Psoriasis is believed to have a hereditary tendency and affects both sexes at an early age. Although the etiology of psoriasis is unknown, an abnormal epidermal growth rate has been demonstrated. A shortened cell cycle time from the normal 8.5 to 9 days to 1.5 to 4 days in the psoriatic skin[49] suggests that a defect in the germinal layers of the epidermis causes a rapid turnover of cells.[17,54]

Vulvar psoriasis may be part of a generalized process or may be localized, involving especially the outer aspects of the labia majora and the genitocrural areas. Other parts of the body most often affected include the scalp, the skin behind the ear, the extensor aspects of the extremity, the nails, and the torso.

The eruptions have sharply defined margins and dull red surfaces covered by fine silvery scales. Removal of these scales often results in punctate bleeding (Auspitz's sign). This is less apparent, however, in the vulvar area because of minimal scaling. Rubbing and scratching may form new lesions (Koebner's phenomenon).

Characteristic histologic features include parakeratosis, lack of granular layer, thinning of the suprapapillary portions of the stratum malpighii, and elongation of the rete pegs (Fig. 5–1). Another typical feature is the accumulation of neutrophils in the stratum corneum, the so-called Munro microabscesses. When abscesses are grossly visible and conspicuous, the process is designated as pustular psoriasis. The papillary dermis is edematous, and the capillaries are dilated and tortuous. The clinical course is variable; some psoriasis undergo remission, whereas others persist locally or progress to chronic and generalized disease.[27] In chronic psoriasis, the epidermis is markedly parakeratotic and hyperplastic. Neutrophilic infiltrates are rare or absent.

Edwards and Hansen[9] reported a 39-year-old with Reiter's syndrome that was associated with pustular psoriasis of the vulva, cervix, hands, and feet, along with conjunctivitis.

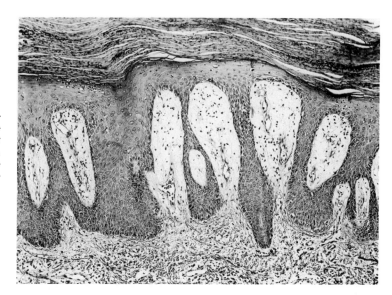

Figure 5–1. Psoriasis. The characteristic changes include marked parakeratosis, thinning of the suprapapillary plate, and elongation of the rete pegs. In the papillary dermis, edema, tortuous capillary, and minimal lymphocytic infiltration are present.

Lichen Planus

Lichen planus is the most common form of desquamative and erosive dermatosis often associated with similar disease in the vagina.[8] It is a chronic inflammatory disease of the skin and mucous membrane (especially of the oral cavity) of unknown cause.[2,10] Most cases occur after the age of 30 years, and women are affected more often than are men. It usually involves the flexor surfaces of the extremity. On the vulva, it appears as well-defined, slightly raised white plaques or interlacing discrete or confluent lines on the labia majora, vestibule, or inner labia mi-

nora. Severe pruritus and scratching cause secondary changes that mimic hypertrophic or atrophic dystrophy. Rarely, lichen planus presents as erosive and desquamative lesions of the gingiva, vagina, and vulva.[31,36]

The histologic changes are characterized by parakeratosis, hyperkeratosis, and wedge-shaped hypergranulosis (Fig. 5–2). Acanthosis manifests as irregular elongation of the rete pegs, with a saw-tooth appearance. Some of the rete pegs have pointed ends. A band-like lymphocytic infiltration immediately beneath the epidermis is characteristic (see Fig. 5–2). When the inflammatory cells extend into the epidermis, the basal

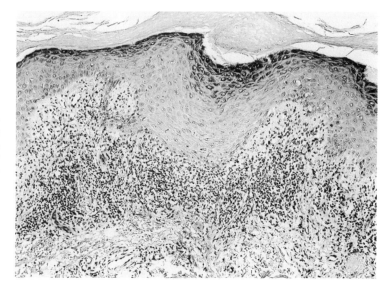

Figure 5–2. Lichen planus. Hyperplastic epidermis demonstrates wedge-shaped hypergranulosis. A band-like, dense, lymphohistiocytic infiltration occurs in the upper dermis.

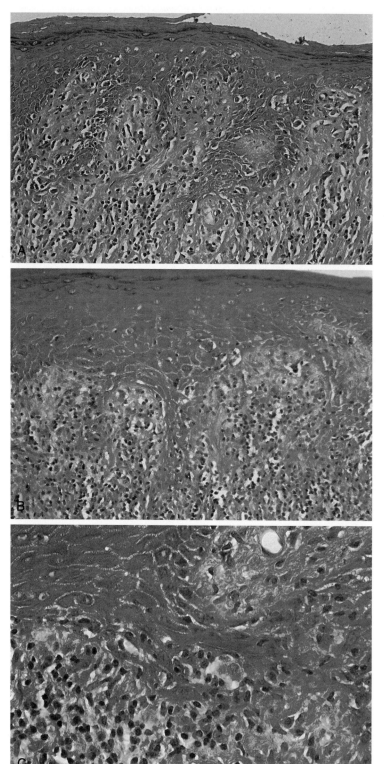

Figure 5–3. Lichen planus. *A,* Elongated rete pegs have a saw-tooth appearance and pointed ends. Scattered degenerated keratinocytes (cytoid bodies) occur in the parabasal layers. Melanophages are mixed with chronic inflammatory cells. *B,* Inflammatory cells obscure the basal cell layer. *C,* Degenerated basal cell with vacuolated cytoplasm are mixed with chronic inflammatory cells.

cell layer becomes obscured (Fig. 5–3). Cytoid bodies of degenerated keratinocytes and dyskeratotic cells occur in the epidermis or the superficial dermis (see Fig. 5–3).[16]

The clinical course of lichen planus is variable. It may be localized to the mucous membrane or the skin or be generalized. Spontaneous regression may be followed by severe exacerbations. Hyperpigmentation usually occurs after resolution.

Bullous Dermatoses

Among the various bullous diseases of the skin, pemphigus, familial benign chronic pemphigus (Hailey-Hailey disease), bullous pemphigoid, benign mucous membrane pemphigoid (cicatricial pemphigoid), juvenile dermatitis herpetiformis (juvenile pemphigoid), and Stevens-Johnson syndrome have predilection for the genital areas.[38] The bullae are intraepidermal in pemphigus vulgaris and its variants. Subepidermal bullae are common in dermatitis herpetiformis, bullous erythema multiforme, and bullous pemphigoid.

Pemphigus

Pemphigus vulgaris, the most common form of pemphigus, occurs most often during the fifth to the eighth decade of life. It usually starts with lesions in the oral cavity, the scalp, and the upper chest and back. In about 50% of women, the disease involves the vulva, vagina, or cervix;

lesions elsewhere on the skin or mucous membrane may be absent. The blisters are flaccid and easily ruptured, leaving a painful, oozing, erythematous, denuded base. The surrounding mucosa or skin has a normal appearance.

Biopsy samples should be taken from the edge of the lesions to reveal the characteristic intraepidermal bullae. In pemphigus vulgaris and pemphigus vegetans, the bullae are located in the suprabasal position (Fig. 5–4), whereas in pemphigus foliaceus and pemphigus erythematosus, they are subcorneal. The bullae contain isolated or loosely aggregated acantholytic cells in which the intercellular bridges (desmosomes) are lost or are not apparent. The epidermis overlying the bullae is usually intact. At the bases of the bullae are upward growths of papillae lined by a few layers of cells (Fig. 5–5). The suprabasal separations often affect the adnexal structures. Scrapings of the lesion often contain degenerated acantholytic cells (as shown by Tzanck test) or regenerating cells with active nuclear features simulating malignant cells.[28]

Immunofluorescent studies are helpful in establishing the diagnosis. Using an indirect immunofluorescent technique, antibodies to intercellular antigens can be detected in the epidermis of approximately 80% of patients with active pemphigus. They are rarely found in other conditions. When direct immunofluorescent techniques are applied to fresh skin biopsies, 90% of patients with active pemphigus are shown to have deposits of IgG and/or C3 in the intercellular spaces of the epidermis.

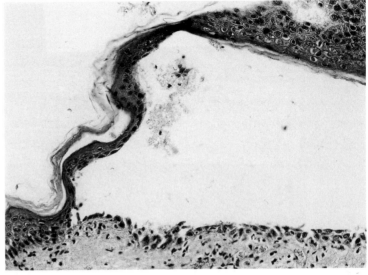

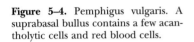

Figure 5–4. Pemphigus vulgaris. A suprabasal bullus contains a few acantholytic cells and red blood cells.

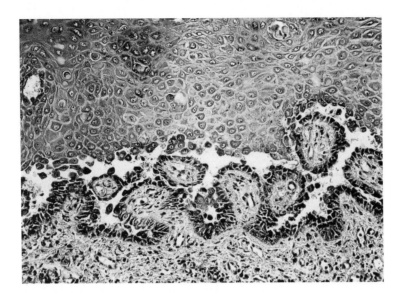

Figure 5–5. Pemphigus vulgaris. The epidermis overlying the bullae is relatively intact. The papillae at the base of the bullae are covered by basal cells.

Such deposits are found in less than 5% of patients with other bullous lesions.[30]

Familial Benign Chronic Pemphigus

Familial benign chronic pemphigus (Hailey-Hailey disease) is a rare, chronic, benign, recurrent, vesiculobullous eruption that is transmitted by a dominant gene. The lesions start to appear in adolescence and tend to involve the neck, axilla, and genitocrural areas as vesicles that become flaccid bullae, rupture, and form crusts.[18] The changes are characterized by bullae in a suprabasal position. The acantholysis is more extensive than the pemphigus vulgaris and affects the epidermis above the bullae. The acantholytic cells in the stratum malpighii are round and

have a homogenized cytoplasm, suggesting premature keratinization and occasionally resembling the corps ronds seen in Darier's disease (Fig. 5–6). The base of the bullae is similar to that seen in pemphigus vulgaris. Unlike pemphigus, however, Hailey-Hailey disease does not involve the adnexal structures of the mucous membrane. The acantholysis in Hailey-Hailey disease rarely progresses to form large bullae but involves most layers of the epidermis.

Hailey-Hailey disease shares certain histologic features with Darier's disease. Darier's disease (keratosis follicularis), transmitted by an autosomal dominant gene, most commonly affects the skin of the face, trunk, and extremities. It is characterized by suprabasal acantholysis and the formation of dyskeratotic cells

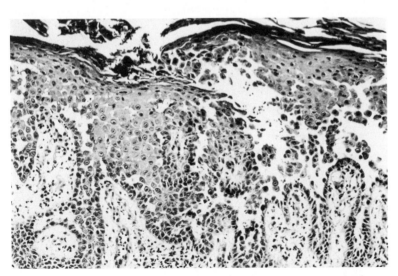

Figure 5–6. Familial benign chronic pemphigus. The epidermis overlying the bullae has undergone severe acantholysis. Some of the acantholytic cells have the appearance of corps ronds.

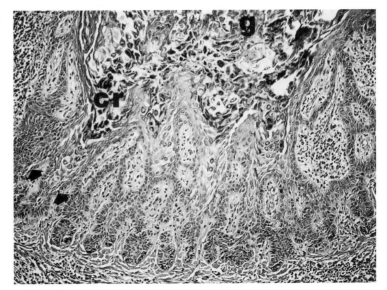

Figure 5–7. Darier's disease is characterized by minimal suprabasal clefts (arrows). Above the clefts, the dyskeratotic, acantholytic cells in the granular and superficial layers have the appearance of corps ronds (cr). Acantholytic parakeratotic cells on the surface are sometimes referred to as grain (g).

(corps ronds) in the upper stratum malpighii, and especially in the granular layer (Fig. 5–7). In addition, the suprabasal separation is often small and slit-like in the form of lacunae rather than bullae. The vulva and vagina may be affected by brownish-crusted papules. The hyperkeratosis and papillomatosis cause the formation of keratotic plugs. Thus, the term *keratosis follicularis* was designated.

Warty Dyskeratoma

Although histologically indistinguishable from Darier's disease, the lesions of warty dyskeratoma or isolated follicular dyskeratosis occur singly in the sun-exposed areas of the skin. No hereditary tendency has been detected. Such a lesion has been reported on the labia majora as an isolated, sharply defined, keratotic nodule measuring a few millimeters.[7] Typically, suprabasal acantholysis involves a cup-shaped keratotic plug. Acantholytic cells intermingled with dyskeratotic cells are found above the regenerating basal cells (Fig. 5–8). Vulvar warty dyskeratoma can be distinguished from viral vesicles, especially herpes, by the lack of nuclear inclusion, multinucleation, and "ground-glass" nuclei. In squamous cell carcinomas, acantholysis occasionally can be prominent, producing a pseudoglandular pattern. Such tumors can be differentiated from benign acantholytic lesions by their confluent or infiltrative

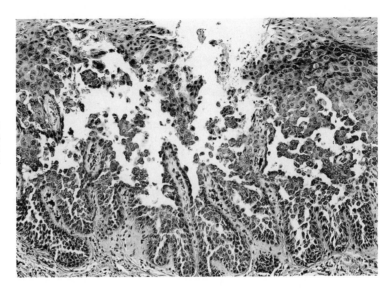

Figure 5–8. Warty dyskeratoma of the vulva presents as a small nodule. This cup-shaped lesion has suprabasal separations, marked acantholysis, and corps ronds in the superficial layers.

growth and nuclear atypism as well as increased mitotic activity of squamous cells.

Pestereli et al.[37] reported a case of multiple papular acantholytic dyskeratotic lesion. This lesion is histologically identical to that of warty dyskeratoma, except that it involves multiple areas of both right and left labia majora. In contrast to Darier's disease and Hailey-Hailey disease, this disorder does not occur elsewhere in the body and has no familiar tendency. In contrast to pemphigus vulgaris, acantholytic dyskeratotic lesions are small and appear in the form of a minor separation in the suprabasal layer.

Bullous Pemphigoid

Bullous pemphigoid occurs in the sixth to eighth decades of life and involves the flexural surfaces of the body, such as the groin and axilla, or of the extremities. Oral lesions occur in 30% of cases. The vaginal mucosa is rarely involved. Involvement of the vulva usually results from extension of the adjacent groin lesions and manifests as subepidermal bullae in an irregular, erythematous base. Within the bullae and dermis, there is an infiltration of neutrophils and eosinophils (Fig. 5–9). Acantholytic cells are absent in the bullae. The development of vulvar pemphigoid secondary to drug hypersensitivity to alpha-adrenergic receptor–stimulating and beta-adrenergic receptor–blocking agents (nadolol [Corgard]) has been reported.[51]

Indirect immunofluorescent study demonstrates circulating antibodies directed to the basement membrane in 70% to 80% of patients with active disease. Direct immunofluorescent studies reveal linear deposits of IgG, IgM, and/or complements at the basement membrane in 90% of cases.[30] Similar deposits are also found in cicatrizing pemphigoid, herpes infection, and systemic lupus erythematosus. The clinical course is chronic and usually benign.

Benign Mucous Membrane Pemphigoid (Cicatricial Pemphigoid)

This bullous disease primarily involves the mucous membrane and has a tendency to heal with scarring. Vulvar disease affects women between 50 and 70 years of age. The involved vaginal or urethral orifice may become stenosed. The initial lesions are small tense bullae that become chronic superficial erosions. The healing process is slow and often results in scarring. Pruritus, loss of the labia minora, and scar formation on the clitoris may simulate lichen sclerosus.

The histologic appearance of the lesion is similar to that of bullous pemphigoid. The subepidermal bulla is devoid of acantholysis. A dermal eosinophilic infiltration and fibrosis may be present. Immunofluorescent studies reveal linear deposits of C3, IgG, and, infrequently, IgM and IgA in the basement membrane.

Erythema Multiforme

The severe form of erythema multiforme, the Stevens-Johnson syndrome, involves the conjunctiva and the mucosal surfaces of the lips. The vagina, anus, and nose are occasionally affected. The lesions change from erythematous macules to frank bullae. Subepidermal separa-

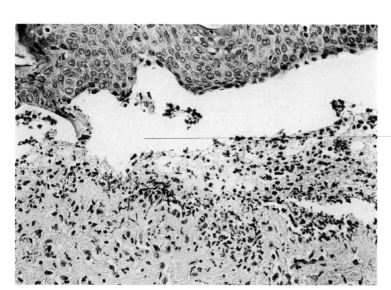

Figure 5–9. Bullous pemphigoid. The bullus is subepidermal and contains neutrophils and fibrin. Infiltration of neutrophils and eosinophils is seen in the upper dermis.

tion is associated with basal cell degeneration. The florid lesions exhibit necrosis of the epidermis and intense inflammatory response in the dermis. Marquette and colleagues[32] report a woman with Stevens-Johnson syndrome involving the vulva and lower vagina. After healing, the vulvar vestibule was covered by a tubal-type glandular epithelium resembling vaginal adenosis. Wilson and Malinak[56] reported sequelae that simulate endometriosis.

Dermatitis Herpetiformis

This chronic, pruritic papulovesicular lesion involves the elbows, knees, scalp, and buttocks. The vulva is rarely affected. Histologically, the subepidermal bullae are associated with perivascular infiltration of lymphocytes, eosinophils, and neutrophils. The presence of IgA at the dermal-epidermal junction by immunofluorescent study is distinctive for this disease.[30]

VULVAR NON-NEOPLASTIC EPITHELIAL DISORDERS

Vulvar Dystrophy

The term *dystrophy of the vulva* was first introduced by Jeffcoate[22] to designate a spectrum of chronic, often pruritic, skin changes with abnormal epithelial growth. Previously, such lesions were designated as leukoplakia vulvae, leukoplakia vulvitis, lichen sclerosus et atrophicus, kraurosis vulvae, primary atrophy, sclerotic dermatosis, atrophic and hypertrophic vulvitis, and neurodermatitis. The term *leukoplakia* was used by Schwimmer[44] to describe a white lesion of the tongue and oral cavity. Later, it was applied clinically to similar changes of the mucous membrane elsewhere in the body. The term *leukoplakia* subsequently was used in different connotations, including a premalignant condition.

The vulvar changes in dystrophy may be white, red, or partly white and red. The epithelium may be hyperplastic or atrophic. The changes may be localized or diffuse. Jeffcoate[22] believes that these changes, despite their varying appearance, do not represent separate entities but rather reactions of the vulvar skin to a variety of systemic or local disorders. Among those identified are achlorhydria, vitamin deficiency, monilial vulvitis, fungus infections in other parts of the body (especially the hands and feet), glucosuria, and allergy.[22] The special environment of the vulva, with its moisture, warmth, and frequent friction, seems to enhance the development of dystrophies.

Whimster[55] observed that when the vulvar "lichen sclerosus and leukoplakia" was grafted to the leg, the lesions cleared spontaneously. The normal skin removed from the leg and transplanted to the vulva developed dystrophy. Because of the confusion of the terminology in the past and the lack of characteristic clinical and pathologic features for the various terms used, the term *chronic vulvar dystrophies* was proposed for "any chronic skin change of uncertain etiology which affects the vulva."[22]

Gardner and Kaufman[17] subdivided dystrophies into three major categories on the basis of histopathologic findings: (1) hypertrophic dystrophies, (2) atrophic dystrophies (lichen sclerosus et atrophicus), and (3) mixed dystrophies (lichen sclerosus with epithelial hyperplasia). Recognizing the importance of cellular atypia, Woodruff and Baens[57] had earlier subdivided hyperplastic vulvitis into grades I, II, and III. Lesions that exhibit no atypia are classified as grade I, those with squamous carcinoma in situ are designated as grade III, and those demonstrating less severe atypia than that of grade III are classified as grade II.

With minor modification of the classification proposed by Kaufman and associates,[23] in 1974 the International Society for the Study of Vulvar Disease[12] recommended the following histologic classification for vulvar dystrophies:

I. Hyperplastic dystrophy, with or without atypia
II. Lichen sclerosus
III. Mixed dystrophy (lichen sclerosus with foci of epithelial hyperplasia), with or without atypia

Most of the hyperplastic dystrophies are believed to represent a form of lichen simplex chronicus or neurodermatitis and were, in the past, called leukoplakias.[17] Lichen sclerosus has previously been referred to as kraurosis vulvae or primary atrophy of the vulva. The word *atrophicus* was deleted, because the epithelium in lichen sclerosus is metabolically active.[13,58]

In 1990, the Nomenclature Committee for the International Society of Gynecological Pathologists[39] proposed the terms of nonneoplastic epithelial disorders (NNED) of skin and mucosa to include:

I. Lichen sclerosus
II. Squamous cell hyperplasia, not otherwise specified (NOS)
III. Other dermatoses

The last section includes specific dermatoses with distinct clinicopathologic features or known etiologic agents. Although the term *lichen sclerosus* is retained, a generic term, *squamous cell hyperplasia*, was selected to reflect the nonspecific histologic changes seen in hyperplastic dystrophy. When the epithelial disorders comprise more than one type, all abnormalities are indicated in the diagnosis, for example, when lichen sclerosus coexists with squamous cell hyperplasia.

In addition, vulvar lesions with atypia or dysplasia are excluded from this category of NNED. Atypical and dysplastic vulvar lesions are classified under the category of vulvar intraepithelial neoplasia (VIN). When lesions of NNED coexist with VIN, the pathologic report should indicate all applicable diagnoses.[29]

Lichen Sclerosus

Lichen sclerosus occurs most often in postmenopausal women, but children and young women may be affected. Compared with hyperplastic dystrophy, lichen sclerosus has distinct gross and microscopic changes that identify it as a separate entity. This variant constitutes about 38% of all dystrophies.[12,23]

Clinical Features

In the early stage, lichen sclerosus appears as multiple small white discolorations of the skin. Later, well-formed plaques develop through coalescence. Further progression produces a typical atrophic, smooth, shiny, parchment-like or "cigarette paper" appearance (Fig. 5–10). The affected labia minora and clitoris may be completely obliterated. Lichen sclerosus may affect any or all areas of the vulva and may extend to the perineum and thigh. The involvement of the perianal skin results in a figure-eight or keyhole configuration.

Of the 107 women studied by Hart and colleagues,[20] 87% had multifocal lesions, and 81% had bilateral lesions. The sites of involvement are the labia minora (68%), the labia majora (60%), the clitoris (51%), the perineum (40%), and the posterior fourchette (36%). Of these, 3% to 5% have extragenital lesions on the neck, trunk, or extremities.[17,20] In males, similar changes, known as balanitis xerotica obliterans, can involve the foreskin and glans penis.

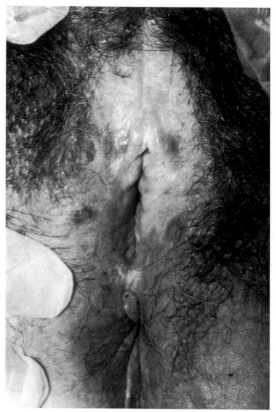

Figure 5–10. Lichen sclerosus. The affected area is symmetrical and has a thin, shiny, atrophic appearance. Extreme atrophy leads to loss of labia minora and a contracted introitus. Several ulcerations result from itching, scratching, and bullous formation. (Courtesy of William Growdon, M.D., Santa Monica-UCLA Medical Center.)

Microscopic Features

Histologically, the epidermis may be normal in thickness or even slightly hyperplastic in the early stage. The dermis is edematous, and fibrous stroma undergoes mild hyalinization and sclerosis (Fig. 5–11A). By elastic stain, the elastic fibers are shown to be decreased in number. The degree of chronic inflammation is mild. The rete pegs are infiltrated by lymphocytes, resulting in so-called epidermotropism (see Fig. 5–11B).

In the advanced stage, the changes are characteristic. The epithelium is thin and atrophic with flattened rete pegs (Fig. 5–12). Focal hydropic degeneration and edema of the basal layer sometimes result in separation of the basal layer from the basement membrane (subepidermal bullae). Hyperkeratosis and a decreased number of melanocytes are common and are responsible for the whitish appearance. Follic-

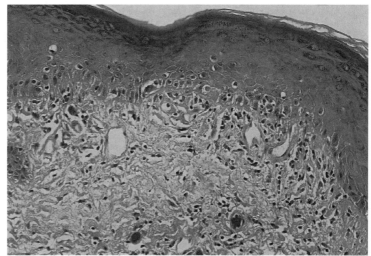

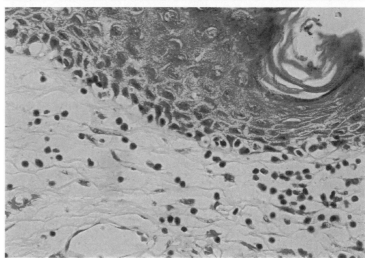

Figure 5–11. Lichen sclerosus in the early stage. *A,* The epidermis is normal in thickness. Hyperkeratosis is evident. Edema, early fibrosis, and hyalinization occur in the papillary and reticular dermis. Chronic inflammation is mild and capillaries are dilated. *B,* Infiltration of lymphocytes in the basal and parabasal layers, so-called epidermotropism. Marked edema is seen in the superficial dermis.

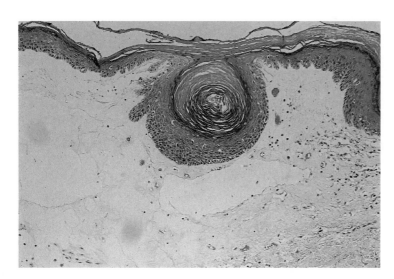

Figure 5–12. Lichen sclerosus in late stage. Atrophy and hyperkeratosis of epidermis with plugging of adnexal ostium is evident.

153

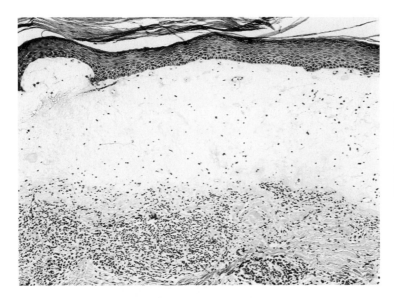

Figure 5–13. Lichen sclerosus. The presence of three distinct zones is diagnostic: (1) hyperkeratosis and atrophy of epidermis with loss of rete pegs, (2) homogenized, acellular dermis, and (3) a band-like infiltration of lymphohistiocytes and plasma cells in the lower dermis.

ular plugging and parakeratosis may also be present.

Immediately beneath the epidermis is hyalinized collagenous tissue with loss of normal collagen and elastic fibers. Below this zone, in the mid-dermis, is a band of chronic inflammatory cells, usually lymphocytes and a few plasma cells (Fig. 5–13).

In the early stage, marked ectasia of the arterioles and capillaries of the papillary dermis is evident. However, with increasing homogenization of the perivascular collagen, the lumens become obliterated (Fig. 5–14). The nerve fibers in the upper dermis undergo degeneration and fragmentation.

In the early stage, lichen sclerosus can be difficult to differentiate from lichen planus, because both lesions have band-like infiltrates of chronic inflammatory cells. Dermal sclerosis and the hyalinization characteristic of lichen sclerosus may be limited. In a comparative study, features indicating early lichen sclerosus include a psoriasiform lichenoid pattern, epidermatropism (lymphocytes in the basal and parabasal layers), decreased elastic fibers as shown by elastic stain, basement membrane thickening, and epidermal atrophy.[16] Basal squamatization, wedge-shaped hypergranulosis, many cytoid bodies, and pointed rete peg ridges, on the other hand, are more typical of

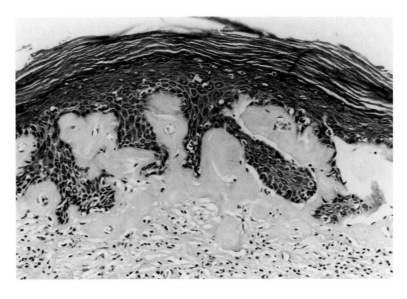

Figure 5–14. Lichen sclerosus. A higher magnification reveals the hyalinized upper dermis, obliterated capillaries, and a bullous formation on the right side of the figure.

lichen planus. Both lesions contain varying numbers of eosinophils and T lymphocytes with expression of CD3, CD8, and OPD4 and TIA-1 without distinct differences.[16]

Carlson et al.[4] compared the histologic features of lichen sclerosus of anogenital sites (121 cases) to those of extragenital sites (20 cases) and found some differences between them. The authors state, "Many of these patients and numerous others also had evidence of superimposed lichen simplex chronicus/lichenification identified by an increased granular layer and an expanded stratum corneum showing a compact orthokeratotic pattern in conjunction with acanthotic (thickening of the spinous layer) or irregular epidermal hyperplasia (elongated rete ridges of variable length with either pointed or rounded ends); these changes of lichenification were found in approximately 75% of vulvar lichen sclerosus cases."[4] In other words, many women with vulvar lichen sclerosus have areas of squamous cell hyperplasia in the form of mixed dystrophy by earlier terminology. In this study, less than 10% of vulvar lichen sclerosus lesions had VIN or human papillomavirus (HPV) changes.[4]

Extragenital lichen sclerosus lesions were more often asymptomatic, more atrophic areas.[4] For the diagnosis of lichen sclerosus, the authors propose the minimal criterion of the presence of a vacuolar interface reaction with a band of sclerosis and lymphocytic infiltration. The prominence of spongiosis and eosinophils in lichen sclerosus resembles allergic contact hypersensitivity.[4]

Squamous Cell Hyperplasia, Not Otherwise Specified

This disorder occurs throughout the reproductive and postmenopausal years and most frequently involves the hood of the clitoris, the labia majora, the interlabial sulci, the outer surface of the labia minora, and the posterior commissure.[10] The adjacent skin of the thighs may be affected. Many lesions are bilateral and symmetrical. They may be localized, elevated, either well or poorly defined, or diffuse (Fig. 5–15). The color depends on the extent of the hyperkeratosis. It is dusky red if hyperkeratosis is minimal, and white if hyperkeratosis is marked. Both red and white areas may be seen in different sites of the same patient. Lichenification, fissures, and excoriations resulting from chronic scratching are often observed. Of all dystrophies, 48% are of the hyperplastic type.[17]

Histologically, varying degrees of hyperkeratosis and acanthosis are present. Sometimes, the granular cell layer is conspicuous. The rete pegs become elongated, widened, branched, and sometimes fused and have smooth borders

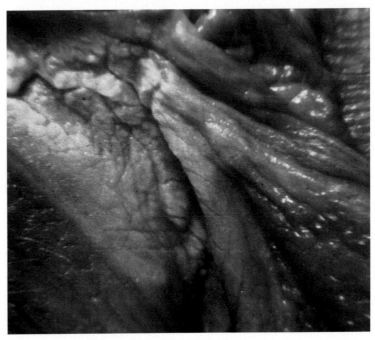

Figure 5–15. Squamous cell hyperplasia with a white, thickened, lichenoid appearance. (Courtesy of Dr. E.G. Friedrich, Jr., and Dr. Edward Wilkinson, University of Florida College of Medicine, Gainesville, Florida.)

(Figs. 5–16 and 5–17A). Parakeratosis may be present. In the dermis, dilated capillaries and an inflammatory infiltration of lymphocytes and plasma cells are present to varying extents (see Fig. 5–16). The orderly maturation and smooth rete pegs are in sharp contrast to the irregular rete pegs associated with desmoplastic stroma in invasive squamous cell carcinoma (see Fig. 5–17B).

Mixed Epithelial Disorders

Approximately 15% of all dystrophies constitute a mixed variant.[17] During the course of follow-up, 27% to 35% of the cases of lichen sclerosus may undergo hyperplastic changes. Histologically, areas of hyperplastic epithelium are found within typical lichen sclerosus (Fig. 5–18A). The stroma demonstrates hyalinization

and chronic inflammation (Figs. 5–18B and 5–19A, B).

In the presence of VIN, the lesions tend to be localized, well-defined, slightly raised, white, and rough and are found most frequently in the fourchette and perineum. Microscopically, the dysplastic cells demonstrate nuclear enlargement, hyperchromasia, irregularity, abnormal or lack of maturation, and an altered nucleocytoplasmic ratio (Fig. 5–20). Normal and abnormal forms of mitoses may be found in varying numbers at different levels of the epithelium. Depending on the extent of these morphologic features, the severity of dysplasia is graded as mild, moderate, or severe. The malignant potential of dystrophy is directly related to the extent and the severity of dysplasia. The majority of VINs are of the simplex type. More detailed dis-

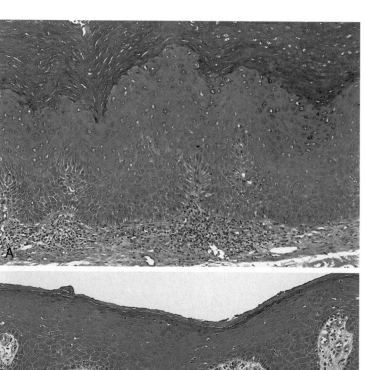

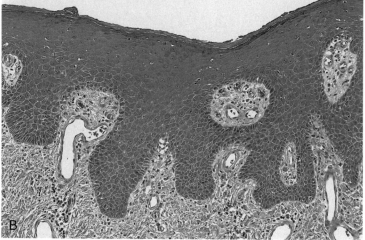

Figure 5–16. Squamous cell hyperplasia. *A,* Marked hyperkeratosis and hypergranulosis. *B,* Plump rete pegs. *C,* Some rete pegs are thin and branching. *D,* Orderly arrangement of parabasal cells without nuclear atypia. Moderate chronic inflammation in the adjacent dermis.

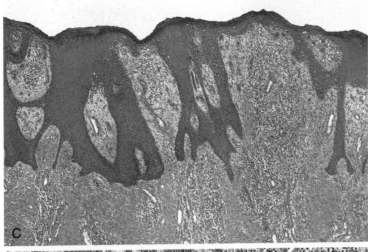

Figure 5–16. *Continued.*

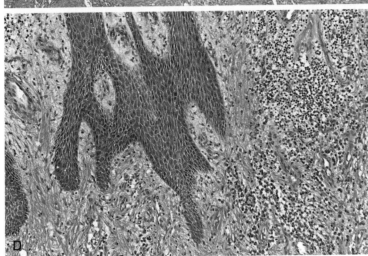

cussions about dysplasia and carcinoma in situ are provided in Chapter 6.

Studies by Special Techniques

Electron-microscopic study of lichen sclerosus reveals an increase of intercellular space between the squamous cells and some degree of acantholysis. The basal cell layer remains intact, and there is no duplication of the basal lamina. The melanocytes are degenerated with few melanosomes. In the dermis, the collagen fibrils vary in thickness and maturity. Between the mature collagen fibrils are abundant thin, immature collagen fibrils. Degenerated collagen fibrils are found in focal areas. Some of the fibroblasts contain collagen fibrils within their cytoplasm, suggesting abnormal collagen formation.[53]

The metabolic activity of the epidermis in lichen sclerosus has been evaluated by triatiated thymidine,[58] acridine-orange fluorescence,[13] and 32P uptake technique.[24] Woodruff and associates[58] and Friedrich and colleagues[13] observed higher metabolic activity in lichen sclerosus than in the normal skin, suggesting that the epidermis in lichen sclerosus is not inactive or degenerative, despite its atrophic appearance on histologic examination. Kaufman and colleagues,[24] on the other hand, found no increase of 32P uptake in lichen sclerosus when compared with normal skin. These contradictory findings suggest that the metabolic activity of lichen sclerosus may be variable, depending on the areas studied and the course of the disease.

In patients with lichen sclerosus, free testosterone and one of its precursors, androstene-

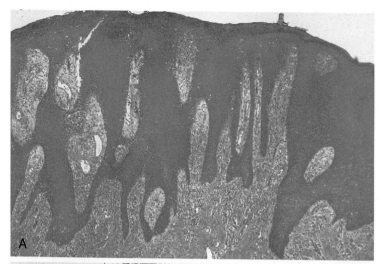

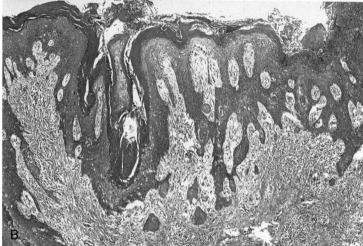

Figure 5–17. Comparison of squamous cell hyperplasia and squamous cell carcinoma. *A*, Squamous cell hyperplasia with smooth rete pegs. *B*, Early invasive squamous cell carcinoma with irregular rete pegs and desmoplastic reaction.

dione, as well as serum dihydrotestosterone were found to be below normal.[14] After the topical application of 2% testosterone propionate, serum dihydrotestosterone and testosterone exceeded the initial and normal ranges. Lichen sclerosus was improved in 80% of patients.[14] Because testosterone is converted to dihydrotestosterone by 5-α-reductase in the skin and soft tissues, a low level of 5-α-reductase in the local tissue may have initiated lichen sclerosus.[14] A restoration of the normal level of 5-α-reductase following topical testosterone therapy may explain the clinical response.[14]

Based on HLA typing, Harrington and Gelsthorpe[19] found a higher than expected frequency of HLA-B40 in 50 white women with lichen sclerosus, suggesting a genetic basis for the development of the disease. In two families

with lichen sclerosus, HLA haplotype A2B44DRW6 was shared by all four generations of one family afflicted by the disease. In the second family, B44DRW6 was identified in one of the members.[15] Because HLA-D alleles are known to affect immune responses, their presence in familial lichen sclerosus supports an autoimmune origin.[48]

In another study, of 68 women with lichen sclerosus, HLA-B21 was found to be significantly increased after correction for the antigens tested, suggesting an immune system disorder.[48]

In a study of 350 women with lichen sclerosus, 21.5% had one or more autoimmune disorders and 42% had elevated autoantibodies.[34] However, in the immunohistochemical stains of lichen sclerosus, the number of CD2+, CD3+, CD4+, and CD8+ lymphocytes was lower than that of the normal controls. B lymphocytes with

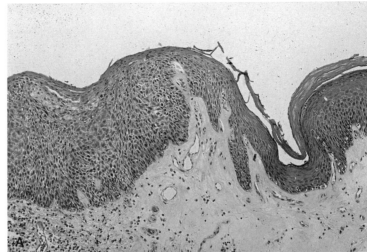

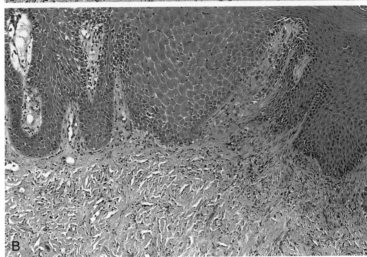

Figure 5–18. *A,* Transition from lichen sclerosus to squamous cell hyperplasia. *B,* Area of squamous cell hyperplasia with plump rete pegs. Stromal fibrosis, hyalinization, and chronic inflammation are similar to those seen in lichen sclerosus.

expression of CD19+ and CD21+ lymphocytes were absent. The number of circulating CD3+ and CD4+ lymphocytes was lower than that of controls. The authors found no evidence of T cell–mediated response.[45]

Berger et al.[1] compared the normal and dystrophic vulvar skin for the expression of retinoic acid receptor (RAR) by immunohistochemistry and nonradioactive in situ hybridization. In the normal vulvar skin, RAR-alpha mRNA was located in the suprabasal cell layers. In contrast, it was found in the basal cell layers of lichen sclerosus. In the case of squamous cell hyperplasia, RAR-alpha mRNA occurred throughout the epithelial cell layers. Quantitatively RAR-alpha expression was lower in lichen sclerosus and in squamous cell hyperplasia than in the normal skin (P value

highly significant). It is interesting that RAR-gamma expression was slightly higher in lichen sclerosus, but no significant difference in squamous cell hyperplasia was apparent when compared with the normal vulvar skin. Based on these abnormal expressions of RAR, the authors suggest that an early differentiation of squamous cells occurs in lichen sclerosus, leading to thinness of the epidermis.[1] These abnormal expressions may also affect the activation of differentiation-specific genes.

Relationship of Vulvar Dystrophy and Cancer

The malignant potential of vulvar dystrophy is difficult to determine because of the different terminologies, nonuniform histologic criteria,

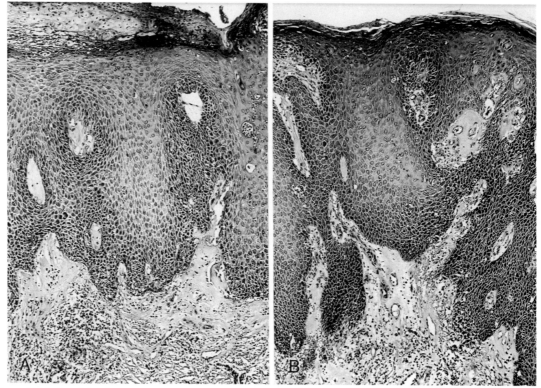

Figure 5–19. *A* and *B,* Mixed epithelial disorder (mixed dystrophy). The dermal hyalinization with chronic inflammation is similar to that seen in lichen sclerosus. The epidermis, however, is markedly hyperplastic with widening and confluence of rete pegs. The surface is hyperkeratotic and parakeratotic. There is no evidence of dysplasia.

and variable follow-up periods.[22,23,33] For these reasons, only some of the more recent studies are included and summarized in Table 5–1.

In 128 women with vulvar dystrophy, atypia was found in none of 48 women with lichen sclerosus, in 10% of women with hyperplastic dystrophy, and in 17% of women with mixed dystrophy.[17] In a study of 92 patients with lichen sclerosus and follow-up data (including 35% with mixed dystrophy using current

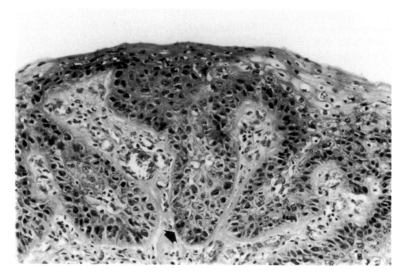

Figure 5–20. Severe dysplasia in a mixed dystrophy. Abnormal cells with nuclear irregularity and hyperchromasia occupy most of the epithelium. Cellular disorganization and occasional mitotic figures (arrow) occur in the deep layers. Toward the superficial layers, squamous maturation is maintained.

Table 5–1. Frequency of Concurrent and Subsequent VIN and Squamous Carcinoma

Lichen Sclerosus	Concurrent	Subsequent
Hart et al.[20], 1975	—	1% Sq. Ca.
Gardner and Kaufman[17], 1981	0%	—
Micheletti et al.[35], 1988	—	1% VIN
Carli et al.[3], 1995	—	0.5% VIN
		1% Sq. Ca.

Squamous Cell Hyperplasia	Concurrent	Subsequent
Gardner and Kaufman[17], 1981	10% VIN	—
Rodke et al.[40], 1988	3% VIN	—
Micheletti et al.[35], 1988	—	17.7% VIN

Mixed Dystrophy	Concurrent	Subsequent
Gardner and Kaufman[17], 1981	17% VIN	—
Rodke et al.[40], 1988	17% Sq. Ca.	—
Micheletti et al.[35], 1988	—	3.6% VIN

VIN, atypia, Vulvar intraepithelial neoplasia; Sq. Ca., squamous carcinoma.

nomenclature), Hart and colleagues[20] found one patient who developed squamous carcinoma 12 years after the initial histologic diagnosis of mixed dystrophy with dysplasia.

In a review of the literature by Hart and colleagues,[20] only 16 of 465 (3%) cases of lichen sclerosus were associated with carcinoma. A report by Wallace[53] indicated that only 12 of 290 patients (4%) with lichen sclerosus followed for a mean of 12.5 years developed carcinoma of the vulva.

In a study by Carli et al.,[3] 211 women with lichen sclerosus were followed for a median of 20 months. One woman developed VIN and two women developed squamous cell carcinoma. The progression rate thus is in the range of 1.4%, which is comparable to that shown by other studies, indicating a low risk of malignant change with lichen sclerosus alone.

A study by Micheletti et al.[35] included 448 women with histologic confirmation of vulvar dystrophy, including 151 (34%) with lichen sclerosus, 214 (48%) with hyperplastic dystrophy, and 83 (19%) with mixed dystrophy. These women were followed 3 to 58 months (median 35 months). One (0.7%) case of lichen sclerosus had atypia. In contrast, 13 (17.7%) women with hyperplastic dystrophy had atypia. Of the 83 women with mixed dystrophies, 3 (3.6%) had atypia. The overall frequency of atypia in this group of women was 9.4%.[35]

In a study by Rodke et al.,[40] biopsies from 50 women with mixed dystrophy were reviewed, including those from 32 women with clinical features of hyperplastic dystrophy and 18 women with mixed dystrophy. The histologic diagnosis of the 32 women with hyperplastic dystrophy included hyperplastic dystrophy in 23 cases, lichen sclerosus with hyperkeratosis in 8 cases, and mixed dystrophy with VIN in 1 case. Among 18 women with a diagnosis of mixed dystrophy, 1 had koilocytosis, 3 had squamous cell carcinoma (17%), 1 had hyperplastic dystrophy, and 2 had mixed dystrophy. This study suggests that mixed dystrophy has a greater malignant potential than does hyperplastic dystrophy.[40]

In a study by Micheletti et al,[35] 11 women were found to have atypia at the time of initial diagnosis. This included eight women with mild atypia, who were all treated medically. Of these, the lesion in six women regressed and in two it progressed. One developed severe atypia with microinvasion 12 months after the initial diagnosis. The other women developed invasive carcinoma 24 months after the initial diagnosis. Three women with severe atypia received wide excision; all were free of atypia at the time of the report. The lichen sclerosus persisted in two women. This study indicates that even mild atypia has potential for progression in 25% of cases.[35]

Kim et al.[25] studied the areas of squamous hyperplasia and normal skin adjacent to 18 vulvar invasive squamous cell carcinomas. Seven (39%) carcinomas were HPV positive. p53 mutations were found in four HPV-negative tumors, but the adjacent normal skin and squamous hyperplasia lacked p53 mutations. The clonality analyzed by polymerase drain reaction for X chromosome inactivation was monoclonal in the carcinoma but polyclonal in the adjacent normal skin and squamous hyperplasia. The authors concluded that squamous hyperplasia is not a direct precursor of HPV-negative squamous cell carcinoma.[25] No VIN is included in this study, however.

OTHER DERMATOLOGIC DISEASES

Acanthosis Nigricans

Acanthosis nigricans typically affects the body folds, especially in the axilla, neck, thigh, submammary, and genital areas, as verrucous, brown patches. Histologically, the lesions are characterized by papillomatosis, hyperkeratosis, and acanthosis. In addition, hyperpigmentation occurs in the basal layer (Fig. 5–21).

Three types of acanthosis nigricans have been recognized by Curth and Aschner.[5] The malignant variant occurs almost exclusively in adults and is associated with visceral malignancies, especially adenocarcinoma of the stomach. The benign variant affects mainly the pediatric age group and is not associated with malignancy or endocrinopathy. Pseudoacanthosis nigricans is associated with obesity, lipodystrophy, endocrinopathy, and autoimmune disorders but not with malignant disease. All three variants have similar histologic features. When acanthosis nigricans is associated with a sudden appearance of pruritic seborrheic keratosis (sign of Leser-Trélat), the chance of having malignant tumor is believed to be high.[21]

Seborrheic Keratosis

Seborrheic keratosis is a slightly raised, well-circumscribed, pigmented, warty lesion that occasionally occurs on the vulva singly or in clusters. Histologically, the lesion has a dome-shaped configuration and consists of basaloid cells in solid sheets and multiple horn cysts. In addition, hyperkeratosis, acanthosis, and papillomatosis of the epithelium and an increase of melanin pigment in the basal and parabasal layers are common findings. Clinically, it may simulate melanocytic lesions.

Roth and Look[41] reported a case of inverted follicular keratosis of the vulva in a 27-year-old woman, whose lesion strongly simulated in situ and invasive squamous cell carcinoma. In the biopsy sample, irregular solid nests of basaloid cells formed squamous eddies, underwent focal acantholysis, and extended into the dermis. These basaloid squamous cells had uniform, slightly enlarged nuclei, small nucleoli, and rare mitotic figures (fewer than one mitotic figure per 10 high-power fields). Although the nuclear cytoplasmic ratios were high, nuclear atypia was minimal. The authors were able to distinguish the lesion from squamous cell carcinoma by the lack of surface in situ carcinoma and desmoplastic stromal reaction.

Plasma Cell Vulvitis

This condition, which is the counterpart of plasma cell balanitis,[50,59] is usually associated with pruritus and dyspareunia. Its classic features include circumscribed, erythematous macules involving the vestibular region, vaginal introitus, or urethral meatus without mucosal erosion. Most women are premenopausal.

The epidermis is usually attenuated with loss of rete pegs and occasionally normal in thickness or hyperplastic. Mild stromal edema and a band-like mild to moderate infiltration of predominantly plasma cells occur in the superficial dermis; telangiectatic vessels and old hemorrhage affect the deeper stroma (Fig. 5–22). The cause is unclear. Infectious organisms are

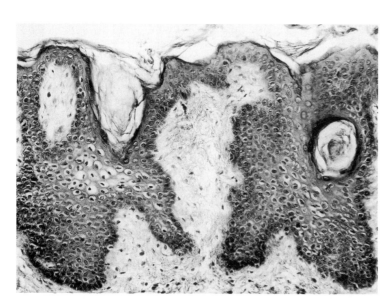

Figure 5–21. Acanthosis nigricans of the vulva associated with mucinous carcinoma of the ovary. Papillomatous proliferation of basaloid cells is accompanied by horn cysts and hyperpigmentation in the basal layer.

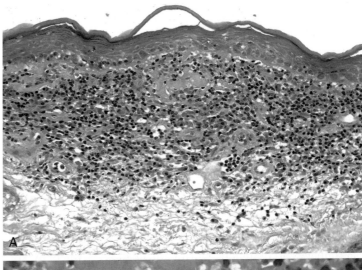

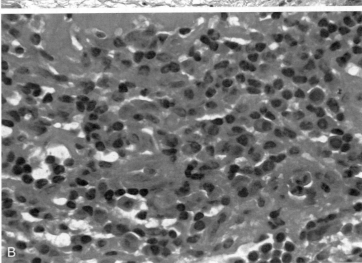

Figure 5–22. Plasma cell vulvitis. *A,* The epidermis is atrophic with no rete pegs. A band-like infiltration of plasma cells and lymphocytes occurs in the superficial dermis. *B,* Abundant plasma cells and stromal fibrosis.

usually absent. The case of a women reported by Yoganathan et al.[59] had positive culture for *Candida albicans.* Thus, infectious agents should be included in the differential diagnosis.

Pyodermas

Pyodermas represent pyogenic infections of the skin, its appendages, or the underlying dermis and subcutaneous tissue. The causative organisms are usually coagulase-positive staphylococcus or hemolytic streptococcus. Less often, they are caused by other bacteria in association with decreasing immunity or other predisposing factors.[11]

Infection of the hair follicles results in folliculitis, furuncle, or carbuncle. In superficial folliculitis, the infection is limited to the upper part of the pilosebaceous duct, whereas deep folliculitis affects the follicle and the sebaceous glands. In furuncle, the infection spreads to perifollicular tissues with localized cellulitis. A deeply situated infection that spreads beneath the deep subcutaneous fascia with communicating and draining sinuses is known as carbuncle.

Pyogenic ulcers of the skin include impetigo, which involves the superficial layer of the skin, and ecthyma, which affects the full thickness of the skin and superficial dermis. Infection of the subcutaneous tissue results in erysipelas and cellulitis.

Hidradenitis Suppurativa

Hidradenitis suppurativa is a chronic suppurative infection of the apocrine glands. It most

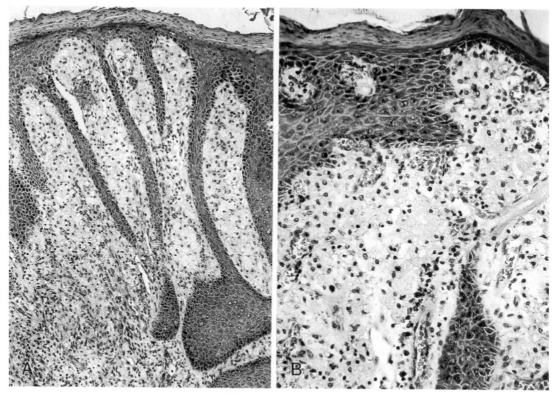

Figure 5–25. Verruciform xanthoma. *A*, The epidermis reveals parakeratosis and pseudoepitheliomatous hyperplasia with elongated rete pegs. Abundant foamy cells are mixed with a small number of lymphocytes and plasma cells. *B*, A higher magnification to demonstrate the foamy character of cytoplasm. (H & E; *A*, ×80; *B*, ×200; Courtesy of Dr. D.J. Santa Cruz, St. Louis, Missouri.)

upper stratum malpighii of verruca vulgaris, are absent in verruciform xanthoma. The cells in the granular cell tumor have abundant eosinophilic, granular cytoplasm, which is PAS-positive. The xanthomatous cells in verruciform xanthoma contain foamy cytoplasm with few or no PAS-positive granules. Bulbous rete pegs, characteristic of verrucous carcinoma, are not found in verruciform xanthoma.[43]

REFERENCES

1. Berger J, Telser A, Widschwendter M, et al. Expression of retinoic acid receptors in non-neoplastic epithelial disorders of the vulva and normal vulvar skin. Int J Gynecol Pathol 19:95, 2000.
2. Bermejo A, Bermejo MD, Roman P, et al. Lichen planus with simultaneous involvement of the oral cavity and genitalia. Oral Surg Oral Med Oral Pathol 69:209, 1990.
3. Carli C, Cattaneo A, De Magnis A, et al. Squamous cell carcinoma arising in vulval lichen sclerosus: A longitudinal cohort study. Eur J Cancer Prev 4:491, 1995.
4. Carlson JA, Lamb P, Malfetano J, et al. Clinocopathologic comparison of vulvar and extragenital lichen sclerosus: Histologic variants, evolving lesions, and etiology of 141 cases. Mod Pathol 11:844, 1998.
5. Curth HO, Aschener BM. Genetic studies on acanthosis nigricans. Arch Dermatol 79:55, 1959.
6. Delke I, Veridiano NP, Trancer ML, et al. Sweet syndrome with involvement of the female genital tract. Obstet Gynecol 58:394, 1981.
7. Duray PH, Merino MJ, Axiotis C. Warty dyskeratoma of the vulva. Int J Gynecol Pathol 2:286, 1983.
8. Edwards L. Desquamative vulvitis. Dermatol Clin 10:325, 1992.
9. Edwards L, Hansen RS. Reiter's syndrome of the vulva. Arch Dermatol 128:811, 1992.
10. Eisen D. The vulvovaginal-gingival syndrome of lichen planus. Arch Dermatol 130:1379, 1994.
11. Friedrich EG Jr. Vulvar Disease. Philadelphia, W.B. Saunders, 1976.
12. Friedrich EG Jr. International Society for the Study of Vulvar Disease: New nomenclature for vulvar disease. Am J Obstet Gynecol 90:1281, 1964.
13. Friedrich EG Jr, Julian CG, Woodruff JD. Acridine-orange fluorescence in vulvar dysplasia. Am J Obstet Gynecol 90:1281, 1964.
14. Friedrich EG Jr, Kalra RS. Serum levels of sex hormones in vulvar lichen sclerosus and the effect of topical testosterone. N Engl J Med 310:488, 1984.
15. Friedrich EG Jr, MacLaren NK. Genetic aspects of vulvar lichen sclerosus. Am J Obstet Gynecol 150:161, 1984.
16. Fung MA, LeBoit PE. Light microscopic criteria for the

diagnosis of early vulvar lichen sclerosus. Am J Surg Pathol 22:473, 1998.

17. Gardner HL, Kaufman RH. Benign diseases of the vulva and vagina, 2nd ed. Boston, G.K. Hall, 1981.

18. Hamm H, Metze D, Brocker EB. Hailey-Hailey disease: Eradication by dermabrasion. Arch Dermatol 130:1143, 1994.

19. Harrington DI, Gelsthorpe K. The association between lichen sclerosus et atrophicus and HLA-B40. Br J Dermatol 104:561, 1981.

20. Hart WR, Norris HJ, Helwig EB. Relation of lichen sclerosus et atrophicus of the vulva to the development of carcinoma. Obstet Gynecol 45:369, 1975.

21. Jacobs MI, Rigel DS. Acanthosis nigricans and the sign of Leser-Trélat associated with adenocarcinoma of the gallbladder. Cancer 48:328, 1981.

22. Jeffcoate TNA. Chronic vulvar dystrophies. Am J Obstet Gynecol 95:61, 1966.

23. Kaufman RH, Gardner HL, Brown DJ, et al. Vulvar dystrophies: An evaluation. Am J Obstet Gynecol 120:363, 1974.

24. Kaufman RH, Gardner HL, Johnson PC. P-32 uptake in lichen sclerosus et atrophicus of the vulva. Am J Obstet Gynecol 98:312, 1967.

25. Kim Y-T, Thomas NF, Kessis TD, et al. P53 mutations and clonality in vulvar carcinomas and squamous hyperplasias: Evidence suggesting that squamous hyperplasias do not serve as direct precursors of human papillomavirus-negative vulvar carcinomas. Hum Pathol 27:389, 1996.

26. Kiryu H, Ackerman AB. A critique of current classifications of vulvar diseases. Am J Dermatopathol 12:377, 1990.

27. Knox JM. Cutaneous inflammations and infections. Clin Obstet Gynecol 21:991, 1978.

28. Krain LS, Rosenthal L, Newcomer VD. Pemphigus vulgaris involving the cervix associated with endometrial carcinoma of the uterus: A case report with immunofluorescent findings. Int J Dermatol 12:220, 1973.

29. Lawrence WD. Non-neoplastic disorders of the vulva (vulvar dystrophies): Historical and current perspectives. Pathol Ann 28(part 2):23, 1993.

30. Lim HW, Bystryn J. Bullous diseases. Clin Obstet Gynecol 21:1007, 1978.

31. Mann MS, Kaufman RH. Erosive lichen planus of the vulva. Clin Obstet Gynecol 34:605, 1991.

32. Marquette GP, Se B, Woodruff JD. Introital adenosis associated with Stevens-Johnson syndrome. Obstet Gynecol 66:143, 1985.

33. McAdams AJ Jr, Kisstner RW. The relationship of chronic vulvar disease, leukoplakia and carcinoma in situ to carcinoma of the vulva. Cancer 11:740, 1958.

34. Meyrick-Thomas RH, Ridley CM, McGibbon DH, et al. Lichen sclerosus and autoimmunity: A study of 350 women. Br J Dermatol 118:41, 1988.

35. Micheletti L, Borgno G, Barbero M, et al. Cellular atypia in vulvar dystrophy. J Repro Med 33:539, 1988.

36. Pelisse M, Leibowitch M, Sedsel D, et al. Un nouveau syndrome vulvo-vagino-ginvival lichen plan erosif pleurimuqueux. Ann Dermatol Venersol 109:797, 1982.

37. Pestereli HE, Karaveli S, Oztekin S, Sorlu G. Benign persistent papular acantholytic and dyskeratotic erup-

tion of the vulva: A case report. Int J Gynecol Pathol 19:374, 2000.

38. Ridley CM. The Vulva. London, W.B. Saunders, 1975.

39. Ridley CM, Frankman O, Jones ISC, et al. New nomenclature for vulvar disease: Report of the committee on terminology of the International Society for the Study of Vulvar Disease. J Reprod Med 35:483, 1990.

40. Rodke G, Friedrich EG Jr, Wilkinson EJ. Malignant potential of mixed vulvar dystrophy (lichen sclerosus associated with squamous cell hyperplasia). J Repro Med 33:545, 1988.

41. Roth LM, Look KY. Inverted follicular keratosis of the vulvar skin: A lesion that can be confused with squamous cell carcinoma. Int J Gynecol Pathol 19:369, 2000.

42. Sanchez NP, Mihm MC. Reactive and neoplastic epithelial alterations of the vulva: A classification of the vulvar dystrophies from the dermatopathologist's viewpoint. J Am Acad Dermatol 6:378, 1982.

43. Santa Cruz DJ, Martin SA. Verruciform xanthoma of the vulva. Am J Clin Pathol 71:224, 1979.

44. Schwimmer E. Die Ideiopathischen Schleim Haut Plaques Der Mumdhohle. Vrtljschr Derm Syph 910:510, 1877–1878.

45. Scrimin F, Rustja S, Radillo O, et al. Vulvar lichen sclerosus: An immunologic study. Obstet Gynecol 95:147, 2000.

46. Scully RE, Bonfiglio TA, Kurman RJ, et al. Histologic Typing of Female Genital Tract Tumors, 2nd ed. New York, Springer-Verlag, 1994, pp 64–79.

47. Shafer WB. Verruciform xanthoma. Oral Surg 31:784, 1971.

48. Sideri M. Rognoni M, Rizzolo L, et al. Antigens of the HLA system in women with vulva lichen sclerosus: Association with HLA-B21. J Repro Med 33:551, 1988.

49. Smith GJ. Psoriasis: New concepts of its pathogenesis. South Med J 70:1030, 1977.

50. Souteyrand P, Wong E, MacDonald DM. Zoon's balanitis (balanitis circum-scripta plasmacellularis). Br J Dermatol 105:195, 1981.

51. Stage AH, Humeniuk JM, Easley WK. Bullous pemphigoid of the vulva: A case report. Am J Obstet Gynecol 150:169, 1984.

52. Sweet RD. An acute febrile neutrophilic dermatosis. Br J Dermatol 76:349, 1964.

53. Wallace HJ. Lichen sclerosus et atrophicus. Transactions of St. John's Hospital Dermatological Society 57:9, 1971.

54. Weinstein FD, Goldfad G, Frost P. Methotrexate. Mechanism of action of DNA synthesis in psoriasis. Arch Dermatol 104:236, 1971.

55. Whimster IW. An experimental approach to the problem of spottiness. Br J Dermatol 77:397, 1965.

56. Wilson EE, Malinak LR. Vulvovaginal sequelae of Stevens-Johnson syndrome and their management. Obstet Gynecol 71:478, 1988.

57. Woodruff JD, Baens JS. Interpretation of atrophic and hypertrophic alterations in the vulvar epithelium. Am J Obstet Gynecol 86:713, 1963.

58. Woodruff JD, Berkowf HI, Holzman GB, et al. Metabolic activity in normal and abnormal vulvar epithelia. Am J Obstet Gynecol 91:809, 1965.

59. Yoganathan S, Bohl TG, Mason G. Plasma cell balanitis and vulvitis (of Zoon): A study of 10 cases. J Reprod Med 39:939, 1994.

6

BENIGN AND MALIGNANT EPITHELIAL TUMORS OF THE VULVA

ADENOCARCINOMA OF UNDETERMINED
   ORIGIN
SMALL CELL CARCINOMA, MERKEL CELL
   TUMOR

BENIGN EPITHELIAL TUMORS

Hidradenoma

Hidradenoma, a benign neoplasm of the sweat gland, has several histologic types. The papillary variant, hidradenoma papilliferum, has a special predilection for the vulva of white women in the reproductive years. In a study by Meeker et al.,[148] 80% of papillary hidradenomas occurred on the vulva; the remaining 20% involved the perianal skin.

Hidradenoma of the vulva usually presents as a small (less than 1 cm), raised cystic or solid dermal nodule.[11] Most hidradenomas are asymptomatic and occur on the labia majora and less often on the labia minora and interlabial groove[216]; with ulceration of the overlying skin, a red, granular, edematous tissue may protrude from the opening. This appearance, although simulating granuloma pyogenicum, is characteristic of hidradenoma.

Histologically, the majority of hidradenomas consist of complex glandular and tubular structures with frequent papillary projections supported by delicate fibrovascular cores (Fig. 6–1). The lining cells are double layered: an inner layer of tall, columnar, secretory cells overlies a layer of myoepithelial cells (Fig. 6–2). Apocrine differentiation and stromal hyalinization with trapped glands simulating invasion are common features. The well-defined border of the lesion on low magnification and the lack of nuclear atypism are indicative of a benign tumor. A cystic variant hidradenoma, cystadenoma papilliferum, also occurs in the vulva, usually originating from the apocrine gland.

Clear cell and mixed tumor variants of hidradenoma, because of their solid growth pattern and the preponderance of clear cells, may be misinterpreted as metastatic carcinoma from the kidney or genital tract. Key features of clear cell hidradenoma include a lobulated arrangement, the lack of an infiltrative irregular border, the presence of hyaline stroma, and small, uniform nuclei lacking pleomorphism and mitotic activity (Fig. 6–3). Mixed tumors (pleomorphic adenomas), which are histologically indistinguishable from those originating in the salivary gland, may arise from the vulvar sweat gland, Bartholin's gland, or ectopic breast tissue.[180] A complete local excision is adequate for these tumors.

Syringoma

Syringoma is an organized tumor with differentiation toward the eccrine sweat ducts. On the vulva, syringoma appears as multiple small (1 to 3 mm) slightly raised, skin-colored papules. These usually become evident after

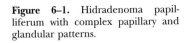

Figure 6–1. Hidradenoma papilliferum with complex papillary and glandular patterns.

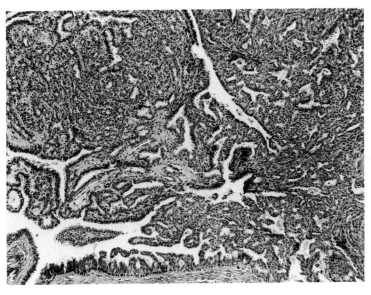

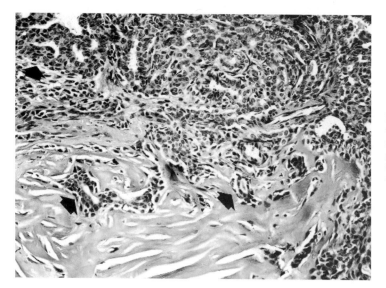

Figure 6–2. Hidradenoma papilliferum with hyalinization and sclerosis of stroma, simulating invasion. The glands are lined by an inner layer of secretory cells and an outer row of myoepithelial cells (*arrows*).

puberty. Most are asymptomatic, but they may be pruritic.[223] Occasional cases are familial, and the patient may have similar lesions on the eyelids, face, or neck.[34,223] A significant increase is seen in individuals with Down syndrome.[32]

Histologically, multiple dilated, comma-shaped ductal structures usually are lined by two layers of cells (Fig. 6–4). Some of the cells are flattened. Histochemical and ultrastructural studies suggest an origin from the intraepidermal eccrine ducts.[97] Despite the growth pattern and the fibrous reaction in the dermis suggestive of an infiltrative growth, syringoma is a benign tumor.

Sebaceous Adenoma

Sebaceous adenoma occurs on the labium minus as raised yellow-tan nodules that are usually 1 to 3 mm in diameter. Histologically, the lesions are well circumscribed. The mature sebaceous cells are arranged in broad sheets and surrounded by several layers of basaloid cells.

Benign Tumor and Tumor-like Conditions of the Bartholin Gland

Because normal Bartholin's glands are not palpable clinically, disease of the Bartholin

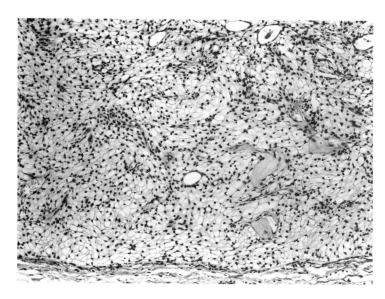

Figure 6–3. Clear cell hidradenoma reveals a well-circumscribed border, solid sheets of polygonal clear cells, and scattered islands of hyalinized stroma.

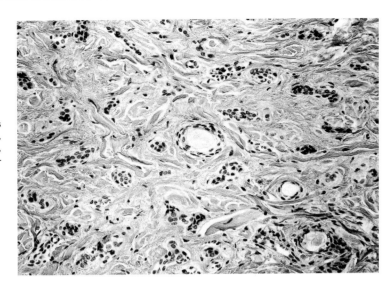

Figure 6–4. Syringoma. Uniform cells form small clusters in the dermis, some of which are comma shaped, whereas others have dilated lumen-containing secretions.

glands is detected primarily by swelling of the gland or by changes in the skin overlying the gland. Most of the diseases are related to inflammation and cystic formation. Benign and malignant neoplasms are less common. In one study of 700 Bartholin's gland lesions treated surgically, only 1% were primary carcinomas; the remainder were cysts, abscesses, and chronic inflammatory conditions.[37] A varicosity of Bartholin's gland may occasionally present as an enlarged gland.[70]

Enlargement of the Bartholin's gland may occasionally be caused by hyperplasia, with or without associated cyst formation. In these cases, the lobules maintain the normal cellular arrangement.[70] Koenig and Tavassoli[124] reported 17 women with nodular hyperplasia (aged 19 to 56 years, mean 35 years). The nodular mass was 1.2 to 4.0 cm in size, predominantly solid, unilateral (only one bilateral), and mucoid to firm and gray-white in appearance. Histologically, the enlarged lobules preserve the normal acinar duct relationship. Mucinous material fills the ducts, some of which become cystic. Mild, chronic inflammation occurs in most cases. Squamous metaplasia usually involves large ducts; less commonly terminal ducts are affected.[124]

Mucocele-like changes of Bartholin's gland were reported in two women who presented with bilateral or unilateral nodules of the vulva.[75] In one patient, the nodules were rubbery, firm, lobulated, and bilateral and measured 4 × 3 × 2 cm and 4 × 2.5 × 2 cm. In the other case, the lesion was partially cystic and nodular and measured 6 × 4 × 2.5 cm. The

histologic appearance was similar to that of an oral mucocele. Pools of mucinous material were surrounded by loose granulation tissue in which scattered foamy, vacuolated macrophages, lymphocytes, eosinophils, and capillaries were present (Figs. 6–5 and 6–6).[75] Traumatic disruption of the excretory duct with extravasation of mucus from the acini is believed to be the cause of mucocele.

Willis[214] described a 4 cm cystadenoma of the Bartholin's gland in a 60-year-old woman. The tumor consisted of ductal and acinar proliferation of mucus-secreting columnar cells in papillary and cribriform patterns. Koenig and Tavassoli[124] reported an adenoma coexisting with adenoid cystic carcinoma in a 45-year-old woman. The adenoma comprised small glands and tubules, which were lined by nonmucinous epithelial and myoepithelial cells. Cells of adenoid cystic carcinoma were basaloid, more atypical than adenomatous cells, and infiltrated into the adjacent structures. An adenomyoma containing both adenomatous tissue and smooth muscle stroma was also described.[124]

VULVAR INTRAEPITHELIAL NEOPLASIA (VIN)

Epidemiology and Carcinogenesis of VIN and Invasive Squamous Cell Carcinoma

Malignant tumors of the vulva constitute about 5.8% of all gynecologic malignancies. The type and frequency of vulvar malignancies observed at Maternity and Barnes Hospital in St. Louis

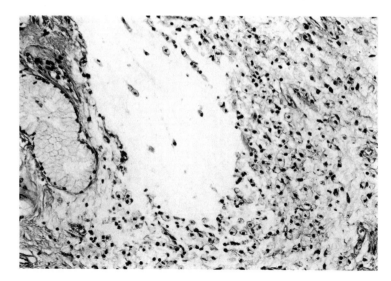

Figure 6–5. Mucocele of Bartholin's gland. Cystic space contains mucus and macrophages with vacuolated cytoplasm.

from 1955 to 1970 included invasive squamous carcinoma, 51%; squamous carcinoma in situ, 25%; metastatic and secondary tumors, 8%; Paget's disease, 8%; malignant melanoma, 3%; adenocarcinoma, 2%; basal cell carcinoma, 2%; and sarcomas, 1%.[50] About three fourths of the vulvar carcinomas were preinvasive and invasive squamous carcinomas.

Based on the data from nine population-based cancer registries in the Surveillance, Epidemiology, and End Results (SEER) program, Sturgeon et al.[187] reported that the incidence of in situ carcinoma from the period 1973 to 1976 until 1985 to 1987 increased from 1.1 to 2.1 per 100,000 white women. The incidence for black women during the same period was 1.6 and 2.3 per 100,000, respectively. The

largest increase was in white women under 35 years of age. Only one of the nine registries included VIN III (vulvar intraepithelial neoplasia, grade III), which accounted for less than 5% of in situ carcinoma cases. The increased incidence thus cannot be explained on the basis of changing terminology to include severe dysplasia. This increase is attributed to changing sexual behavior and human papillomavirus (HPV) infection.[184]

The incidence of invasive carcinoma between 1973 to 1976 and 1985 to 1987, respectively, was stable at 1.3 and 1.2 for 100,000 white women, and 1.7 and 1.1 for black women per 100,000.[187]

The SEER data included 2,948 (50%) women with in situ carcinoma and 2,346 (39%) women

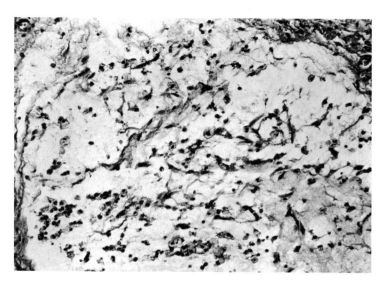

Figure 6–6. Mucocele of Bartholin's gland. Part of the cyst wall consists of myxoid granulation tissue with proliferation of capillaries and scattered lymphocytes and plasma cells.

with invasive squamous cell carcinoma. The remaining 11% of vulvar malignancies are of the nonsquamous type, including 205 basal cell carcinomas, 203 malignant melanomas, 123 cases of Paget's disease, 61 adenocarcinomas, 34 sarcomas, and 28 others.[187]

The overall incidence rate of vulvar carcinoma in the United States is about 1.8 per 100,000 women, which is one eighth that of cervical carcinoma. Although cervical squamous carcinoma reaches a plateau between the ages of 40 and 69 years,[101,149] vulvar carcinoma continues to increase. After the age of 75 years, the incidence rate is 20 per 100,000 women, which is comparable to that of cervical carcinoma.[42]

Crum[42] proposed two models for the development of vulvar squamous cell carcinoma. The first group included women between the ages of 35 and 65 years, an age range frequently associated with VIN. The invasive carcinoma is basaloid or poorly differentiated. Patients have a high frequency of clinical condyloma and HPV DNA in the malignant tumor. In the second group, the women are usually 55 to 85 years, and the condition is associated with lichen sclerosus, squamous cell hyperplasia, and vulvar atypia. Invasive carcinoma is well differentiated, keratinizing, and infrequently associated with HPV DNA.[42]

In the study by Trimble et al.,[194] the histologic features of high-grade VIN and invasive squamous cell carcinoma were correlated with the age of the women and their HPV status. The HPV DNA was determined by in situ hybridization using the Digene Omniprobe.

Among 54 women with high-grade VIN, 89% had detectable HPV DNA. The mean age was 49 years, and 65% of women were younger than 55 years. Among the 21 women with the warty or basaloid type of squamous carcinoma, 86% had detectable HPV DNA, the mean age was 60.8 years, and 38% were younger than 55 years. In contrast, of the 48 women with keratinizing squamous cell carcinoma, only 6.3% had detectable HPV DNA, the mean age was 65.1 years, and only 17% were younger than 55 years (*P* value highly significant).[194] Among the squamous cell carcinomas that were positive for HPV, 71% were type 16, 1% were type 18, and the remaining tumors were of an unknown type.[194]

These findings strongly support at least two pathways. First is the development of high-grade VIN and warty or basaloid squamous carcinoma through the effect of HPV. The other pathway is non–HPV-related factors in women with keratinizing squamous cell carcinoma.

To further confirm this hypothesis, the type of squamous cell carcinoma is correlated with the adjacent epithelial changes. Of the 48 women with keratinizing squamous cell carcinoma, 9 had lichen sclerosus, 16 had squamous hyperplasia, and 2 had VIN. In contrast, of the 21 women with warty or basaloid squamous cell carcinoma, only 1 had lichen sclerosus, 4 had squamous hyperplasia, and 17 had high-grade VIN. Essentially 52% of women with keratinizing squamous cell carcinoma had lichen sclerosus or squamous hyperplasia. In contrast, 81% of the women with warty or basaloid squamous cell carcinoma had high-grade VIN in the vicinity.[194]

In an investigation of risk factors associated with VIN and warty or basaloid carcinoma (as compared with keratinizing squamous cell carcinoma), the risk factor for the former group is similar to those of cervical carcinoma, including the number of sexual partners, age at first intercourse, association with abnormal Papanicolaou smears, and cigarette smoking. Thus, the study by Trimble et al.[194] also supports at least two different causes for the development of vulvar squamous cell carcinomas.

Toki et al.[193] investigated the epithelial changes adjacent to invasive vulvar carcinoma by correlating the morphology and HPV status using in situ hybridization and polymerase chain reaction (PCR). Of women with keratinizing squamous cell carcinoma, 74% had squamous hyperplasia in the vicinity. Of those with squamous cell hyperplasia, 10% also had areas of lichen sclerosus (mixed vulvar dystrophy). All lesions of squamous hyperplasia were negative for HPV DNA. Only 10% of epithelial hyperplasias had the warty or basaloid type of VIN.[193]

A study by Hording et al.[106] also supports two different pathways. Lichen sclerosus was found adjacent to keratinizing squamous cell carcinoma in 71% of cases and epithelial hyperplasia in less than 10%. Differentiated type of VIN III was found in 75% of keratinizing squamous cell carcinomas with only 4% harboring HPV DNA. HPV DNA was identified in 81% of warty or basaloid carcinomas, as compared with 10% in the keratinizing squamous cell carcinoma.

In their study, Lee et al.[136] found missense point mutation of p53 in five (24%) of 21 vulvar squamous cell carcinomas. Of these five, four (80%) were HPV negative. These findings support the concept that p53 mutation may occur either with incorporation with HPV E6 oncoprotein or in the absence of HPV. Kim et al.[120] investigated 18 vulvar squamous cell carcinomas to correlated p53 mutation and HPV status. Four tumors were found to have p53 mutation and all were HPV negative. P53 mutation was not detected in the normal or adjacent hyperplasia. Further PCR study for X chromosome inactivation demonstrated monoclonality in squamous cell carcinoma and polyclonality in the adjacent normal or hyperplastic lesions. The authors concluded that squamous cell hyperplasia itself is not a direct precursor of HPV negative squamous cell carcinoma.[120]

Vulvar Intraepithelial Neoplasia of Squamous Type

Terminology

Many terms have been designated for potential precursors of vulvar squamous carcinoma, including atypical hyperplasia, dysplasia, atypia, Bowen's disease,[23] erythroplasia of Queyrat,[175] carcinoma in situ,[217] carcinoma in situ simplex,[2,3] intraepithelial carcinoma, and intraepithelial neoplasia.[43]

In 1912, Bowen[23] described two cases of red, scaly, oozing lesions on the buttock and thigh, respectively. Because of the cellular atypism and the persistence of recurrence, he termed the disease *precancerous dermatosis* and believed that invasive carcinoma would eventually occur. The erythroplastic lesion, described first by Queyrat[175] in 1911, occurred on the glans penis. It has a striking clinical and histologic resemblance to Bowen's disease. However, there is no increase in the frequency of internal malignancy.[90]

Abell and Gosling[3] recognized a simplex type of carcinoma in situ, whose "cytologic features of malignancy, although definite, were more subtle and not nearly as striking as those of Bowen's disease. The bizarre nuclear aberrations of Bowen's disease were absent, and maturation was maintained in the superficial layers." This variant in their series comprised 24% of intraepithelial carcinomas; the remaining carcinomas were of Bowen's type. The simplex type is often associated with lichen sclerosus[3] and invasive squamous cell carcinomas.[224] Koilocytosis and dyskeratosis are uncommon. In 1976, the International Society for the Study of Vulvar Disease (ISSVD) proposed the terms *carcinoma in situ* for all variants of intraepithe-

lial carcinoma and *atypia* for changes less severe than those in carcinoma in situ.[78]

The term *vulvar intraepithelial neoplasia* (VIN) later was proposed to reflect the morphologic and biologic continuum of atypia (dysplasia) and carcinoma in situ.[44,46] The morphologic spectrum starts with lesions resembling atypical condyloma and extends to those made up entirely of immature basaloid cells. The majority of VINs express varying degrees of koilocytosis, dyskeratosis, squamous maturation, nuclear pleomorphism, and mitotic aberrations. A minority of VINs may fulfill the clinical features of multicentric pigmented Bowen's disease or bowenoid papulosis. Because of the controversy regarding the specificity of this entity, it is discussed in a separate section.

The Terminology Committee of the ISSVD in 1986[212] and the International Society of Gynecological Pathologists recommended that all intraepithelial abnormalities having neoplastic potential be grouped together and graded according to the degree of cellular disorganization, maturation disturbances, and mitotic activity as mild dysplasia (VIN I), moderate dysplasia (VIN II), or severe dysplasia or carcinoma in situ (VIN III). Recent studies have shown at least two distinct types of VIN: warty or basaloid and simplex type. This discussion follows this concept.

Warty and Basaloid VIN

Clinical Features

Because the majority of VINs detected clinically are severe dysplasia or carcinoma in situ, the clinical and gross features of less severe changes are poorly documented. For this reason, most available information concerns the VIN III category.

Vulvar carcinoma in situ may be seen in persons of any age group. In earlier studies, it was described as a disease affecting women after the fourth decade of life.[217] However, in recent years, it has been seen in women in their twenties and, on rare occasions, in females in their teens.[30,103] As many as 40% of the cases now occur in women younger than 40 years of age.[30,81] The mean age of the patients in one series involving cases from 1958 to 1978 was 47 years.[30] In two studies that included cases from 1967 to 1977 and 1971 to 1975, the mean age was 39 years.[69,81] In a study conducted in New Zealand, the mean age during the period 1961 to 1980 was 52.7 years, as compared with that of 35.8 years during 1980 to 1992.[116] This difference in mean age reflects the changing nature of the disease in recent years.

Pruritus is the most common complaint, occurring in 50% of symptomatic women. The presence of a visible lesion or mass and vaginal bleeding are less frequent.[79] In one series, 48% of the women were asymptomatic. The lesion was detected by a careful inspection of the vulva during routine examination.[81] Some of these patients had prior cervical dysplasia or carcinoma in situ.

In 70% of the cases, the lesion involves the labia majora and minora or perineum.[113] In addition, the lesion may extend to the anal canal (22%), clitoris (18%), vagina (10%), and urethra (2%).[81] About 70% of VINs are multifocal.[81]

Associated findings include genital warts in 15% to 30% of patients and a history of herpes genitalis in 10% to 12%.[30,33,69,81,119,165,172,183] Condylomas are particularly common in women who are younger than 40 years and who have multifocal VIN. Overall, 20% to 25% of these women had previous, concurrent, or subsequent cervical dysplasia or carcinoma in situ.[5,30,81]

In the study by Herod et al.,[102] 133 women with VIN I to VIN III, from Birmingham, United Kingdom, were reviewed. The clinical findings by colposcopic examination included hyperkeratosis (41%), acetowhitening after application of 3% acetic acid (40%), vulvar warts (24%), leukoplakia (21%), erythematous or inflammatory changes (15%), and ulcers (5%).[102]

Gross Appearance

The gross appearance of the lesions is highly variable. The typical lesions are slightly raised from the adjacent normal skin or squamous mucosa. They are usually sharply defined and round or irregular in shape. The surface may be lichenoid and hyperkeratotic (white), eczematoid and scaly (pink), or erythematous (red; Fig. 6–7). The lesions usually have a dull red background with white epithelial islands, but any combination of the aforementioned patterns may occur. Foci of hyperpigmentation are common. In one study, 34% of the lesions were hyperpigmented.[81] Less frequently, the lesions are polypoid or verrucous, resembling condyloma. Ulceration is rare in vulvar carcinoma in situ unless it is associated with invasive carcinoma or secondary inflammation.

The lesion may be discrete or coalescent and single or in multiples[215,216] (Figs. 6–7 and 6–8A and B). Most of the lesions are 1 to 3 cm in

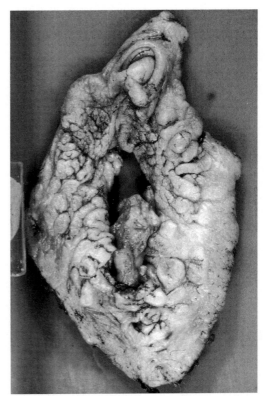

Figure 6–7. Multifocal squamous cell carcinoma in situ. Multiple raised plaques involve most of the vulvar skin. The surface usually appears smooth and white; less commonly, it is warty and pigmented.

size. Others are larger or involve the entire vulva. Nuclear staining, using 1% toluidine blue, is positive in 60% of cases.[81] Abnormal foci with increased cellularity are stained deep blue, whereas the normal skin shows little or no uptake of the dye (see Fig. 6–8A). However, false-positive and false-negative rates are high. A neoplasm having marked hyperkeratosis will be only slightly stained, whereas a benign ulcer may be deeply stained.[86] It is more practical to use a handheld magnifying lens to identify the abnormal areas for cytologic or histologic study. Colposcopic examination in experienced hands is helpful in localizing the abnormal area and visualizing the vascular patterns.

For cytologic evaluation, first the lesions should be moistened with saline. After removal of the surface debris, the scraped material is transferred to the glass slide and fixed promptly to avoid drying artifact. For biopsy, a dermatologic or Keyes punch is recommended.

Because of the variable gross appearance and the lack of symptoms in 50% of women with in situ carcinomas, a high index of suspicion, care-

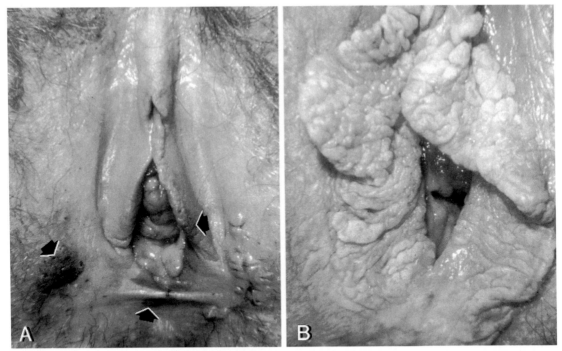

Figure 6–8. *A,* Multifocal squamous cell carcinoma in situ of the vulva after toluidine blue staining. A large papule is noted on the lower right labium majus; a smaller, flatter lesion is seen on the left labium minus; and separate lesions are noted at the fourchette. *B,* Confluent carcinoma in situ of the vulva involving the labia minora bilaterally and the fourchette. (From Wilkinson EJ, et al. Multicentric nature of vulvar carcinoma in situ. Obstet Gynecol 58:69, 1981, Figs. 1 and 2; used with permission by the American College of Obstetricians and Gynecologists.)

ful inspection, and frequent biopsy of abnormal areas are essential for early diagnosis.

Microscopic Features

In a study by Herod et al.,[102] the severity of VIN on the basis of grades I, II, and III is 19%, 12%, and 69%, respectively. Histologic evidence of HPV effect is seen in 78%. Those with HPV change were younger, with a mean age of 38.1 years as compared with 52.8 years among those without HPV change ($P = 0.001$). Viral change was also more common during the period 1988 to 1992 than 1978 to 1987 (85% versus 55%).

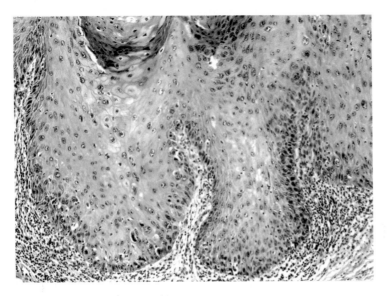

Figure 6–9. VIN I, mild squamous dysplasia. It maintains squamous maturation and cellular polarity, but nuclear atypism and cellular proliferation occur in the deep layers of the epithelium.

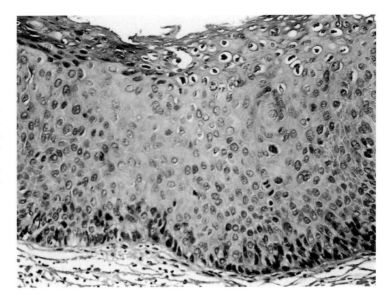

Figure 6–10. VIN I, mild squamous dysplasia with koilocytosis. This lesion has some of the features of papillomavirus infection, such as koilocytosis, parakeratosis, and cellular proliferation. The degree of nuclear atypia and cellular disorganization, however, exceeds that of ordinary condyloma.

Warty and basaloid dysplasia and carcinoma in situ share most of the following characteristics: (1) surface hyperkeratosis, parakeratosis, and koilocytosis; (2) proliferation of immature cells with an increased nucleocytoplasmic ratio, nuclear hyperchromasia, multinucleation, and atypism; (3) maturation disturbances (dyskeratosis); and (4) mitotic abnormalities. Based on the severity of these changes, the lesions are subclassified into mild dysplasia (VIN I) (Figs. 6–9 and 6–10), moderate dysplasia (VIN II) (Fig. 6–11), se-

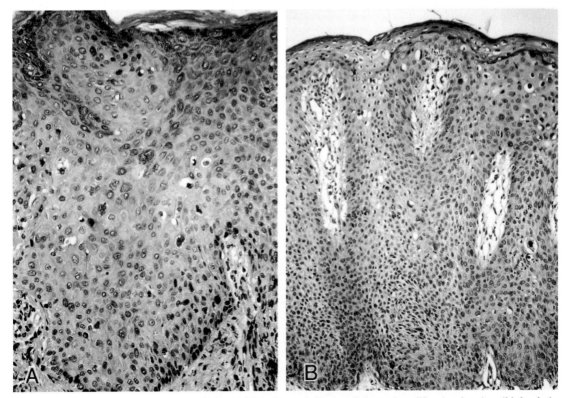

Figure 6–11. VIN II, moderate squamous dysplasia. This change is more cellular and proliferative than in mild dysplasia. Individual cells also appear less mature. Binucleated and multinucleated cells are present. Koilocytosis is seen in the superficial layers.

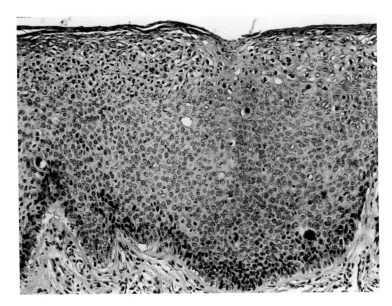

Figure 6–12. VIN III, severe squamous dysplasia. This highly cellular lesion comprises immature cells with a relatively uniform nuclear size and shape. Scattered corps ronds and mitotic figures are present.

vere dysplasia (Fig. 6–12), and carcinoma in situ (Fig. 6–13).

VIN I has the appearance of flat condyloma or atypical condyloma, in which koilocytosis is evident in the intermediate and superficial layers. In the lower third of the epithelium, mitotic activity is increased and mild nuclear atypia is evident. The basal cell layer is often maintained (see Figs. 6–9 and 6–10).

In VIN II, a greater degree of cellular proliferation occurs in the lower two thirds of the epithelium. The proliferating cells appear parabasal-like and present with increased mitotic activity and often are associated with abnormal mitotic figures (see Fig. 6–11).

In VIN III, abnormal cells with severe nuclear atypia, increased mitotic activity, and abnormal mitotic figures extend almost through the entire thickness of the epithelium with varying degrees of surface abnormality (see Figs. 6–12 and 6–13).

Skipped areas of uninvolved squamous epithelium are sometimes found within the lesions. The transition from normal to abnormal epithelium is generally sharp.

In all grades of VIN, abnormal epithelium has hyperkeratotic and parakeratotic layers, beneath which the keratinocytes often contain coarse and numerous keratohyaline granules (see Figs. 6–9, 6–10, and 6–11A). The degree

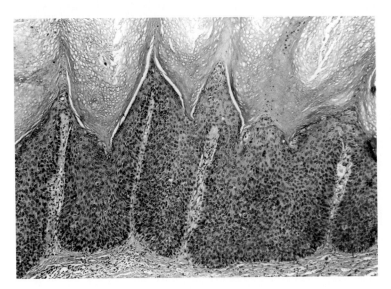

Figure 6–13. VIN III, warty squamous cell carcinoma in situ. The surface is papillomatous, hyperkeratotic, and parakeratotic. Immature cells occupy the entire thickness of the epithelium. (H&E, ×80)

of squamous maturation, manifested by the amount of eosinophilic cytoplasm and the nucleocytoplasmic ratios, varies considerably from lesion to lesion and even within the same lesion. Most mild and moderate dysplasias retain squamous differentiation (see Figs. 6–9, 6–10, and 6–11). Even in severe dysplasia and carcinoma in situ, maturation is apparent in the superficial layers (see Figs. 6–12 and 16–13). Scattered throughout the epithelium are dyskeratotic cells with pyknotic nuclei and densely eosinophilic homogeneous cytoplasm (Fig. 6–14). Some have the appearance of corps ronds, with a central, round pyknotic nucleus, a clear halo, and an outer eosinophilic shell (see Fig. 6–14). Mitotic figures are abundant and found at all levels of the epithelium (Fig. 6–15). Abnormal forms can be found in a majority of cases.[83]

In some lesions, a majority of the atypical cells are vacuolated or "pagetoid," with clear, slightly granular acidophilic cytoplasm (see Fig. 6–15).[89] Such cells can be distinguished from Paget's cells by the lack of mucin on histochemical stains. Also present are giant mononucleated and multinucleated cells. Small epithelial pearls comprising well-differentiated cells arranged in concentric whorls are sometimes found, especially in the deep layers (Fig. 6–16). These epithelial pearls are found in 16% of in situ carcinomas,[81] and 25% of these contain foci of early stromal invasion. When this feature is present, it is prudent to search for invasive foci in the specimen.

Warty and basaloid VIN III have certain distinct features. However, the two types often overlap in the majority of VINs. For this reason, warty and basaloid VINs are discussed together.

In the warty type of VIN III, the surface is spiky owing to hyperkeratosis and parakeratosis. The proliferating cells are more mature than are the basaloid type and have more abundant eosinophilic cytoplasm, distinct cell borders, and large nuclei that are sometimes multinucleated. Mitotic activity is high. The nuclear cytoplasmic ratios are increased.

In contrast, the basaloid type of VIN III has

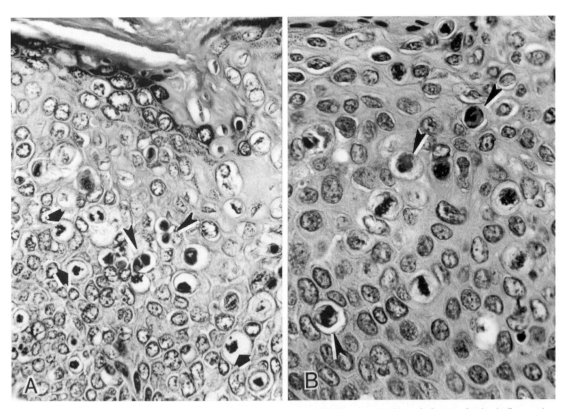

Figure 6–14. VIN III. *A* and *B*, Note the various forms of dyskeratotic cells (*arrowheads*) and abnormal mitotic figures (*arrows*). Corps ronds and dyskeratotic cells have pyknotic, homogeneous nuclei and densely eosinophilic cytoplasm. The cytoplasm sometimes has a thin rim of eosinophilic material between the perinuclear halo and outer clear space (*B*, left lower corner). Several abnormal metaphase mitoses are present (*arrows*).

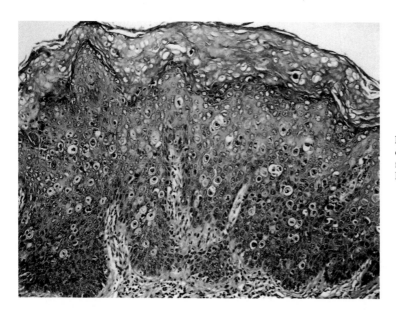

Figure 6–15. VIN III, warty squamous cell carcinoma in situ. Scattered corps ronds and dyskeratotic cells simulate Paget's disease.

a smooth surface with a variable amount of keratin debris. The proliferating cells are immature and resemble parabasal cells. In many cases, they resemble classic carcinoma in situ of the cervix (Fig. 6–17).

Features Shared by Warty and Basaloid VIN III

An increase of melanin pigment is found in the basal and parabasal layers of the epithelium, either focally or extensively, in a majority of cases (Fig. 6–18). Involvement of the pilosebaceous structures is found in two thirds of cases.[2,3] Basally located atypical cells extend into the

outer root sheath and eventually replace the sebaceous glands (Fig. 6–19A and B). Depending on the plane of sectioning, hair shafts and the lobular pattern of the involved pilosebaceous units may still be recognizable (see Fig. 6–19C). Equally common is the finding that the involved units are completely separated from the epidermis, leaving only isolated nests of atypical cells located in the deep dermis (see Fig. 6–19C). In such cases, an erroneous interpretation of invasive carcinoma may occur. Multiple, deeper cuts are often helpful to confirm the connection with pilosebaceous units or lack of stromal invasion. Depending on the

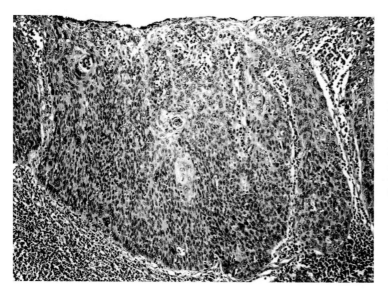

Figure 6–16. VIN III, squamous cell carcinoma in situ. A few clusters of better-differentiated cells having eosinophilic cytoplasm and forming small whorls occur in the background of immature cells. Serial sections reveal an early invasive squamous cell carcinoma adjacent to this focus.

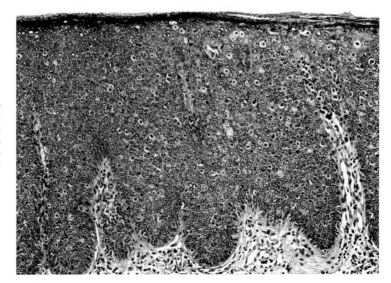

Figure 6–17. VIN III, basaloid squamous cell carcinoma in situ. It is made up entirely of small, primitive cells with scanty cytoplasm. Numerous corps ronds, dyskeratotic cells, and mitotic figures are found throughout the epithelium.

anatomic location of the lesion, direct extension into the periurethral glands and Bartholin's gland can occur (see Fig. 6–19D).

Tangential sections of epithelial clefts and folds at the base of a polypoid lesion often result in irregular clusters of atypical cells within the dermis (Fig. 6–20). The rete pegs may likewise appear irregular in size and shape (Fig. 6–21) and may be mistaken for invasive carcinoma. However, a careful examination of the dermis reveals no desmoplastic reaction to support stromal invasion. Lymphocytes, histocytes, and sometimes plasma cells are present in the dermis in 90% of cases.[81] The capillaries in the papillary layer are dilated and tortuous. Fibrosis may be present in varying degrees.

Baggish et al.[8] measured the thickness of vulvar carcinoma in situ. The epidermal thickness varies from 0.35 to 1.66 mm (mean 0.93 ± 0.37 mm). Thirty-six percent of the lesions involve skin appendages and measure 1.53 ± 0.77 mm. This study implies that to eradicate 95% of carcinoma in situ, the depth of tissue destruction needs to reach 2.5 mm by laser evaporation.

In a study by Wright and Chapman,[220] the normal skin had a mean thickness of 0.31 ± 0.11 mm. In the nonhairy area involved by VIN,

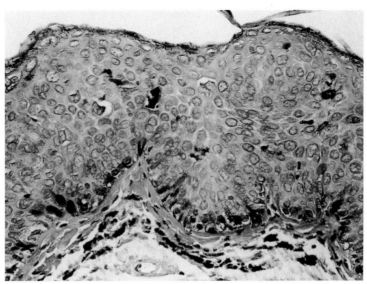

Figure 6–18. An increase of dendritic cells, hyperpigmentation of the basal cells, and melanophages in the dermis contribute to the pigmented appearance of squamous cell carcinoma in situ.

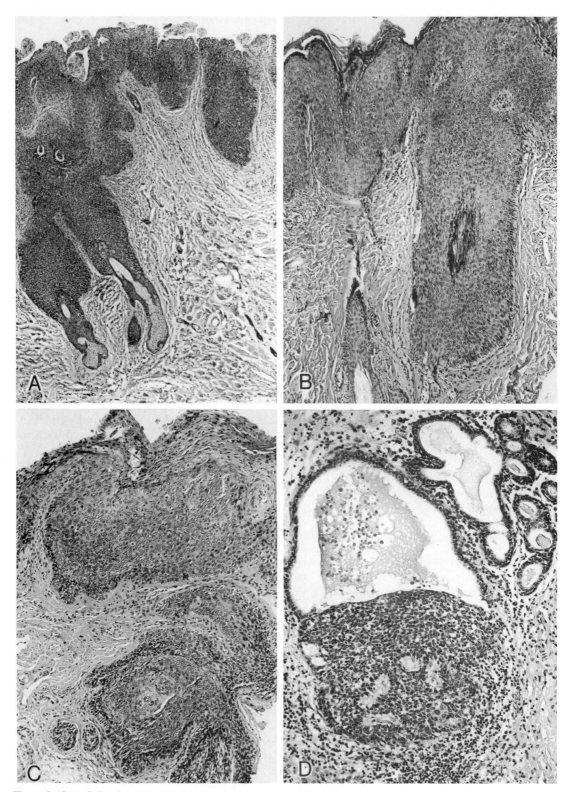

Figure 6–19. *A,* Cells of squamous cell carcinoma in situ extend into the hair follicle and sebaceous gland. *B,* They have replaced the hair sheath cells, leaving only the hair shaft in the center. *C,* An oblique cut of the involved pilosebaceous unit results in isolated nests and bulky, solid sheets of neoplastic cells. The lobular and branching patterns correspond to the pre-existing sebaceous ducts and glands. Note the lack of desmoplasia in the adjacent stroma. *D,* Cells of squamous cell carcinoma in situ extend into the duct of the Bartholin's gland.

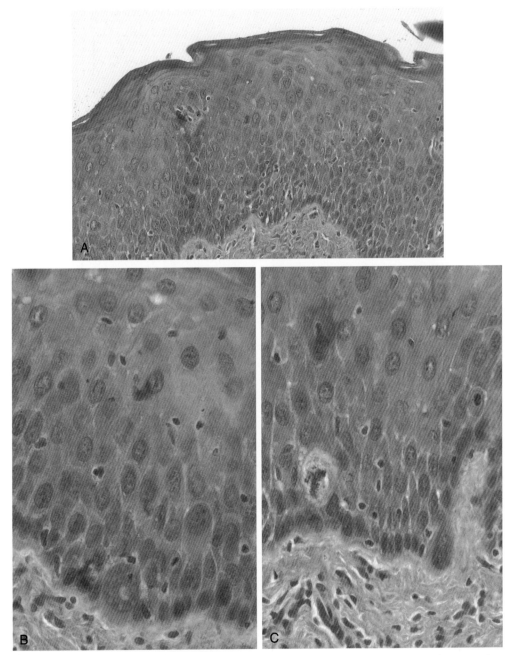

Figure 6–23. Simplex type of VIN I. *A*, Low-power view resembles mild hyperplasia. *B*, On closer examination of deep layers, atypical cells with large nuclei occur in the basal and parabasal layers. *C*, Atypical mitotic figures and atypical cells occur in the deep layers.

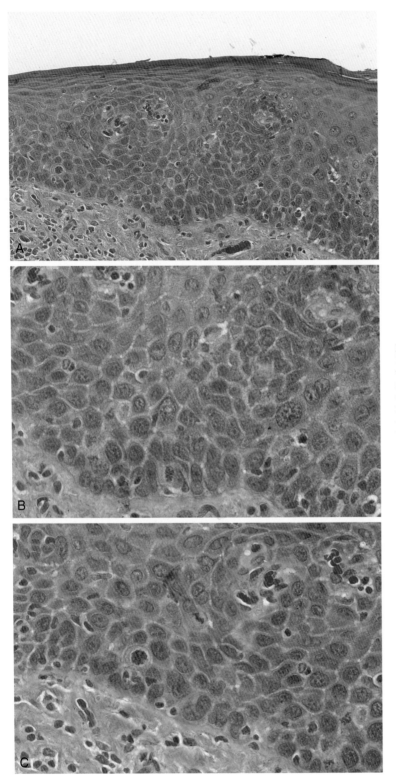

Figure 6–24. Simplex type of VIN II. *A,* Low-power view resembles hyperplasia with hyperkeratosis. *B* and *C,* Higher magnification reveals atypical immature cells occupying the lower half of the epithelium. A distinct layer of normal basal cells is replaced by a disorderly arrangement of atypical cells.

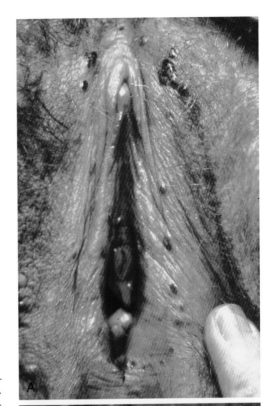

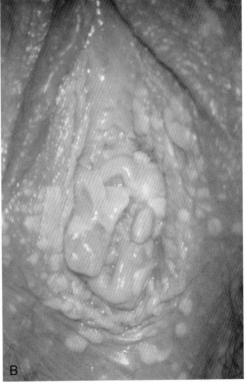

Figure 6–28. Clinical appearance of bowenoid papulosis. *A,* Multiple small, raised, dark brown nodules about 1 to 3 mm in size. *B,* Multiple small, warty, gray-white lesions in the lower vulva. (Courtesy of Edward J. Wilkinson, M.D., University of Florida, College of Medicine, Gainesville, Florida.)

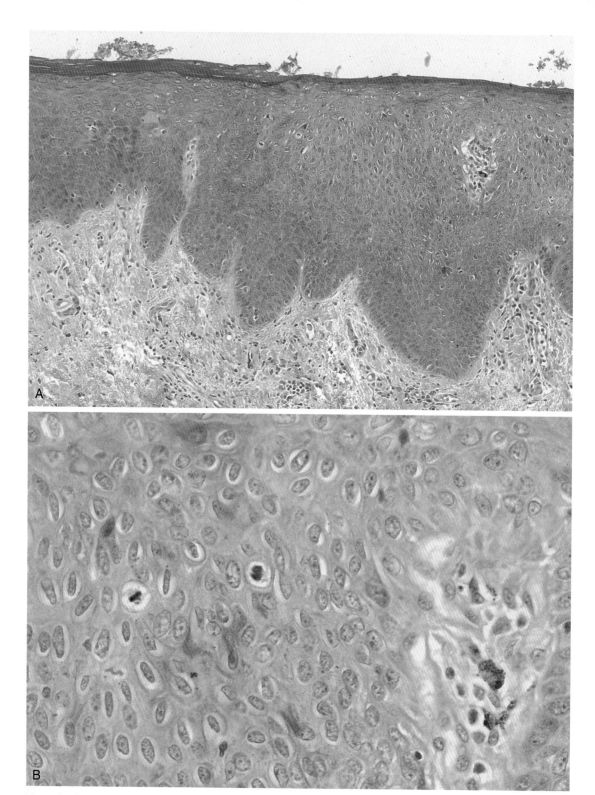

Figure 6–29. VIN I, mild squamous dysplasia, biopsy of bowenoid papulosis. *A,* A comparison of normal epidermis on the left and abnormal epithelium on the right. In the latter, proliferation of monotonous squamous cells can be seen. *B,* Higher magnification to demonstrate proliferating cells with mild nuclear atypia and scattered mitotic figures. Melanophages occur in the papillary dermis.

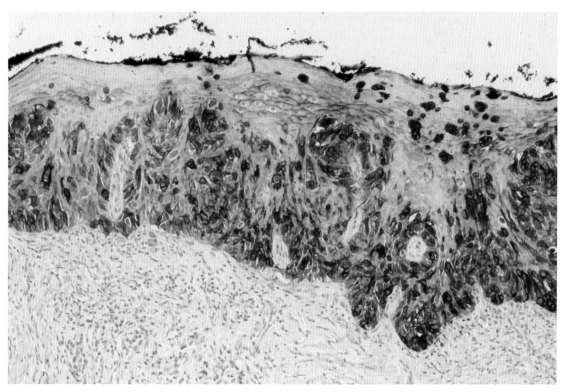

Figure 6–36. Paget's disease with immunohistochemical stain for carcinoembryonic antigen. Paget's cells are strongly positive for CEA and migrate through the epidermis.

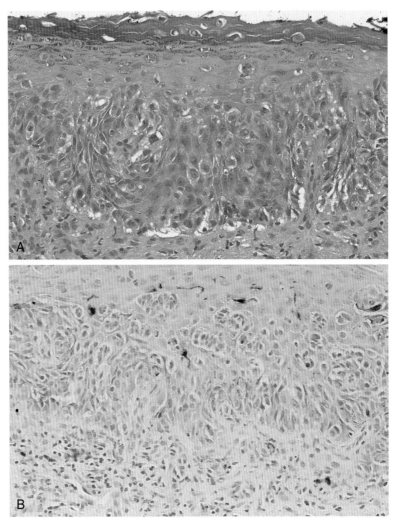

Figure 6–37. *A*, Paget's disease with dendritic cell hyperplasia simulating superficial spreading melanoma. *B*, Immunohistochemical stain for S-100 protein demonstrates dendritic cells with multipolar processes. Paget's cells are negative for S-100 protein, which rules out melanoma.

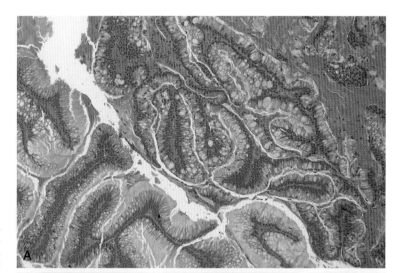

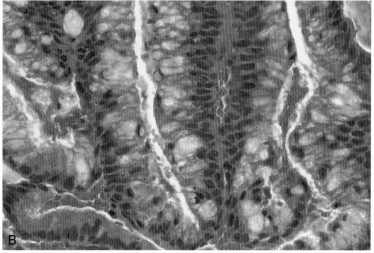

Figure 6–54. Well-differentiated mucinous adenocarcinoma of Bartholin's gland. *A*, Tumor cells form villous projections. *B*, Tall columnar cells demonstrate one to two layers of nuclear stratification and mild nuclear atypia resembling colonic adenoma.

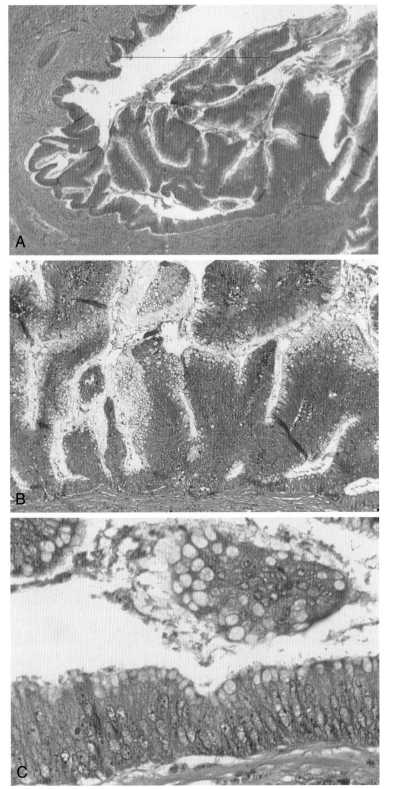

Figure 6–55. Well-differentiated papillary adenocarcinoma of Bartholin's gland. *A,* Papillary cystic tumor. *B,* Multiple papillary projections. *C,* Tumor cells present with nuclear stratification, moderate nuclear atypia, and multiple nucleoli.

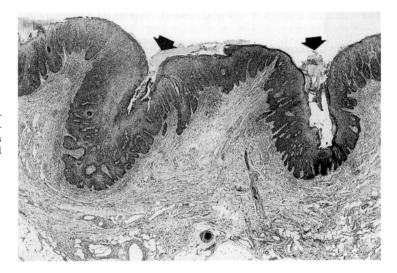

Figure 6–20. A polypoid, raised squamous carcinoma in situ with deep epithelial clefts (*arrows*). Tangential cuts of the clefts often produce bulky and irregular rete pegs.

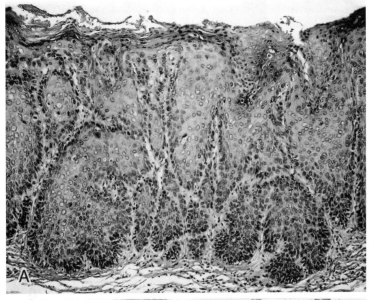

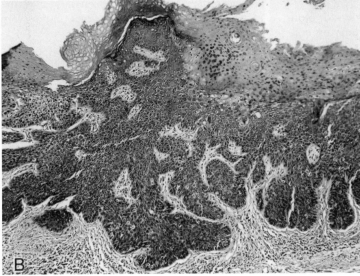

Figure 6–21. Squamous cell carcinoma in situ cut obliquely through the rete pegs (*A*) and a hair follicle (*B*). Note the well-defined base of epithelium, smooth configuration of the rete pegs, and a lack of desmoplasia in the dermis.

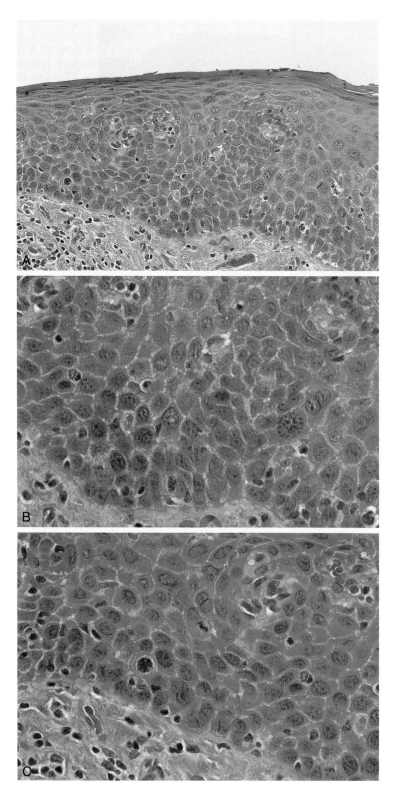

Figure 6–24. Simplex type of VIN II. *A*, Low-power view resembles hyperplasia with hyperkeratosis. *B* and *C*, Higher magnification reveals atypical immature cells occupying the lower half of the epithelium. A distinct layer of normal basal cells is replaced by a disorderly arrangement of atypical cells. (See color section.)

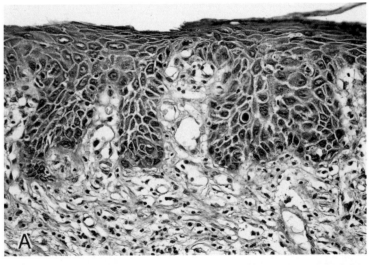

Figure 6–25. Simplex type of VIN III. The abnormal cells in the superficial layers retain a mature appearance. In the deep layers, cellular proliferation and increased mitotic activity occur. The rete pegs are prominent. The degree of nuclear atypia and cellular disorganization is mild (*A*), moderate (*B*), and severe (*C*). An island of better-differentiated cells with early whorl formation can also be seen in *C*.

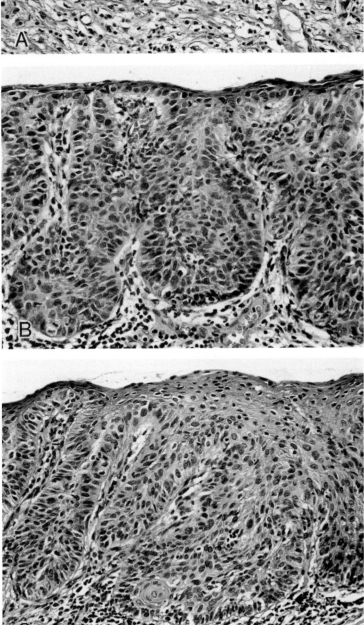

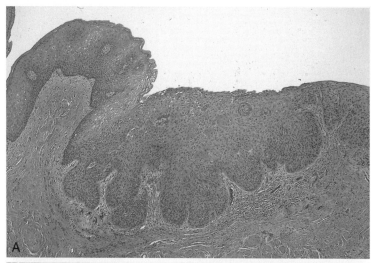

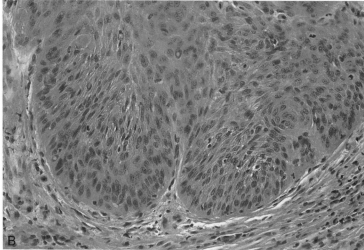

Figure 6–26. Simplex type of VIN III that progressed to invasive squamous carcinoma. *A,* VIN III with bulky rete pegs. *B,* Immature atypical cells in the deep layers. *C,* Early stromal invasion by multiple branching rete pegs, some of which contain keratin pearls. *D,* Another focus of stromal invasion consisting of irregular nests of tumor cells extending into the stroma.

Micheletti et al.[151] Of the 21 lesions previously diagnosed histologically as hyperplastic dystrophy with mild atypia or VIN I, only 4 (19%) were accepted by the reviewers as such. It is important to carefully assess the nuclear atypia, mitotic activity, and cellular polarity to distinguish reactive hyperplasia from VIN.

In a study by McLachin et al.,[147] 12 cases had the appearance of multinucleated atypia of the vulva. Multinucleated giant cells occurred in the middle and lower third of the epithelium. The nuclei were generally 2 to 10 in number, slightly hyperchromatic, and irregular and contained nucleoli. The mean age of the women was 37 years (range 22 to 56 years). They presented with leukoplakia, irritation, or pigmented lesion of the vulva.

The multinucleated atypia of the vulva do not contain atypical cells with hyperchromatic nuclei or abnormal mitotic figures typically seen in VIN. In addition, the binucleated or multinucleated giant cells in condyloma typically occur in the intermediate and superficial layers. In this atypia, giant cells were found in the middle and lower thirds of the epithelium. It is believed to be a reactive change.[134]

Ultrastructural Features

In the cells of Bowen's disease, the tonofilaments are scanty, whereas cytoplasmic organelles, including polyribosomes, mitochondria, and Golgi complexes, are abundant,[140,141,163] The nuclei contain coarse, irregularly shaped chromatinic clumps. The chromatin material beneath the nuclear membrane is irregular in thickness (see Fig. 6–23). Nuclear bodies and inclusions are often present. The cell mem-

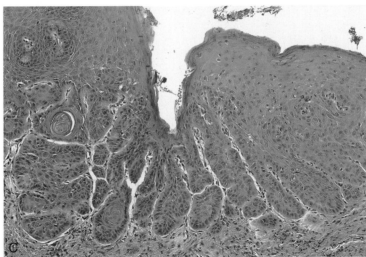

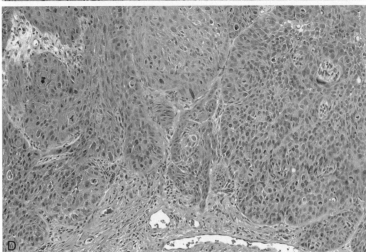

Figure 6–26. *Continued*

branes exhibit microvillus processes projecting into dilated intercellular spaces (see Fig. 6–23). The desmosomes are few in number, small, and poorly developed.[140,141,163] These ultrastructural features suggest an increase in cellular activity and lack of maturation.

Also present are scattered, degenerated abnormal cells engulfed by neighboring cells (Fig. 6–27). The corps ronds are characterized by multiple membrane-bound vacuoles around the pyknotic nucleus. Aggregates of thick, condensed tonofibrils account for the strong eosinophilia in the cytoplasm of dyskeratotic cells and corps ronds (see Fig. 6–27).[140,141,163] These vacuoles and aggregates of tonofibrils, as well as pyknotic nuclei, are signs of degeneration.

The basal lamina is usually intact.[140,141] However, foci of disrupted basal lamina with extension of cytoplasmic processes into the un-

derlying stroma have been observed in Bowen's disease and in bowenoid papulosis.[121,163] Whether this feature has any clinical significance remains to be clarified.

Multifocal and Confluent Bowen's Carcinoma In Situ

The multifocal nature of vulvar carcinoma in situ is supported by the clinical finding of multiple, discrete lesions and the development of new lesions at different sites after the initial complete excision. In a study by Japaze et al.,[113] 45% of the lesions were multifocal. In a study by Forney et al.,[69] the disease was unifocal in 14 cases, multifocal in 15 cases, and extended beyond the true vulva onto the perianal mucosa in 5 cases. Multifocal lesions had a tendency to become confluent. The patients were

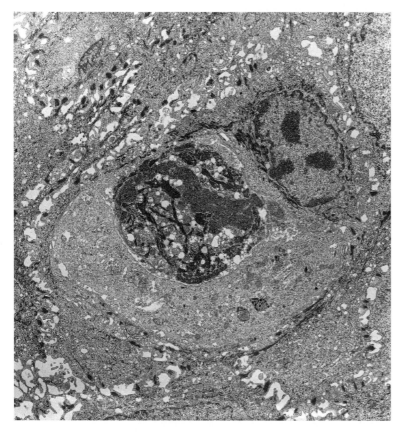

Figure 6–27. Ultrastructural appearance of a dyskeratotic cell characterized by condensed masses of chromatin corresponding to the pyknotic nucleus and coarse bundles of tonofib-rils, which attribute to the densely eosinophilic cytoplasm seen in H&E slide. The adjacent well-preserved cells contain varying amounts of tonofilaments, and their peripheral cell membranes exhibit complex, microvillus processes. The nuclear chromatin forms coarse aggregates. This feature is characteristic of immature cells with high proliferative activities. (×5880)

young, with a mean age of 31 years,[69] and cervical or vaginal intraepithelial neoplasia was found in 38% of the cases.[55] In a study by Friedrich et al.,[81] 70% of the vulvar carcinomas in situ were multifocal (see Fig. 6–8A) or large, confluent (see Fig. 6–8B) lesions.

According to nuclear DNA ploidy analysis, 80% of the multifocal carcinomas in situ had different stem cell lines.[210] In addition, stem cell lines in two recurrent lesions also differed from those of the original neoplasia, supporting the clinical observation of multicentric origin.[81] Among the confluent lesions, analysis of DNA ploidy in different areas of the same lesions demonstrated distinct stem cell lines in four of six specimens. This finding can be explained by the development of new stem cell lines in confluent lesions or the merger of several lesions having variable stem cell lines to become a confluent lesion.[210]

Van Beurden et al.[198] applied PCR and reverse transcriptase-PCR to detect E6/E7 transcripts in multifocal VIN III samples. These VINs included 46% warty type, 17% basaloid type, 35% mixed type, and 2% differentiated type. HPV DNA was detected in 92%, including 83% with type 16.

In a subsequent study, 27 women with VIN III and concomitant CIN or vaginal intraepithelial neoplasia (VAIN) were studied.[198] Twenty-five (93%) cases of lesions had HPV type 16, one had HPV type 33, and one had type 45. The HPV type was similar in 78%, but different in 22% (six cases). The latter included three women with HPV 16 in VIN and HPV 31 in CIN. The other had HPV 16 in VIN and unidentified type in CIN. One had HPV 16 in VIN and unidentified type in VAIN. One had HPV 45 in VIN and HPV 31 in CIN. The authors found HPV type 16 to be the predominant type and suggested immune deficiency against this infection as a possible explanation for the development of multicentric disease in the lower genital tract.[199]

Despite a high frequency of multicentric vulvar carcinoma in situ, only 2 of 86 invasive vulvar carcinomas were multifocal in origin.[113] It has been suggested that not all vulvar carcinomas in situ have the same potential for undergoing invasion.[113]

Incidence of Second In Situ and Invasive Malignant Neoplasm

In a study by Herod et al.,[102] 37% of the women studied had concurrent or previous CIN, 6% had vaginal intraepithelial neoplasia, and 4% had anal intraepithelial neoplasia.

Overall, one third of the women with vulvar squamous carcinoma in situ had previously, or subsequently, developed in situ or invasive neoplasms elsewhere in the genital tract (18% to 38%) or extragenital organs (4% to 5%).[2,30,69,81,113,218] In the female genital tract, in situ and invasive squamous carcinomas of the uterine cervix are most common.[2,30,55,69,81,113,218]

Multicentric Pigmented Bowen's Disease (Bowenoid Papulosis)

The term *multicentric pigmented Bowen's disease* was used initially by Lloyd.[138] Subsequently, Wade et al.[203,204] adapted the term *bowenoid papulosis* for similar lesions. In most instances, bowenoid papulosis affects the anogenital areas of both sexes, especially the penile glans and shaft, and vulvar skin. It occasionally in-volves the skin of the abdomen, axilla, and nipple.[16,19,121,190,203,204] A slight predominance occurs in females.[92,171] It is likely that some reported cases of regressed vulvar atypia and multifocal carcinomas in situ[76,81,186] meet the criteria of bowenoid papulosis.

Bowenoid papulosis affects women between 6 and 55 years of age (mean 32 years). The peak incidence occurs in the third decade (50%), followed by the fourth decade.[171] Approximately 10% of patients are pregnant at the time of diagnosis. The lesions are known to exist from 2 months to 11 years (median 9 months).[171] Earlier reports emphasized the high frequency of multiplicity and small size (2 to 10 mm; mean 4 mm)[19,81,204] In a subsequent series, only two thirds of cases were multiple, and some lesions reached 3.3 cm (median 0.7 cm) in size.[171]

Typical lesions are slightly elevated, reddish-brown to violaceous papules, and some have slight scaling (Fig. 6–28). The papules may become confluent and form small plaques. On the vulva, the most common clinical impressions are condyloma, verrucae vulgaris, nevi, seborrheic keratosis, lichen planus, and psori-

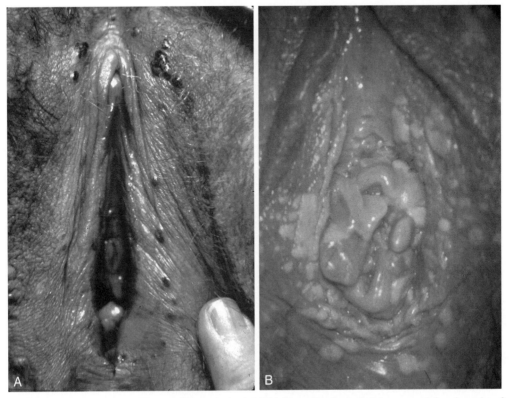

Figure 6–28. Clinical appearance of bowenoid papulosis. *A*, Multiple small, raised, dark brown nodules about 1 to 3 mm in size. *B*, Multiple small, warty, gray-white lesions in the lower vulva. (Courtesy of Edward J. Wilkinson, M.D., University of Florida, College of Medicine, Gainesville, Florida.) (See color section.)

asis.[171] A varying number of patients had had recent genital herpes or condyloma.

Despite the benign clinical appearance of these lesions, the histologic findings are those of mild dysplasia (Fig. 6–29), moderate dysplasia (Fig. 6–30), and carcinoma in situ (Fig. 6–31). Dyskeratotic cells and atypical cells with mitotic figures, including abnormal forms, are easily detected. Round, basophilic, inclusion-like bodies are often seen in the stratum corneum and granular cell layer. Several authors have emphasized the cellular uniformity,[196] the lack of follicular involvement (90%),[171,196] a frequent involvement of acrosyringium (88%),[171] normal mitotic figures[171] as distinctive features of bowenoid papulosis. Others have found abnormal mitotic figures and severe nuclear pleomorphism in bowenoid papulosis and are unable to distinguish bowenoid papulosis from typical carcinoma in situ based on clinical or morphologic criteria.[92] Bowenoid papulosis is an intraepithelial neoplasia that lacks distinct morphologic features to be recognized as a separate entity. The term *bowenoid papulosis* is best used to describe a clinical condition having a typical appearance.

Immunoperoxidase technique revealed that 5%[92] to 10%[25] of cases of bowenoid papulosis had demonstrable HPV capsid antigens. Hybridization technique showed that all 12 specimens had HPV type 16 DNA,[92] a high-risk group.[44,87] Fang et al. identified a variant of HPV 16 in a bowenoid papulosis.[59]

The clinical behavior of these lesions has been benign, with the majority controlled by local excision, local destruction, or topical 5-FU. However, 20% (15/74) of the patients had local recurrence,[171] and a few cases pro-

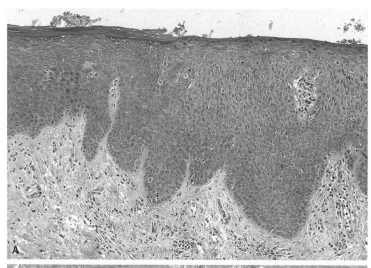

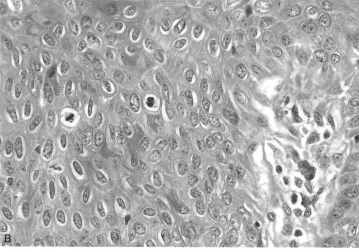

Figure 6–29. VIN I, mild squamous dysplasia, biopsy of bowenoid papulosis. *A,* A comparison of normal epidermis on the left and abnormal epithelium on the right. In the latter, proliferation of monotonous squamous cells can be seen. *B,* Higher magnification to demonstrate proliferating cells with mild nuclear atypia and scattered mitotic figures. Melanophages occur in the papillary dermis. (See color section.)

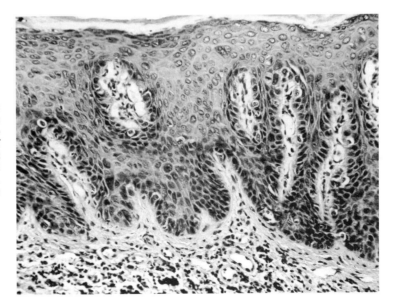

Figure 6–30. Biopsy of a vulvar lesion from a 23-year-old woman who has the multiple 3 to 5 mm pigmented lesions of the vulva clinically typical of bowenoid papulosis. Histologically, it demonstrates moderate dysplasia and hyperpigmentation of the basal layer. Melanophages are present in the dermis.

gressed to in situ or invasive carcinoma.[15,51] Thus, patients with bowenoid papulosis require adequate local treatment and close follow-up.

Prognosis of VIN

Depending on the size, number, and location of VIN, most patients receive some form of therapy, ranging from local excision to laser therapy, topical 5-fluorouracil (5-FU), or vulvectomy.[7,62,69,81] Persistent or recurrent disease occurs in 7% to 25% of patients following surgical excision.[2,45,116] Extension into the anal mucosa is a major source of treatment failure. The response to topical 5-FU is highly variable, perhaps influenced by the thickness of the keratin layer and involvement of pilosebaceous structures. In one study, local recurrence was higher with laser vaporization than with local excision (75% versus 40%, P <0.001).[102]

In surgically excised specimens for VIN III, occult invasive squamous carcinoma was found in 8% (3/37) of cases. These carcinomas were all less than 1 mm in depth. All patients were disease free at the time of report.[81]

In a study by Chafe et al.,[36] 69 women with

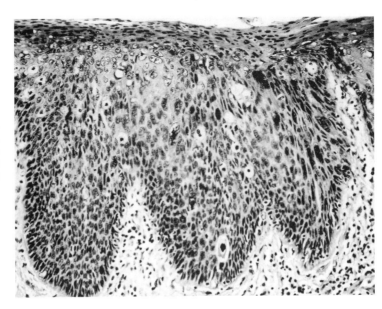

Figure 6–31. Biopsy from a young female of a vulvar lesion with clinical features of bowenoid papulosis. The histologic findings are indistinguishable from those of squamous cell carcinoma in situ.

VIN III underwent surgical excision. Thirteen (18.8%) had coexisting invasive carcinoma. Of these, eight (62%) tumors were less than 1 mm and four (31%) were more than 1 mm, and one had a verrucous carcinoma. Raised lesions with an irregular surface in elderly women are particularly likely to have occult invasive carcinoma.[36] The mean age for VIN only is 36 years, as compared with 58 years for invasive carcinoma ($P \leq 0.0034$).[36]

Following surgical excision for VIN III, 3.8%,[116] 7%,[102] 8%,[81] and up to 12%[45] of women subsequently developed invasive squamous cell carcinoma. All of these women were immunosuppressed or older than 45 years.[29,45,81,116]

What would happen if VIN grade III lesions were left untreated? In a study by Jones and Rowan,[116] eight women had only biopsy or grossly incomplete excision. Seven (88%) of them developed invasive carcinoma in 2 to 8 years.[116] The lesion of the eighth woman regressed without further treatment.[116]

In a study by Herod et al.,[102] 19 women were followed medically without surgical excision, including eight cases of VIN I, five of VIN II, and six of VIN III. During a mean follow-up period of 30 months, none progressed to invasive carcinoma, but eight women required surgical treatment.[102]

Spontaneous regression without treatment for VIN III was noted in 10% (5 of 50) of women.[81] All five women were young, with a mean age of 21.2 years, and had multifocal, raised lesions.[81] These lesions most likely represent bowenoid papulosis.

In summary, for women with VIN III the recurrent or persistent rate following various treatment modalities is in the range of 25%. Following surgical resection, 3.8% to 12% of women developed invasive squamous cell carcinoma. Based on a few untreated VIN III lesions, as many as 88% of VIN III lesions were reported to have progressed to invasive carcinoma. Spontaneous regression of VIN III lesions was most likely bowenoid papulosis in young women.

Vulvar Intraepithelial Neoplasia of Glandular Type

Paget's Disease

Since the initial report by Sir James Paget in 1874, Paget's disease of the nipple has become a well-recognized clinical and pathologic entity. It has also been described in extramammary sites, including the eyelid, axilla, perianal region, mons pubis, glans penis, and vulva. Although the histologic features of Paget's disease of various sites are similar, their natural history and morphogenesis differ.

Clinical Features

Most patients with Paget's disease of the vulva are white and postmenopausal. Among the reported series, the ages varied from 38 to 87 years, with an average of 58.5 to 67 years.[41,61,126,135,195] Sixty-five percent of patients were older than 60 years of age.[84] Pruritus, irritation, a burning sensation, and discomfort were the primary complaints and usually had been present for many years.

The lesions appear as erythematous, eczematous, and indurated, with scattered islands of hyperkeratosis giving a white, speckled appearance (Fig. 6–32). They frequently are ulcerated, moist, and oozing, and they bleed readily on contact. The margins are generally well demarcated and sometimes irregular. The presence of induration or a palpable mass suggests an underlying carcinoma. The affected skin ranges from less than 1 cm to more than 10 cm in dimension. The labia majora are most frequently affected, and multiple sites of involvement are common among extensive lesions. The extent of the disease is closely correlated with the duration of symptoms.[135]

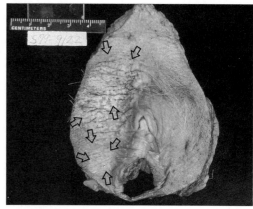

Figure 6–32. Paget's disease of the right vulva. Two thickened plaque-like lesions with a granular, whitish appearance.

Pathologic Features

The diagnostic features of Paget's disease are isolated or aggregated large, pale cells in the epidermis. Their pale-staining, sometimes clear, vacuolated cytoplasm is readily recognized under low-power magnification. Paget's cells are most numerous in the deep layers and rete pegs. Nests of Paget's cells are separated from the dermis by an attenuated layer of basal squamous cells and an intact basement membrane. Glandular lumens with their secretory products are reported in 50% to 90% of cases.[126,135] In the upper epidermis, Paget's cells tend to become isolated and fewer in number and often exhibit an ameboid migration pattern that resembles that of superficial spreading malignant melanoma (Fig. 6–33A and B).

Individual Paget's cells are characterized by abundant pale, foamy, vacuolated cytoplasm, which is less frequently finely granular or clear.

The nuclei are large and eccentrically located. A signet-ring appearance is occasionally seen. The nucleoli are usually prominent. Cells obtained by imprint or scraping of the lesion also retain these features.[14]

In about 50% of cases, hyperkeratosis and parakeratosis with a verrucous papillomatous appearance are apparent. Rare corps ronds and even nuclear atypia of squamous cells may be seen.[170] These features may lead to an erroneous diagnosis of Bowen's disease. Hawley et al.[98] reported a case of VIN III associated with invasive Paget's disease.

Involvement of the outer sheath of the hair follicles and pilosebaceous units is found in 80% of cases (see Fig. 6–33C).[126] This may extend to a considerable depth in the dermis. Involvement of the sweat ducts and, less frequently, the sweat glands may be observed. The reported frequency, however, is highly variable. In the dermis, a varying degree of chronic in-

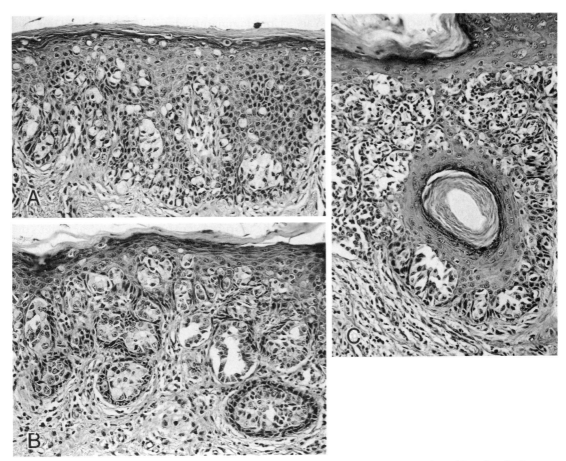

Figure 6–33. *A,* Paget's cells migrate through the epidermis in an ameboid pattern. The number of Paget's cells decreases from the basal layer to the superficial layer. *B,* Paget's cells appear in single form or in clusters with glandular lumen. They have abundant clear, vacuolated cytoplasm and atypical nuclear features. *C,* Involvement of the hair follicle is common.

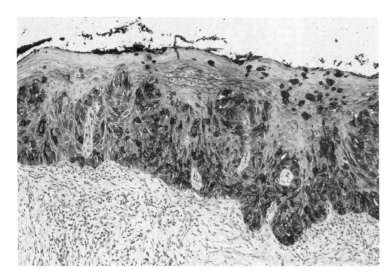

Figure 6–36. Paget's disease with immunohistochemical stain for carcinoembryonic antigen. Paget's cells are strongly positive for CEA and migrate through the epidermis. (See color section.)

Figure 6–37. *A,* Paget's disease with dendritic cell hyperplasia simulating superficial spreading melanoma. *B,* Immunohistochemical stain for S-100 protein demonstrates dendritic cells with multipolar processes. Paget's cells are negative for S-100 protein, which rules out melanoma. (See color section.)

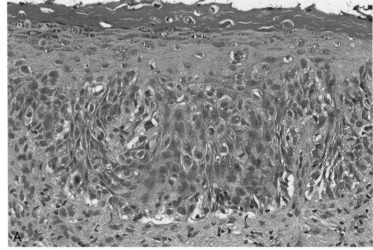

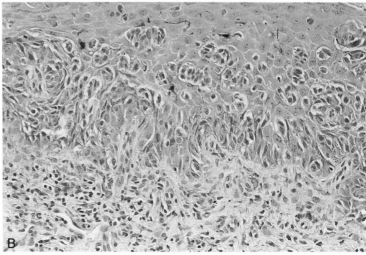

Ultrastructural Features

Ultrastructural studies of vulvar Paget's cells reveal glandular differentiation with membrane-bound secretory granules, well-developed Golgi membranes, profiles of endoplasmic reticulum, and occasionally mucinous droplets (Fig. 6–38).[125] Glandular lumens and intercellular spaces lined by microvilli are also present. A small number of cells do not contain secretory vacuoles and have scanty cytoplasmic organelles, occasional glycogen particles, and microfilaments. Paget's cells are joined by tight junctions or small, poorly developed desmosomes. The latter are also found between the Paget's cells and neighboring squamous cells.[125,159] Although most of the Paget's cells do not contain tonofibrils, Fetherston and Friedrich[64] reported tonofibrils and desmosomes in some Paget's cells, suggesting squamous differentiation. These findings of both glandular and squamous features in Paget's cells suggest to these researchers that Paget's disease may have originated from multipotential basal cells.[64]

The cells of invasive carcinoma of the sweat glands share the same features as those of Paget's cells. The invasive cells, however, contain fewer secretory granules than those of epidermal Paget's cells.[125,135]

Morphogenesis

In mammary Paget's disease, almost all cases have associated intraductal or invasive ductal carcinoma of the breast. Rarely, the malignant cells are confined to the lactiferous ducts.[168] Consequently, most authors believe that Paget's disease of the nipple results from migration of underlying malignant cells through the existing mammary and lactiferous ducts that subsequently results in invasion of the epi-

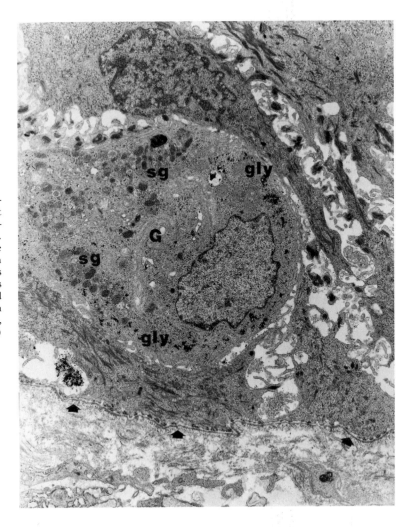

Figure 6–38. This electron micrograph shows a Paget's cell just above a basal cell, which is ensheathed by basal lamina (*arrows*). The Paget's cell contains multiple secretory granules (sg), glycogen particles (gly), and Golgi complexes (G). The adjacent squamous cells have abundant tonofilaments and desmosomes. (×11,250; From Roth LM, et al. Am J Surg Pathol 1:193, 1977, Fig. 7; used with permission.)

dermis. Similarly, perianal Paget's disease frequently coexists with underlying sweat gland or anorectal carcinomas. In contrast, only 30% of patients with vulvar Paget's disease have demonstrable in situ or invasive adnexal carcinoma, and the remaining 70% have purely intraepidermal carcinoma (see Table 6–1).

Two major viewpoints on the morphogenesis of Paget's disease have been expressed. The first hypothesis suggests an origin from the basal or suprabasal layer of the epidermis and its appendages, including the intraepidermal sweat ducts.[84,100] Embryologically, the cells of stratum germinativum, which give rise to the epidermis and various adnexal tissues, are believed to be multipotential. Anatomically, the ducts of the apocrine sweat gland are connected to the pilosebaceous unit and rarely drain directly onto the skin surface. The eccrine sweat ducts open to the epidermis at the rete pegs through intraepidermal ducts; therefore, eccrine and apocrine structures are closely related to the epidermis and hair follicle.[100]

Pathologically, a higher concentration of Paget's cells in the parabasal layers, compared with the upper epidermis, supports an origin from cells located deep in the epidermis and pilosebaceous unit or the adnexal tissue. The latter possibility seems to be unlikely in four vulvectomy specimens subjected to total sectioning in which coiled portions of sweat glands were not involved.[93]

The second hypothesis suggests that Paget's cells are derived from the carcinoma of the sweat gland or Bartholin's gland.[126,135,191] Paget's cells reach the epidermis by upward migration through the pre-existing ducts. Demonstration of underlying malignancy requires extensive sampling and serial sections. Unlike the long, dilated lactiferous ducts of the nipple, the sweat glands are small and the course of intraepidermal sweat ducts is short. Inflammation often obscures or destroys the sweat ducts. By total embedding and semiserial sectioning of five vulvectomy specimens, it was observed that all had demonstrable in situ carcinoma of the sweat glands. In addition, two had invasive carcinoma.[135] In another report of six specimens studied by "ample" sections, four had in situ carcinoma and one had invasive carcinoma of the sweat gland.[126] Other authors considered in situ carcinoma of the sweat gland to represent downward extension of intraepithelial Paget's disease.[84,100]

It is of interest that extramammary Paget's disease has a tendency to occur in areas rich in apocrine sweat glands, such as the axilla, perianal region, vulva, scrotum, nasal vestibule, and eyelid (Moll's gland). In vulvar Paget's disease, only some of the in situ and invasive carcinomas of the sweat glands are clearly of the apocrine type.[135] Electron-microscopic studies suggest an origin from the eccrine sweat glands in some cases[63,126] and an equivocal origin in most disease.[84,159,181]

In normal skin, the presence of carcinoembryonic antigen and milk fat globules in eccrine and apocrine sweat has been demonstrated by the immunoperoxidase technique.[157,202] It is not surprising that these antigens are also expressed in mammary and extramammary Paget's disease.[157,202] Gross cystic disease fluid protein-15, which is reactive with apocrine but nonreactive with the eccrine sweat gland, has been demonstrated in six of seven cases of extramammary Paget's disease, including all five vulvar cases.[145] These immunostains, in addition to supporting an apocrine origin, are useful diagnostically.

It is reasonable to conclude that approximately 30% of women with vulvar Paget's disease have underlying carcinoma. The remaining 70% of cases are intraepithelial carcinomas. Despite repeated recurrences over long periods of time, the disease has remained intraepithelial, and no underlying carcinoma can be detected in most of these patients.[84] Only rarely does Paget's disease progress to invasive carcinoma.

Prognosis

The prognosis of vulvar Paget's disease depends on the extent of epidermal involvement and whether invasive carcinoma is present. In lesions confined to the epidermis, the clinical course is often protracted, with frequent recurrences even after seemingly adequate surgical resection. In a review of reported cases, 28% to 38% of patients developed recurrence after surgery.[84,195] The recurrence in more than half of the cases appeared within 18 months of initial treatment.[84]

In attempting to explain this high recurrence rate, four vulvectomy specimens were studied by subserial total sectioning.[93] It was found that the extent of histologic involvement in each case was far greater than the clinical appearance of the lesion indicated. Paget's cells spread horizontally into the grossly normal skin to a considerable distance. The outline of the lesion is irregular, making detection of involved margins difficult unless the peripheral aspect of the process is studied comprehensively. Furthermore, multicentric, discrete, separate foci are found in all cases. These findings—that is, multicentricity, irregular borders, and undetected cellular involvement—are the basis of frequent recurrences. Examination of the entire surgical margins by frozen section, although time-consuming, is recommended by some authors.[135]

Fishman et al.[68] reported the accuracy of frozen section diagnosis on vulvar Paget's disease. Of the frozen sections on excision margins, 38% were reported as negative; however, the permanent sections were positive. Two of five (40%) with positive margins recurred, as compared to three of nine (33%) with negative margins. The authors question the value of frozen section diagnosis on the excision margins.[68]

Direct extension of Paget's disease into the hair follicles, sweat ducts, and sweat glands does not appear to have prognostic significance.[135] These cases can be treated in the same manner as those confined to the epidermis, that is, with partial, total, or simple vulvectomy with adequate margin, and especially the perineal margin. Recurrences are re-excised for careful histologic study, because intraepithelial Paget's disease of the vulva may occasionally become invasive and metastasize.

DiSaia et al.[54] reported a case of recurrent Paget's disease in a split-thickness graft. The authors favor the theory of migration of the tumor cells from the adjacent skin with Paget's disease as causing local recurrence.

In the presence of underlying invasive adnexal carcinoma, the prognosis is poor because of the high recurrence rate and the propensity for lymph node metastasis.[65] Of the 28 patients with invasive carcinoma collected from the literature, 23 had follow-up information. Of these, 14 patients (61%) had a total of 22 local recurrences, and 11 (48%) had lymph node metastases. All 11 died in less than 5 years.[21] Of the 38 cases of anogenital Paget's disease reported by Helwig and Graham,[100] 13 had invasive adenocarcinoma. Of these, 11 had lymph node metastasis, and all died of the disease. Because of the poor prognosis in association with invasive adnexal carcinoma, radical vulvectomy with bilateral inguinal lymphadenectomy is recommended.[195]

Progression from intraepithelial Paget's disease to invasive adenocarcinoma, although rare, has been well documented.[88] Minimally invasive Paget's disease is defined as having a depth of invasion of less than 1 mm from the basement membrane.[67] Even with this depth of invasion, local recurrence and lymph node metastasis were reported.

Fine et al.[67] reported an invasive Paget's disease with a 1 mm depth and 10 mm size. After the hemivulvectomy, multiple bilateral inguinal lymph node metastases developed and were removed by lymphadenectomy.

I have seen two cases of Paget's disease in which invasive carcinoma occurred directly from the epidermis (Fig. 6–39). In both patients, the tumor had a depth of 3 mm, measuring from the base of epidermis. One patient had metastasis to an inguinal lymph node. In view of the lack of any underlying Paget's disease and a long history of vulvar symptoms, these 2 cases are interpreted as invasive Paget's disease.

Hart and Millman[96] described the development of an invasive Paget's disease (1 cm size, 4 to 5 mm depth) that metastasized to 2 of 30 inguinal lymph nodes 10.8 years after the initial simple vulvectomy for intraepithelial Paget's disease.

Kodama et al.[123] reported on 30 cases of vulvar Paget's disease, including 10 intraepithelial cases, 9 with minimally invasive carcinoma, and 11 with underlying carcinoma. Of the 10 women with intraepithelial Paget's disease, 3 had local recurrence. Of the nine women with minimally invasive carcinoma, one had local recurrence, one died of lung carcinoma, and the other eight were free of disease. Of the 11 women with underlying carcinoma, 7 died of disease, 1 was alive with disease, 2 showed no evidence of disease, and 1 died of cervical cancer.[123]

Association with Other Malignancies

Like Bowen's disease of the vulva, Paget's disease of the vulva is associated with an increased incidence of malignancies at other sites. In a review of eight reports, 30% of patients had carcinoma at other sites (see Table 6–1), a frequency greater than normally expected. Malignancy sites include the breast, rectum, cervix, urinary bladder, gallbladder, skin, and other sites. Among these, breast carcinoma is the most frequent. In one series 18% (14 of 78) had had breast carcinoma before, concomitant with, or after diagnosis of vulvar Paget's disease.[82] Although the development of breast and vulvar carcinoma do not appear to be related, it is interesting to note that both sites are in the "milk line." It is suggested that patients with Paget's disease of the

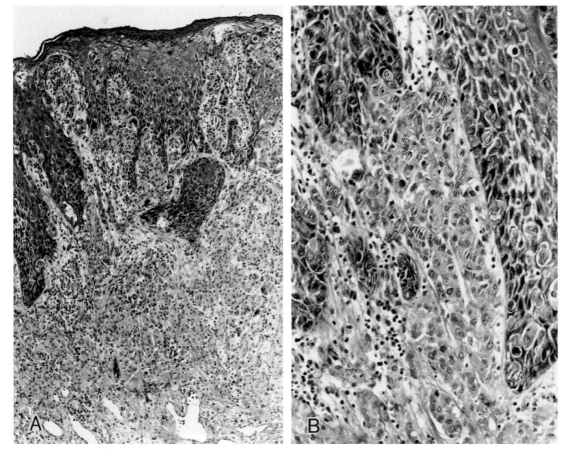

Figure 6–39. Invasive Paget's disease. *A,* The tumor cells arise from the base of epithelium and invade the dermis. *B,* A higher magnification demonstrates solid nests of poorly differentiated malignant cells with vacuolated cytoplasm. No carcinoma is found in the underlying sweat glands. Although the lesion is only 3 mm in depth, there is metastasis in the inguinal lymph nodes.

vulva should undergo a careful examination of the breasts.[82]

INVASIVE CARCINOMAS

Clinical Staging System

To assess the extent of vulvar malignancy, the International Federation of Gynecologists and Obstetricians (FIGO; Table 6–2) developed a clinical staging system.[39,40] The staging system is based on the extent of the tumor (T), the clinical status of the inguinal lymph node (N), and the presence or absence of distant metastasis (M).

Stage I tumors are less than 2 cm in diameter without suspicious groin lymph nodes. T1 tumors are subdivided into T1a, with stromal invasion of less than 1 mm, and T1b, with greater than 1 mm invasion. Stage II tumors in-

clude those greater than 2 cm in size, confined to the vulva, and not associated with suspicious groin lymph nodes. Stage III tumors extend beyond the vulva with involvement of the urethra, vagina, perineum, or anus. The groin lymph nodes may be nonpalpable or suspicious but are not clinically positive for metastasis. Any tumors with clinically positive groin lymph node, involvement of urinary bladder or rectum, fixation to bone, or metastasis to distant sites are classified as Stage IV tumors (see Table 6–2).

Other authors have proposed a postoperative staging system incorporating the site (clitoral versus labial) and histologic findings of lymph nodes into the classification system.[80,129,185]

Conventional Squamous Cell Carcinoma

Invasive squamous cell carcinoma constitutes approximately 80% of all primary vulvar ma-

Table 6–2. TNM Surgical Staging System for Squamous
Cell Carcinoma of the Vulva[39,40,107]

Primary Tumor (T)

TX	Primary tumor cannot be assessed
TO	No evidence of primary tumor
Tis	VIN IIII
TI	Tumor confined to the vulva/perineum, $\leq$2 cm in greatest dimension
	T1a as for T1 and with $\leq$1 mm of stromal invasion*
	T1b as for T1 and with >1 mm of stromal invasion†
T2	Tumor confined to vulva/perineum, >2 cm in greatest dimension
T3	Tumor of any size with adjacent spread to lower urethra or vagina or anus
T4	Tumor invades upper urethral mucosa, bladder mucosa, or rectal mucosa or is fixed to pubic bone

Regional Lymph Node(s)(N)

NX	Regional lymph nodes cannot be assessed
NO	No regional lymph node metastasis
NI	Unilateral regional lymph node metastasis
N2	Bilateral regional lymph node metastasis

Distant Metastasis (M)

MX	Distant metastasis cannot be assessed
MO	No distant metastasis
M1	Distant metastasis (including pelvic lymph node metastasis)

*Also applies to verrucous carcinoma, Paget's disease of the vulva, adenocarcinoma not otherwise specified, basal cell carcinoma, and Bartholin's gland carcinoma, but not to malignant melanoma.
†The depth of invasion is defined as the measurement of the tumor from the epitheial stromal junction of the adjacent most superficial dermal papilla to the deepest point of invasion.

lignant tumors. The remaining 20% are basal cell carcinomas, malignant melanomas, sarcomas, and carcinoma of the Bartholin's gland or sweat glands. Despite the readily accessible location for examination, delay in diagnosis and treatment for vulvar cancer remains a significant problem.[154]

Clinical Features

Carcinoma of the vulva affects women in the third to tenth decades of life, with the peak incidence occurring between 70 and 79 years of age.[13,91,154] More than 70% of the patients studied were older than 60 years.[13,66,91,207] The mean age of the patients in the reported series was 63 to 67 years,[13,66,154] which is about 15 to 20 years older than that of carcinoma in situ.[74,111] In one series, the mean age for patients with Stage I, II, and III tumors was 62.5, 71.2, and 70.5 years, respectively.[109] Approximately 75% of patients presented with a tumor mass.[66,154] Pruritus, pain, perineal bleeding, and the presence of a groin mass were less common. In patients with Stage I tumors, however, 75% complained of pruritus, 55% noted ulcerated lesions, and only 41% presented with a tumor mass (Fig. 6–40).[143]

Local vulvar diseases were frequently found in association with vulvar cancer. Clinical features of leukoplakia and dystrophies were found in 43% to 70% of cases.[27,66,143,154] Most dystrophies were of the hypertrophic type with or without atypia. Mixed dystrophies and lichen sclerosus were less common (Fig. 6–41).[27,224] After surgical treatment for vulvar carcinoma, 10% of patients had recurrence or persistence of dystrophies.

Other diseases reported to be associated with vulvar cancer include arsenic exposure,[18,77] syphilis,[154] and diabetes,[66,91] as well as obesity, hypertension, and arteriosclerosis.[91,160] Rarely, hypercalcemia was reported to occur in women with vulvar squamous cell carcinoma without bone metastasis. The serum calcium level returned to normal after removal of tumor.[161]

Gross Appearance

The majority of vulvar carcinomas involve the labia majora or minora, especially the upper labia majora.[66] Approximately 11% to 24% of tumors predominantly involve the clitoris.[13,66,113,206] Some authors believe that these tumors should be distinguished from other vulvar carcinomas because of the direct lymphatic drainage from the clitoris to the pelvic lymph nodes.[129] However, an increase in

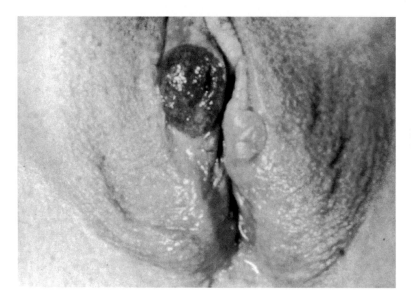

Figure 6–40. An early squamous carcinoma of the right labium minus presents as a raised, reddish nodule with mucosal ulceration.

pelvic lymph node metastasis from clitoral carcinoma has not been proved.

The gross appearance of the tumor is variable. Most tumors are ulcerated lesions with firm raised, rolled edges or indurated plaques. The tumors sometimes are nodular (see Fig. 6–40) or exophytic with a verrucous appearance. The gross appearance of the tumor does not correlate with the histologic type, degree of differentiation, or frequency of nodal metastasis.[73]

The size of the tumor varies from less than 1 cm in diameter to greater than 8 cm.[73] Tumor size is closely related to the lymph nodal metastasis and prognosis. Table 6–3 summarizes the frequency of groin lymph node metastasis in relation to the clinical tumor size. In most studies, the frequency of lymph node involvement is based on groin node dissection. Several series have also included patients who have not undergone groin dissection. If no tumor recurred during the follow-up period, the groin lymph nodes were considered to be uninvolved. The mean follow-up period varied from 3 to 5 years.

Of cases involving tumors less than 1 cm in size, a total of 103 cases were reported in four

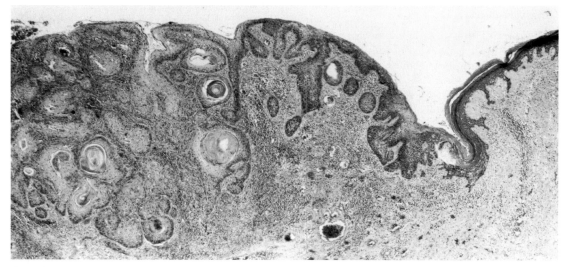

Figure 6–41. A gradual transition from the lichen sclerosus (*right*) to dysplasia and a well-differentiated, keratinizing squamous invasive carcinoma (*left*).

Table 6–3. Correlation of Tumor Size and
Frequency of Groin Node Metastasis

Tumor Less Than 1 cm in Size	
Franklin and Rutledge[73]	1/18 (5.5%)
Magrina et al.[143]	2/20 (10%)
DiSaia et al.[53]	2/20 (10%)
Sedlis et al.[184]	6/45 (13%)
Total	11/103 (10.7%)

Tumor 1–2 cm in Size	
Magrina et al.[143]	9/86 (10.4%)
Sedlis et al.[184]	12/83 (14.5%)
Total	21/169 (12.4%)

Tumor Less Than 2 cm in Size	
Krupp and Bohn[129]	3.8% (36.4% if greater than 2 cm)
Parker et al.[169]	5.0%
Binder et al.[20]	10.4% (43.5% if greater than 2 cm)
Figge and Gandenz[66]	10.5% (37.5% if greater than 2 cm)
Iversen et al.[109]	10.5%
Wharton et al.[207]	11.1%
Margina et al.[143]	12.3%
Sedlis et al.[184]	14.1% (26.6% if greater than 2 cm)
Homesley et al.[105]	18.9% (41.6% if greater than 2 cm)

Tumors Less Than 3 cm in Size	
Krupp and Bohn[129]	9.7% (42.5% if greater than 3 cm)
Cassidy et al.[35]	14% (39% if greater than 3 cm)
Sedlis et al.[184]	18.2% (29.3% if greater than 3 cm)

series.[53,73,143,184] Of these cases, 11 (10.7%) patients had groin lymph node metastasis, including 2 women who developed groin recurrence postoperatively.[143]

Of tumors between 1 and 2 cm in size, 12.4% of women had lymph node metastasis.[143,184] Of tumors less than 2 cm in size, regardless of the depth of invasion, the reported groin lymph node involvement varies from 3.8%[129] to 18.9%.[105] Of tumors greater than 2 cm in size, 26.6% to 43.5% of cases involved lymph node metastasis (see Table 6–3).[20,66,105,129,184] The 5-year survival rate for patients with tumors less than 2 cm in size was 91%, compared with 63% for tumors greater than 2 cm.[129]

In tumors smaller than 3 cm, 9.7% to 18.2% had lymph node metastasis compared with 29.2% to 42.5% when tumors were greater than 3 cm.[35,129,184] The 5-year survival rate for patients with tumors less than 3 cm was 86% compared with a 57% survival rate if the tumors were greater than 3 cm.[129] A comparison of two series is summarized in Table 6–4.

Although the tumor size correlates to a certain extent with the groin node metastasis and prognosis, considerable heterogeneity exists within the group of tumors of comparable tumor size, especially regarding the depth of invasion and degree of differentiation.

Histologic Features

Growth Patterns

Early invasive carcinoma of the vulva invades the underlying stroma by three different growth patterns: pushing, mixed pushing and infiltrative, and diffusely infiltrative. In our study of 63 Stage I carcinomas, 34 (54%) tumors formed well-defined, round to oval-

Table 6–4. Tumor Size and Frequency of
Groin Node Metastasis of Resectable Vulvar
Squamous Cell Carcinoma

	Binder et al.[20]	Homesley et al.[105]
≤1.0 cm	0%	18%
1.1–2.0 cm	19%	19.4%
2.1–3.0 cm	44%	31.4%
3.1–4.0 cm	42%	54.3%
>4.1 cm	44%	47.4%
Total	29%	34.2%

shaped nests with smooth pushing borders (Fig. 6–42A and B). The desmoplastic reaction was inconspicuous or mild. In 18 (29%) neoplasms, the rete pegs sent out multiple tongue-like processes and additional small nests and isolated cells (see Fig. 6–42C). The remaining 11 (17%) tumors diffusely infiltrated the stroma in a so-called spray pattern (see Fig. 6–42D). Desmoplastic stromal response was apparent. With increasing tumor size and stromal invasion, the growth patterns changed from pushing type to mixed or diffusely infiltrative type.

In a small biopsy, the diagnosis of invasive carcinoma can usually be made on properly oriented specimens with adequate depth. Pitfalls of overdiagnosing squamous in situ carcinoma as invasive neoplasm, particularly in relation to tangential cuts, have been discussed previously (see Figs. 6–19 and 6–21).

It is more difficult to distinguish well-differentiated squamous carcinoma with pushing borders from benign hyperplasia. In determining the invasive nature, the configuration of the epithelial nests and the stromal response are most helpful. At the point of invasion, the epithelial cells protrude into the stroma with a smooth or pointed border. These cells often form whorls or epithelial pearls, contain eosinophilic cytoplasm, and appear better differentiated than the neighboring cells. This eosinophilia is attributed to the accumulation of actin filaments, which facilitate cell motility. The interfacing stroma reveals layers of fibroblasts, keratin debris, lymphocytes, plasma cells, and dilated capillaries and lymphatics. The presence of additional isolated, atypical cells in the stroma, either singly or in small nests, further supports the diagnosis of invasive carcinoma.

In pseudoepitheliomatous hyperplasia, the rete pegs have an elongated and irregular shape. Individual cells, including those in the overlying epithelium, maintain cellular maturation and a uniform appearance without nuclear atypia (Fig. 6–43). The cells appear active and have prominent nucleoli and occasional mitotic figures. Keratin pearl formation rarely occurs.

Degree of Differentiation

Using Broders' criteria, 85% of the vulvar cancers are well or moderately differentiated; the remaining 15% are poorly differentiated.[154] The former have cells with prominent intercellular bridges, cytoplasmic keratinization, and frequent formation of concentrically laminated keratin pearls. Their nuclei demonstrate a mild to moderate degree of atypism and infrequent mitotic figures (Fig. 6–44). In poorly differentiated tumors, a high nucleocytoplasmic ratio, nuclear pleomorphism, and abundant mitoses are evident (Fig. 6–45). Individual cells sometimes exhibit keratinization. Rarely, spindle-shaped tumor cells predominate (Fig. 6–46). Such tumors require differentiation from those of mesenchymal origin.

Several studies have shown that the degree of differentiation is related to lymph node metastasis and prognosis. Of well-differentiated tumors, 35% have lymph node involvement compared with 62% of anaplastic carcinomas. Of undifferentiated tumors, 70% are Stage III or IV. In contrast, only 10% of well-differentiated tumors are Stage III or IV.[66]

By Broders' grading method, 15%, 30%, and 48%, respectively, of grade 1, grade 2, and grade 3 resectable vulvar squamous carcinomas were found to involve groin nodal disease (Table 6–5).[20] In a study of 637 vulvar squamous cell carcinomas by Homesley et al.,[105] the frequency of lymph node metastasis using the standard grading method is 26.8%, 36.1%, and 54.8% for grade 1, grade 2, and grade 3 tumors, respectively ($P < 0.00005$; see Table 6–5).

The histologic grading method of the Gynecologic Oncology Group is based on the amount of undifferentiated component. The "undifferentiated" cells are defined as small cells with scant cytoplasm, which often appear in cords and small nests invading the stroma.[105] Well-differentiated grade I tumor has no undifferentiated elements. Grade II contains 1% to 30%, grade III 31% to 50%, and grade IV more than 50% of undifferentiated components. The frequency of nodal metastasis from grade I to grade IV tumors is 2.8%, 15.1%, 41.2%, and 59.7%, respectively.[105] This method appears better than the Broders' method in identifying tumors with low risk for metastasis.

Histologic Type

Using the World Health Organization (WHO) classification, Stage I vulvar squamous carcinoma can be divided into the keratinizing type, 75% to 85%; large cell nonkeratinizing type, 10% to 20%; and small cell type, 5%.[109,143,169] In a study by Binder et al.,[20] the frequency of nodal metastasis is 36% for the keratinizing type and 10% for the nonkeratinizing type ($P = 0.0066$). Several studies have found no corre-

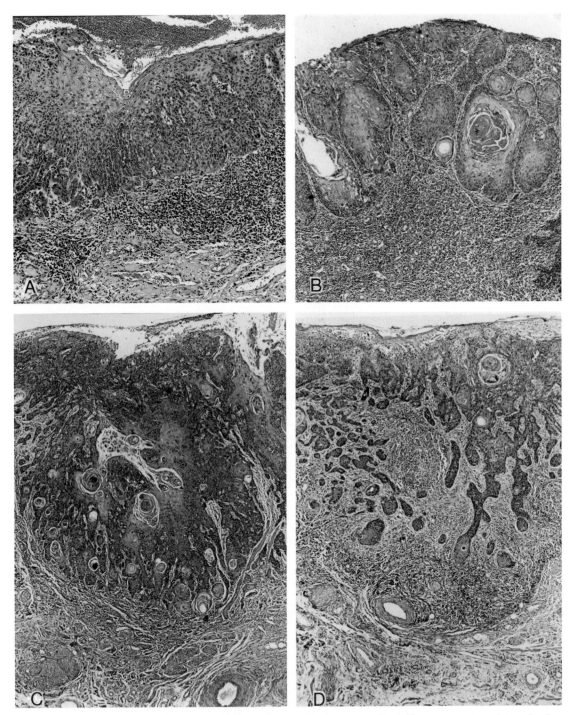

Figure 6–42. Different patterns of stromal invasion. *A,* Pushing borders; expansile, bulky rete pegs extend into the dermis. *B,* Pushing borders; isolated nests of invasive carcinoma have a round, smooth configuration. A heavy lymphocytic infiltration without desmoplasia is common for tumors with pushing border. *C,* A mixed pattern of tongue-like pushing processes and small, irregular, infiltrating nests. *D,* Diffusely infiltrating pattern with irregular nests and cords surrounded by desmoplastic stroma.

207

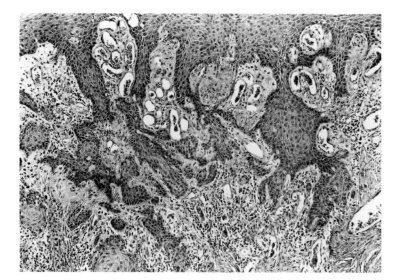

Figure 6–43. Pseudoepitheliomatous hyperplasia with irregular nests of cells in the dermis. The cells maintain orderly maturation. The overlying epithelium is hyperplastic but not dysplastic. Fibroids and chronic inflammation are common.

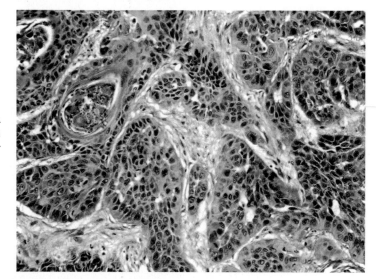

Figure 6–44. Keratinizing, moderately differentiated squamous cell carcinoma with individual cell keratinization and occasional keratin pearls.

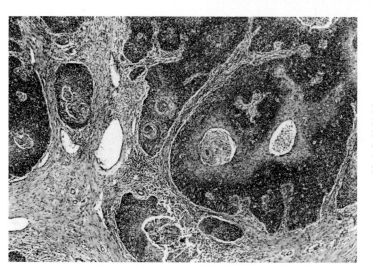

Figure 6–45. Poorly differentiated squamous cell carcinoma consists largely of immature "undifferentiated" cells with scanty cytoplasm. Foci of squamous differentiation sometimes occur near the center of invasive nests.

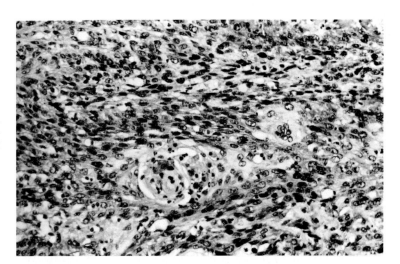

Figure 6–46. Poorly differentiated squamous cell carcinoma with predominantly spindle cells simulating sarcoma.

lation between histologic type and lymph node metastasis, tumor recurrence, or prognosis.[110,143,169] A higher frequency of vascular invasion is found in large cell nonkeratinizing carcinoma (30%) than in keratinizing (12.7%) and small cell (12.5%) tumors.[109] These differences are not statistically significant, however.

In a study by Kurman et al.,[131] 100 vulvar squamous cell carcinomas were classified as keratinizing type (65%), basaloid type (28%), and warty type (7%). Patients with basaloid type or warty type were younger than those with keratinizing tumors. These two types had a strong association with HPV infection. In contrast, 68% of keratinizing type were associated with squamous cell hyperplasia. The tumor size, depth of stromal invasion, and frequency of groin node metastasis were not correlated with tumor type. In terms of prognosis, women with basaloid type had a slightly better outcome than those with keratinizing type.

The keratinizing type is characterized by the presence of individual cell keratinization and keratin pearl formation. The basaloid carcinoma consists of sheets of small, immature squamous cells with round to oval nuclei, coarsely granular chromatin, and scant cytoplasm and resemble the cells of basaloid type of VIN. An occasional keratin pearl may be seen (see Fig. 6–45).

Warty type of tumor is similar morphologically to papillary or papillotransitional carcinoma seen in the cervix, vagina, and head and neck region. This type of carcinoma is characterized by a papillary growth pattern with a hyperkeratotic surface. The tumor cells form irregular nests at the base (Fig. 6–47). The proliferating cells are immature in appearance, resembling basal cells. They have uniform oval nuclei containing coarsely granular chromatin, high nuclear cytoplasmic ratios, and increased mitotic activity. The degree of nuclear atypia is variable from mild to severe. There are occasional multinucleated cells and cells resembling koilocytes. Occasional keratinized cells occur in the center of the nests.

Table 6–5. Comparison of Different Grading Methods and Groin Node Metastasis of Resectable Vulvar Squamous Cell Carcinoma

| | Standard Broders' Method | | GOG Method | |
	Binder et al.[20]	Homesley et al.[105]	Homesley et al.[105]	
Grade 1	15%	26.8%	Grade 1	2.8%
Grade 2	30%	36.1%	Grade 2	15.1%
Grade 3	48%	54.8%	Grade 3	41.25%
Total	29%	34.5%	Grade 4	59.7%
	$P = 0.0038$	$P = 0.00005$	Total	34.8%
			$P = 0.0001$	

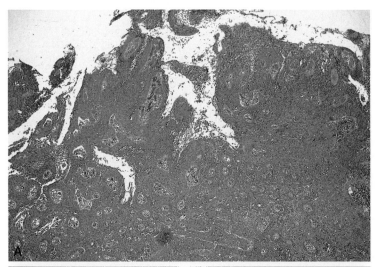

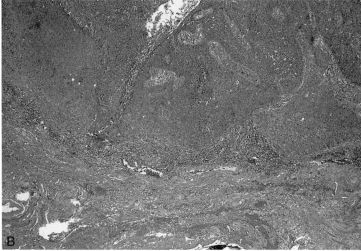

Figure 6–47. Warty type of squamous cell carcinoma. *A,* The surface is exophytic and papillomatous in appearance. *B,* At the base, solid sheets of tumor cells grow by pushing borders.

Rastkar et al.[177] reported 18 warty invasive squamous carcinomas, which were generally greater than 2 cm in size. About one third of the lesions were multifocal. A history of cervical and vulvar malignancies was common. The depth of invasion in the majority of cases was less than 1 mm, as measured from the basement membrane. Only a few reach to 4 mm in depth.

Depth of Invasion

The methods for measuring the depth of invasion varied in the early reports. Although all investigators agree that the end point of measurement is the deepest focus of invasion, some investigators measured from the surface of the epithelium (thickness),[52,57,118,143,184,222] the deepest rete pegs,[28] the most superficial dermal papillae,[94,211,213] or the base of the epithelium.[10,162] In several studies, the method of measurement was not indicated.[73,122,155,158] The Nomenclature Committee of the International Society of Gynecological Pathologists and FIGO recommend that measurement be made with the use of a calibrated eyepiece micrometer. The depth of invasion represents the vertical distance from the most superficial dermal papilla adjacent to the tumor to the deepest point of tumor. Tumor thickness is measured from the granular layer, excluding the hyperkeratotic layers, a method also applied to skin melanoma measurement. The results of the two methods differ only slightly, with an average of 0.3 mm.

Table 6–6 summarizes the reported frequency of inguinal lymph node metastasis in Stage I carcinomas of less than 2 cm in size based on the

Table 6–6. Frequency of Groin Node Metastasis and Depth of Stromal Invasion (measured from base of dermal papillae) in Stage I Squamous Carcinoma

Up to 1.0 mm, <2 cm Maximal Dimension

Wilkinson et al.[213]	0/5
Hoffman et al.[104]	0/24
Hacker et al.[94]	0/34
Magrina et al.[144]	0/40*
Total	0/103

0–3 mm, <2 cm Maximal Dimension

Wilkinson et al.[213]	2/29 (7.0%)
Hoffman et al.[104]	2/60 (3.3%)
Hacker et al.[94]	4/70 (5.7%)
Total	8/159 (5%)

0–5 mm, <2 cm Maximal Dimension

Parker et al.[169]	3/58 (5.2%)
DiSaia et al.[53]	1/19 (5.3%)
Barnes et al.[10]	2/18 (11.1%)
Wilkinson et al.[213]	2/30 (6.7%)
Hoffman et al.[104]	10/75 (13.3%)
Hacker et al.[94]	5/77 (6.5%)
Total	23/277(8.3%)

3–5 mm, <2 cm Maximal Dimension (base of dermal papillae)

Hoffman et al.[104]	8/15 (53.3%)
Hacker et al.[94]	1/7 (14.3%)
Total	9/22 (41%)

*Two women developed local recurrence, and the third developed groin metastasis.

depth of stromal invasion. When the tumor was less than 1 mm in depth or thickness, none of the 103 tumors metastasized to the groin lymph node (see Table 6–6).[94,104,144,213]

Among the 159 cases reported with tumor infiltration up to 3 mm, the overall frequency of nodal metastasis was 5.0% (see Table 6–6). When the vertical dimension increased to 5 mm, the overall risk of nodal metastasis was 8.3% (see Table 6–6). With stromal invasion between 3.1 and 5.0 mm, 41% of women had lymph node metastasis (see Table 6–6)[94,104]; however, the number of cases was small.

A comparison of the depth of invasion and tumor thickness in relation to groin nodal metastasis is summarized in Table 6–7. For surgically resected vulvar squamous carcinoma of all stages, the risk for groin metastasis started to increase with stromal invasion of greater than 2 mm. In contrast, a marked increase in metastasis was seen with tumor thickness greater than 4 mm.[20]

Vascular Space Invasion

Several authors have investigated other morphologic features in an attempt to better define the behavior of early carcinoma. In a study of Stage I carcinoma by Magrina et al.,[143] two of nine patients with vascular invasion had nodal metastasis. However, seven patients with nodal involvement did not have vascular penetration. The authors concluded that vascular invasion is not significantly related to metastasis, recurrence, or prognosis.[143]

On the other hand, Iversen et al.[110] found lymphovascular invasion to be significant in relation to lymph node metastasis. In their series of Stage I cancers, 6 of 15 patients with vascular invasion had nodal metastasis, compared with only 2 of 61 tumors without vascular involvement but with nodal involvement ($P <$ 0.005).[110] In a study by Heaps et al.,[99] when all stages of vulvar squamous carcinomas were combined, local recurrence developed in 12% of patients without vascular lymphatic space invasion, as compared to 39% when this invasion was present ($P = 0.0031$).

Mode of Spread and Prognosis

The clinical stage, as recommended by FIGO, provides a general guide for prognosis and treatment. The crude 5-year survival rates following radical surgery for patients with Stage I tumors range from 77.6% to 87.5%[91,109,154]; with Stage II tumors, 75% to 87%[91,154]; with Stage III tumors, 39.5% to 56.3%[91,154]; and with Stage IV tumors, 8.3%.[91] The corrected or actuarial 5-year survival rates for Stage I tumor are 86% to 97%[109,143,154]; for Stage II tumors, 75 to 95%[109,154]; and for Stage III tumors, 44% to 50%. The overall 5-year survival rate is in the range of 67%.[109,154]

Table 6–7. Comparison of Stromal Invasion, Tumor Thickness, and Groin Nodal Metastasis of Clinically Resectable Vulvar Squamous Cell Carcinoma

	Stromal Invasion Binder et al.[20]	Tumor Thickness Binder et al.[20]
≤1.0 mm	0%	0%
1.1–2.0 mm	0%	0%
2.1–3.0 mm	21%	11%
3.1–4.0 mm	25%	6%
4.1–5.0 mm	22%	42%
>5.1 mm	56%	57%

All P values ≤0.0001.

In a study by Magrina et al.,[144] 40 women had stage IA1 tumor with stromal invasion up to 1 mm, representing 17% of all stages of vulvar squamous carcinomas. The treatment modalities included 10% local excision, 22.5% wide local excision, 7.5% hemivulvectomy, 17.5% simple vulvectomy, and 42.5% radical vulvectomy.

Two women developed local recurrence. The first women had a 1 × 1 cm tumor with a 0.2 mm depth. Tumor recurred 2 years following a wide local excision. She was alive and well following re-excision at 6 years. The second patient had a 2 × 1.5 cm tumor with a depth of 0.1 mm located on the left clitoral region. Four years following local excision, a 2 × 1.1 cm tumor, 3 mm in depth, recurred in the right paraurethral region. It was treated by wide local excision. There was no palpable groin disease. However, 3.5 years later this patient developed right groin, pelvic, and para-aortic metastases. She died 3 months later.[144]

Of the ten women who received groin lymphadenectomy, none developed groin recurrence. However, 1 of 30 women without groin dissection developed groin metastases 7.5 years following initial excision. She died of disease 7.7 years after the detection of groin metastases. The overall 5 and 10 cause-specific survival rates were 100% and 94.7%, respectively, for patients with stage IA1 tumor.[144]

Most carcinomas of the vulva spread first to the ipsilateral groin lymph node. More advanced tumors involve the contralateral groin lymph node or pelvic lymph nodes. The frequency of lymph node metastasis is closely related to tumor size, depth, and extent. The reported frequency of groin lymph node involvement in all stages of vulvar carcinoma varies from 28% to 37%.[91,129,154,182] In unilateral carcinomas, the majority of groin lymph node metastasis occurred in the ipsilateral side, and less than 10% had bilateral groin lymph node involvement. In contrast, patients with bilateral or midline tumors had a higher risk of bilateral nodal disease. Among the Stage II, III, and IV bilateral tumors, 24% were associated with unilateral and 33% with bilateral groin lymph node metastasis.[108]

The reported frequency of pelvic lymph node metastasis of all stages varies from 7.8%[13] to 14.3%[66] to 16%.[74] With few exceptions,[35] pelvic lymph node metastasis, if present, is always associated with groin lymph node involvement.[47,91,108,154] The risk of developing pelvic lymph node metastasis is closely related to the number and bilaterality of groin node

metastasis. Although no patients with fewer than four unilateral groin node metastases had pelvic node involvement, 26% of patients with bilateral groin involvement and 50% of those with more than four unilateral groin lymph node metastases had pelvic node metastasis.[47] Therefore, patients with bilateral involvement or more than four unilateral groin lymph node metastases had a high risk of developing pelvic metastasis and a worse prognosis.[47]

Whether or not clitoral carcinomas have a higher frequency of groin and pelvic lymph node metastasis remains controversial. In one series, 41% of clitoral lesions had groin node involvement, compared with 30% for all vulvar carcinomas.[47] In another series of Stage II, III, and IV tumors, 66.7% of clitoral lesions had groin lymph node metastasis, compared with 50% for all carcinomas.[108] Pelvic metastasis occurred in 11% of clitoral tumors, in contrast to 8.3% for all tumors. However, these numbers are not statistically significant.[108] The author concluded that clitoral carcinomas demonstrated no higher rate of groin or pelvic metastasis than tumors located elsewhere.[108]

If vulvar carcinomas extend locally to involve the vagina, urethra, urinary bladder, or anorectum, the risk of lymph node metastasis and local recurrence increases. The lymphatics in these sites may drain directly into the pelvic lymph node in addition to the groin lymph node via the usual channels and the hemorrhoidal plexus. Metastasis to distant sites rarely occurs, mainly in advanced cases.

In a study by Homesley et al.,[105] 588 cases of resectable squamous cell carcinoma from 1977 to 1984 were followed. In women with normal groin nodes by clinical examination, 23.9% were found to have metastasis. In the absence of groin or pelvic lymph node metastasis, the reported 5-year survival rates following surgery vary from 84%[154] to 86%,[13,109] 87%,[91] and 93%.[129] If lymph nodes are involved, the 5-year survival rates decrease to 24%,[129] 33%,[91] 38%,[154] 52%,[109] and 55.6%.[13] Discrepancies observed in these series can be explained by the sample size, variations in the population surveyed, and possibly the modes of treatment.

The number of groin lymph node metastases and extracapsular extension further affect the prognosis.[200] Although no difference exists in survival among patients with one to three ipsilateral groin node metastases, the prognosis is adversely affected in the presence of more than three ipsilateral groin metastases, bilateral groin metastasis, and pelvic metastasis.[47] The absolute survival rate for patients with pelvic metastasis at 3 years is 12.5%[91] to 25%[109] and, at 5 years, 18%.

Recurrences at local or distant sites are related to the status of resection margins, the extent of the disease, and lymph node status.[99,109,146,154] When the tumor involves the lines of resection, local recurrence develops in 50% of cases.[109] Of patients with proven groin node metastases, 20% have recurrence in the thigh or groin. Among patients with clinically suspicious or positive groin lymph nodes before surgery, 40% have local recurrence.[182] In patients with no nodal metastasis, tumor recurrence is usually local (73.3%) and, less frequently, distant (20%). If the groin nodes are involved, the recurrence is almost equally distributed between the local and distant sites.[146]

In a study by Heaps et al.,[99] 135 women with vulvar squamous cell carcinoma from Stage I to Stage IV were investigated for the factors associated with local recurrence. This study identified the status of the resection margin as the most important predictor of local recurrence. Of 91 patients who had a tumor clearance of 8.0 mm or more as measured on tissue section, none developed local recurrence. Of the 44 women with less than 8.0 mm of clearance, 21 (48%) had local recurrence and 23 (52%) did not ($P < 0.0001$). Among the latter, 14 (61%) remained free of disease and 9 (39%) had advanced disease, declining health, or short follow-up. Increasing depth of stromal invasion was associated with greater local recurrence. Using the threshold of 9.1 mm, the outcome of the patient was correctly predicted in 81.5% of cases. Other factors that increased local recurrence included infiltrative (as compared with pushing) growth pattern, the presence of vascular lymphatic space invasion, and mitotic activity of greater than 10 mitoses per 10 high-power fields.[99] The majority of local and distant recurrences occurred within the first 2 years following treatment,[73] resulting in a high death rate during this period.[6]

In a study by Mariani et al.,[142] 44 vulvar squamous cell carcinomas from Stage I to Stage IV were studied by flow cytometry for ploidy pattern. Thirty-four percent of the tumors were found to have an aneuploid pattern. The aneuploidy was correlated with histologic grade. Of grade I well-differentiated tumors, 12% were aneuploid, as compared with 63.2% for grade II and grade III tumors ($P = 0.0004$). Aneuploidy was also associated with poor prognostic factors, such as advanced stage, deep stromal invasion, and positive inguinal lymph node metastasis. Using a multivariate regression model, FIGO stage was the most important predictor of survival rates. Ploidy pattern was not an independent prognostic factor.[142]

Incidence of Second Malignancies

Patients with invasive vulvar carcinoma, such as those with vulvar carcinoma in situ, have a significant risk of developing second malignancies. Previous or subsequent malignant lesions are found in 18% to 20% of patients.[67,92,143] The uterine cervix, vagina, breast, and endometrium are most frequently involved. Carcinomas of the ovary, lung, colon, and other sites are less common.[91,143]

Verrucous Squamous Carcinoma

Buschke and Löwenstein,[31] in 1925, described a cauliflower-like growth of the penis, which, despite the morphologic resemblance to benign condyloma acuminatum, was locally aggressive. Since then, similar changes have been reported in the vulva, rectum, scrotum, penis, and perineum as giant condyloma, carcinoma-like condyloma, and Buschke-Löwenstein tumor by various authors.[48,117] These tumors, although appearing benign histologically, may extend into the anorectum, form sinus tracts, and recur deep in the pelvic soft tissue.[48,117]

In 1948, Ackerman[4] reported a variant of squamous carcinoma, called verrucous carcinoma, which involved the oral cavity. He emphasized its distinct pathologic features, its indolent course, and the rarity of metastasis. Such tumors were subsequently reported in the larynx, nasal cavity, paranasal sinuses, penis, anorectum, and female genital tract.[128,139] The similarity in the natural history and pathologic features of giant condyloma and verrucous carcinoma leads to the conclusion that they represent the same disease entity.[128,139,174]

A total of 44 verrucous carcinomas of the female genital tract were reported up to 1978,[173] with 17 involving the vulva; 14 the cervix, 10 the vagina, and 3 both the cervix and vagina.

Clinical Features

Verrucous carcinoma of the vulva affects women after the fifth decade of life. Most patients present with a long-standing, slow-growing, warty lesion. At the time of diagnosis, the lesion, in most cases, is extensive. Inguinal lymph nodes are enlarged owing to reactive hyperplasia. In one study, 50% of the patients had histologically confirmed condyloma 3 to 10 years before the diagnosis of vulvar verrucous carcinoma.[114]

Gross Appearance

The neoplasms are invariably described as warty, fungating, or cauliflower-like masses that range from 0.8 to 10 cm in size.[71] They vary in color from gray-pink to yellow to white and have a raised, polypoid appearance (Fig. 6–48). With ulceration and secondary inflammation, the tumor may become indurated and have a firm consistency. On cut surface, the thickness of the lesion varies from a few millimeters to 10 mm. Characteristically, the base is smooth and well demarcated from the underlying tissue.

Microscopic Features

The tumor comprises exophytic papillary fronds with hyperkeratosis and parakeratosis on the surface. The larger and more extensive verrucous carcinomas, in addition, have a lobular configuration and a smooth surface. Between the lobules, the epithelium often extends deep into the stroma in an endophytic manner. Between the papillary fronds, long rete pegs compress the fibrovascular stroma (Fig. 6–49). A central fibrous stalk, characteristic of condyloma acuminatum, is absent. Branching and fusion of rete pegs is frequently found, especially in tangential sections. The individual tumor cells have abundant eosinophilic, keratinizing cytoplasm and intercellular bridges. In the deep portion of the tumor, keratin pearls and keratin cysts are sometimes present. The nuclei are relatively uniform. Nuclear atypia, when present, is mild (Fig. 6–50A). Mitoses are rare and confined to the parabasal and basal layers. Most important, the base of the tumor is well defined and smooth. Bulky rete pegs have blunt, regular, pushing borders. The basement membrane appears to be intact. Within the stroma, a band-like infiltration of lymphocytes, plasma cells, and occasional eosinophils is invariably present. During the course of multiple recurrences and subsequent radiotherapy, nuclear atypia and mitotic activity may increase (Fig. 6–50B).

Differential Diagnosis

Verrucous carcinoma should be distinguished from pseudoepitheliomatous hyperplasia, condyloma acuminatum, and well-differentiated squamous carcinoma with a papillary or verrucous appearance.

Pseudoepitheliomatous hyperplasia usually occurs at the edge of chronic ulcers and lacks an exophytic appearance. The rete pegs are narrow, elongated, sharp-pointed, and jagged, unlike the bulky solid masses seen in verrucous carcinoma (see Fig. 6–43).[128]

Condyloma acuminatum is smaller and usually multiple and has a central fibrovascular core supporting individual papillary fronds.[50,128] In verrucous carcinoma, this fibrous core is absent. More likely to be seen are the fibrous septa compressed by the long rete pegs.

Some conventional squamous carcinomas of the vulva can have a verrucous growth pattern

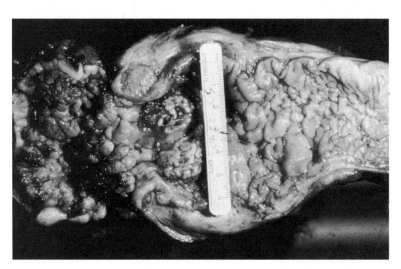

Figure 6–48. Verrucous carcinoma of the vulva and perianal skin extends into the anorectum (*right*). This polypoid, nodular mass has well-defined borders. (Courtesy of Peter Tang, M.D., Cleveland, Ohio, and from Judge JR. Giant condyloma acuminatum involving vulva and rectum. Arch Pathol 88:46, 1969.)

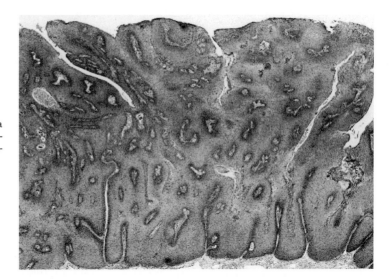

Figure 6–49. Verrucous carcinoma made up of bulky, mature squamous epithelium clearly separated from the underlying dermis.

with marked hyperkeratosis. In the presence of marked nuclear atypia or invasion, they should not be classified as verrucous carcinoma.

In a superficial and poorly oriented biopsy, a verrucous carcinoma is often underdiagnosed as some type of hyperplastic squamous papilloma or condyloma acuminatum. A well-oriented deep biopsy, which includes the base of tumor, should be accompanied by a description of tumor size and clinical appearance. Multiple biopsies are sometimes required before a definitive diagnosis of verrucous carcinoma can be made.

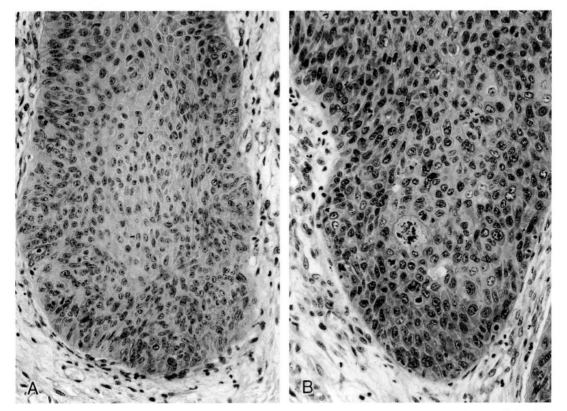

Figure 6–50. *A*, Verrucous carcinoma before radiotherapy. *B*, After radiotherapy, nuclear pleomorphism, cellular disorganization, and mitotic activity are markedly increased. (H&E; *A* and *B*, ×250)

Studies with the Use of Special Techniques

Electron-microscopic studies of verrucous carcinoma demonstrate well-differentiated squamous cells with abundant tonofilaments and glycogen particles in the cytoplasm. Numerous desmosomes and microvillous projections extend into the intercellular spaces. The overall architecture and maturation process resemble those of normal epidermis. The basal lamina is continuous and sometimes multilayered.[127] By immunofluorescent study, the basement membrane follows the borders of the rete pegs. It is focally thickened and only rarely thinned or absent.[174]

Autoradiographic study following incubation with titrated thymidine reveals that the labeled cells are confined to the three deepest basal and parabasal layers. This is in contrast to nonverrucous squamous carcinomas, in which the labeled S-phase cells are more abundant and found throughout the tumor. These ultrastructural and autoradiographic features confirm an orderly maturation and proliferation of tumor cells from the basal and parabasal layers, which are ensheathed by an intact basement membrane.[174] These characteristics possibly can explain the lack of metastatic potential in verrucous carcinoma.

Rondo et al.[176] have identified an HPV type 6 in a rapidly growing verrucous carcinoma of the vulva. The viral genomes, although similar to a variant of HPV type 6 (type 6b) found in a condyloma, differ in a special region that is thought to control viral replication and cell transformation. This difference in the viral DNA sequences may explain an intermediate behavior of verrucous carcinoma between that of genital warts and conventional squamous carcinomas.

Prognosis

Although a limited number of vulvar verrucous carcinomas have been reported, their behavior is similar to those occurring elsewhere. The tumor tends to be slow growing but extends into the adjacent perineum, anorectum, and inguinal region over a period of months and sometimes several years.[117,139] Local recurrences are common following incomplete excision. Recurrence in ischiorectal and gluteal fossa and rectum often requires abdominoperineal resection or pelvic exenteration. The tumor does not respond to topical application of podophyllin or 5-FU. A complete, en bloc resection of the tumor is the treatment of choice.

The need for groin lymph node dissection is debatable. Of the patients with vulvar verrucous carcinoma who underwent groin lymph node dissection, none had lymph node metastasis.[85,139,173] The lesion does not respond to irradiation; furthermore, irradiation can cause accelerated growth and anaplastic transformation.[86,139] Among the three large series of verrucous carcinomas of various sites, only 7 of 103 patients with lymph node dissection had metastasis. Three of these patients received prior irradiation to the primary tumor.[4,128] Other tumors may have contained foci of conventional invasive carcinoma. Death is primarily related to extensive uncontrolled local recurrences. Groin and distant metastases occur rarely.

In view of the distinct natural history and different mode of therapy for verrucous carcinoma, distinction from nonverrucous squamous carcinoma should be made.

Basal Cell Carcinoma

Clinical Features

Basal cell carcinoma of the vulvar skin constitutes 2% to 3% of all vulvar malignancies.[46] It is a disease of postmenopausal women in their sixth to eighth decades of life, with an average age of 65 years.[167] Black women are rarely affected. The presence of a mass associated with pruritus, bleeding, or ulceration is the most common complaint. The clinical appearance is highly variable. An ulcer of a nodular mass is the most frequent manifestation, but a lesion may also appear as papillomatous, erythematous plaque, leukoplakic, or cystic. Hyperpigmentation is occasionally present, leading to the diagnosis of nevus or malignant melanoma. The size varies from a few millimeters to 10 cm and is usually about 1 cm in diameter. In a review of 58 cases reported in the literature, the frequency of location was as follows: 42 (71%) involved the labium majus, 5 (9%) involved both the labium majus and labium minus, 4 (7%) involved the labium minus, 4 (7%) involved the clitoris, 3 (5%) involved the urethra, and 1 (2%) involved the fourchette.[167]

In a study by Benedet et al.,[12] of 28 women with vulvar basal cell carcinoma,[13] they ranged in age from 44 to 95 years (mean 74 years). The most common location was the anterior half of the vulva. Eighty-two percent had T1 disease with a lesion of 2.0 cm or less in size. The remaining 18% had T2 tumors. Following a wide local excision, three women developed local recurrence, including one who also developed metastasis in the left neck and died 2 years later. This woman's tumor was 2.0 cm in size and deeply invasive to subcutis with perineural invasion. Ten women also had other basal cell carcinomas in the body. Eleven women had additional malignancies. Overall, 39% of women had another basal cell carcinoma or other malignancy.[13]

Pathologic Features

The histologic appearance of basal cell carcinomas of the vulva is similar to that of lesions at other sites. The tumor consists of solid nests of closely packed, uniform basaloid cells. The cytoplasm is scanty, and the nuclei are small and hyperchromatic with a round or oval shape. The most distinctive feature is the radial, vertical, or parallel arrangement of the cells in the outermost layer of the epithelial nest, so-called peripheral palisading (Fig. 6–51). Mitoses vary in number; generally, they are not numerous. Cystic degeneration and necrosis are common in large tumors. Subtypes of basal cell carcinoma with adenoid cystic pattern and dense sclerotic stroma (morphea type) have been described in the vulvar region.[46,150] One basal cell carcinoma is reported to have originated from a fibroepithelial tumor.[46]

A study by Feakins and Lowe[60] described several growth patterns in vulvar basal cell carcinoma, including superficial, compact lobular, infiltrative, adenoid, and morphea types. The differential diagnosis includes basaloid squamous cell carcinoma, which is often associated with high-grade VIN and includes numerous mitotic figures and a greater degree of nuclear atypia.

In Benedet's literature review of 153 cases in 1997, 18 (12%) cases recurred and only one woman died of tumor. Of seven metastatic basal cell carcinomas, five were larger than 6 cm, one was a 2.5 cm shallow ulcer, and the other was a 2.0 cm deeply invasive tumor. All metastasized initially to the groin, except one to the left neck.[115,188] Subsequently, Feakins and Lowe[60] reported 9% recurrence, and one metastatic tumor to the groin that caused death in 23 months.

In a vulvar biopsy in which basaloid cells are arranged in glands and cribriform pattern, the differential diagnosis should include adenoid basal cell carcinoma, adenoid cystic carcinoma of the sweat gland and of the Bartholin's gland, and metastatic carcinoma, especially from the uterine cervix. Similarly, it is crucial to distinguish between a basal cell carcinoma of the skin and a basaloid, cloacogenic carcinoma of the anorectum. A superficial location, an origin from the basal layer of the epidermis, and the presence of peripheral palisading strongly support the diagnosis of basal cell carcinoma.

Because basal cell carcinoma rarely metastasizes to the regional lymph nodes, a wide local excision with adequate margins is considered to be adequate.[26]

Adenosquamous Carcinoma

Vulvar carcinomas, designated and reported as adenosquamous type, have included squamous carcinoma with acantholysis and pseudoglan-

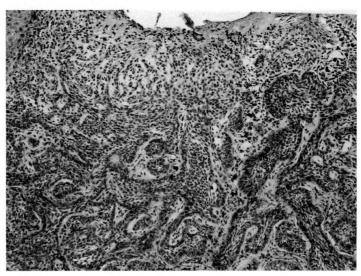

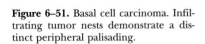

Figure 6–51. Basal cell carcinoma. Infiltrating tumor nests demonstrate a distinct peripheral palisading.

dular pattern (Fig. 6–52) and true adenosquamous carcinoma (Fig. 6–53), which may arise from the skin appendages and Bartholin's gland.[178]

In a series of 50 squamous cell carcinomas of the vulva, pseudoglandular pattern with acantholytic cells is present in 34% of the cases, with 4% extensive, and 30% focal.[133] There is no difference in the clinical presentation and the frequency of nodal metastasis between squamous cell carcinoma with and without adenoid pattern.[133] At the time of the report, 38% of the patients with adenoid squamous carcinoma had died from their disease, compared with 18% who had ordinary squamous cell carcinoma. This is not statistically significant.[132]

Underwood et al.,[197] on the other hand, noted statistically significant differences in the clinical stage, inguinal nodal metastasis, and prognosis between 18 adenosquamous carci-

nomas and 77 ordinary squamous cell carcinomas of the vulva. Patients with adenosquamous carcinoma had more advanced T4 lesions (FIGO classification, 67% versus 39% for ordinary squamous carcinomas), a higher frequency of groin metastasis (72% versus 23% for ordinary squamous carcinomas), and a poorer 5-year survival rate (5.5% versus 62.3% for ordinary squamous cell carcinoma).[197]

Differences in the two series can be explained by the better differentiated keratinizing squamous carcinoma in the cases of Lasser et al.[133] The squamous component is less differentiated and often comprises spindle-shaped cells in the tumors studied by Underwood et al.[197] In addition, cells lining the glandular spaces have basophilic granular cytoplasm suggestive of mucoid production.[197] In the groin metastasis, glandular component is absent in the Lasser et al. series[133] but is present in 4 of 13 patients in

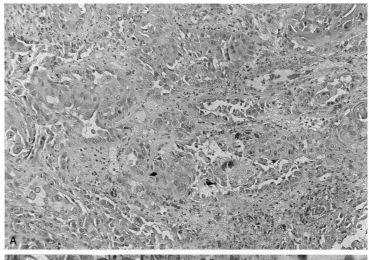
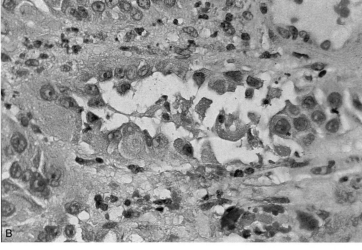

Figure 6–52. *A,* Moderately differentiated squamous cell carcinoma with pseudoglandular pattern and acantholysis. *B,* Higher magnification to illustrate necrotic and degenerated tumor cells.

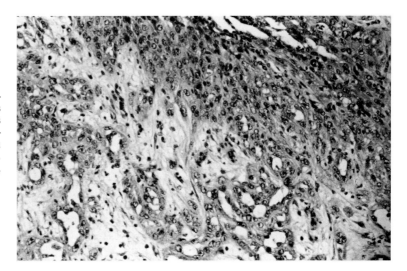

Figure 6–53. Adenosquamous carcinoma. This carcinoma consists of poorly differentiated squamous carcinoma (*upper right*) and adenocarcinoma with luminal formation and mucous secretion (*lower left*). (Courtesy of Takashi Okagaki, M.D., Minneapolis, Minnesota.)

the Underwood et al. cases.[197] These findings suggest that squamous carcinomas with acantholysis and pseudoglandular pattern should be distinguished from those with true glandular differentiation demonstrable by histochemical reactions, such as mucicarmine and PAS stains.

Ultrastructural study can further confirm the diagnosis of adenosquamous carcinoma by finding squamous cells, glandular cells, and intermediate cells between squamous and glandular cells.[197] The squamous cells have small to moderate amounts of microfilaments, glycogen particles, and a few desmosomal junctions. The glandular cells form glandular lumens with microvilli projecting into them. Secretory granules similar to those of endocervical or goblet cells are present. Thus, the study by Underwood et al.[197] suggests that the entity of adenosquamous carcinoma, when confirmed by strict criteria and histochemical and ultrastructural studies, has a worse prognosis than do conventional squamous carcinoma and squamous carcinoma with acantholysis.

Of the three adenosquamous carcinomas of the vulva described by Rhatigan and Mojadidi,[178] two were clinically related to the area of the Bartholin's gland, although this gland was not contiguous to the tumor histologically. In addition to glandular cells, squamous and transitional cell carcinomas were observed. The authors suggest a possible origin from the Bartholin's gland or from cloacogenic or müllerian epithelium. At the time of the report, one patient was lost to follow-up after 3 years, another patient was living without tumor after 12 years, and the third patient, who had groin metastasis, died of uremia 1 year later. These

cases seem to have a different histologic appearance from that of adenosquamous carcinoma of the skin appendages. The glands in these tumors are well formed and lined by tall columnar cells. Mucinous material was present in two of the three cases.[178]

Sweat Gland Carcinoma

Sweat gland carcinoma of the vulvar region is exceedingly rare. Eichenberg[58] in 1934, reported a 0.5 cm tumor on the labium majus of a 30-year-old woman. The tumor was described as a solid and intracystic papillary carcinoma with local invasion and with metastasis to inguinal lymph nodes. The patient was well 2 years after surgery. Novak and Stevenson[162] illustrated two vulvar adenocarcinomas of probable sweat gland origin and commented that some of the cases reported earlier as sweat gland carcinoma were, in fact, hidradenomas.

Rich et al.[179] reported a poorly differentiated adenocarcinoma of the sweat glands occurring in the posterior fourchette of a 53-year-old woman who had received external irradiation and intracavitary radium application for a Stage III-B squamous cell carcinoma of the cervix 7 years earlier. There was no evidence of recurrence of the cervical malignancy. The vulvar lesion was 2×3 cm in size, partially ulcerated, erythematous, and pruritic. Histologically, the tumor cells are arranged in cords, small acini, and solid nests resembling ductal carcinoma of the breast. The cytoplasm is finely granular and negative for PAS and mucinous material. Under the electron microscope, the cells are seen to be joined by a few poorly formed desmosomes. The cytoplasm contains abundant ribosomes, a small number of glycogen-like granules, and bundles of tonofilaments in the perinuclear region. Secretory granules are not identified. The lesion was removed by a wide excision and invaded 5 mm into the dermis. Follow-up information was not available.

Wick et al.[209] reported on five patients with vulvar sweat gland carcinoma, including two coexisting with extramammary Paget's disease. Three patients were known to have died of recurrent tumor after surgery. Key histologic features that support a malignant rather than benign sweat gland tumor include nuclear anaplasia, high mitotic activity, necrosis, and infiltration of the adjacent tissue, blood vessels, or nerves.

Sweat gland carcinomas of the skin demonstrate a spectrum of histologic patterns ranging from ductal, acinar, cylindromatous, papillary, mixed solid and papillary, or mucin-secreting to a clear cell hidrademonatous appearance. Among the 39 reported cases from various sites, 19 patients (49%) developed one or more recurrences, 28 (72%) eventually developed metastasis, and 11 (28%) were known to have died of disease at the time of the report.[153] These findings suggest that sweat gland carcinomas are highly aggressive and require adequate wide excision.

Benign and Malignant Mixed Tumor of Salivary Gland Type

Benign and malignant mixed tumors resembling those originating from the salivary gland have been reported.[164,215] Ordonez et al.[164] reported a mobile nodule in the left labium majus of a 65-year-old patient who previously had been treated with intracavitary radium for Stage I-B squamous carcinoma of the cervix. The nodule was 1 cm in size and had the histologic appearance of a benign mixed tumor.

Ordonez et al.[164] reported that a malignant mixed tumor was observed in a 69-year-old patient who presented with a polypoid mass protruding from the vagina and involving the left lower lateral vaginal wall, the rectovaginal septum, the left labium majus, and the periurethral area. After biopsy, a pelvic exenteration was followed by radiotherapy. The tumor mass measured 7 cm and contained benign mixed tumor with foci of adenoid cystic carcinoma, undifferentiated carcinoma, and malignant cells arranged in single rows resembling those observed in breast carcinoma. Multiple nodules were noted on chest x-ray examination 14 months after the surgery.[164] A case of salivary gland adenoma mixed with adenoid cystic carcinoma and epithelial-myoepithelial carcinoma was reported.[166]

An undifferentiated carcinoma presumably arising from the sweat gland of the vulva was reported to simulate epithelioid sarcoma and malignant rhabdoid tumor.[130]

Carcinoma of the Bartholin Gland

Clinical Features

Carcinoma of the Bartholin gland is rare, constituting 2% to 7% of all vulvar malignancies.[56] Women between 40 and 70 years of age are most often affected. The average age is 49.5 years. Approximately one third of the patients are younger than 40 years of age. The youngest patient reported was 15 years old.[156] For some unknown reason, there is a predilection for the left side. The most common symptom includes a palpable mass in the vulva, vagina, or introitus, usually associated with pain or a burning sensation.[24] Dyspareunia is common, and pruritus may be present. The mass is hard, tender, indurated, and often cystic. In one series, 50% of the patients were diagnosed and treated initially for a benign cystic or inflammatory lesion. Poor wound healing, persistent infection, or distant metastases eventually lead to histologic study and correct diagnosis.[37]

To avoid delay in the detection of carcinoma, it is recommended that an excision, rather than marsupialization of a Bartholin gland lesion, be performed in patients older than 40 years and that, at the time of marsupialization, the drainage of a Bartholin gland abscess be sent for culture and cytologic smears.[56]

Pathologic Features

Several histologic variants have been reported. In a review of 152 reported cases, adenocarcinoma and squamous cell carcinoma each constituted 45% of the cases. The remaining 10% were undifferentiated carcinoma, sarcoma, or malignant melanoma.[9] Transitional cell carcinoma and adenoid cystic carcinoma also occur in the Bartholin gland.[1,201,205]

Adenocarcinomas present with different growth patterns, from papillary, cystic, or cribriform to solid (Figs. 6–54 to 6–56). The majority of tumors secrete mucin, including some very well differentiated mucinous adenocarcinomas that simulate colonic adenoma (see Fig. 6–54). Biopsy of hidradenoma papilliferum from the posterior vulva may raise the question of Bartholin's gland carcinoma. The former is made up of two cell types, epithelial and myoepithelial. The latter with local infiltration, single cell type, and nuclear atypia should lead to a correct diagnosis of Bartholin's gland carcinoma (see Fig. 6–56).

Squamous cell carcinomas, in general, are associated with varying degrees of keratin formation. Transitional cell carcinoma resembles that occurring in the urinary tract. Adenoid cystic carcinomas have the same histologic appearance as those originating in the salivary gland. The basaloid cells are arranged in nests with microcystic and cribriform patterns (Fig. 6–57). Acellular hyaline or mucinous material in the glandular lumens produces a characteristic cylindromatous appearance (Fig. 6–58). Perineural invasion is sometimes present.

Milchgrub et al.[152] reported two adenoid cystic carcinomas consisting entirely of tubules and less than 5% of cribriform glands. One patient had residual tumor following hemivulvectomy and developed bone metastases and died 6 years after diagnosis. The other patient had residual tumor following hemivulvectomy and unilateral inguinal femoral lymphadenectomy, and no follow-up data were available.

Review of the literature of adenoid cystic carcinoma of Bartholin's gland did not reveal a correlation between the growth patterns (tubular, cribriform, solid) and survival.

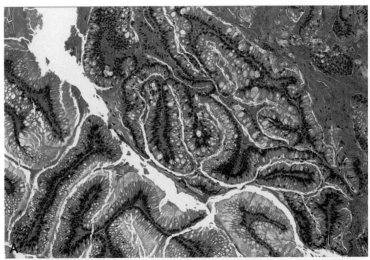
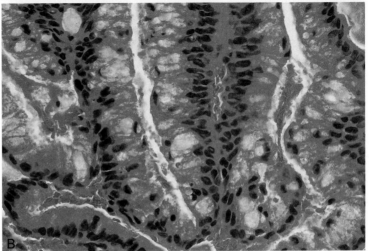

Figure 6–54. Well-differentiated mucinous adenocarcinoma of Bartholin's gland. *A,* Tumor cells form villous projections. *B,* Tall columnar cells demonstrate one to two layers of nuclear stratification and mild nuclear atypia resembling colonic adenoma. (See color section.)

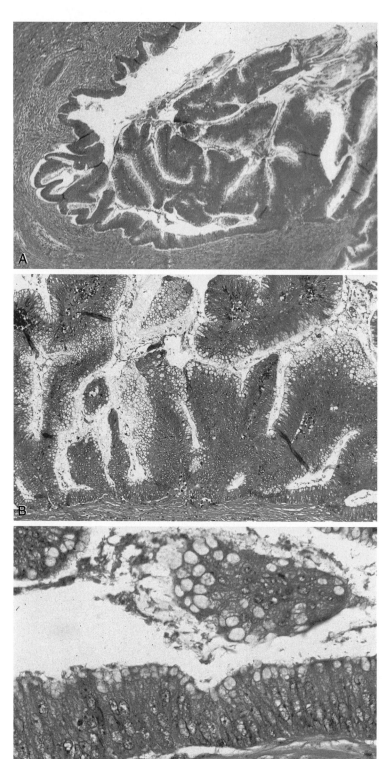

Figure 6–55. Well-differentiated papillary adenocarcinoma of Bartholin's gland. *A*, Papillary cystic tumor. *B*, Multiple papillary projections. *C*, Tumor cells present with nuclear stratification, moderate nuclear atypia, and multiple nucleoli. (See color section.)

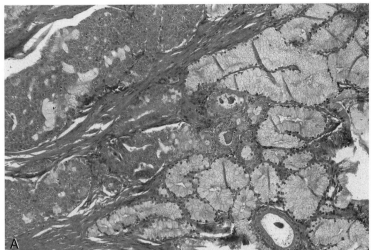

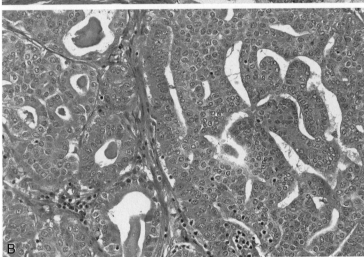

Figure 6–56. Moderately differentiated adenocarcinoma of Bartholin's gland. *A,* Local infiltration of Bartholin's gland. *B,* Complex papillary glands and moderate nuclear atypia further support adenocarcinoma.

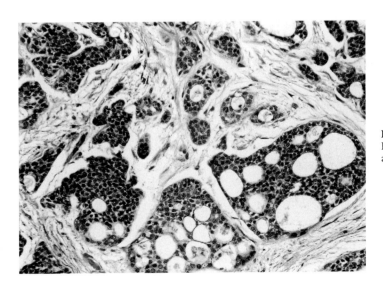

Figure 6–57. Adenoid cystic carcinoma of Bartholin's gland. Uniform basaloid cells are arranged in cribriform pattern.

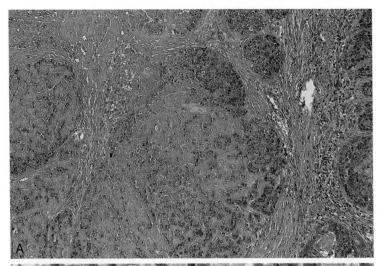

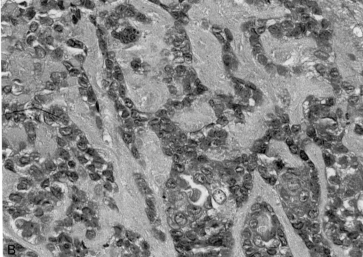

Figure 6–58. Adenoid cystic carcinoma of Bartholin's gland, poorly differentiated. *A,* Solid nests of basaloid cells undergo necrosis. Abundant eosinophilic hyalinized stroma accumulates in the stroma. *B,* Tumor cells are surrounded by basement-like eosinophilic material. Two types of tumor cells are suggested. The larger epithelial cells and the smaller and darker cells resembling myoepithelial cells.

Because none of the tumor types are unique for Bartholin's gland carcinoma, the pathologic findings should be considered relative to the anatomic location and clinical information. When a squamous cell carcinoma of Bartholin's gland involves the overlying skin, it may not be distinguished from that arising from the vulvar epithelium. We agree with Chamlain and Taylor,[37] who have set the criteria for carcinoma of Bartholin's gland as follows: (1) the transition from normal to neoplastic elements must be demonstrated histologically, (2) the tumor must involve a major portion of Bartholin's gland and be histologically compatible with Bartholin's gland, and (3) there must be no evidence of a primary tumor elsewhere.

Ultrastructural Features

The ultrastructural findings of Bartholin's gland carcinoma correspond to the degree of differentiation as observed by light microscopy. In well-differentiated adenocarcinomas, the tumor cells contain abundant rough endoplasmic reticulum, well-developed Golgi membranes, and secretory vacuoles. The latter include small, electron-dense granules 200 nm in diameter that resemble those found in the normal acinar cells of Bartholin's gland, large mucous vacuoles of goblet cells, and large, irregularly shaped granules of moderate electron density seen in the eccrine sweat gland.[132] The cells form glandular lumens and are joined by desmosomes and tight junctions. In poorly differentiated carcinomas,

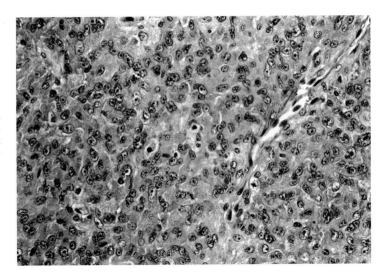

Figure 6–59. This poorly differentiated carcinoma of Bartholin's gland consists of solid sheets of cells having abundant eosinophilic cytoplasm, pleomorphic nuclei, and prominent nucleoli.

the glandular formation is less apparent, and secretory granules are few (Figs. 6–59 and 6–60).[156] In the case of a 15-year old patient, the demonstration of glandular lumen by electron microscopy enabled the authors to rule out an alveolar rhabdomyosarcoma.[156]

Prognosis

The prognosis for patients with carcinoma of the Bartholin gland has improved in recent years, with 5-year survival rates in the 40% to 50% range following radical surgery.[137,208] Important prognostic features include tumor size, degree of differentiation, extent of local invasion, and inguinal and pelvic lymph node status.[156] Close to 50% of patients with carcinoma of Bartholin's glands have inguinal node metastasis,[208] and 18% of these patients have additional metastasis in the pelvic lymph nodes.[137] Tumor recurrences are mostly local and pelvic and, less frequently, distant.[208]

Adenoid cystic carcinomas, making up approximately one third of the adenocarcino-

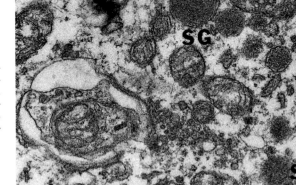

Figure 6–60. Under the electron microscope, the cells contain numerous mitochondria, well-developed Golgi complexes, and secretory granules (SG), supporting the diagnosis of a poorly differentiated adenocarcinoma. ($\times 37,700$)

mas of the Bartholin gland, have a slow, insidious course with local recurrence and perineural spread and do not metastasize to the lymph node.[17] Metastasis is predominantly via vascular channels, usually after local recurrence, to the lung, liver, and bone. The clinical course seems to be less aggressive than that of squamous or adenocarcinoma of Bartholin's gland. It is crucial that adenoid cystic carcinoma not be confused with basal cell carcinoma of the skin, with adenoid cystic pattern.[1]

Adenocarcinoma of Undetermined Origin

Primary adenocarcinoma of the vulva most often originates from glands normally present in the vulva, including Bartholin's glands, sweat glands, sebaceous glands, paraurethral glands, and the minor vestibular glands. Rarely, adenocarcinoma may arise from aberrant breast tissue, endometriosis, or misplaced cloacal remnant. In some cases, the exact site of origin is unknown. Tiltman and Knutzen[192] described a well-differentiated mucinous adenocarcinoma occurring in the vulvar vestibule adjacent to the external urethral meatus, which metastasized to the left inguinal lymph node. After ruling out all possible sources, the authors suggested an origin from misplaced cloacal renmants.[192]

Small Cell Carcinoma, Merkel Cell Tumor

Merkel cell tumors occur most frequently in the skin of the head, neck, and extremities of elderly persons. A diffuse infiltrative growth pattern often simulates a malignant lymphoma or leukemia. The uniformly round to oval nuclei have a distinct punctate chromatin pattern, high nucleocytoplasmic ratio, and mitotic activity. Vascular lymphatic invasion is common. Metastasis occurs most frequently (about 50% of cases) to the regional lymph nodes and to the visceral organs in 15% of cases.[22] Occasionally, Merkel cell tumor and squamous cell carcinoma coexist.[189]

Bottle et al.[22] reported a Merkel cell tumor in the labium majus of a 73-year-old woman. It had a nodular erythematous appearance and measured 3 cm × 2 cm in size. The ipsilateral inguinal lymph nodes were suspicious for metastasis. Postoperatively, the patient died of acute myocardial infarction. Autopsy confirmed the presence of metastases in the inguinal and para-aortic lymph nodes, vertebral bodies, liver, and pulmonary vessels. The lungs and uterine cervix revealed no primary tumors. In this and the other reported case of vulvar Merkel cell tumor, squamous carcinoma in situ was found adjacent to but separated from the Merkel cell tumor.[22,189] Whether any pathogenetic relationship exists between the two lesions has not been established.

DeMola et al.[49] reported a case of vulvar Merkel cell carcinoma. The 2 cm polypoid nodule near the left posterior fourchette was excised locally. Re-excision and left inguinal lymphadenectomy showed no residual tumor. Liver metastases were confirmed 6 months later by FNA, and the patient died a year later. Tumor cells expressed cytokeratin and neuron-specific enolase but were negative for chromogranin, S-100 protein, and neurofilaments. Until 1993, five cases were reported in the vulva. All patients had regional or distant metastases, four died in 2 years, and one was lost to follow-up.

A combination of surgical excision, radiation therapy, and chemotherapy is recommended.[38,49]

REFERENCES

1. Abell MR. Adenocystic (pseudoadenomatous) basal cell carcinoma of vestibular glands of vulva. Am J Obstet Gynecol 86:470, 1963.
2. Abell MR. Intraepithelial carcinomas of epidermis and squamous mucosa of vulva and perineum. Surg Clin North Am 45:1179, 1965.
3. Abell, MR, Gosling JRG. Intraepithelial and infiltrative carcinoma of vulva: Bowen's type. Cancer 14:318, 1961.
4. Ackerman LV. Verrucous carcinoma of the oral cavity. Surgery 23:670, 1948.
5. Anders KH, Hall TL, Fu, YS. Epidemiologic and histopathologic studies of female genital warts. In Fenoglio CM, Wolff, MW, Rilke F (eds). Progress in Surgical Pathology. Philadelphia, Woods & Field, 1986, pp 33–47.
6. Anderson JA, Philips PR, Senthilselvan A, et al. Preoperative prognosis for cancer of the vulva. Obstet Gynecol 58:365, 1981.
7. Baggish MS, Dorsey JH. CO_2 laser for the treatment of vulvar carcinoma in situ. Obstet Gynecol 57:371, 1981.
8. Baggish MS, Sze EHM, Adelson MD, et al. Quantitative evaluation of the skin and accessory appendages in vulvar carcinoma in situ. Obstet Gynecol 74:169, 1989.
9. Barclay DL, Collins CG, Macey HB. Cancer of the Bartholin gland: A review and report of eight cases. Obstet Gynecol 24:329, 1964.
10. Barnes AE, Crissman JD, Schellhas HF, et al. Microinvasive carcinoma of the vulva: A clinicopathologic evaluation. Obstet Gynecol 56:234, 1980.
11. Basta A, Madej JG Jr. Hydradenoma of the vulva: Incidence and clinical observations. Eur J Gynae Oncol 11:185, 1990.

12. Benedet JL, Miller DM, Ehlen TG, Bertrand MA. Basal cell carcinoma of the vulva: Clinical features and treatment results in 28 patients. Obstet Gynecol 90:765, 1997.

13. Benedet JL, Turko M, Fairey RS, et al. Squamous carcinoma of the vulva: Results of treatment, 1938 to 1976. Am J Obstet Gynecol 134:201, 1979.

14. Bennington JL, Smith DC, Figge DC. Detection of cells from extramammary Paget's disease of the vulva in a vaginal smear. Obstet Gynecol 27:772, 1966.

15. Bergenon C, Naghashfar Z, Canaan C, et al. Human papillomavirus type 16 in intraepithelial neoplasia (bowenoid papulosis) and coexistent invasive carcinoma of the vulva. Int J Gyn Pathol 6:1, 1987.

16. Berger BW, Hori Y. Multicentric Bowen's disease of the genitalia. Arch Dermatol 114:1698, 1978.

17. Bernstein SG, Voet RL, Lifshitz S. Adenoid cystic carcinoma of Bartholin's gland. Am J Obstet Gynecol 147:385, 1975.

18. Bettley FR, O'Shea JA. The absorption of arsenic and its relation to carcinoma. Br J Dermatol 92:563, 1975.

19. Bhawan J. Multicentric pigmented Bowen's disease: A clinically benign squamous cell carcinoma in situ. Gynecol Oncol 10:201, 1980.

20. Binder SQ, Huang I, Fu YS, et al. Risk factors for the development of lymph node metastasis in vulvar squamous cell carcinoma. Gynecol Oncol 37:9, 1990.

21. Boehm F, Morris JML. Paget's disease and apocrine gland carcinoma of the vulva. Obstet Gynecol 38:185, 1971.

22. Bottle K, Lacey CG, Goldberg J, et al. Merkel cell carcinoma of the vulva. Obstet Gynecol 63:61, 1984.

23. Bowen JT. Precancerous dermatosis: A study of two cases of chronic atypical epithelial proliferation. J Cut Dis 30:241, 1912.

24. Bowing HH, Fricke RE, Kennedy TJ. Radiation therapy for carcinoma of Bartholin's gland. Am J Roentgenol 61:517, 1949.

25. Braun L, Farmer ER, Shah KV. Immunoperoxidase localization of papilloma virus antigen in cutaneous warts and bowenoid papulosis. J Med Virol 12:187, 1983.

26. Breen JL, Neubecker RD, Greenwald E, et al. Basal cell carcinoma of the vulva. Obstet Gynecol 46:122, 1975.

27. Buscema J, Stern JL, Woodruff JD. The significance of histologic alterations adjacent to invasive vulvar carcinoma. Am J Obstet Gynecol 137:902, 1980.

28. Buscema J, Stern JL, Woodruff JD. Early invasive carcinoma of the vulva. Am J Obstet Gynecol 140:563, 1981.

29. Buscema J, Woodruff JD. Progressive histobiologic alterations in the development of vulvar cancer. Am J Obstet Gynecol 138:146, 1980.

30. Buscema J, Woodruff JD, Parmley TH, et al. Carcinoma in situ of the vulva. Obstet Gynecol 55:225, 1980.

31. Buschke A, Löwenstein L. Uber carcinoma-ahnliche Condylomata Acuminata des Penis. Klin Wochensche 4:1726, 1925.

32. Butterworth T, Strean LP, Beerman H. Syringoma and mongolism. Arch Dermatol 90:483, 1964.

33. Caglar H, Tamer S, Hreshchysmn MM. Vulvar intraepithelial neoplasia. Obstet Gynecol 60:346, 1982.

34. Carneiro SJ, Gardner L, Knox M. Syringoma: Three cases with vulvar involvement. Obstet Gynecol 39:95, 1972.

35. Cassidy RE, Braden FR, Cerha HT. Factors that might influence prognosis in malignancies of the vulva. Am J Obstet Gynecol 74:361, 1957.

36. Chafe W, Richards A, Morgan L, Wilkinson E. Unrecognized invasive carcinoma in vulvar intraepithelial neoplasia (VIN). Gynecol Oncol 31:154, 1988.

37. Chamlain DL, Taylor HB. Primary carcinoma of Bartholin's gland. Obstet Gynecol 39:489, 1972.

38. Chen KTK. Merkel's cell (neuroendocrine) carcinoma of the vulva. Cancer 73:2186, 1994.

39. American Joint Committee on Cancer. ACC Cancer Staging Manual, 5th ed. Philadelphia, Lippincott-Raven, 1997.

40. Creasman WT. New gynecologic cancer staging. Obstet Gynecol 75:287, 1990.

41. Creasman WT, Gallager HS, Rutledge F. Paget's disease of the vulva. Gynecol Oncol 3:133, 1975.

42. Crum CP. Carcinoma of the vulva: Epidemiology and pathogenesis. Obstet Gynecol 79:448, 1992.

43. Crum CP, Braum LA, Shah KV, et al. Vulvar intraepithelial neoplasia: An analysis of nuclear DNA content and human papilloma virus antigens. Cancer 49:468, 1982.

44. Crum CP, Ikenberg H, Richart RM, et al. Human papillomavirus type 16 and early cervical neoplasia. N Engl J Med 310:3812, 1984.

45. Crum CP, Liskow A, Petras P, et al. Vulvar intraepithelial neoplasia (severe atypia and carcinoma in situ). Cancer 54:1429, 1984.

46. Cruz-Jiminez PR, Abell MR. Cutaneous basal cell carcinoma of vulva. Cancer 36:1860, 1975.

47. Curry SL, Wharton T, Rutledge F. Positive lymph nodes in vulvar squamous carcinoma. Gynecol Oncol 9:63, 1980.

48. Dawson DF, Duckworth JK, Bernhart H, et al. Giant condyloma and verrucous carcinoma. Gynecol Oncol 9:63, 1980.

49. DeMola IRL, Hudock PA, Steinetz C, et al. Merkel cell carcinoma of the vulva. Gynecol Oncol 51:272, 1993.

50. Dehner LP. Metastatic and secondary tumors of the vulva. Obstet Gynecol 42:47, 1973.

51. Devillez RL, Stevens CS. Bowenoid papules of the genitalia: A case progressing to Bowen's disease. J Am Acad Dermatol 3:149, 1980.

52. DiPaola GR, Gomez-Rueda N, Arrighi L. Relevance of microinvasion in carcinoma of the vulva. Obstet Gynecol 45:647, 1975.

53. DiSaia PJ, Creasman WT, Rich WM. An alternate approach to early cancer of the vulva. Am J Obstet Gynecol 133:825, 1979.

54. DiSaia PJ, Dorion GE, Cappuccini F, Carpenter PM. A report of two cases of recurrent Paget's disease of the vulva in a split-thickness graft and its possible pathogenesis-labeled "retrodissemination." Gynecol Oncol 57:109, 1995.

55. DiSaia PJ, Rich WM. Surgical approach to multifocal carcinoma in situ of the vulva. Am J Obstet Gynecol 35:578, 1970.

56. Dodson MG, O'Leary JA, Averette HE. Primary carcinoma of Bartholin's gland. Obstet Gynecol 35:578, 1970.

57. Dvoretsky P, Bonfiglio T, Helmkamp F, et al. The pathology of superficially invasive, thin vulvar squamous cell carcinoma. Int J Gynecol Pathol 3:331, 1984.

58. Eichenberg HE. Hidradenoma vulvae. Ztschr Geburtsh Gynak 109:358, 1934.

59. Fang BS, Guedes AC, Munoz LC, Villa LL. Human papillomavirus type 16 variants isolated from vulvar bowenoid papulosis. J Med Virol 41:49, 1993.

152. Milchgrub S, Wiley EL, Vuitch F, Albores-Saavedra J. The tubular variant of adenoid cystic carcinoma of the Bartholin's gland. Am J Clin Path 101:204, 1994.
153. Miller WL. Sweat-gland carcinoma. Am J Clin Pathol 47:767, 1967.
154. Morley GW. Infiltrative carcinoma of the vulva: Results of surgical treatment. Am J Obstet Gynecol 124:874, 1976.
155. Morley GW. Cancer of the vulva: A review. Cancer 48:597, 1981.
156. Mossler JA, Woodard BH, Addison A, et al. Adenocarcinoma of Bartholin's gland. Arch Pathol 104:523, 1980.
157. Nadji M, Ganjei P, Penneys NS, et al. Immunohistochemistry of vulvar neoplasms: A brief review. Int J Gynecol Pathol 3:41, 1984.
158. Nakao CY, Nolan JF, DiSaia PJ, et al. "Microinvasive" epidermoid carcinoma of the vulva with an unexpected natural history. Am J Obstet Gynecol 120:1122, 1974.
159. Neilson D, Woodruff JD. Electron microscopy in in situ and invasive vulvar Paget's disease. Am J Obstet Gynecol 113:719, 1972.
160. Newcomb PA, Weiss NS, Daling JR. Incidence of vulvar carcinoma in relation to menstrual, reproductive, and medical factors. J Natl Cancer Inst 73:391, 1984.
161. Nichols CE, Bonney WA. Carcinoma of the vulva producing hypercalcemia. Obstet Gynecol 42:58, 1973.
162. Novak E, Stevenson RR. Sweat gland tumors of the vulva, benign (hidradenoma) and malignant (adenocarcinoma). Am J Obstet Gynecol 50:641, 1945.
163. Olson RL, Nordquist R, Everett MA. An electron microscopic study of Bowen's disease. Cancer Res 28:2078, 1968.
164. Ordonez NG, Manning JR, Luna MA. Mixed tumor of the vulva: A report of two cases probably arising in Bartholin's gland. Cancer 48:181, 1981.
165. Oriel JDD, Whimster IW. Carcinoma in situ associated with virus-containing anal warts. Br J Dermatol 84:71, 1971.
166. Padmanabhan V, Cooper K. Concomitant adenoma and hydrid carcinoma of salivary gland type arising in Bartholin's gland. Int J Gynecol Pathol 19:377, 2000.
167. Palladino VS, Duffy JL, Bures GL. Basal cell carcinoma of the vulva. Cancer 24:460, 1969.
168. Paone JF, Baker RR. Pathogenesis and treatment of Paget's disease of the breast. Cancer 48:341, 1975.
169. Parker RT, Duncan I, Rampone J, et al. Operative management of early invasive epidermoid carcinoma of the vulva. Am J Obstet Gynecol 123:349, 1975.
170. Parmley TH, Woodruff JD, Julina CG. Invasive vulvar Paget's disease. Obstet Gynecol 46:341, 1975.
171. Patterson JW, Kao GF, Graham JH, et al. Bowenoid papulosis: A clinicopathologic study with ultrastructural observations. Cancer 57:823, 1986.
172. Pilotti S, Delle Torre G, Rilke F, et al. Immunohistochemical and ultrastructural evidence of papilloma virus infection associated with in situ and microinvasive squamous cell carcinoma of the vulva. Am J Surg Pathol 8:751, 1984.
173. Powell JL, Franklin EW III, Nickerson JF, et al. Verrucous carcinoma of the female genital tract. Gynecol Oncol 6:565, 1978.
174. Priorleau PG, Santa Cruz DJ, Meyer JS, et al. Verrucous carcinoma. Cancer 45:2849, 1980.
175. Queyrat L. Erythroplasie du gland. Bull Soc Fr Dermatol Sympt 28:378, 1911.
176. Rando RF, Sedlacek TV, Hung J, et al. Verrucous carcinoma of the vulva associated with an unusual type 6 human papillomavirus. Obstet Gynecol 67:70S, 1986.
177. Rastkar G, Ojagaki T, Twiggs LB, et al. Early invasive and in situ warty carcinoma of the vulva: Clinical, histologic, and electron microscopic study with particular reference to viral association. Am J Obstet Gynecol 143:814, 1982.
178. Rhatigan RM, Mojadidi O. Adenosquamous carcinoma of the vulva and vagina. Am J Clin Pathol 59:208, 1973.
179. Rich PM, Okagaki R, Clark B, et al. Adenocarcinoma of the sweat gland of the vulva: Light and electron microscopic study. Cancer 47:1352, 1981.
180. Rorat E, Wallach RC. Mixed tumors of the vulva: Clinical outcome and pathology. Int J Gyneco Pathol 3:323, 1984.
181. Roth LM, Lee SC, Ehrlich CE. Paget's disease of the vulva—A histogenetic study of five cases, including ultrastructure observations and review of the literature. Am J Surg Pathol 1:193, 1977.
182. Rutledge F, Smith JP, Franklin EW. Carcinoma of the vulva. Am J Obstet Gynecol 106:1117, 1970.
183. Schwartz PE, Naftolin F. Type 2 herpes simplex virus and vulvar carcinoma in situ (Editorial). N Engl J Med 305:517, 1981.
184. Sedlis A, Homesley H, Bundy BM, et al. Positive groin lymph nodes in superficial squamous cell vulvar cancer. Am J Obstet Gynecol 156:1159, 1987.
185. Shanbour KA, Mannel RS, Morris PC, et al. Comparison of clinical vs. surgical staging systems in vulvar cancer. Obstet Gynecol 80:927, 1982.
186. Skinner MS, Sternberg WH, Ichinose H, et al. Spontaneous atypia of the vulva. Obstet Gynecol 42:40, 1973.
187. Sturgeon SR, Brinton LA, Devesa SS, Kurman RJ. In situ and invasive vulvar cancer incidence trends (1973 to 1987). Am J Obstet Gynecol 166:1482, 1992.
188. Sworn MJ, Hammond GT. Metastatic basal cell carcinoma of the vulva: Case Report. Br J Obstet Gynecol 86:332, 1979.
189. Tang CK, Toker C, Nedwich A, et al. Unusual cutaneous carcinoma with features of small cell (oat cell-like) and squamous cell carcinomas: A variant of Merkel cell neoplasm. Am J Dermatopathol 4:537, 1982
190. Taylor PT, Stenwig JT, Clausen H. Paget's disease of the vulva. Gynecol Oncol 3:46, 1975.
191. Tchang F, Okagaki T, Richart RM. Adenocarcinoma of the Bartholin's gland associated with Paget's disease of vulvar area. Cancer 31:221, 1973.
192. Tiltman AJ, Knutzen VK. Primary adenocarcinoma of the vulva originating in misplaced cloacal tissue. Obstet Gynecol 51:308, 1978.
193. Toki T, Kurman RJ, Park JS, et al. Probable nonpapillomavirus etiology of squamous cell carcinoma in older women: A clinicopathologic study using in situ hybridization and polymerase chain reaction. Int J Gynecol Pathol 10:107, 1991.
194. Trimble C, Hildesheim A, Brinton LA, et al. Heterogeneous etiology of squamous carcinoma of the vulva. Obstet Gynecol 87:59, 1996.
195. Tsukada Y, Lopez RG, Pickren JW, et al. Paget's disease of the vulva: A clinicopathologic study of eight cases. Obstet Gynecol 45:73, 1975.
196. Ulbright TM, Stehman FB, Roth LM, et al. Bowenoid dysplasia of the vulva. Cancer 50:2910, 1982.
197. Underwood JW, Adcock LL, Okagaki T. Adenosquamous carcinoma of skin appendages (adenoid squa-

mous cell carcinoma, pseudoglandular squamous cell carcinoma, adenoacanthoma of sweat gland of Lever) of the vulva: A clinical and ultrastructural study. Cancer 42:1851, 1978.

198. Van Beurden M, ten Kate FJW, Smits H, et al. Multifocal vulvar intraepithelial neoplasia grade III and multicentric lower genital tract neoplasia is associated with transcriptionally active human papillomavirus. Cancer 75:2879, 1995.

199. Van Beurden M, ten Kate FJW, Tjong-A-Hung SF, et al. Human papillomavirus DNA in multicentric vulvar intraepithelial neoplasia. Int J Gynecol Pathol 17:12, 1998.

200. Van der Velden J, van Lindert ACM, Lammes FB, et al. Extracapsular growth of lymph node metastases in squamous cell carcinoma of the vulva. Cancer 75:2885, 1995.

201. Van Nagell JR, Tweeddale DN, Roddick JW. Primary adenoacanthoma of the Bartholin gland. Obstet Gynecol 34:87, 1969.

202. Vanstapel MJ, Gatter KC, Dewolf-Peeters D, et al. Immunohistochemical study of mammary and extra-mammary Paget's disease. Histopathology 8:1013, 1984.

203. Wade TR, Kopf AW, Ackerman AB. Bowenoid papulosis of the genitalia. Arch Dermatol 115:306, 1979.

204. Wade TR, Kopf AW, Ackerman AB. Bowenoid papulosis of the penis. Cancer 42:1890, 1978.

205. Wahlstrom T, Vesterlinen E, Saksela E. Primary carcinoma of Bartholin's glands: A morphological and clinical study of six cases including a transitional cell carcinoma. Gynecol Oncol 6:354, 1978.

206. Way S, Benedet JL. Involvement of inguinal lymph nodes in carcinoma of the vulva. Gynecol Oncol 1:119, 1973.

207. Wharton JT, Gallager S, Rutledge FN. Microinvasive carcinoma of the vulva. Am J Obstet Gynecol 118:159, 1974.

208. Wheelock JB, Goplerud DR, Dunn LJ, et al. Primary carcinoma of the Bartholin's gland: A report of ten cases. Obstet Gynecol 63:820, 1984.

209. Wick MR, Goeliner JR, Wolfe JT, et al. Vulvar sweat gland carcinomas. Arch Pathol Lab Med 109:43, 1985.

210. Wilkinson EJ, Friedrich EG Jr, Fu YS. Multicentric nature of vulvar carcinoma in situ. Obstet Gynecol 58:69, 1981.

211. Wilkinson EJ. Superficial invasive carcinoma of the vulva. Clin Obstet Gynecol 28:188, 1985.

212. Wilkinson EJ, Kneale B, Lynch PJ. Report of the ISSVD Terminology Committee. J Reprod Med 31:973, 1986.

213. Wilkinson EJ, Rico MJ, Pierson KK. Microinvasive carcinoma of the vulva. Int J Gynecol Pathol 1:29, 1982.

214. Willis RA. Pathology of Tumors. London, Butterworths, 1960, p 556.

215. Wilson D, Woodger BA. Pleomorphic adenoma of the vulva. J Obstet Gynecol Br Comm 81:1000, 1974.

216. Woodruff JD. Vulvar atypia and carcinoma in situ. J Reprod Med 17:155, 1976.

217. Woodruff JD, Hilderbrandt EE. Carcinoma in situ of the vulva. Obstet Gynecol 12:414, 1958.

218. Woodruff, JD, Julian CG, Puray T, et al. The contemporary challenge of carcinoma in situ of the vulva. Am J Obstet Gynecol 115:677, 1973.

219. Woodworth H, Dockerty MB, Wilson RB, et al. Papillary hidradenoma of the vulva: A clinicopathologic study of 69 cases. Am J Obstet Gynecol 110:501, 1971.

220. Wright VC, Chapman WB. Colposcopy of intraepithelial neoplasia of the vulva and adjacent sites. Cont Colposcopy 20:231, 1993.

221. Yang B, Hart WR. Vulvar intraepithelial neoplasia of the simplex (differentiated) type. Am J Surg Pathol 24:429, 2000.

222. Yazigi R, Piver MS, Tsukada Y. Microinvasive carcinoma of the vulva. Obstet Gynecol 51:368, 1978.

223. Young AW Jr, Herman EW, Tovell HMM. Syringoma of the vulva: Incidence, diagnosis, and cause of pruritus. Obstet Gynecol 55:515, 1980.

224. Zaino RJ, Husseinzadeh N, Nahhas W, et al. Epithelial alterations in proximity to invasive carcinoma of the vulva. Int J Gynecol Pathol 1:173, 1982.

7

BENIGN AND MALIGNANT EPITHELIAL NEOPLASMS OF THE VAGINA

BENIGN EPITHELIAL NEOPLASMS AND TUMOR-LIKE CONDITIONS

Fibroepithelial Polyp

Fibroepithelial polyps of the vagina are uncommon. They are of interest to the pathologist because they may be confused with sarcoma botryoides. They may represent hamartomas and have been referred to as fibrous polyps, pseudosarcoma botryoides,[34] sarcoma botryoid–like lesions,[92] fibroepithelial polyps,[12,21] and vaginal polyps.[26] Although vaginal bleeding was observed in 4 of 18 cases,[26] in other women there was evidence of a vaginal growth, which, in some instances, was an incidental finding. Polyps rarely develop in infants but are more common in adults. The median age at detection is 48.5 years, with a range of 18 to 86 years.[26] They have been observed during pregnancy.[92] In a series of 18 cases, only two polyps were detected in gravid women.[26]

Polyps usually occur singly, measuring about 1.5 cm in greatest dimension. Only rarely are larger polyps observed. In one case, the polyp measured 3.6 cm in greatest dimension.[21] In only 3 of 15 cases was the lesion characterized as pedunculated,[26] and it was more likely to be polypoid or nodular.

Mucitelli et al.[88] reported on 18 cases of vulvovaginal polyps in women aged 24 to 72 years. The polyps were 0.6 to 4.5 cm in size and appeared as polypoid, nodular, pedunculated lesions or skin tags. Nine were vaginal (six anterior wall, two lateral wall, one posterior wall), four were of unknown site, and five were vulvar (three labium minus, two labium majus). The surface of fibroepithelial polyps is smooth or irregular and rarely ulcerated. Polyps may have a rubbery consistency or may be soft. They are covered by stratified squamous epithelium similar to that of the normal vaginal epithelium (Fig. 7–1). Within the stroma, there are variable amounts of myxoid or edematous connective tissue.

Blood vessels are usually abundant (see Fig. 7–1). In about half of cases within the stroma, there are a variable number of spindle cells containing large pleomorphic nuclei (Fig. 7–2).[26] The nuclei are hyperchromatic and are usually single and only rarely are multiple. Mitoses are infrequent. Multinucleated giant cells are common (Fig. 7–3). There is no tendency for the atypical stromal cells to be distributed in a "cambium layer." Cross striations are not observed in the cytoplasm. A variable number of leukocytes may occur within the stroma.

The origin of the atypical stromal cells is unknown; some investigators have suggested the possibility of hormonal stimulation.[21,34,92] A subepithelial myxoid connective tissue zone from 0.5 to 5 mm in width extending from the cervix to the vulva in normal women has been described.[27,33] In about 25% of cases, atypical cells with bizarre, hyperchromatic nuclei are present within the connective tissue of this zone.[33] Abnormal mitoses may occur.[117]

Nucci et al.[93] retrieved 33 cases of vulvovaginal fibroepithelial polyps from a consultative service. They described unusual histologic fea-

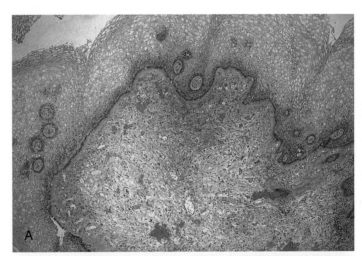

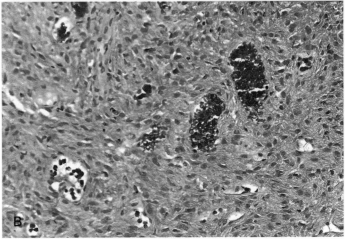

Figure 7–1. Fibroepithelial polyp. *A*, Glycogenated mature vaginal squamous mucosa and the underlying fibrous stroma with myxoid change. *B*, Moderate increase in cellularity and vascularity in part of the stroma.

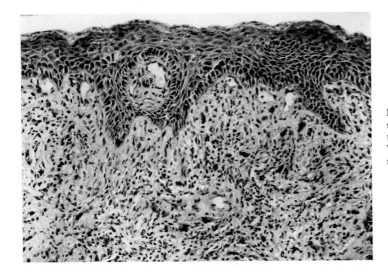

Figure 7–2. Lamina propria beneath the surface of fibroepithelial polyp. Note scattered giant cells. (H&E, ×200; courtesy of William M. Christopherson, M.D., University of Louisville.)

tures, such as hypercellularity, nuclear pleomorphism, increased mitotic activity, and abnormal mitotic figures. Twelve of 33 fibroepithelial polyps contained three or more of the features just listed. Local recurrences were identified in three of 21 women with follow-up, including two pregnant women and one postmenopausal woman. These local recurrences were not associated with local destruction or infiltrative behavior. Several pregnant women had multiple polyps. No metastasis was noted in any of these women. Thus, despite these unusual histologic features, none of these fibroepithelial polyps behaved in a malignant fashion.

Stromal cells and multinucleated giant cells are positive for vimentin (8 of 12 cases) and desmin (5 of 12 cases) (Fig. 7–4) and negative for S-100 protein, cytokeratin, α-1-antitrypsin,

and epithelial membrane antigen.[88] Hartmann et al.[51] also demonstrated estrogen and progesterone receptor proteins by immunohistochemistry. With electron microscopy, stromal cells resemble fibroblasts and myofibroblasts. After simple excision, there was no recurrence.

Benign Müllerian Papilloma

This benign tumor of the vagina and cervix has been identified by several different terms, including *benign mesonephric papillary* and *polypoid tumors*,[66] *mesonephric papilloma of childhood*,[4] and *intramural papilloma*.[136] It typically occurs in children aged 14 months to 9 years and usually in 2 to 5 years. Most patients present with vaginal bleeding or discharge. Pelvic examination

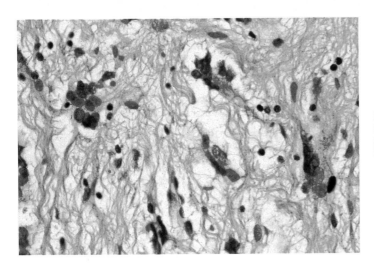

Figure 7–3. High-power view of stroma of fibroepithelial polyp with multinucleated giant cells. Some of the nuclei are irregular and hyperchromatic.

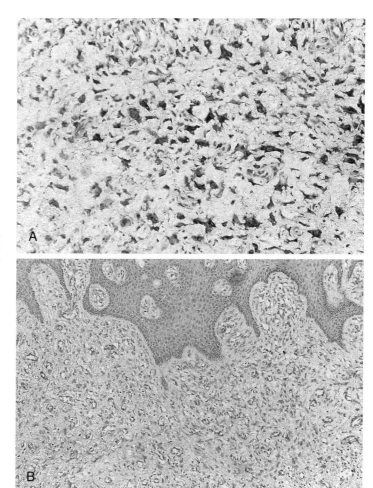

Figure 7–4. Stromal cells of fibroepithelial polyp are positive for desmin (*A*) and negative for actin (*B*) by immunohistochemical stains.

reveals an exophytic, papillary, polyp-like tumor involving the mucosal surface of the ectocervix or upper vagina that measures 1 to 3.5 cm in size, has a red, granular appearance, and bleeds readily on touch. Ulbright et al.[136] described one such tumor located in the muscularis of the vagina, to which they applied the term *intramural papilloma.*

Histologically, the polypoid tumor forms multiple papillary fronds supported by myxomatous to densely fibrous stroma. The surface is covered by several layers of columnar or low cuboidal cells (Fig. 7–5). Some have mucinous cytoplasm, resembling endocervical cells; others have cytoplasm varying from densely eosinophilic to vacuolated (Fig. 7–6). Cilia and glycogen particles are generally absent. The nuclei are uniformly round to oval, basally located, and low in mitotic activity. Foci of squamous metaplasia are found in most cases (Fig. 7–7). Hobnail cells are found occasionally.[4]

Near the base of stalks, the epithelium may form complex, cribriform glands. Osseous metaplasia is occasionally seen in the stroma.[136]

Histochemical and ultrastructural findings vary from tumor to tumor. Some authors, having failed to detect any mucin, glycogen, or mucopolysaccharide in the tumor cells, favor a mesonephric origin.[4,66] Others have found features supporting a müllerian origin, including mucopolysaccharides in the glandular lumens, numerous microvilli, conspicuous lysosomes, and abundant perinuclear microfilaments resembling endometrial cells.[136] A müllerian origin is favored on the basis of positive cytokeratin, epithelial membrane antigen, and weak carcinoembryonic antigen.[80]

It is important to recognize this rare tumor because of the possibility of confusing it with clear cell carcinoma. Hobnail cells and complex papillary and glandular patterns can be seen in polypoid tumor, clear cell carcinoma,

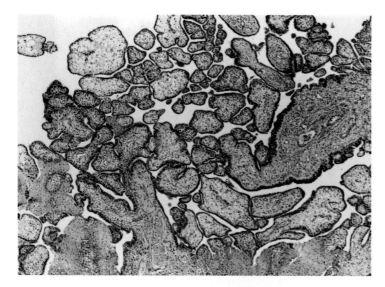

Figure 7–5. Müllerian papilloma presents with multiple papillary fibrovascular cores that are covered by epithelial cells.

Figure 7–6. Müllerian papilloma. Some of the glands are lined by endocervical-type cells with mucinous, clear cytoplasm. Others are nonciliated, low columnar to cuboidal cells with eosinophilic cytoplasm. A layer of reserve cell hyperplasia can be seen in some of the glands.

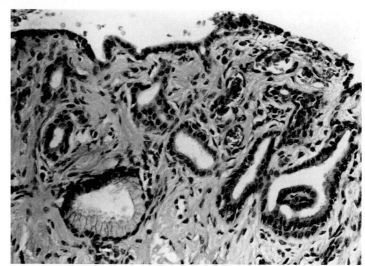

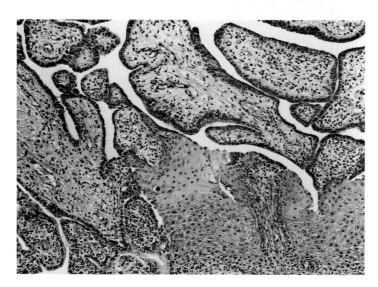

Figure 7–7. Müllerian papilloma. The glandular cells often undergo squamous metaplasia.

and endodermal sinus tumor (yolk sac) tumor. The latter two tumors demonstrate a greater degree of nuclear atypism and mitotic activity. Clear cell carcinoma, in addition, contains abundant glycogen, which is scanty or absent in müllerian papilloma. In endodermal sinus tumor, primitive cells often form the central capillary core and Schiller-Duval body. The müllerian papilloma is superficial in location and consists of benign-appearing cells with frequent squamous metaplasia.

All patients who have undergone complete local excision have been free of disease 2 to 10 years later.[65,124] Of more than 50 cases reported in the literature, there was no recurrence after treatment by complete local excision.[26] Local recurrence can occur following incomplete excision.[80] A 5-year-old girl presented with vaginal spotting and was found to have a 0.8 cm polypoid mass in the right vaginal wall, which was removed by forceps. Two years later, tumor recurred at the previous excision site and measured 1.8 cm in size.[80]

Benign Mixed Tumor

Benign mixed tumors resembling those of the salivary gland are rare in the vagina. In 1953, Brown[18] reported a single case. Whelton[141] reported a case classified as a mixed tumor; however, the nature of this neoplasm is uncertain on the basis of the limited description and illustrations. Komiya et al.,[71] Chen,[25] and Buntine et al.[19] reported isolated cases. Sirota et al.[132] described eight cases classified as mixed tumors.

The neoplasms occurred in women aged 20 to 53 years, with a mean age of 31 years.[132] Infrequently, the tumors presented as slowly enlarging, painless masses; more commonly, they were identified on routine pelvic examination.[141] In the reported cases, the neoplasms often originated in or near the hymenal ring. Of 11 cases, four originated from the posterior vaginal wall, two arose from the lateral vaginal wall, one was related to the anterior vaginal wall, and in four cases the site of origin was unclear.[132]

The preoperative diagnosis was cyst in three cases and a solid neoplasm or polyp in six cases; in two cases, it was unstated.[132] The tumors were usually discrete, often were submucosal in location, and ranged from 1.5 to 5 cm in greatest dimension.[132] On gross examination, the tumors were discrete, soft, and usually not encapsulated. The cut surface was pale gray or pink.

Branton and Tavassoli (16) reported on 28 women aged 20 to 69 years (mean 40.5). Most of the mixed tumors were located in the introitus, posterior vaginal wall, and close to the hymenal ring. The tumors were 1.0 to 6.0 cm (mean 2.6) in size, well circumscribed but nonencapsulated, gray-white, and sometimes gelatinous.

On histopathologic examination, the neoplasms are composed predominantly of sheets of spindle cells and less commonly of mature stratified squamous epithelium and glands. The spindle cells have small round, oval, or spindle-shaped nuclei (Figs. 7–8 and 7–9). The chromatin is finely granular, and nucleoli are indistinct. Only two of eight cases involved sig-

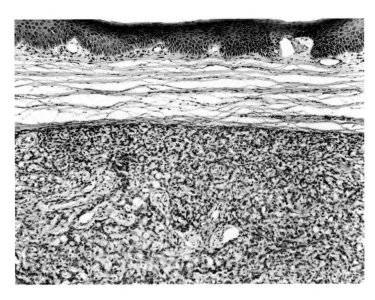

Figure 7–8. Benign mixed tumor of the vagina. The tumor lies beneath the surface of the vagina. In this site, the stroma has a whorled pattern. (From Sirota RL. Am J Surg Pathol 5:413, 1981; used by permission.)

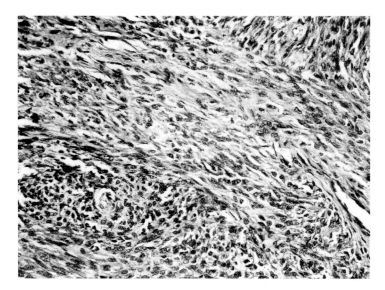

Figure 7–9. Benign mixed tumor of the vagina. In this portion of the tumor, spindylate are cells arranged in bundles. (From Sirota RL, et al. Am J Surg Pathol 5:413, 1981; used by permission.)

nificant numbers of mitoses.[132] The spindle cells are arranged in a poorly defined whorled pattern (see Fig. 7–8) or intersecting fascicles (see Fig. 7–9). In most cases, stains for mucin were weakly positive in intercellular locations.[132] In seven of eight cases, stratified squamous epithelium (Fig. 7–10) was well glycogenated with a variable content of keratin and arranged in well-circumscribed nests.[132]

Droplets or pools of mucin are sometimes observed in the squamous epithelium. In three of eight cases, glands were lined by mucin-containing epithelium, and in an additional case, the glands were lined by a simple cuboidal or flat epithelium. The glandular epithelium merges with the squamous epithelium. Less frequently, the stromal cells contain spaces with globular deposits of hyalin material. However, chondroid tissue had not been reported.[25]

Branton et al.[16] reported the spindle cells to have small, oval, hyperchromatic nuclei, scant cytoplasm, and indistinct cell borders. These cells are sometimes mixed with fibroblasts. The background stroma may contain myxoid areas, hyalin globules, and small blood vessels. Twenty-one of 28 (75%) tumors contain rare glands, which are lined by a layer of columnar to cuboidal cells. Nests of glycogenated mature squamous cells occurred in 15 (54%) tumors. Immunohistochemical stains further demon-

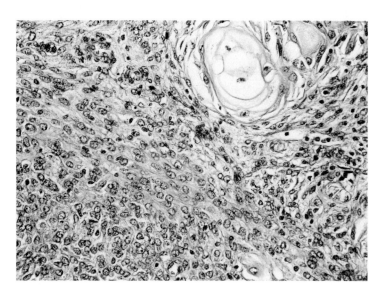

Figure 7–10. Benign mixed tumor of the vagina. A squamous component is present in this portion of the tumor. (From Sirota RL, et al. Am J Surg Pathol 5:413, 1981; used by permission.)

strated cytokeratin in the spindle cells of 9 of 10 tumors and smooth muscle actin in all tumors, at least focally.

Progesterone receptor protein was found in all five tumors tested, and estrogen receptor protein was negative or weak. S-100 protein and glial filament acidic protein were negative.[16]

By electron microscopic examination, spindle cells contain tonofilaments but do not have the characters of myoepithelial cells, such as myofibrils, pinocytic vesicles, and basal lamina. These authors favored an epithelial origin, especially the urogenital sinus epithelium, and proposed the term *vaginal spindle cell epithelioma.*[16]

Of the 22 women with follow-up data, three developed local recurrence at 5 months, 3 years, and 8 years, all at the earlier excision sites. None of the tumors had metastasized. A complete surgical excision should be curative.[16] Wright et al.[144] reported on a 61-year-old woman who presented with a mass in the posterior vaginal wall. Eight years earlier she had undergone a local excision of vaginal tumor and total abdominal hysterectomy with bilateral salpingo-oophorectomy. The recurrent mass was covered by smooth mucosa, firm in consistency, and oval in shape. There was no tumor recurrence 3 years after reexcision.

Brenner Tumor

Chen[24] described a polypoid 1.5 cm solid nodule in the midvagina of a 67-year-old woman. Histologically, it resembled Brenner tumor of the ovary and consisted of cellular fibrous stroma and islands of transitional cells. Most of the latter had clear or eosinophilic cytoplasm and uniform, grooved nuclei. In addition, mucus-secreting, endocervical-type cells were found contiguous with the transitional cells or formed isolated glands. The author favored a müllerian origin.[24] There was no evidence of recurrence 7 years after excision.

Buntine et al.[19] reported on a 5 cm polypoid tumor in the posterior vaginal wall of a 53-year-old woman. The tumor was designated as benign müllerian mixed tumor, but histologically it resembled Brenner tumor. The differential diagnosis includes vaginal mixed tumor, which occurs predominantly in premenopausal women, presenting with a mass in the lower vagina adjacent to the hymenal ring and 1 to 6 cm in size. The proliferating cells have the appearance of squamous cells and

are associated with densely cellular fibrous stroma with hyaline spherules.

Vaginal Brenner tumor affects postmenopausal women. The mass varies from 0.5 to 2.0 cm in size and is located in the mid to upper vaginal wall. Clusters of transitional cells are surrounded by cellular fibrous stroma.

VAGINAL INTRAEPITHELIAL NEOPLASIA (VAIN)

Epidemiology and Carcinogenesis of VAIN and Squamous Cell Carcinoma

Owing to a close anatomic relationship between the vagina and the cervix and uterus superiorly, the vulva inferiorly, the rectum posteriorly, and the bladder anteriorly, 80% to 90% of vaginal malignancies are secondary neoplasms, originating from the adjacent sites. They involve the vagina by direct extension and lymphatic or hematogenous spread. Primary malignant neoplasms of the vagina are uncommon, accounting for 1% to 2% of the malignant tumors observed in the female genital tract. Of vaginal malignancies, 90% to 95% are of epithelial origin. Of these, 90% are in situ or invasive squamous cell carcinomas. The remaining 2% to 4% of tumors include adenocarcinomas, malignant melanoma, sarcoma, embryonal rhabdomyosarcoma in children, and others.[87,101,126]

Based on information obtained in the Third National Cancer Survey, covering the period 1969 to 1971,[29] the incidence for in situ cancer of the vagina was 0.20 case per 100,000 white women and 0.31 case per 100,000 black women. The incidence for invasive squamous cell cancer of the vagina was 0.42 case per 100,000 white women and 0.93 case per 100,000 black women. In this survey, invasive cancer of the vagina accounts for 2.7% of the cancers observed in the lower genital tract of white women and 2.5% of those found in black women.[52] The annual incidence rate of VAIN (dysplasia and carcinoma in situ) is 0.3 case per 100,000 women as compared to 38 per 100,000 for CIN, 1 per 100,000 for vulvar intraepithelial neoplasia, and 0.6 per 100,000 for invasive vaginal carcinoma.[117]

The age-specific incidence rates observed for in situ and invasive cancer of the vagina are unlike those associated with cancer of the uterine cervix. In both white and black women, the highest incidence rates observed for in situ and invasive vaginal cancers occur after the age of 60 years. Only 11% of vaginal cancers are detected before the age of 50 years, compared with 43% of primary cervical cancers. Cancer of the uterine cervix is detected at an earlier age than is vaginal cancer, and the incidence rates increase more rapidly in young women.[52]

It has been postulated that cancer of the lower genital tract develops in response to a stimulus or stimuli affecting the uterine cervix, vagina, and vulva. In keeping with this hypothesis, it has been noted that cancer of the vagina may develop simultaneously with cancer of the uterine cervix, although some authors maintain that this should be distinguished from cancers confined to the vagina.[47]

Risk factors for the development of in situ and invasive vaginal squamous carcinomas are previously reported abnormal Pap smears, vaginal discharge and irritation, or prior hysterectomy. Genital warts were associated with carcinoma in situ but not invasive carcinoma. Smoking status and the number of sexual partners, important risk factors for cervical and vulvar carcinomas, are not identified in vaginal carcinoma.[17]

Agents implicated in vaginal carcinogenesis have included viruses, immunosuppression, and ionizing radiation. Both human papillomavirus (HPV) and herpes simplex virus infections often produce multiple lesions in one anatomic site (multifocal) or involve multiple sites (multicentric) in the lower genital tract. Among women with vaginal condyloma, 85% had additional lesions in the cervix or vulva or both.[3] Malignant change can occur in condyloma.[76,79] HPV types 16 and 18 are important etiologic agents.

Immunosuppressive therapy has clearly increased the risk of HPV infection and squamous neoplasia. Radiation therapy to cervical cancer exposes the vagina to a sublethal dose of irradiation. This may predispose the vagina to the development of postradiation dysplasia.[82,84,143] Whether in utero diethylstilbestrol exposure leads to an increase in vaginal and cervical squamous neoplasia remains controversial.

Since the majority of preinvasive and early invasive vaginal neoplasms are clinically silent, routine cervicovaginal cytology remains the most effective means of detecting these changes. Women who have had prior genital neoplasia or hysterectomy for benign conditions especially need continuous surveillance. When such women develop vaginal carcinoma, it is clinically more advanced and carries a poorer prognosis than

that which occurs in women who have had a hysterectomy for cervical neoplasia.[135] This difference is probably related to infrequent cytologic screening after hysterectomy for benign disease.

VAIN without Prior Radiation

Clinical and Gross Features

VAIN includes dysplasia and carcinoma in situ (CIS).[103] In one study, the severity of VAINs were mild dysplasia (VAIN 1) 50%, moderate dysplasia (VAIN 2) 20%, and severe dysplasia and CIS (VAIN 3) 30%.[117]

Mean age for vaginal carcinoma in situ is 46.9 years, as compared with 57 years for invasive carcinoma. In a study of 82 women with squamous dysplasia of the vagina, 56% had cervical neoplasia (33% intraepithelial and 23% invasive), and 16% had vulvar neoplasia (10% intraepithelial and 6% invasive).[62] Only 37% (30 patients) had neither cervical nor vulvar neoplasia. Of the 45 women with squamous CIS, 78% had cervical neoplasm (49% intraepithelial and 29% invasive), and 27% had vulvar neoplasia (18% CIS and 9% invasive). Several patients had both cervical and vulvar disease. Only 11% (five women) had neither cervical nor vulvar neoplasm. In women with vaginal dysplasia or CIS, one third had had prior ionizing radiation.[62]

The associated cervical dysplasia or CIS was detected concurrently (within 1 year) with vaginal dysplasia and CIS in 53% of cases, prior to the vaginal lesion in 37%, and subsequent to the vaginal disease in 10%. The invasive cervical carcinoma occurred concurrently with vaginal dysplasia or CIS in 19% of cases, 1 to 5 years earlier in 25%, and more than 5 years previously in 56%.[62] From a clinical standpoint, concurrent vaginal lesions are generally regarded as the extension, persistence, or recurrence of the adjacent malignancy.

The average age at detection of CIS is reported to range from 31 to over 70 years of age, with a mean age of 53 years.[64] Patients with synchronous cervical and vaginal neoplasia are approximately 45 years of age, which is younger than those who develop vaginal lesions after hysterectomy for cervical cancer or those having primary vaginal in situ cancers.[64] In a UCLA series, the mean age of patients with dysplasia was 49.7 years. Those who had had no prior radiation were an average of 7 years younger than those who did have prior radiation (47.5 versus 54.8 years). Patients with squamous CIS had a mean age of 52.5 years, and there was a difference of 7 years between those with and without prior radiation (57.4 versus 50.1 years).[62] The difference in age can be explained by the older mean age for cervical invasive rather than intraepithelial carcinoma and the development of dysplasia several years following radiation.

Patients with vaginal dysplasia and CIS are generally asymptomatic, and the changes are initially detected by cytology. In a series by Hernandez-Linares et al.,[61] the cytology was positive in 80% of patients with vaginal CIS. When symptoms are present, they include postcoital spotting, dyspareunia, burning, and leukorrhea. The majority of changes occur in the upper vagina or apex[8] and less frequently involve the middle or lower third of the vagina.[45,73,78,87] Multicentric foci of neoplastic involvement are observed in 10% to 17% of cases.[8,61]

Vaginal squamous CIS is usually described as white and well defined.[6] Gray and Christopherson[49] reported a pink "blush" or a slightly granular appearance. The Schiller's test may aid in localizing the abnormality, and colposcopy may detect or localize the change. In patients previously treated for cancer of the uterine cervix or vulva, the possibility of CIS of the vagina should be considered.

Microscopic Features

Criteria for the classification of vaginal dysplasia and CIS are generally similar to those used for the cervix. The degree of cellular differentiation, maturation sequence and cellular po-

larity, mitotic activity, and nuclear atypism are most important.

In VAIN 1, mild dysplasias, the cells maintain orderly maturation from the parabasal to the superficial layers. However, hypercellularity, disorganization, and increased mitotic activity occur, especially in the deep layers (Fig. 7–11). In the intermediate and superficial layers, the nuclei are enlarged, hyperchromatic, and slightly irregular (see Fig. 7–11).

In VAIN 2, moderate dysplasias, squamous differentiation in the upper third of the epithelium is maintained. However, there is a greater degree of proliferation, higher mitotic activity, and loss of polarity in the lower two thirds of the epithelium when compared with that of mild dysplasias (Figs. 7–12 and 7–13). Koilocytosis is a common feature in mild and moderate dysplasias.

In VAIN 3, severe dysplasia and CIS, immature cells with scanty cytoplasm, hyperchromatic and irregular nuclei, and coarse chromatin pattern have a disorderly arrangement (Figs. 7–14 and 7–15). Mitotic figures, including abnormal forms, are found in all levels. Squamous differentiation is absent or limited to the most superficial layers (see Figs. 7–14 and 7–15). Some of the lesions in the distal vagina closely resemble those of Bowen's disease of the vulva. In association with squamous cell CIS of the vagina, microinvasion or early invasion has been reported.[49] The cellular changes associated with vaginal carcinoma in situ resemble those observed in the presence of intraepithelial cancer of the uterine cervix.[72]

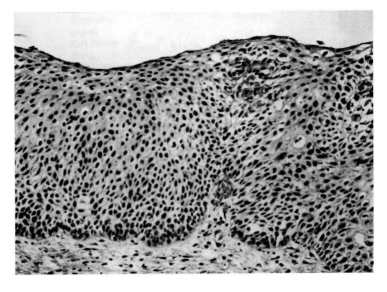

Figure 7–11. VAIN 1, mild squamous dysplasia, with increased cellularity and minor nuclear changes. Note the intact basal cell layer.

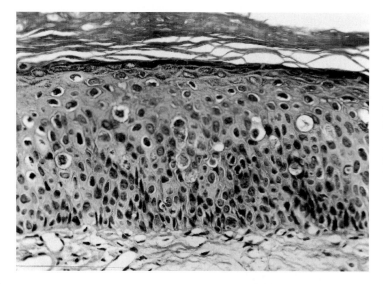

Figure 7–12. VAIN 2, moderate dysplasia. Although the maturation is maintained in the superficial layers, considerable disorganization and mitotic activity are present in the lower two thirds.

Figure 7–13. VAIN 2 to 3, moderate to severe dysplasia. This dysplastic epithelium reveals squamous maturation and koilocytosis in the superficial layers. The lower two thirds of epithelium, however, demonstrates nuclear atypism, loss of polarity, and several mitotic figures, including abnormal forms.

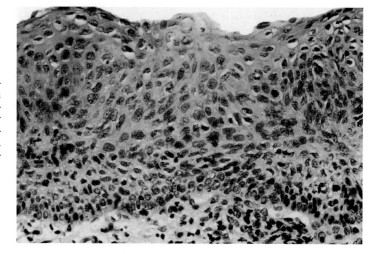

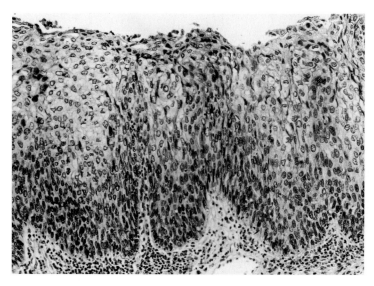

Figure 7–14. VAIN 3, severe dysplasia, composed almost entirely of immature cells. Squamous differentiation is limited to the superficial layers.

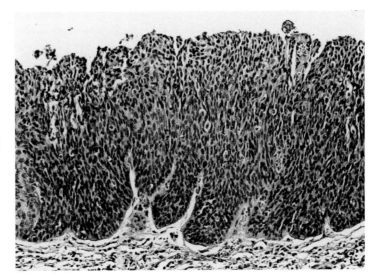

Figure 7–15. VAIN 3, squamous cell carcinoma in situ. The entire epithelium is replaced by neoplastic cells. Mitoses are evident.

Sherman and Paull[128] reported that the diagnosis of VAIN is often hampered in postmenopausal women due to mucosal atrophy and the location in the vaginal cuff following prior hysterectomy or radiotherapy for intraepithelial or invasive cervical carcinoma. In their series of 45 women with VAIN, the median age was 60.5 years. Twenty-seven women (60%) had a prior history of cervical or vulvar intraepithelial or invasive squamous neoplasia. An additional eight (18%) women had ovarian, endometrial, or hematopoietic malignancies. The agreement between the cytologic and histologic diagnoses was 56% for VAIN 2 and VAIN 3 lesions combined. The authors proposed to classify VAIN into low- and high-grade groups. Cytologic screening is important for the detection of VAIN.[128]

Radiation Changes and Postradiation Dysplasia

Vaginal discharge is usually observed within a week after the initiation of radiotherapy.[15] This is the result of trauma associated with the applicators used, the direct effects of ionizing radiation, and the altered physiology of the vagina. Contact or spontaneous bleeding may occur after removal of the radium applicators. Spotting may result from the atrophic vagina or induced abrasions or from telangiectasia. Dyspareunia may be related to the state of the epithelium or to the narrowing of the introitus and shortening or constriction of the vagina.[5,46]

Abrasion and erythema of the vaginal vault may be observed early. Erythema may persist for weeks or months. The vaginal mucosa may be covered by a white membrane. Ultimately, the vaginal mucosa becomes pale. Telangiectasia may become evident in the upper vagina. On palpation, the tissue is firm. This is more pronounced in the apex of the vagina. Adhesions may form between the cervix and the vagina or between apposing vaginal surfaces.[46]

Histopathologic examination may show a loss of the vaginal epithelium and vascular dilatation and hyperemia.[5] Re-epithelialization of the vaginal mucosa ultimately occurs.[147] As compared with the normal mucosa, the irradiated mucosa is thin and atrophic and lacks distinct basal and parabasal layers. The nuclei appear slightly larger than normal, the cytoplasm is abundant and sometimes vacuolated, and small nucleoli may be seen (Fig. 7–16). There is hyalinization in the underlying connective tissue, and minute areas of necrosis and bizarre fibroblasts may occur. The walls of many of the vascular spaces are thickened owing to replacement by connective tissue, and the lumens are reduced in size. An infiltration of lymphocytes and plasma cells may be observed in the lamina propria. This becomes less pronounced with the passage of time. These epithelial and stromal changes may persist many years following radiation.

In cellular samples of the cervix and vagina, the early radiation changes include cellular and nuclear enlargement, cytoplasmic polychromasia, and multinucleation and vacuolization of the cytoplasm.[15,72] Regeneration is reflected in the cells, and atrophic cells ultimately become

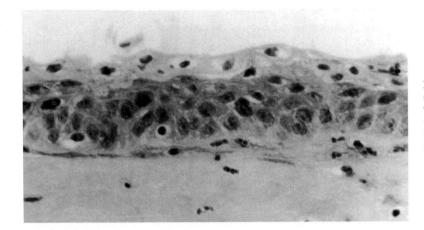

Figure 7–16. Chronic radiation changes of vaginal mucosa revealing atrophy, slight nuclear enlargement, and vacuolated cytoplasm. Cell borders are ill defined.

dominant, replacing the mature glycogenated cells.[70]

Dysplastic changes in the vaginal or cervical mucosa have been described following radiotherapy for carcinoma of the uterine cervix.[70,99,147] These changes occur after a latent period of several months to more than 10 years.[140] The abnormality is usually detected by cytology in the absence of clinically evident recurrent cancer. In 28 cases of postradiation dysplasia, 15 (53.6%) involved the vagina, 7 (25%) involved the cervix and vagina, and only 6 (21.4%) were confined to the cervix.[99]

The dysplastic epithelium is composed of cells that retain, to varying degrees, their ability to differentiate at the surface of the epithelium. Depending on the severity of dysplasia, the cellular polarity may be inconstant in only the lower one third or in the entire epithelium (Figs. 7–17 to 7–19). The cell cytoplasm is usually acidophilic or indeterminant in staining and less often is basophilic. The nuclei are enlarged, hyperchromatic, and occasionally binucleated or multinucleated (see Fig. 7–18). Mitoses are infrequent. Hyperkeratosis may occur over the surface of the altered epithelium, along with the development of a well-defined granular cell layer.

The cells originating in the altered epithelium are distinctive.[99] They are of variable size, with a mean area of 593 square microns. The cells are usually round, oval, or polygonal in form and less frequently are irregular in shape. The cytoplasm stains eosinophilic in 40% of the cells, is cyanophilic in 14% of the cells, and indeterminate in 46% of cells. The nuclei have a

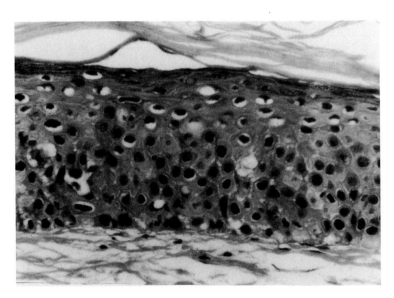

Figure 7–17. Postradiation mild dysplasia with hyperkeratosis, nuclear enlargement, hyperchromasia, and perinuclear vacuoles.

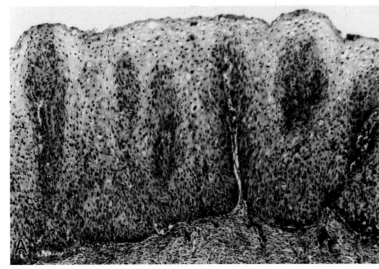

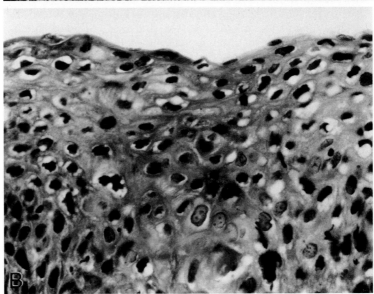

Figure 7–18. Postradiation moderate dysplasia. *A,* Increased cellularity and marked proliferation occur in the lower two thirds of epithelium. *B,* A higher magnification to show binucleation and poorly stained chromatin with a smudgy appearance. Perinuclear halo is common in radiated epithelium.

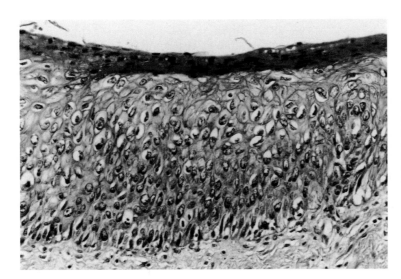

Figure 7–19. Postradiation severe dysplasia. Dysplastic cells in a disorderly arrangement occupy the entire thickness of epithelium. There is parakeratosis on the surface. Cells in the intermediate layers contain perinuclear halos to simulate koilocytes.

mean area of 138 square microns and are round or oval and less frequently are irregular in configuration. The nuclei are hyperchromatic. The nuclear chromatin is finely granular and often associated with irregular clumping. Chromocenters are evident in some cells; however, nucleoli are uncommon.

Of 84 women with confirmed postradiation dysplasia, 47 (56%) ultimately had a recurrence of their cervical carcinomas.[140] A relationship exists between the time of detection of postradiation dysplasia and the likelihood of cancer recurrence. Of 71 women found to have had postradiation dysplasia 1 to 3 years after the initial diagnosis of cancer, 71% developed recurrence within 3 years, compared with 44% of women who had developed the intraepithelial change after an interval of 3 years. Using microspectrophotometric analysis of the cells originating in postradiation dysplasia, Okagaki et al.[95] found that there was an 86% probability rate of recurrence when the abnormal cells had an aneuploid DNA distribution. There was no correlation between the diploid or polyploid DNA content of the cells and the likelihood of cancer recurrence.

The presence of dysplasia indicates that there is an increased probability of recurrence of the previously treated cervical cancer. This is more likely to occur when the interval between the diagnosis of cancer and the detection of the intraepithelial change is short or when the altered cells have an aneuploid DNA distribution. The ultimate fate of the vaginal change is unclear.

Squamous Neoplasia in Diethylstilbestrol-Exposed Progeny

There is concern about the increased frequency and malignant potential of squamous dysplasia and CIS in the vaginas and cervices of young women exposed to diethylstilbestrol (DES) in utero.[85] Some investigators believe that a large area of the squamous metaplasia associated with vaginal adenosis and cervical ectropion is predisposed to the development of neoplasia.[35,36,85,96]

Prevalence

With the exception of a few studies that reported a high prevalence of dysplasia and CIS,[35,36,85] the occurrence of vaginal dysplasia varied from 1.3% to 4.8%, and cervical dysplasia occurred in less than 1% to 6% of cases.[11,20,50,111,112,116,127,146] In general, the transition to cancer is low.[53,110]

Discrepancies are attributable, in part, to the different morphologic criteria used by the investigators. There is a tendency to misdiagnose immature squamous metaplasia as dysplasia and to overevaluate dysplasia as CIS.[43,114,115,116] This is especially true in some of the earlier reports. Crush artifacts and reparative inflammatory changes may also lead to overinterpretation.

Another important factor is bias in patient selection, which is clearly demonstrated in a report by the National Cooperative Diethylstilbestrol Adenosis (DESAD) Project.[116] In this study involving 4,589 women, vaginal dysplasia was found in 0.9% of the participants identified through record review, in 0.7% of self-referrals, in 1.5% of physician referrals, and in 1.6% of those with DES-type changes without a confirmed DES exposure. All changes were mild to moderate in severity and were located in the upper third of the vagina.

In the cervix, dysplasia was found in 1.4% of the record review group, in 2.0% of self-referrals, in 2.1% of physician referrals, and in 2.6% of those having DES changes without confirmed DES exposure.[116] Most changes were mild to moderate in severity. The severe dysplasia and CIS that did exist tended to occur in the latter two groups. In general, the incidence rates for dysplasia and CIS were higher for the cervix than for the vagina. If the rates were tabulated by patient rather than by site, 1.83% of the record review group had dysplasia in the vagina or cervix during the initial DESAD examination. This frequency is believed to reflect most closely the overall DES population. Each of the other two groups had a higher rate. These findings may explain the higher frequency of dysplasia reported by several medical centers that receive a significant number of referral cases.[115,116]

The DESAD study has further documented that the prevalence rate of vaginal dysplasia in the record review group was nearly equal to that observed in well-matched controls (1.42% versus 1.08%).[116] The rate of cervical dysplasia was greater in the controls than in the record review group (3.96% versus 1.27%).

When the incidence rates for dysplasia and CIS were expressed by the number of cases per 1,000 women-years of follow-up, the record review group and controls had 15.7 versus 7.9 cases diagnosed by cytology or biopsy ($P < 0.01$).[113] When the mild dysplasias were excluded, the incidence rates remained higher for the exposed group. The increased incidence rates were apparently correlated with the extent of squamous metaplasia, that is, when it reached to the outer half of the cervix or into the vagina.[117] One potential difficulty is the histologic distinction between condylomatous and dysplastic changes. This factor inevitably has some influence on the data.[109] The role of venereal transmission in the development of squamous dysplasia and CIS is suggested by the presence of HPV structural antigens and HPV DNA in these lesions.[13,38] The rates of genital herpes are also reported to be increased in the exposed group when compared with matched controls (11.8% versus 6.3%).[1,113]

Microscopic Features

In general, the histologic and cytologic features of dysplasia are similar among the DES-exposed and non–DES-exposed population.[10,30,39,40,42,116] In histologic sections, the severity of dysplasia and carcinoma in situ is graded by the degree of maturation, variation in nuclear size and shape, nuclear cytoplasmic ratio, polarity, and mitoses.

Among the intraepithelial neoplasms of the cervix and vagina, 70% have koilocytosis. Using the immunoperoxidase technique, HPV capsid antigens were detected in 43% of cervical and vaginal squamous dysplasias[38] (Figs. 7–20 and 7–21). In a subsequent update of our cases, 48% of cervical dysplasia and CIS expressed HPV capsid antigens, especially in mild and moderate dysplasias. Similarly, 57% of the vaginal intraepithelial abnormalities contained HPV capsid antigens. By in situ hybridization technique, HPV DNA was detected in the vaginal lesions of all five DES-exposed progeny, including type 6 in four women and type 16 in the fifth patient.[13]

In cytologic smears, dysplastic cells derived from mild dysplasia retain the mature appearance of superficial or intermediate squamous cells. The enlarged hyperchromatic nuclei have finely granular chromatin. Cells of moderate and severe dysplasia resemble metaplastic or

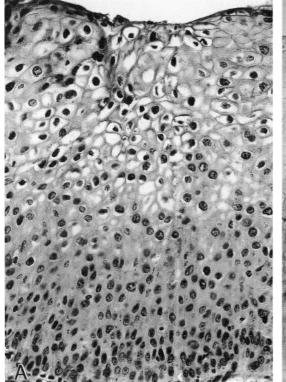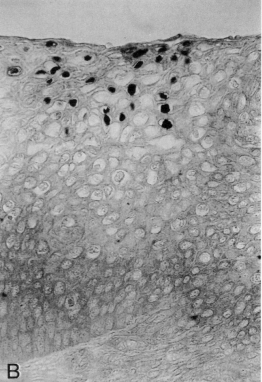

Figure 7–20. *A*, Mild dysplasia of the cervix with koilocytosis in the upper third of the epithelium and proliferation of parabasal cells. *B*, Comparable area as in *A*, stained by the immunoperoxidase stain for papillomavirus structural antigens. Nuclei, which contain structural antigens, appear dark brown. (From Fu et al. Obstet Gynecol 61:59, 1983, Fig. 1; used with permission from the American College of Obstetricians and Gynecologists.)

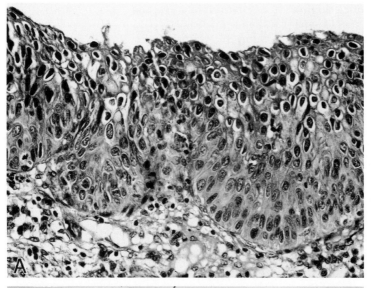

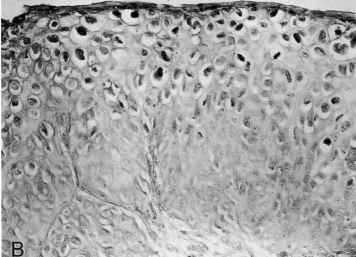

Figure 7–21. *A*, Moderate dysplasia of the cervix. *B*, Same area as in *A* stained with immunoperoxidase stain for papillomavirus structural antigens. Darkly stained antigen-positive nuclei are scattered in the upper third of the epithelium. (From Fu et al. Obstet Gynecol 61:59, 1983, Fig. 2; used with permission from the American College of Obstetricians and Gynecologists.)

parabasal cells. The nucleocytoplasmic ratio is increased and the nuclear atypism is more apparent than that of mild dysplasia. Cells of CIS have high nucleocytoplasmic ratios and coarsely granular chromatin. The dysplastic cells of all grades derived from DES-exposed women tend to appear in aggregates, whereas the dysplastic cells from non–DES-exposed women are predominantly isolated. Robboy et al.[112] reported a lack of correlation between the cellular and histologic samples in many of the DES-exposed women. This may be related to the difficulty of detecting a small lesion within a broad area of squamous metaplasia and the low-grade nature of dysplasia found in most cases.

Differential Diagnosis

Vaginal squamous mucosa in association with atrophy, inflammation, and squamous metaplasia often has the appearance of increased cellularity and nucleocytoplasmic ratio because of the loss of glycogen in the cytoplasm (Figs. 7–22 and 7–23). The normal cellular polarity, in contrast to that of dysplastic epithelium, is maintained. Mitotic activity, although it may be increased in response to an inflammation, is rare and limited to the deep layers. In a reactive, reparative epithelium, slight nuclear atypism and prominent nucleoli can occur. In dysplasia, a greater degree of cellular atypicality and heterogeneity is present.

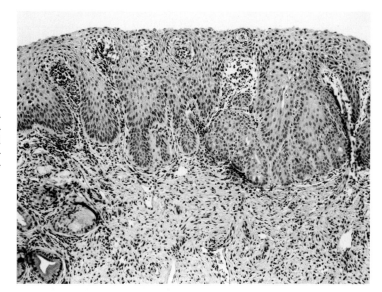

Figure 7–22. Immature squamous metaplasia of the vagina. (From Fu et al. Obstet Gynecol 52:129, 1978, Fig. 2; used with permission from the American College of Obstetricians and Gynecologists.)

It is important to distinguish immature squamous metaplasia, a frequent occurrence in DES-exposed women, from the more significant intraepithelial abnormalities.[91] By using rigid histologic criteria, it should be possible to consistently differentiate squamous metaplasia from neoplasia. Immature squamous metaplasia, despite its apparent lack of maturation, consists of uniform cells without nuclear atypism or any increase in mitotic activity.[41,43] Vaginal condyloma retains a distinct basal layer and mild increase of proliferation in the parabasal layers. Nuclear atypia is limited to the superficial layers, with nuclear hyperchromasia and enlargement. Orderly maturation is maintained. When more significant nuclear atypism is identified, the lesion is classified according to the criteria for dysplasia and CIS (Figs. 7–24 to 7–28).

The abnormal mitotic figures most commonly identified include abnormal metaphases, such as two-group metaphase (a small group of chromosomes detached from the metaphase plate), three-group metaphase (detached chromosomes on either side of the metaphase plate), and V-shaped metaphase (partially split metaphase in a V-shape). Other abnormal forms include ring-form mitosis, giant mitosis (an obvious increase in chromosomes), multipolar mitosis, and bizarre forms (Fig. 7–29).[43] Al-

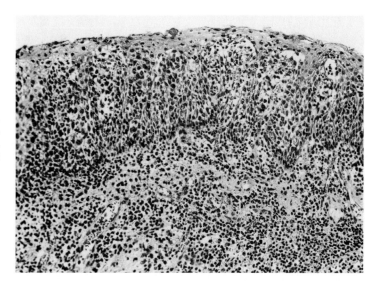

Figure 7–23. Chronic vaginitis. In response to inflammation, the vaginal mucosa often becomes nonglycogenated and hypercellular. Rare mitotic figures can be seen.

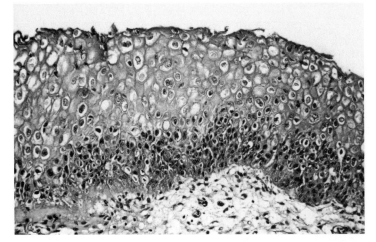

Figure 7–24. VAIN 1, mild dysplasia with koilocytosis in the upper two thirds of the epithelium and excessive cellular proliferation in the parabasal layers. (From Fu et al. Obstet Gynecol 52:129, 1978, Fig. 3; used with permission from the American College of Obstetricians and Gynecologists.)

Figure 7–25. VAIN 1, mild dysplasia with orderly maturation. Cells with mild nuclear enlargement, irregularity, and hyperplasia occur in the upper third of epithelium. (From Fu et al. Obstet Gynecol 52:129, 1978, Fig. 7; used with permission from the American College of Obstetricians and Gynecologists.)

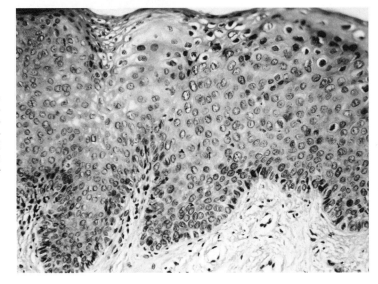

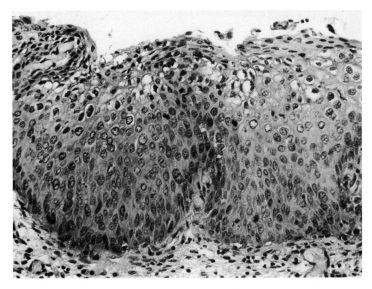

Figure 7–26. VAIN 2, moderate dysplasia with proliferation of immature cells in the lower two thirds of epithelium. Koilocytes occur in the upper third of epithelium (From Fu et al. Am J Clin Pathol 72:502, 1979, Fig. 8; used with permission from the American Society of Clinical Pathologists.)

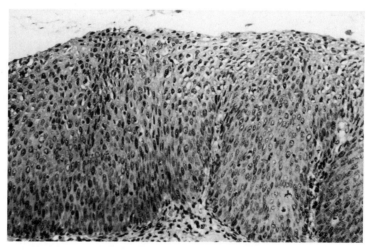

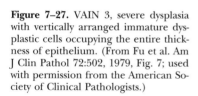

Figure 7–27. VAIN 3, severe dysplasia with vertically arranged immature dysplastic cells occupying the entire thickness of epithelium. (From Fu et al. Am J Clin Pathol 72:502, 1979, Fig. 7; used with permission from the American Society of Clinical Pathologists.)

though the technique of nuclear DNA analysis is not used routinely, it is a useful adjunct to assess changes that are difficult to classify histologically. These abnormal mitotic figures are usually found in moderate or more severe dysplasias.

INVASIVE CARCINOMAS

FIGO Clinical Staging

The clinical staging of vaginal cancer is similar to that used in classifying cancers of the uterine cervix. Stage 0 cancers are confined to the vaginal mucosa. Stage I cancers are limited to the vaginal wall. Stage II cancers involve the subvaginal tissues without extension to the pelvic wall. In Stage III disease the neoplasm extends

to the pelvic wall, and in Stage IV cancer the neoplasm spreads beyond the true pelvis or involves the mucosa of the bladder or rectum. There is spread to the adjacent organs in Stage IV-A and to distant sites in Stage IV-B.[142]

Conventional Squamous Cell Carcinoma

Because the majority of patients with vaginal cancer have had prior or concurrent histologically similar cervical or vulvar cancer, strict criteria have been proposed for a diagnosis of primary vaginal carcinoma. In some instances, it may not be possible to determine with certainty whether the vaginal squamous neoplasia represents a new primary or recurrent disease of cervical and vulvar origin.

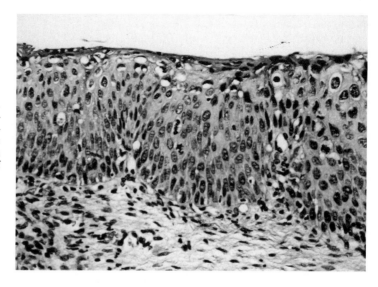

Figure 7–28. VAIN 3, severe dysplasia. Dysplastic cells with nuclear pleomorphism occur in the entire thickness of epithelium. (From Fu et al. Am J Clin Pathol 72:502, 1979, Fig. 10; used with permission from the American Society of Clinical Pathologists.)

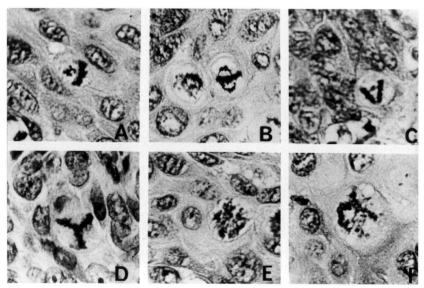

Figure 7–29. Various abnormal mitotic figures are illustrated. *A*, Two-group metaphase. *B*, Three-group metaphase (*right*) and ring-form mitosis (*left*). *C*, V-shaped metaphase. *D*, Tripolar mitosis. *E*, Giant mitosis. *F*, Bizarre mitosis. (From Fu et al. Am J Clin Pathol 72:502, 1979, Fig. 1; used with permission from the American Society of Clinical Pathologists.)

Criteria for Primary Vaginal Carcinoma

According to the FIGO staging method, a primary vaginal tumor must be in the vagina without involvement of the cervix or vulva as demonstrated by clinical or histologic examination.[74] For example, a neoplasm that involves both the cervix and vagina is classified as cervical primary. In the presence of prior cervical or vulvar cancer, a specified time interval should have elapsed to rule out the possibility that the vaginal tumor is a recurrence of the previous site. According to Peters et al.,[102] the disease-free period should be a minimum of 5 years for invasive cervical carcinoma and 2 years for cervical CIS. In the series by Pride and Buchler,[105] only 1.26% of the patients who received radiotherapy for cervical cancer developed recurrent disease after 10 years. For this reason, these investigators suggest that a 10-year disease-free period should follow pelvic irradiation for cervical carcinoma.

Clinical and Gross Features

In the UCLA series,[62] invasive squamous carcinoma involved the vagina of 164 patients. Of these patients, 116 (71%) had prior or concurrent invasive cervical carcinoma, 10 (6%) had cervical dysplasia or CIS, 25 (15%) had invasive vulvar carcinoma, and three (2%) had vulvar CIS. Only 19 women (12%) had no prior cervical or vulvar neoplasia. Of the 116

women with invasive squamous cell carcinoma of the cervix and vagina, 52 (45%) had concurrent disease (within 1 year of each other), and 47 (41%) had vaginal tumor 1 to 5 years following cervical disease. The remaining 21 (18%) developed vaginal tumor 6 or more years following cervical neoplasia. One patient had vaginal carcinoma more than 10 years prior to cervical carcinoma. Using the criteria of Pride and Buchler,[105] 44 (27%) of 164 patients had primary vaginal squamous carcinoma.[62]

Most patients are postmenopausal, 58 to 65 years of age, and about 10 years older than cervical carcinoma patients. Bleeding and discharge are reported to be the most common symptoms of vaginal cancer,[2,139] although bladder pain and frequent voiding may be early symptoms.[139] Vaginal cancer may be initially detected by cellular studies, by pelvic examination, or by means of colposcopy. When limited in extent, the squamous cell cancer may present as an ulcerated nodule or as a localized exophytic growth.[81] In more advanced cancers, induration and ulceration occur, and the friable nature of the tissue is evident. Fistulas may be associated with advanced cancers.[106,126] Most carcinomas involve the upper posterior vagina and tend to spread upward and extend into the cervix. The second most common site of origin is the lower anterior vagina. The third most common site is the middle third of the vagina.[7]

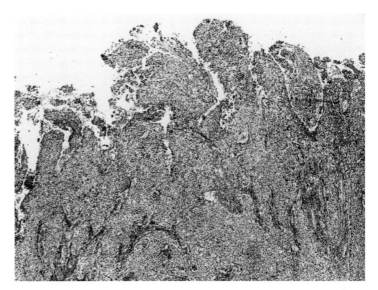

Figure 7–30. Primary squamous cell carcinoma of the vagina of the large-cell nonkeratinizing type.

Microscopic Features

On histologic examination, vaginal cancer resembles its counterpart in the uterine cervix (Fig. 7–30). Using the terminology proposed by the World Health Organization, most cancers are of the large cell type, and keratinizing cancers are less common.[62] This is also reflected in studies using the Broders classification.[106] Most of the squamous cell cancers are moderately differentiated and less frequently are well differentiated.[75] The spindle cell variant of squamous cell carcinomas has also been reported to occur in the vagina.[134] There is no apparent correlation between the histologic grade and the prognosis, except for verrucous and poorly differentiated carcinomas.[97,100] Epidermal growth factor was strongly expressed, but HER-2/neu was not overexpressed in vaginal, cervical, or vulvar carcinomas.[9]

Microinvasive Squamous Cell Carcinoma

Vaginal microinvasive squamous carcinoma is defined by some authors as stromal invasion less than 2.5 mm in depth. It is characterized by tongue-like projections extending into the stroma. At the point of invasion, the cells contain abundant eosinophilic cytoplasm, appearing more mature than the adjacent cells (Fig. 7–31). The associated stromal responses, in-

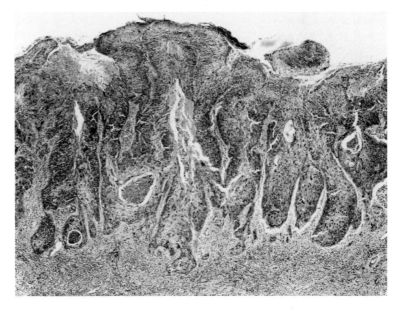

Figure 7–31. Early microinvasive cancer of the vagina with irregular infiltrating processes at the base. Its thickness is 2.25 mm, measuring from the surface to the deepest point of invasion.

cluding lymphocytic infiltration and desmo-plasia, are helpful for recognizing the invasive nature of the disease. Squamous pearls may be present elsewhere in the intraepithelial neo-plasia. In the presence of this finding or the cellular changes suggestive of an invasive car-cinoma, serial section of the biopsy is recom-mended (Fig. 7–32).

Of six women who developed invasive carci-noma less than 2.5 mm in thickness, the lesion in one woman followed hysterectomy for CIN by 59 months. The other five women developed invasive carcinoma 82 to 246 months after treat-ment for cervical cancer by pelvic radiotherapy. Four women were alive and well, one died of disease 35 months after surgery, and one died of other causes.[32]

Prognosis

The vaginal wall and the adjacent organs are readily infiltrated by the neoplasm. Neoplasms arising in the posterior vaginal wall may invade the rectovaginal septum or rectum. Cancers that develop in the anterior vaginal wall may invade the vesicovaginal septum or urinary bladder. The extent of disease as defined by the FIGO clinical staging correlates with survival. According to the review of literature, Benedet and colleagues[7] reported 5-year disease-free survival rates of 71% (50% to 84%) for Stage I patients, 47% (41% to 65%) for Stage II, 25% (15% to 50%) for Stage III, and 8% (0% to 25%) for Stage IV, with an overall 5-year sur-vival rate of 45%.

Malignant cells may spread to a different group of regional lymph nodes according to the site of origin. Tumors in the upper third of the vagina tend to metastasize to the pelvic lymph nodes (external iliac, obturator, and hypogastric nodes) and occasionally to the ureteral node.[83] Lower vaginal carcinomas drain to the inguinal nodes and occasionally to the medial group of external iliac nodes. Pos-terior wall lesions may spread to the rectovagi-nal septum and presacral nodes.[83]

Treatment modalities have included surgery (lo-cal excision to radical vaginectomy with hysterec-tomy) or radiotherapy, or both.[37,67,75,81,121,133] Treatment is individualized according to the stage of the disease, location, size, prior radia-tion treatment, and general medical status of the patient.

Verrucous Squamous Carcinoma

Only 1 of 105 cases of verrucous cancer de-scribed by Kraus and Perez-Mesa[77] involved the vagina. It is difficult to determine the precise number of cases with vaginal involvement, since similar if not identical processes have been classified as pseudoepithelial hyperplasia, giant condyloma of Buschke-Löwenstein, well-differentiated squamous cell carcinoma, or atypical squamous papilloma. Ramzy et al.[107] reported two cases classified as verrucous can-cer with vaginal involvement and cite two pre-viously reported cases. This diagnostic problem is also reported by Robertson et al.[118] On re-

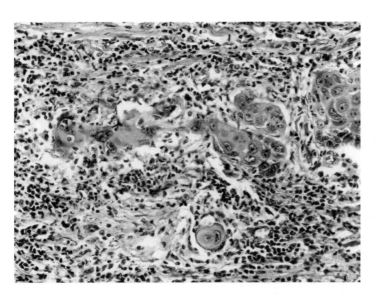

Figure 7–32. Early microinvasive cancer of the vagina found beneath surface epithe-lium after serially sectioning tissue.

view of the histologic slides of verrucous carcinoma of the genital tract, five cases were reclassified as giant condyloma, eight cases as intraepithelial neoplasia with or without condylomatous change, and five cases as conventional invasive squamous cell carcinoma. The authors stress the importance of accurate diagnosis in the presence of HPV changes for verrucous carcinoma.[118]

Verrucous cancer is an exophytic growth with numerous excrescences, some of which are friable. Early in its evolution, verrucous cancer is readily demarcated from the uninvolved epithelium, and this may be misinterpreted as evidence of its benign nature. On histopathologic examination, the multiple processes are covered by stratified squamous epithelium and lack a central core of vascularized connective tissue. The tips of the processes may be blunt rather than pointed, and confluence of the villus processes may occur. The squamous epithelium is relatively mature, although premature keratinization and epithelial pearls may occur. Parakeratosis or hyperkeratosis may exist over the surface of the processes. Mitoses are uncommon and are more likely to be observed in the lower levels of the process. At its base, the verrucous cancer is sharply demarcated from the stroma, and there may be bulbous epithelial masses (Fig. 7–33).

The neoplasm grows by direct extension and rarely spreads to the lymph nodes. Most studies indicate that verrucous cancer does not respond to ionizing radiation. Surgical excision is more likely to eradicate the neoplasm.

Papillary Squamous (Squamotransitional) Cell Carcinoma

This variant of squamous cell carcinoma is rarely reported to occur in the vagina (Fig. 7–34). Rose et al.[119] reported on an 82-year-old woman who had had a hysterectomy for cervical dysplasia 20 years earlier and presented with vaginal bleeding. A 4 cm mass was found in the anterior distal vagina and distal urethra. A superficial biopsy revealed papillary squamotransitional cell carcinoma with no evidence of stromal invasion. HPV type 16 was detected by in situ hybridization and polymerase chain reaction (PCR) techniques. Immunohistochemical stain was positive for CK-7, but CK-20 negative, consistent with squamous cell carcinoma with transitional cell features. No follow-up data were reported.[119]

In contrast, transitional cell carcinomas of the urinary tract usually express either CK-7 or CK-20, or both. Singer et al.[131] reported on a case of vaginal transitional cell carcinoma, which was positive for both CK-7 and CK-20. This tumor occurred in a 59-year-old woman with stress urinary incontinence. A right trigone papillary tumor was found and removed by transurethral resection. The bladder transitional cell carcinoma was predominantly low grade but focally high grade. A recurrent lesion was treated similarly 6 months later. A vaginal tumor was found in the dorsal wall 4 years later. It was a noninvasive low-grade transitional cell carcinoma. However, it spread to the adjacent mucosa by pagetoid pattern. No follow-up information was available.[131]

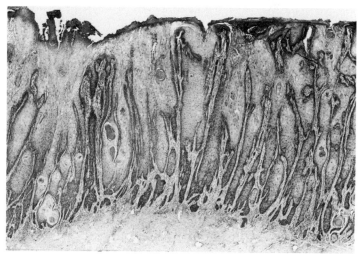

Figure 7–33. Verrucous squamous carcinoma. In addition to its well-differentiated appearance, the base of carcinoma reveals pushing borders.

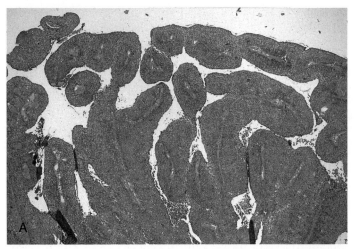

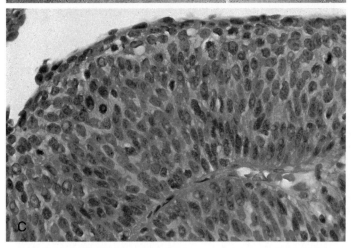

Figure 7–34. Papillary squamotransitional cell carcinoma of the vagina. *A*, Low power showing multiple papillary fronds on the surface. *B*, Pushing border at the base. *C*, High magnification to demonstrate tumor cells with severe nuclear atypia, nuclear grooves, and increased mitotic activity.

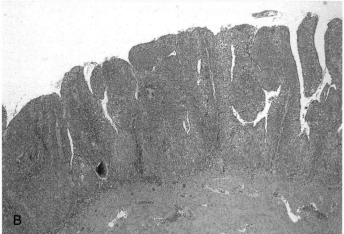

Clear Cell Adenocarcinoma

Seven cases of vaginal clear cell adenocarcinoma occurring in adolescent females were described in 1970.[59] It was later reported that six of these seven patients had been exposed to

DES in utero.[60] A registry was established to study these neoplasms, and 346 cases had been accessioned into the registry by 1978. An analysis of these cases was reported in 1975 and 1979.[56,57] Of the accumulated cases, 189 (55%) were designated as vaginal, 145 (42%) were cervical, and 12 (3%) were unclassified as to site of origin. In a subsequent update of 519 cases of vaginal and cervical clear cell carcinoma recorded in the registry,[86] 60% had positive exposure to DES, 23% were negative for hormones and other medication, and 12% had a positive history for another hormone or an unidentified medication. In the remaining 5%, the history of medication was unknown. Among the DES-exposed women, the risk of developing clear cell carcinoma from birth to age 34 years was estimated at 0.1%.[86]

The relative risk for the development of vaginal clear cell adenocarcinoma in DES-exposed progeny with and without maternal vaginal bleeding is 365.6 and 459.0, respectively. The relative risk for vaginal adenosis with and without maternal vaginal bleeding was 15.4 and 92.8, respectively. A strong association between DES exposure and vaginal adenosis and clear cell adenocarcinoma was demonstrated. However, vaginal bleeding did not sufficiently reduce the risk for vaginal adenosis and clear cell adenocarcinoma.[125] Investigation of postnatal factors by case study method demonstrated no increase for the development of clear cell adenocarcinoma with the use of oral contraceptive or pregnancy.[98] Vaginal adenosis and clear cell adenocarcinoma of the vagina were also reported in women who had 5-fluorouracil and/or carbon dioxide laser treatment for vaginal condyloma.[14,48]

Clinical and Gross Features

In the cases accumulated in the registry, the median age at detection was 19.0 years, with a range of 7 to 34 years.[86] The incidence of clear cell carcinoma among DES-exposed women increases from age 15 years, reaches a plateau from 17 to 22 years, and declines sharply afterward. At diagnosis, 91% of DES-exposed women were 15 to 27 years of age.[86] In most cases, there was a history of abnormal bleeding or discharge. However, 20% of the women were asymptomatic.

The pathologic findings are well described in several studies.[53,58,123] The neoplasms usually occur in the anterior vaginal wall, most frequently in the upper one third of the vagina. Involvement of the lower two thirds of the vagina is uncommon, although rarely the neoplasm extends from the cervix to the vulva. The neoplasms vary from 0.2 to 10 cm in greatest dimension and may be polypoid, nodular, or ulcerated. Some adenocarcinomas are confined to the lamina propria and are recognized solely on the basis of induration of the vaginal wall. These are usually localized and may be covered by intact stratified squamous epithelium. The apposing vaginal wall is rarely involved by a "kissing lesion."

Microscopic Features

On histopathologic examination, three major growth patterns are described: a tubulocystic type, a solid type, and a papillary type. The tubulocystic type is reported to be the most common, whereas the papillary type occurs least frequently. In the tubulocystic type (Fig. 7–35), spaces of varying size are lined by a simple flat, cuboidal, or columnar epithelium. In many columnar cells, the nucleus is enlarged

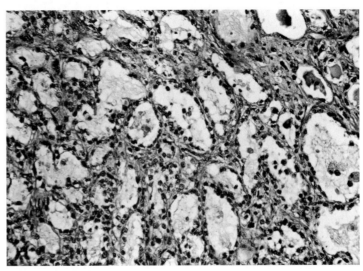

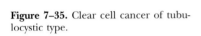

Figure 7–35. Clear cell cancer of tubulocystic type.

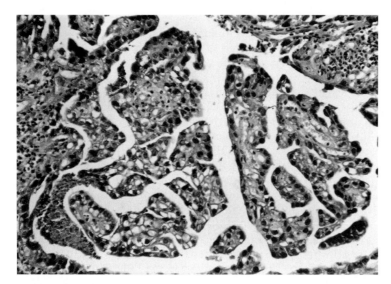

Figure 7–36. Clear cell carcinoma of papillary type.

and appears to protrude into the lumen beyond the limits of the cytoplasm. This is referred to as a hobnail cell. In other cases, the glands are lined with a nonglycogenated columnar epithelium somewhat like that associated with endometrial cancer. Mucin may occur within the gland lumens, but only rarely is it demonstrated within the cytoplasm.

In papillary variants (Fig. 7–36), the epithelium lining the glands or cysts is characterized by numerous papillary projections. The epithelium is similar to that observed in the tubulocystic type. Psammoma bodies may be observed. In the solid type (Fig. 7–37), the cells are polygonal in form and are arranged in solid nests or masses. The nuclei are enlarged and

often have an eccentric location and are surrounded by abundant clear cytoplasm. Under electron microscopic examination, malignant cells of clear cell carcinomas in different patterns share similar characteristics. The cytoplasm contains pools of glycogen particles, which are dissolved by tissue processing for light microscopy and result in a clear appearance. The microvilli, although numerous, are short and blunt. Mitochondria and Golgi complexes are abundant, but lipid droplets are scanty.[31] These ultrastructural features are similar to those of clear cell carcinomas that occur in the endometrium and ovary and support a müllerian origin.[31] In cells of renal cell carcinoma, the clear appearance results from accu-

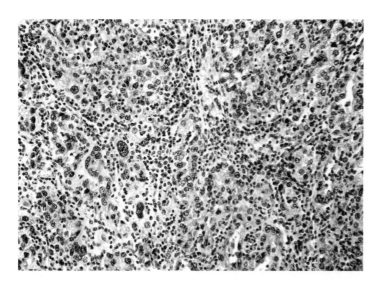

Figure 7–37. Clear cell carcinoma of solid type.

mulation of both lipid and glycogen particles. The microvilli are long, thin, numerous, and regularly spaced.

The cells derived from clear cell adenocarcinoma may occur in aggregates or in an isolated state. Variation in cell size is conspicuous in some neoplasms. In other cases, this is less evident. The cytoplasm is variable in amount, poorly stained, and sometimes vacuolated. There is an altered nucleocytoplasmic ratio. The nuclei are round or oval. Variation in nuclear size may be observed; however, it is not prominent in many neoplasms. There is hyperchromasia, and the nuclear chromatin is aggregated and irregularly distributed. A chromatinic membrane is observed in many cells. One or more nucleoli may be observed.

Assessing the accuracy of the cellular technique in detecting clear cell adenocarcinoma is difficult. In a study of 95 proven clear cell adenocarcinomas, only 74% of the samples were reported to be "suspicious" or "positive." In this study, the source of the specimen was often unknown. A sample obtained from the uterine cervix would not be optimal for detecting a vaginal neoplasm. Sputum or vaginal samples may aid in detecting metastatic lesions or local recurrent disease.[10]

Prognosis

Both clinical and pathologic features have a bearing on the ultimate prognosis. Patients who are asymptomatic at the time of detection are more likely to have smaller neoplasms, offering a better prognosis. The prognosis is more favorable in women older than 19 years compared with those younger than 15 years of age,[123] which may be a reflection of the type of tumor. The tubulocystic type of clear cell adenocarcinoma offers the best prognosis and is reported to be four times more common in women older than 19 years. The solid and papillary types have a less favorable prognosis. Although size and depth of penetration are related to the frequency of lymph node spread, occasionally a small neoplasm with limited infiltration may be associated with lymph node involvement.[23] Mitoses are less frequent in vaginal than in cervical neoplasms. Clear cell adenocarcinoma may spread locally or may metastasize by way of lymph or blood vascular channels.[59] The neoplasm is more likely to metastasize to sites outside the abdominal cavity than is squamous cell cancer of the vagina. Persistent or recurrent disease has been observed in more than one fourth of the cases accumulated in the registry.[56]

The overall survival rate is reported to be better than that associated with primary vaginal squamous cell cancer. Of 185 vaginal clear cell adenocarcinomas, the 5-year actuarial survival was 87% for women with clinical Stage I neoplasms, 76% for women with clinical Stage II tumors, and 30% for women with clinical Stage III cancers.[56] Tumor recurred sometimes more than 20 years after treatment.[55]

The prognosis and biologic behavior of vaginal clear cell adenocarcinom are different among those with and without DES exposure. DES-exposed progeny had better survival rates and lower para-aortic lymph node metastasis, lung metastasis, and supraclavicular lymph node metastasis than did non–DES-exposed women. The 5- and 10-year survival rates for DES exposed women were 84% and 78%, respectively, as compared with 69% and 60% for those without DES exposure. Only 9% of DES-exposed patients developed lung metastasis, as compared to 24% for non–DES-exposed women. Overall, 21% of DES-exposed women died of the disease as compared with 30% for those without DES exposure.[54]

Other Adenocarcinomas and Argentaffin Carcinoma

The majority of primary adenocarcinomas of the vagina are of the clear cell type. Their precursors are thought to be atypical adenosis or glandular dysplasia.[42] Well-documented vaginal adenocarcinomas of mesonephric origin are rare.[63,145] Rare examples of vaginal endometrioid or non–clear cell carcinoma have been reported.[108,122,130]

An example of adenocarcinoma in situ of the vagina was reported by Clement and Benedet.[28] The change was observed in a patient previously treated with hysterectomy for cervical in situ carcinoma with squamous and glandular components. Although no squamous component was identified in the vaginal lesion, the neoplastic columnar cells formed complex glands and cribriform pattern, appeared focally as signet-ring cells, and migrated through the adjacent squamous mucosa in a pagetoid fashion.[28] The lesion resembled a typical cervical adenocarcinoma in situ, but its origin from benign adenosis could not be demonstrated histologically.

A neoplasm described as a mixed intestinal adenocarcinoma of the vagina with argentaffin

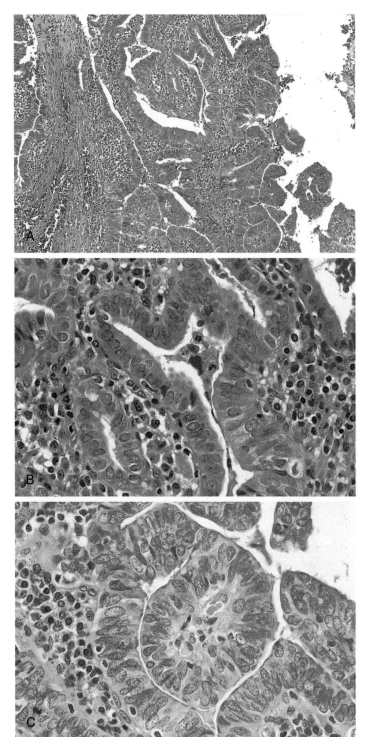

Figure 7–39. Vaginal adenocarcinoma, endometrioid type. *A,* Complex papillary glands associated with chronic inflammation in the stroma. *B* and *C,* Endometrioid cells with nuclear stratification and moderate nuclear atypia.

Synovioid Tumor of Vagina

Okagaki et al.[94] described a neoplasm arising in the left lateral vaginal fornix of a 24-year-old woman. The neoplasm was believed to be of mesenchymal origin and had features suggestive of synovial sarcoma. The neoplasm was submucosal in origin and measured 3 cm in greatest dimension. In part, the tumor comprised flattened epithelioid cells in the acinar

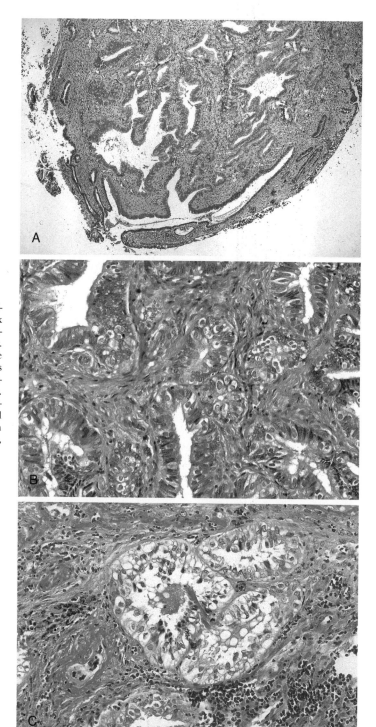

Figure 7–40. Prolapsed fallopian tube following vaginal hysterectomy. *A*, Complex branching papillary and cystic glands simulate glandular neoplasm on low power. *B*, The glandular cells are ciliated. Notice that the background smooth muscle cells differ from the desmoplastic stroma expected to occur in an invasive carcinoma. *C*, Mucosal erosion, hemorrhage, and reactive nuclear atypia in tubal epithelial cells. (Courtesy of Dr. Virginia H. Smith and Dr. David Lawrence, San Luis Obispo, California.)

or tubular component (Fig. 7–41). The cells had round or oval nuclei and contained one to three nucleoli. Mitoses were infrequent. Some acini contained proteinaceous material (Fig. 7–42). At the periphery of the tumor were sheets of elongated cells that infiltrated the surrounding tissue. Mucin was evident within the acinar cells and their lumens and within the spindle-shaped cells at the periphery. Electron microscopy suggested that the

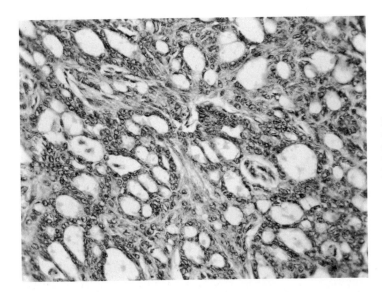

Figure 7–41. Vaginal synovial-like sarcoma. Among the glandular spaces are spindle-shaped sarcomatous cells. (From Okagaki T. Cancer 37:2306, 1976; used by permission.)

epithelioid and spindylate cells were of common origin. The tumor cells had cytoplasmic vacuoles limited by a smooth membrane and amorphous material of low to medium density resembling the vacuoles in synovial tissue. Slender, long microvilli protruding into the acinar lumens were similar to those observed in synovial cells. Intracytoplasmic bundles of short microfilaments, observed in mesothelioma and adenomatoid tumor, were not observed. The findings also differed from those of endodermal sinus tumor.

Later, a similar tumor was reported by Shevchuk et al.,[129] who favored an origin from the mesonephric duct on the basis of well-formed basement membranes, distinct desmosomes, scanty cytoplasmic filaments, and abundant telolysosomes. The latter are usually absent in synovial sarcoma.[129] In addition, PAS-positive and disease-resistant material was found in the tumor and in the adjacent mesonephric rests. These synovioid tumors may be similar to the female adnexal tumor, which was initially reported in the broad ligament and paraovarian region.[69] Similar tumors were reported to occur in the paravaginal area under the designation of "Gartner's duct or wolffian duct adenocarcinoma."[63,145] After local excision, these tumors occasionally recur or metastasize.

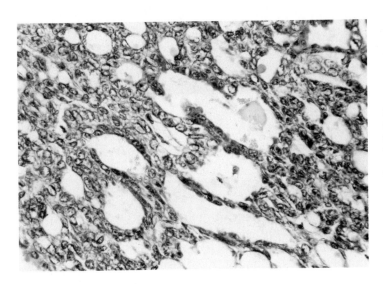

Figure 7–42. Vaginal synovial-like sarcoma. Glandular and stromal cells have a similar nuclear appearance. The glandular lumens contain secretory material. (From Okagaki T. Cancer 37:2306, 1976; used by permission.)

REFERENCES

1. Adam E, Kaufman RH, Adler-Storthz K, et al. A prospective study of association of herpes simplex virus and human papillomavirus infection with cervical neoplasia in women exposed to diethylstilbestrol in utero. Int J Cancer 35:19, 1985.
2. Al-Durdi M, Monaghan JM. Thirty-two years experience in management of primary tumors of the vagina. Brit J Obstet Gynecol 127:513, 1977.
3. Anders KH, Hall TL, Fu YS. Epidemiology and histopathologic studies of female genital warts. In Fenoglio CM, Wolff MW, Rilke F (eds). Progress in Surgical Pathology. Philadelphia, Field and Wood, 1986, pp 33–47.
4. Andrews CF, Jourdain L, Damjanov I. Benign cervical mesonephric papilloma of childhood: Report of a case studied by light and electron microscopy. Diag Gynecol Obstet 3:39, 1981.
5. Arbitol MM, Davenport JH. The irradiated vagina. Obstet Gynecol 44:249, 1974.
6. Audet-Lapointe P, Body G, Vauclair R, et al. Vaginal intraepithelial neoplasia. Gynecol Oncol 36:232, 1990.
7. Benedet JL, Murphy KJ, Fairey RN, et al. Primary invasive carcinoma of the vagina. Obstet Gynecol 62:715, 1983.
8. Benedet JL, Sanders BH. Carcinoma in situ of the vagina. Am J Obstet Gynecol 148:695, 1984.
9. Berchuck A, Rodriguez G, Kamel A, et al. Expression of epidermal growth factor receptor and HER-2/neu in normal and neoplastic cervix, vulva, and vagina. Obstet Gynecol 76:381, 1990.
10. Bibbo M, Ali I, Al-Naqeeb M, et al. Cytologic findings in female and male offspring of DES treated mothers. Acta Cytol 19:568, 1975.
11. Bibbo M, Gill WR, Azizi F, et al. Follow-up study of male and female offspring of DES-exposed mothers. Obstet Gynecol 49:1, 1977.
12. Blaustein A. Pathology of the Female Genital Tract. New York, Springer-Verlag, 1977, p 70.
13. Bornstein J, Kaufman RH, Adam E, et al. Human papillomavirus associated with vaginal intraepithelial neoplasia in women exposed to diethylstilbestrol in utero. Obstet Gynecol 70:75, 1987.
14. Bornstein J, Sova Y, Atad J, et al. Development of vaginal adenosis following combined 5-fluorouracil and carbon dioxide laser treatments for diffuse vaginal condylomatosis. Obstet Gynecol 81:86, 1993.
15. Boschann HW. Radiation changes in benign cells. In Wied GL (ed). Compendium on Diagnostic Cytology, 4th ed. Chicago, Tutorials of Cytology, 1976.
16. Branton PA, Tavassoli FA. Spindle cell epithelioma, the so-called mixed tumor of the vagina: A clinicopathologic, immunohistochemical, and ultrastructural analysis of 28 cases. Am J Surg Pathol 17:509, 1993.
17. Brinton LA, Nasca PC, Mallin K, et al. Case-control study of in situ and invasive carcinoma of the vagina. Gynecol Oncol 38:49, 1990.
18. Brown CE. Mixed epithelial tumor of vagina. Am J Clin Pathol 23:237, 1953.
19. Buntine DW, Henderson PR, Biggs JSG. Benign müllerian mixed tumor of the vagina. Gynecol Oncol 8:21, 1979.
20. Burke L, Antonioli D, Rosen S. Vaginal and cervical squamous cell dysplasia in women exposed to diethylstilbestrol in utero. Am J Obstet Gynecol 132:537, 1978.
21. Burt RL, Pritchard RW, Kim BS. Fibroepithelial polyp of the vagina: A report of five cases. Obstet Gynecol 47:525, 1976.
22. Chafe W. Neuroepithelial small cell carcinoma of the vagina. Cancer 64:1948, 1989.
23. Chambers J, Rogers LW, Julian CG. Minute clear cell adenocarcinoma with early metastasis to pelvic lymph nodes. Am J Obstet Gynecol 131:228, 1978.
24. Chen KTK. Brenner tumor of the vagina. Diag Gynecol Obstet 3:255, 1981.
25. Chen KTK. Benign mixed tumor of the vagina. Obstet Gynecol 57:89S, 1981.
26. Chirayil SJ, Tobon H. Polyps of the vagina: A clinicopathologic study of 18 cases. Cancer 47:2904, 1981.
27. Clement PB. Multinucleated stromal giant cells of the uterine cervix. Arch Pathol Lab Med 109:200, 1985.
28. Clement PB, Benedet JL. Adenocarcinoma in situ of the vagina: A case report. Cancer 43:2479, 1979.
29. Cutler S, Young JL. Third National Cancer Survey: Incidence Data. National Cancer Institute Monograph No. 41, 1975.
30. Daly JW, Ellis GF. Treatment of vaginal dysplasia and carcinoma in situ with topical 5-fluorouracil. Obstet Gynecol 55:350, 1980.
31. Dickersin GR, Welch WR, Erlandson R, et al. Ultrastructure of 16 cases of clear cell adenocarcinoma of the vagina and cervix in young women. Cancer 45:1615, 1980.
32. Eddy GL, Singh KP, Gansler TS. Superficially invasive carcinoma of the vagina following treatment for cervical carcinoma: A report of six cases. Gynecol Oncol 36:376, 1990.
33. Elliott GB, Elliott JDA. Superficial stromal reactions of lower genital tract. Arch Pathol 95:100, 1973.
34. Elliott GB, Reynolds HA, Fidler HK. Pseudosarcoma botryoides of the cervix and vagina in pregnancy. J Obstet Gynecol Br Comm 74:728, 1976.
35. Fowler WC, Edelman DA. In utero exposure to DES: Evaluation and followup of 199 women. Obstet Gynecol 51:459, 1978.
36. Fowler WC, Schmidt G, Edelman DA, et al. Risks of cervical intraepithelial neoplasia among DES-exposed women. Obstet Gynecol 58:720, 1981.
37. Frick HC II, Jacox HW, Taylor MC Jr. Primary carcinoma of the vagina. Am J Obstet Gynecol 101:695, 1968.
38. Fu YS, Lancaster WD, Richart RM, et al. Cervical papillomavirus infection in diethylstilbestrol-exposed progeny. Obstet Gynecol 61:59, 1983.
39. Fu YS, Reagan JW, Hawliczek S, et al. The use of cellular studies in the investigation of the DES-exposed woman. In Herbst AL (ed). Intrauterine Exposure to Diethylstilbestrol in the Human. Chicago, American College of Obstetricians and Gynecologists, 1978, p 34.
40. Fu YS, Reagan JW, Richart RM. Cytologic diagnosis of diethylstilbestrol-related genital tract changes and evaluation of squamous cell neoplasia. In Herbst AL, Bern HA (eds). Development Effects of Diethylstilbestrol (DES) in Pregnancy. New York, Thieme-Stratton, 1981, p 46.
41. Fu YS, Reagan JW, Richart RM, et al. Nuclear DNA and histologic studies of genital lesions in diethylstilbestrol-exposed progeny. I: Intraepithelial squamous abnormalities. Am J Clin Pathol 72:503, 1979.
42. Fu YS, Reagan JW, Richart RM, et al. Nuclear DNA and histologic studies of genital lesions in diethyl-

stilbestrol-exposed progeny. II: Intraepithelial glandular abnormalities. Am J Clin Pathol 72:515, 1979.

43. Fu YS, Robboy SJ, Prat J. Nuclear DNA study of vaginal and cervical squamous cell abnormalities in DES-exposed progeny. Obstet Gynecol 52:129, 1978.

44. Fukushima M, Twiggs LB, Okagaki T. Mixed intestinal adenocarcinoma-argentaffin carcinoma of the vagina. Gynecol Oncol 23:387, 1986.

45. Gallup DG, Morley GW. Carcinoma in situ of the vagina: A study and review. Obstet Gynecol 46:334, 1975.

46. Gardner HL, Kaufman RH. Benign Diseases of the Vulva and Vagina, 2nd ed. Boston, G.K. Hall, 1981.

47. Geelhoed GW, Henson DE, Taylor PT, et al. Carcinoma in situ of the vagina following treatment for carcinoma of the cervix: A distinctive clinical entity. Am J Obstet Gynecol 124:510, 1976.

48. Goodman A, Zukerberg LR, Nikrui N, Scully RE. Vaginal adenosis and clear cell carcinoma after 5-fluorouracil treatment for condylomas. Cancer 68:1628, 1991.

49. Gray LA, Christopherson MM. In-situ and early invasive carcinoma of the vagina. Obstet Gynecol 34:226, 1969.

50. Hart WR, Zaharov I, Kaplan BJ, et al. Cytologic findings in stilbestrol-exposed females with emphasis on detection of vaginal adenosis. Acta Cytol 20:7, 1976.

51. Hartmann CA, Sperling M, Stein H. So-called fibroepithelial polyps of the vagina exhibiting an unusual but uniform antigen profile characterized by expression of desmin and steroid hormone receptors but no muscle-specific actin or macrophage markers. Am J Clin Pathol 93:604, 1990.

52. Henson D, Tarone R. An epidemiologic study of cancer of the cervix, vagina and vulva based on the Third National Cancer Survey in the United States. Am J Obstet Gynecol 129:525, 1977.

53. Herbst AL. Diethylstilbestrol exposure—1984. N Engl J Med 311:1433, 1984.

54. Herbst AL. Behavior of estrogen-associated female genital tract cancer and its relation to neoplasm following intrauterine exposure to diethylstilbestrol (DES). Gynecol Oncol 76:147, 2000.

55. Herbst AL, Anderson D. Clear cell adenocarcinoma of the vagina and cervix secondary to intrauterine exposure to diethylstilbestrol. Sem Surg Oncol 6:343, 1990.

56. Herbst AL, Norusis MJ, Rosenow PJ, et al. An analysis of 346 cases of clear cell adenocarcinoma of the vagina and cervix with emphasis on recurrence and survival. Gynecol Oncol 7:111, 1979.

57. Herbst AL, Poskanzer DC, Robboy SJ, et al. Prenatal exposure to stilbestrol: A prospective comparison of exposed female offspring with unexposed controls. N Engl J Med 292:334, 1975.

58. Herbst AL, Robboy SJ, Scully RE, et al. Clear cell adenocarcinoma of the vagina and cervix in young females: An analysis of 170 registry cases. Am J Obstet Gynecol 119:713, 1974.

59. Herbst AL, Scully RE. Adenocarcinoma of the vagina in adolescence: A report of 7 cases including 6 clear cell carcinomas (so-called mesonephromas). Cancer 25:745, 1970.

60. Herbst AL, Ulfelder H, Poskanzer DC. Adenocarcinoma of the vagina: Association of maternal stilbestrol therapy with tumor appearance in young women. N Engl J Med 284:878, 1971.

61. Hernandez-Linares W, Puthawala A, Nolan JF, et al.

Carcinoma in situ of the vagina: Past and present management. Obstet Gynecol 56:356, 1980.

62. Hilborne LH, Fu YS. Intraepithelial, invasive and metastatic neoplasms of the vagina. In: Wilkinson EJ (ed). Pathology of the Vulva and Vagina. New York, Churchill Livingstone, 1987, pp 181–207.

63. Hinch WM, Silva EG, Guarda LA, et al. Paravaginal wolffian duct (mesonephros) adenocarcinoma: A light and electron microscopic study. Am J Clin Pathol 80:539, 1983.

64. Hummer WK, Mussey E, Decker DG, et al. Carcinoma in situ of the vagina. Am J Obstet Gynecol 108:1109, 1970.

65. James T. A benign polypoid tumor of the cervix uteri in a girl three years old. J Obstet Gynecol Br Emp 58:762, 1951.

66. Janovski NA, Kasdon EJ. Benign mesonephric papillary and polypoid tumors of the cervix in childhood. Pediatrics 63:211, 1963.

67. Johnston GA, Klotz J, Boutselis JG. Primary invasive carcinoma of the vagina. Surg Gynecol Obstet 156:34, 1983.

68. Kaminski PF, Maier RC. Clear cell adenocarcinoma of the cervix unrelated to diethylstilbestrol exposure. Obstet Gynecol 62:720, 1983.

69. Kariminejad MH, Scully RE. Female adnexal tumor of probable wolffian origin: A distinct pathologic entity. Cancer 31:671, 1973.

70. Kaufman RH, Topek NH, Wall JA. Late irradiation changes in vaginal cytology. Am J Obstet Gynecol 81:859, 1961.

71. Komiya H, Kawahara T, Nagata H, et al. A case of rare vaginal mixed tumor. Iryo 19:171, 1965.

72. Koss LG. Diagnostic Cytology and Its Histopathologic Bases, 2nd ed. Philadelphia, J.B. Lippincott, 1968.

73. Koss LG, Melamed MR, Daniel WN. In situ epidermoid carcinoma of cervix and vagina following radiotherapy for cervical cancer. Cancer 14:353, 1961.

74. Kottmeier HL. The classification and clinical staging of carcinoma of the uterus and vagina: A report by the Cancer Committee of the International Federation of Gynecology and Obstetrics. J Int Fed Gynecol Obstet 1:83, 1963.

75. Kottmeier HL, Kolstad P. Annual Report on Results of Treatment in Carcinoma of Uterus, Vagina, and Ovary. Stockholm, Sweden, Radiumhemmet, 1976.

76. Kovi J, Tillmann RL, Lee SM. Malignant transformation of condylomata acuminata: A light microscopic and ultrastructural study. Am J Clin Pathol 61:702, 1974.

77. Kraus FT, Perez-Mesa C. Verrucous carcinoma: Clinical and pathologic study of 105 cases involving oral cavity, larynx and genitalia. Cancer 19:26, 1966.

78. Lee RA, Symmonds RE. Recurrent carcinoma in situ of the vagina in patients previously treated for in situ carcinoma of the cervix. Obstet Gynecol 7:61, 1976.

79. Levy DL, Kelly JM. Primary multifocal carcinoma in situ of the vagina and vulva in a young woman. Am J Obstet Gynecol 127:327, 1977.

80. Luttges JE, Lubke M. Recurrent benign Müllerian papilloma of the vagina: Immunohistochemical findings and histogenesis. Arch Gynecol Obstet 255:157, 1994.

81. Marcus RV, Million RR, Daly JW. Carcinoma of the vagina. Cancer 42:2507, 1978.

82. Marcus SL. Multiple squamous cell carcinomas involving the cervix, vagina, and vulva: The theory of multicentric origin. Am J Obstet Gynecol 80:802, 1960.

83. Marcus SL. Primary carcinoma of the vagina. Obstet Gynecol 15:673, 1960.

84. Marino MJ. Vaginal cancer: The role of infectious and environmental factors. Am J Obstet Gynecol 165:1255, 1991.

85. Mattingly RE, Stafl A. Cancer risk in diethylstilbestrol-exposed offspring. Am J Obstet Gynecol 126:543, 1976.

86. Melnick S, Cole P, Anderson D, et al. Rates and risks of diethylstilbestrol-related clear-cell adenocarcinoma of the vagina and cervix: An update. N Engl J Med 316:514, 1987.

87. Moran JP, Robinson HJ. Primary carcinoma in situ of the vagina: Report of 2 cases. Obstet Gynecol 20:405, 1962.

88. Mucitelli DR, Charles EZ, Kraus FT. Vulvovaginal polyps: Histologic appearance, ultrastructure, immunocytochemical characteristics, and clinicopathologic correlations. Int J Gynecol Pathol 9:20, 1990.

89. Mudhar HS, Smith JHF, Tidy J. Primary vaginal adenocarcinoma of intestinal type arising from an adenoma: Case report and review of literature. Int J Gynecol Pathol 20:204, 2001.

90. Naves AE, Monti JA, Chichoni E. Basal-like carcinoma in the upper third of the vagina. Am J Obstet Gynecol 137:136, 1980.

91. Ng ABP, Reagan JW, Nadji M, et al. Natural history of vaginal adenosis in women exposed to diethylstilbestrol in utero. J Reprod Med 18:1, 1977.

92. Norris HJ, Taylor AB. Polyps of the vagina: A benign lesion resembling sarcoma botryoides. Cancer 19:207, 1966.

93. Nucci MR, Young RH, Fletcher CDM. Cellular pseudosarcomatous fibroepithelial stromal polyps of the lower female genital tract: An underrecognized lesion often misdiagnosed as sarcoma. Am J Surg Pathol 24:231, 2000.

94. Okagaki T, Ishida T, Hilgers RD. A malignant tumor of the vagina resembling synovial sarcoma: A light and electron microscopic study. Cancer 37:2306, 1976.

95. Okagaki T, Meyer AA, Sciarra JJ. Prognosis of irradiated carcinoma of cervix uteri and nuclear DNA in cytologic postirradiation dysplasia. Cancer 33:647, 1974.

96. Orr JW Jr, Shingleton HM, Gore H, et al. Cervical intraepithelial neoplasia associated with exposure to diethylstilbestrol in utero: A clinical and pathologic study. Obstet Gynecol 58:75, 1981.

97. Palmer JP, Biback SM. Primary cancer of the vagina. Am J Obstet Gynecol 67:377, 1954.

98. Palmer JR, Anderson D, Helmrich SP, Herbst AL. Risk factors for diethylstilbestrol-associated clear cell adenocarcinoma. Obstet Gynecol 95:814, 2000.

99. Patten SF, Reagan JW, Obenauf M, et al. Postirradiation dysplasia of uterine cervix and vagina: An analytical study of the cells. Cancer 16:173, 1963.

100. Perez CA, Arneson AN, Dehner LP, et al. Radiation therapy in carcinoma of the vagina. Obstet Gynecol 44:862, 1974.

101. Perez CA, Arneson AN, Galakatos A, et al. Malignant tumors of the vagina. Cancer 31:36, 1973.

102. Peters WA, Kumar NB, Morley GW. Carcinoma of the vagina: Factors influencing treatment outcome. Cancer 55:892, 1985.

103. Petrilli ES, Townsend DE, Morrow CP, et al. Vaginal intraepithelial neoplasia: Biologic aspects and treatment with topical 5-fluorouracil and the carbon dioxide laser. Am J Obstet Gynecol 138:321, 1980.

104. Prasad CJ, Ray JA, Kessler S. Primary small cell carcinoma of the vagina arising in a background of atypical adenosis. Cancer 70:2484, 1992.

105. Pride GL, Buchler DA. Carcinoma of the vagina 10 or more years following pelvic irradiation therapy. Am J Obstet Gynecol 127:513, 1977.

106. Pride GL, Scholtz AE, Chuprevich TW, et al. Primary invasive squamous carcinoma of the vagina. Obstet Gynecol 53:218, 1978.

107. Ramzy I, Smout MS, Collins JA. Verrucous carcinoma of the vagina. Am J Clin Pathol 65:644, 1976.

108. Ray J, Ireland K. Non–clear-cell adenocarcinoma arising in vaginal adenosis. Arch Pathol Lab Med 109:781, 1985.

109. Richart R. The incidence of cervical and vaginal dysplasia after exposure to DES. JAMA 255:36, 1986.

110. Robboy SJ. Risk of cancer, dysplasia for DES daughters found "very low." JAMA 241:1555, 1979.

111. Robboy SJ, Friedlander LM, Welch WR, et al. Cytology of 575 young females exposed prenatally to diethylstilbestrol (DES). Obstet Gynecol 48:511, 1976.

112. Robboy SJ, Keh PC, Nickerson RJ, et al. Squamous cell dysplasia and carcinoma-in-situ of the cervix and vagina after prenatal exposure to diethylstilbestrol: Examination and followup of 1424 females. Obstet Gynecol 51:528, 1978.

113. Robboy SJ, Noller KL, O'Brien P, et al. Increased incidence of cervical and vaginal dysplasia in 3,980 diethylstilbestrol-exposed young women. Experience of the National Collaborative Diethylstilbestrol Adenosis Project. JAMA 252:2979, 1984.

114. Robboy SJ, Prat J, Welch WR, et al. Squamous cell neoplasia controversy in the female exposed to diethylstilbestrol. Human Pathol 8:483, 1977.

115. Robboy SJ, Scully RE, Welch WR, et al. Intrauterine diethylstilbestrol exposure and its consequences. Arch Pathol Lab Med 101:1, 1977.

116. Robboy SJ, Szyfelbein WM, Goellner JR, et al. Dysplasia and cytologic findings in 4,589 young women enrolled in diethylstilbestrol adenosis (DESAD) project. Am J Obstet Gynecol 140:579, 1981.

117. Robboy SJ, Welch WR. Selected topics in the pathology of the vagina. Hum Pathol 22:868, 1991.

118. Robertson DI, Maung R, Duggan MA. Verrucous carcinoma of the genital tract: Is it a distinct entity? Can J Surg 36:147, 1993.

119. Rose PG, Stoler MH, Abdul-Karim FW. Papillary squamotransitional cell carcinoma of the vagina. Int J Gynecol Pathol 17:372, 1998.

120. Rusthoven JL, Daya D. Small-cell carcinoma of the vagina. Arch Pathol Lab Med 114:728, 1990.

121. Rutledge F. Cancer of the vagina. Am J Obstet Gynecol 97:635, 1967.

122. Scannell RC. Primary adenocarcinoma of the vagina. Am J Obstet Gynecol 38:331, 1939.

123. Scully RE, Robboy SJ, Welch WR. Pathology and pathogenesis of diethylstilbestrol-related disorders of the female genital tract. In. Herbst AL (ed). Intrauterine Exposure to Diethylstilbestrol in the Human. Chicago, American College of Obstetrics and Gynecology, 1978, p 8.

124. Selzer I, Nelson HM. Benign papilloma (polypoid tumor) of the cervix uteri in children. Am J Obstet Gynecol 84:165, 1962.

125. Sharp GB, Cole P. Vaginal bleeding and diethylstilbestrol exposure during pregnancy: Relationship to genital tract clear cell adenocarcinoma and vagi-

nal adenosis in daughters. Am J Obstet Gynecol 162:994, 1990.

126. Sheets JL, Dockerty MB, Decker MB, et al. Primary epithelial malignancy in the vagina. Am J Obstet Gynecol 89:121, 1964.

127. Sherman AI, Goldrath M, Berlin A, et al. Cervical-vaginal adenosis after in utero exposure to synthetic estrogens. Obstet Gynecol 44:531, 1974.

128. Sherman ME, Paull G. Vaginal intraepithelial neoplasia: Reproducibility of pathologic diagnosis and correlation of smears and biopsies. Acta Cytol 37:699, 1993.

129. Shevchuk MM, Fenoglio CM, Lattes R, et al. Malignant mixed tumor of the vagina probably arising in mesonephric rests. Cancer 42:214, 1978.

130. Shingleton HM, Younger JB, Beasley WE, et al. Adenocarcinoma of the vagina in a patient with gonadal dysgenesis. Obstet Gynecol 53:92S, 1979.

131. Singer G, Hohl MK, Hering F, Anabitarte M. Transitional cell carcinoma of the vagina with pagetoid spread pattern. Hum Pathol 29:299, 1998.

132. Sirota RL, Dickersin GR. Mixed tumors of the vagina: A clinicopathologic analysis of eight cases. Am J Surg Pathol 5:413, 1981.

133. Smith WG. Invasive cancer of the vagina. Clin Obstet Gynecol 24:503, 1981.

134. Steeper TA, Piscioli F, Rosai J. Squamous cell carcinoma with sarcoma-like stroma of the female genital tract. Cancer 52:890, 1983.

135. Stuart GCE, Allen HH, Anderson RJ. Squamous cell carcinoma of the vagina following hysterectomy. Am J Obstet Gynecol 139:311, 1981.

136. Ulbright TM, Alexander RW, Kraus FT. Intramural papilloma of the vagina: Evidence of müllerian histogenesis. Cancer 48:2260, 1981.

137. Ulich TR, Liao SW, Layfield L, et al. Endocrine and tumor differentiation markers in poorly differentiated small cell carcinoids of the cervix and vagina. Arch Pathol Lab Med 110:1054, 1986.

138. Wagner D, Sprenger E, Merkle D. Cytophotometric studies in suspicious cervical smears. Acta Cytol 20:366, 1976.

139. Way S. Primary carcinoma of the vagina. Am J Obstet Gynecol 55:739, 1948.

140. Wentz WB, Reagan JW. Clinical significance of post-irradiation dysplasia of the uterine cervix. Am J Obstet Gynecol 106:812, 1970.

141. Whelton JA. Mixed tumor arising in vagina. Obstet Gynecol 19:803, 1962.

142. Wilkinson EJ. Pathology of the vagina. Curr Opin Obstet Gynecol 3:553, 1991.

143. Woodruff JD. Carcinoma in situ of the vagina. Clin Obstet Gynecol 24:485, 1981.

144. Wright RG, Buntine DW, Forbes KL. Recurrent benign mixed tumor of the vagina. Gynecol Oncol 40:84, 1991.

145. Yosem HL. Adenocarcinoma of Gartner's duct cyst presenting as a vaginal lesion: A case report. Sinai Hosp J 10:112, 1961.

146. Zerner J, Fu YS, Taxiarchis LN, et al. A clinicopathologic study of vagina and cervix in DES-exposed progeny. Am J Diag Obstet Gynecol 2:245, 1980.

147. Zimmer TS. Late irradiation changes: Cytological study of cervical and vaginal smears. Cancer 12:193, 1959.

8

BENIGN AND MALIGNANT EPITHELIAL LESIONS OF THE UTERINE CERVIX

BENIGN TUMORS AND TUMOR-LIKE CONDITIONS OF SQUAMOUS EPITHELIUM

Hyperplasia, Atrophy, Hyperkeratosis, Parakeratosis, and Pagetoid Dyskeratosis

In response to chronic irritation and inflammation, the ectocervical squamous epithelium undergoes hyperplasia. The epithelium becomes thickened through elongation and widening of the rete pegs (Fig. 8–1A). The mitotic activity may be increased in the parabasal layers. With the cessation of estrogenic stimulation, the squamous mucosa undergoes atrophy. This is manifested by flattening of rete pegs, loss of glycogen in the intermediate layers, and a decrease in thickness (Fig. 8–1B). The atrophic mucosa is susceptible to trauma and infection.

In hyperkeratosis, acellular keratin material overlies a thickened, prominent granular cell layer (Fig. 8–2). The parakeratosis, on the other hand, retains pyknotic nuclei in the superficial layers of miniature squamous cells (Fig. 8–3). Hyperkeratosis and parakeratosis produce a raised, white appearance. They are common in the cervical mucosa of prolapsed uterus, as well as in hyperplastic and neoplastic squamous epithelia. For this reason, a biopsy should be performed on any unexplained white epithelium.

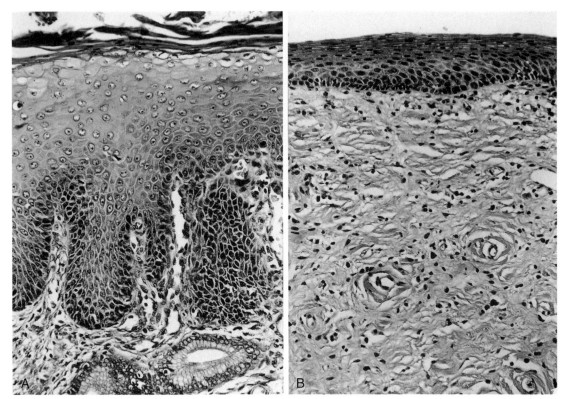

Figure 8–1. *A,* Marked hyperplasia with elongated and plump rete pegs. Surface hyperkeratosis and parakeratosis are present. *B,* Atrophic squamous mucosa, characterized by a decrease in thickness, scanty cytoplasm, and lack of rete pegs.

Van-Bernal et al.[360a] described pagetoid dyskeratosis of the cervical squamous mucosa. These pagetoid cells occur singly and in clusters. They have abundant pale, clear cytoplasm. The nuclei are often pyknotic and surrounded or compressed by perinuclear halos with a signet-ring appearance. There are intercellular bridges between the pagetoid cells and adjacent squamous cells. These pagetoid cells most commonly occur in the parabasal and intermediate layers (Fig. 8–4). These cells do not contain mucinous material. By immunohistochemical stain, the cytoplasm contains high molecular weight cytokeratin. Low molecular weight cytokeratin, CEA, and HPV DNA were all negative.[360a]

This pagetoid dyskeratosis was identified in 37% of the consecutive prolapsed uteri. The mean age of women was 66.9 years. In the second group of 100 women with uterine leiomyoma with a mean age of 44.8 years, only 5% had pagetoid dyskeratosis. The authors concluded that these pagetoid cells represent premature keratinization. Such pagetoid cels should be distinguished from koilocytes, which typically occur in the intermediate and superficial layers. In addition, nuclear atypia is evident. In contrast, pagetoid dyskeratosis occurs primarily in the lower half of ectocervical mucosa.

Fibroepithelial Polyp, Ectocervical Polyp, and Squamous Papilloma

Fibroepithelial polyp or ectocervical polyp is a polypoid, raised lesion on the ectocervix or at the squamocolumnar junction. It rarely exceeds 1 to 2 cm in size. The nodule is made up of fibrous tissue with telangiectasia and sometimes proliferation of blood vessels. The overlying squamous mucosa may be hyperplastic, hyperkeratotic, or ulcerated. The latter often leads to acute and chronic inflammation.

Squamous papilloma is a papillary proliferation of mature squamous epithelium supported by fibrovascular stalks. The squamous epithelium is thickened, hyperplastic, and hyperkeratotic but lacks koilocytosis and nuclear atypia. The cause is unknown but possibly related to viral infection, trauma, or irritation.

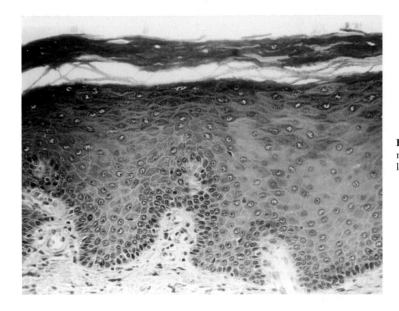

Figure 8–2. Hyperkeratosis of squamous mucosa with prominent granular layers in a prolapsed uterus.

CERVICAL INTRAEPITHELIAL NEOPLASIA (CIN)/SQUAMOUS INTRAEPITHELIAL LESIONS (SIL) AND RELATED LESIONS

Terminology

The concept of carcinoma in situ (CIS) as a precursor of invasive carcinoma was recognized by Broders[55] in 1932. The term *dyskaryosis* was used by Papanicolaou[266] to characterize the nuclear changes seen in the early cervical malignancy. In 1949, Papanicolaou used the term *dysplasia* for "such cytologic changes as would be suggestive of but not conclusive of malignancy."[266] Reagan et al.,[288] in 1953, applied the term *dysplasia and*

atypical hyperplasia for cervical epithelial changes that "are somewhat similar to, but generally less extensive than, those characterizing carcinoma in situ." Reagan and coworkers[285–287] established the cell morphology of dysplasia and CIS by detailed analyses and planimetric measurements. Richart,[295] based on the findings of chromosome karyotyping, DNA ploidy analysis, tissue culture, and clinical follow-up, proposed the term *cervical intraepithelial neoplasia* (CIN) to encompass dysplasia and carcinoma in situ. CIN is subdivided into the following categories: CIN 1 for mild dysplasia, CIN 2 for moderate dysplasia, and CIN 3 for both severe dysplasia and CIS.

In 1994, the term *epithelial cell abnormalities* (ECAs) was proposed in the Bethesda System

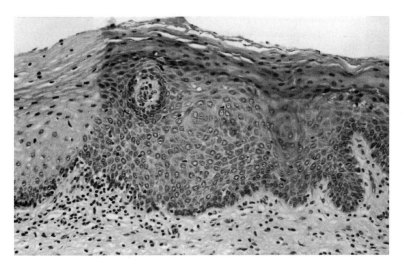

Figure 8–3. Parakeratosis overlying a nonglycogenated mature squamous metaplasia. Compare with normal native cervical squamous mucosa on the left.

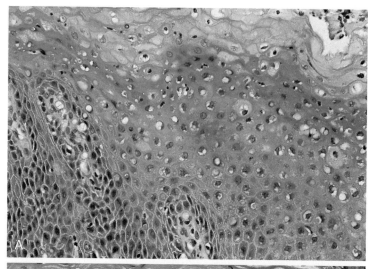

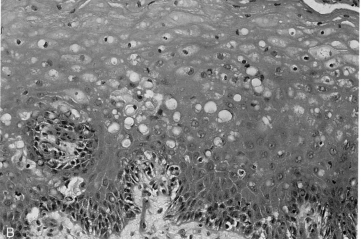

Figure 8–4. Pagetoid dyskeratosis. *A,* Scattered clear cells in the intermediate layer. *B,* Small pyknotic nuclei and abundant clear cytoplasm around the nuclei. *C,* Some clear cells have a signet-ring appearance, but no nuclear atypia is seen.

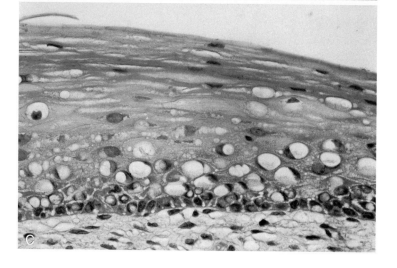

for reporting cervical and vaginal smears.[199] Squamous cell ECAs include atypical squamous cells of undetermined significance (ASCUS), low-grade SIL (LGSIL, including flat condyloma and CIN 1), and high-grade SIL (HGSIL, including CIN 2 and CIN 3). Condyloma acuminatum is a benign neoplasm, not included in the CIN/SIL. The term *SIL* has been widely used for cytologic diagnosis. Some authors also have accepted SIL as a histologic diagnosis. In this chapter, both CIN and SIL are used interchangeably.

ASCUS is defined as "cellular abnormalities that are more marked than those attributable to reactive changes but that quantitatively or qualitatively fall short of a definitive diagnosis of squamous intraepithelial lesion (SIL). Because the cellular changes in the ASCUS category may reflect an exuberant benign change or a potentially serious lesion, which cannot be unequivocally classified, they are interpreted as being of undetermined significance."[199] Although clearly defined cytologic criteria exist for the diagnosis of ASCUS, the diagnostic consistency remains problematic. Colposcopically directed biopsies of women with ASCUS vary from normal to inflammatory to reactive atypia to CIN/SIL. Some changes are related to HPV effects. Many cervical biopsies are performed because of abnormal cervical smears. For these reasons, ASCUS is discussed along with CIN/SIL.

Epidemiology of Squamous Intraepithelial Lesions and Invasive Carcinoma

Incidence and Mortality Rates

In the United States, currently about 50 million Papanicolaou (Pap) smears are estimated to be performed annually; of these, 2 million Pap smears are in the category of atypical squamous cells of undetermined significance (ASCUS), 300,000 smears are CIN 1 or CIN 2, and 65,000 smears are CIN 3.[333] About 12,800 women develop invasive cervical carcinoma, and 4000 women die of this tumor annually.[270] Worldwide 400,000 new cervical cancers are diagnosed each year.

In the last 5 decades, the incidence of invasive cervical cancer in the United States has fallen by at least 75%,[94] from 38.3 per 100,000 in 1947 to 1948 to 15.1 per 100,000 white women in 1969 to 1971. Among non-white women during the same time period, the incidence declined from 74.6 to 31.3 per 100,000.[94]

The SEER (Surveillance, Epidemiology, and End Results) Program of the National Cancer Institute reveals that from 1973 to 1977 the age-adjusted incidence of invasive cervical cancer for white women is three times the mortality (10.9 and 3.5 per 100,000 women); it is 2.5 times for black women (25.7 and 10.5 per 100,000 women). The ratio of carcinoma in situ (CIS) to invasive carcinoma incidence is 3:1 for white women and 2.5:1 for non-white women. The peak incidence of CIS is in the 25- to 29-year-old age group.

According to Kessler,[185] the mortality rates fell from 9.6 to 3.8 per 100,000 white women between 1950 and 1975, representing a 60% reduction. For non-whites, a reduction of 53% occurred (from 22.0 to 10.3 per 100,000 women). During the same time period, no demonstrable improvement was shown in survival rates for 5 or more years. The decrease in mortality is attributed to detection and treatment at earlier, curable states.[185] A cytologic screening program is the single most important factor that leads to early detection of cervical cancer and its precursors. American women who have never had a Pap smear or have not had one in the previous 5 years have a 3.7 to 4.3 times higher risk of developing squamous carcinoma when compared with women who have had a Pap smear within the last 2 years.[53]

In a northern California study conducted by Kaiser Permanente, 455 women who had enrolled in this HMO plan for more than 30 months during 1988 to 1994 developed invasive cervical carcinoma. Of these, 53% had no Pap smear performed, 28% had a normal smear, 9% had an abnormal smear and were followed, 4% had an abnormal smear but were not investigated further, and the smear results of 6% were unclear. Thus, failure to have cervical smears or to follow guidelines remains the most common problem among those who developed cervical cancer, followed by false-negative smears. The overall frequency of squamous carcinoma in this population is 68%, and the remaining 32% are nonsquamous types. Women who never had cervical smears performed have the highest frequency of squamous cell carcinoma (77%). In contrast, women who had normal smears have the lowest frequency of squamous cell carcinoma (56%) ($P < 0.05$).[344] This implies that cervical cancer screening is more effective in the detection of squamous cell cancer than of glandular neoplasm.

The incidence of cervical cancer worldwide varies from 6.0 per 100,000 women in Israel to 87.8 per 100,000 women in Cali, Colombia.[185] In countries that lack screening programs, cervical cancer causes more deaths than any other pelvic malignancy.

Weiss et al.[373] surveyed the incidence of in situ and invasive cervical cancer in the metropolitan Detroit area from 1973 to 1991. This registry is part of the SEER Program. During this period, among women 15 to 39 years of age, an increasing frequency of in situ cervical cancer was most notable among single white women. This was in contrast to a nonlinear decrease among black women, especially married women, of 75%. In 1991, the incidence rate for in situ carcinoma was 121.05 per 100,000 white females, as compared with 74.33 per 100,000 black females. Although the number of invasive cervical cancer cases is small, there is an increase among single white females. The authors attribute this increasing incidence of carcinoma in situ to a greater exposure to risk factors. Other contributing factors are differences in accessibility of diagnostic and therapeutic services for white and black females.[373] In situ carcinoma in white females was diagnosed at an earlier age than that in black women.[373]

Risk Factors and Potential Etiologic Agents

Before the use of HPV DNA testing, the most consistent risk factors for the development of cervical cancer included early age at first intercourse, especially younger than 20 years; early age of first pregnancy; multiple sexual partners; marital instability; and exposure to high-risk males.[186,301,300] Women married to men whose previous wives had in situ or invasive cervical squamous carcinoma have a 2.7-fold higher risk of developing cervical cancer than that noted in matched controls.[185] The development of cervical cancer in women who are married to men with penile cancer also underscores the importance of the male factor.[225]

It has long been suspected that certain carcinogenic agents are transmitted through sexual contact. In early studies, a variety of infectious, physical (trauma, irradiation), and chemical agents (sperm DNA, protamine and histone in semen, sex hormones) were suspected to cause cervical cancer.[291] In the 1960s and 1970s, herpes simplex virus type 2 (HSV-2) was linked to cervical squamous dysplasia and carcinoma in situ.[251,252] Seroepidemiologic surveys revealed that 31% of women with cervical dysplasia or carcinoma in situ and 52% of women with invasive squamous cell carcinoma had detectable neutralizing antibodies against HSV-2, as compared with 22% in the controls.[5a] In many geographic areas, the incidence of cervical cancer showed a linear relationship with the occurrence of HSV-2 antibodies.[284]

Specific antigens and various structural and nonstructural specific polypeptides were isolated in tissue culture cells transformed by HSV-2. Using antisera against HSV-2–specific antigens (AG-4) and immunofluorescent technique, 61% to 82% of dysplasia and 92% to 100% of invasive carcinomas had demonstrable antigens.[16] Similarly, ICP 10 (infected cell-specific protein) and VP-143 (virus-specific protein) were found in dysplastic and malignant cells but not in normal cells.[16,65] However, no further molecular evidence has become available in recent years to prove that HSV-2 initiates or enhances the development of cervical cancer.

On the other hand, the relationship between human papillomavirus (HPV) and female lower genital cancers has been extensively investigated and substantiated. In a study by Ho et al.,[158] high-risk HPV types were determined by polymerase chain reaction (PCR) and Southern blot hybridization from the cervicovaginal lavage of 608 college students who were followed for 3 years by annual Pap smear. The mean age of this population was 20 years. The annual incidence of HPV infection was 14%, and the cumulative incidence at 3 years was 43%. The mean duration of infection was 8 months. At the end of 12 and 24 months, 30% and 9% of women had persistent infection, respectively.[158] Persistent infection is defined as the presence of the same type of HPV detected at least two times over 1 or more years.[60,158]

Those who were HPV positive at baseline were three times more likely to develop SIL than HPV-negative subjects. Among those who were HPV-positive, 29 (11%) developed low-grade SIL and 2 (0.8%) high-grade SIL. The women who developed SIL all had persistent HPV infection for 6 months or more. Persistence was associated with older age, types of HPV, and infection with multiple types. The development of SIL was related to persistent HPV infection of high-risk types.[158]

When HPV DNA testing is used, the importance of earlier risk factors has been revised. In a study by Herrero et al.,[154] the odds ratios (OR) for the development of CIN and cervical carcinoma having HPV infection, especially HPV type 16, exceeded 200, when compared with normal population.[154] In the study by Nobbenhuis et al.,[257] 353 women with an initial diagnosis of mild, moderate, or severe dysplasia were followed by cytology, colposcopy, and HPV testing by PCR for 14 high-risk types every 3 to 4 months for a median of 33 months. The end point of the progression is defined as the development of CIN 3. Thirty-three (9.3%) women had progression of their disease, and all had high-risk HPV types. The cumulative 6-year incidence of progression was 40%. Of the 103 women who developed CIN 3, 98 (95%) had HPV infection of high-risk type at the baseline study. No women with a negative HPV test demonstrated clinical progression.

Nobbenhuis et al.[257] calculated the odds ratio for the development of CIN 3 with persistent high-risk HPV infection as 3231 (95% confidence range 42–2468) when compared with those without HPV infection. In this study, age, smoking history, age at first sexual intercourse, and more than two sexual partners did not influence the development of CIN 3.[257] This study demonstrates the importance of persistent HPV infection as the strongest factor in the progression of CIN.

The importance of persistent HPV infection was also shown in a study by Wallin et al.[370] They studied cells extracted from the archival most recent normal Pap smear before the detection of invasive carcinoma for HPV DNA types 16 and 18 by PCR. This baseline study included 104 women (85 with squamous cell carcinoma and 19 with adenocarcinoma). A similar test was performed on tissue from cervical biopsy with carcinoma. An age-matched control group did not have cervical carcinoma. HPV DNA was detected in 30% of Pap smears and 77% of tumor samples, as compared with only 3% positive baseline smears in the control. The odds ratio was 15:1 when the baseline was positive and the tumor sample negative for HPV DNA; 122.6 when baseline was negative and tumor positive; and 213.4 when both baseline and tumor were positive for HPV DNA.[370] Persistent HPV infection is a definitive risk for the development of cervical cancer.

In an earlier study by Bosch et al.,[45] HPV DNA was detected by PCR, and the OR for the development of cervical cancer when compared with controls was 23.8:1. Among HPV-positive cases, only the use of oral contraceptives was significant, with an OR of 6.5:1. Among HPV-negative cases, the OR for early age at first intercourse was 4.3:1 and that for early age at first birth was 5.0:1. A lower OR for HPV infection found in this study is likely a result of the less sensitive HPV detection technique used as compared with that used in the newer studies.

The question of cervical cancer and oral contraceptive use was investigated by a case-control study of 759 invasive cervical cancer patients and 1430 controls in Panama, Costa Rica, Columbia, and Mexico. The relative risk was 1.3 for recent use, 1.2 for nonrecent use, and 1.7 for more than 5 years of use. The risk was significant for adenocarcinoma at 2.2 and minimal for squamous cell carcinoma at 1.1.[51] Earlier studies also found only a mild increase of relative risk for oral contraceptive users.[367]

Metabolites of cigarettes, including nicotinine, nicotine, and other mutagenic agents, have been detected in the cervical mucus of smokers.[159,310] Cigarette smoking may also cause immunosuppression and promote the oncogenicity of HSV and HPV.[394] However, when compared with high-risk type HPV infection, smoking history becomes an insignificant risk factor.[257]

Wylie-Rosett et al.,[385] in a case control study, found that women with severe dysplasia or CIS were more likely to have a total vitamin A intake below the pooled median of 3450 IU and/or a beta-carotene intake below the median 2072 IU than that of normal controls ($P < 0.05$). The retinol-binding protein was detectable in 78.8% of the dysplastic samples, compared with 23.5% of the normal tissue samples ($P < 0.005$). In a study by Brock et al.,[54] plasma beta-carotene reduced risk by 80% and vitamin C by 60% in the development of CIS. Immunosuppressive therapy and radiotherapy to the pelvis are significant predisposing factors for the development of neoplasia.

Human Papillomavirus

The techniques for the detection of HPV have undergone remarkable changes in the last 3 decades.[108,112,214,215,217,235,292,332] The development of antisera against genus-specific HPV capsid structural antigens derived from bovine papillomavirus or human skin warts was an important early step leading to the visualization of HPV antigens in the cytologic and tissue samples by immunoperoxidase technique.[109,166,234] In a study by Kurman et al.,[198] 43% (65 of 152) of mild dysplasia, 15% (12 of 82) of moderate dysplasias, and 4% (2 of 47) of severe dysplasias had demonstrable HPV structural antigens. An additional 13% (6 of 47) of severe dysplasias and 10% (4 of 41) of CIS contained antigens in the adjacent mild or moderate dysplasia.[198] The use of in situ hybridization by radioactive or biotin-labeled probes has improved the sensitivity and detection rates. However, inherent technical limitations preclude widespread use.

Detection of HPV DNA by PCR and hybrid capture I and II has been well established and highly sensitive.[293] These techniques were used in clinical trials for primary cervical cancer screening and for improvement of conventional cervical smears.[321,333,384]

More than 100 types of HPV have been identified, of which more than 30 types occur in the genital tract. Ten to 15 types cause genital cancers.[86,395] It is well known that invasive cervical cancer is preceded by dysplasia and carcinoma in situ. High-grade SILs (CIN 2 and CIN 3) are associated with high-risk HPV types, including 16, 18, 31, 33, 35, 39, 45, 51, 52, 56, 58, 59, 68, and others. Low-grade SILs (condyloma and CIN 1), however, are linked to both low-risk (types 6, 11, 42, 43, and 44) and high-risk types.[292,293,395,396] With few exceptions, most invasive cervical cancers contain high-risk HPV DNA subtypes, especially 16 and 18. HPV type 18 has a propensity to occur in glandular neoplasms, small cell carcinoma, and neuroendocrine carcinomas.[85]

The HPV genomes of different types consist of three basic elements (Fig. 8–5). First is the noncoding region of so-called long controlling region (LCR) or upstream regulatory region, which contains a steroid-responsive promoter. It regulates viral replication and transcription. The coding regions with protein sequences, also referred to as open reading frames (ORFs), consist of early (E) and late (L) regions in relation to gene production in a course of infection. The ends of early and late regions connect to the noncoding sequences, LCR (see Fig. 8–5).

Once HPV reaches to the basal cells through defects in the epithelial surface, early ORFs are expressed in a nonproductive, episomal state. There are six ORFs in the early region, E1 to E7. E3 was found only in bovine papillomavirus. E1 and E2 gene products are related to viral replication. E2 gene products of high-risk HPV types also repress the expression of oncogenes E6 and E7. E4 and E5 gene products are related to the cytokeratin disruption and host immune responses, respectively.

The late regions, L1 and L2, code for viral capsid proteins. As the affected squamous cells move up to the superficial layers, thousands of viral copies are replicated and viral capsid structures are expressed in the nuclei of mature squamous cells.

The differences in the oncogenicity of HPV are most likely related to the function of E6 and E7 of high-risk types and the ability of HPV to integrate into the host cells. It is estimated that

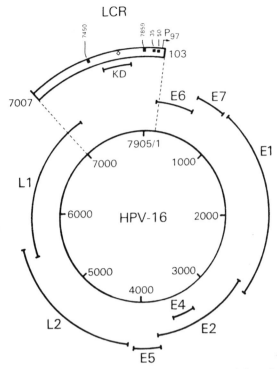

Figure 8–5. Human papillomavirus structure consisting of a long controlling region (LCR), which is connected to early (E) and late (L) opening reading frames. (Used with permission from Fig. 49–19. Fu YS, Sherman ME. Chapter 49. The Uterine Cervix. In: Principles and Practice of Surgical Pathology and Cytopathology. Silverberg SG [ed]. New York, Churchill Livingstone, 1997, pp 2343–2409.)

HPV DNA type 16 is integrated in 75% of invasive squamous carcinomas, and HPV DNA type 18 is integrated in most carcinomas.[86]

After viral DNA is integrated into the human chromosome DNA, viral genomes are unable to replicate. It is suggested that viral DNA forms in the late region and between E1 and E2 ORFs are disrupted. This eliminates the normal expression of certain regulatory genes, such as E2. Reduction of E2 is believed to lead to overexpression of E6 and E7. The viral integration apparently occurs at random fragile sites without a consistent pattern of intrachromosomal localizations.

The E6 and E7 regions of HPV 6/11 appear to bind either less actively or not at all to the host cell proteins. On the other hand, E6 and E7 oncoproteins of HPV 16 and 18 are found to bind with p53 and retinoblastoma (Rb) gene, respectively.

P53 and Rb gene are gatekeepers to regulate cell cycle. P53 in the normal cells binds with DNA to stimulate the expression of transcriptional genes to inhibit growth. Rb protein binds with a transcriptional complex, E2F. Phosphorylation of Rb by cyclin-D/cyclin–dependent kinase 4 (CDK4) complex releases E2F, which links to DNA sites and begins transcription and expression of genes required for DNA synthesis and chromosome replication. When cellular DNA damage occurs, p53 and Rb proteins are increased to arrest cells at the G1 or G2 phase for repair of DNA. Cyclin-dependent kinases (CDKs) regulate the cell cycle to make sure G2 nuclei do not replicate until going through mitosis. Cyclins D and E move cells from the G0 into the G1 phase, cyclins E and A affect the S-phase, and cyclins A and B control mitosis. D type is sensitive to growth factors and degraded by the ubiquitin-proteasome proteolytic pathway.[14] CDKs can be inactivated by CDK inhibitors (CKI). One of the CKIs is p16[INK4,] also known as CDKN2 (cyclin D kinase inhibitor 2) or CK12. P16 protein antagonizes the functions of CDK 4 and CDK 6. As is discussed later in the section on specialized techniques, cyclin E and p16 are both biomarkers of HPV lesions.[184a]

When E6 oncoprotein of HPV type 16 and 18 binds with p53, DNA is free of regulation. When E7 oncoprotein binds to Rb protein, the E2F is released to interact with DNA. Loss of both copies of p53 or Rb by binding to E6 and E7 or through allelic loss causes increased proliferation by loss of cell cycle regulation. A loss of p53 function may also be caused by deletion or mutation. P53 mutations also increase genomic instability and drug resistance of tumor cells. Somatic mutations of the p53 gene are infrequent in HPV-positive cervical and vulvar carcinomas but are more common in HPV-negative vulvar carcinomas.[379]

Multiple oncogenic events and mutations take place from the initiation of CIN to the eventual development of invasive cancer. Molecular studies have enhanced our understanding of how HPV infections initiate excessive cellular proliferation. Persistent HPV infections cause CIN/SIL to progress.[267] Based on loss of heterozygosity (LOH) studies, multiple deletions occur in the chromosomes of CIN; some are monoclonal, and others are polyclonal.[138]

Rader et al.[282] compared the chromosomal changes in CIN 3 and the adjacent invasive squamous cell carcinoma. Areas of CIN 3 and invasive carcinoma were microdissected from the tissue section. PCR technique with oligonucleotide primers was used to detect microsatellite polymorphism in six chromosome sites. LOH of 3p 14.1–12 was detected in 30% of CIN 3 (versus 37% of invasive carcinomas); LOH of

6p23 in 21% of CIN 3 (versus 33% of invasive carcinomas); LOH of 2q33–37 in 14% of CIN 3 (versus 27% of invasive carcinomas), LOH of 11q23.3 in none of CIN 3 (versus 33% of invasive carcinomas); and LOH of 19q13.4 in 4% of CIN 3 (versus 13% of invasive carcinomas).[282] These findings suggest that mutations in 3p and 6p are steps in the early stage of cervical carcinogenesis, whereas 11q and 6q are related to tumor progression.[282]

In a subsequent study of 49 stage IB invasive squamous cell carcinomas by O'Sullivan et al.,[264a] LOH of 11q23.3 was found in 38.8% of tumors and none in the adjacent CIN 3. Of the 36 tumors with vascular space invasion, 39% had LOH of this site. This was also observed in 20% of tumor cells dissected from lymph node metastasis. LOH of this site was also associated with 5.5 times greater tumor recurrence than carcinomas without this mutation. The authors suggest that LOH of 11q23.3 is an important step in tumor progression of cervical, breast, and ovarian cancers.[264a]

Atypical Squamous Cells of Undetermined Significance (ASCUS)

In the ASCUS/LSIL Triage Study (ALTS), 3388 women with the cytologic diagnosis of ASCUS were randomized for immediate colposcopy, HPV testing for high-risk HPV types by hybrid capture II, and conservative management. These ALTS cases were enrolled from the clinic centers of the University of Alabama, the Magee-Women's Hospital in Pittsburgh, the University of Oklahoma, and the University of Washington.[333]

After review of the original index smears by the panel members, 31% of the smears were revised as negative, 55% remained as ASCUS, 11% were upgraded to low-grade SIL, and 3% were upgraded to high-grade SIL. It is interesting that the positive rates for high-risk HPV types were 32.7% for the negative group, 50.6% for ASCUS, 88.7% for low-grade SIL, and 97.0% for high-grade SIL.[333]

Based on the colposcopic directed biopsies of women with ASCUS, 1.7% of biopsies were classified as atypia, 14.5% as CIN 1, 6.3% as CIN 2, and 5.1% as CIN 3. Close to three quarters (72.3%) of women had no lesion to biopsy or no abnormality was found in the biopsy. The overall frequency of atypia and CIN is 28%, which is higher than that of other studies.

In a study by Grenko et al.,[136] five pathologists working in the same department reviewed 124 biopsies removed for the cytologic diagnosis of ASCUS. The diagnostic categories included normal, squamous metaplasia, reactive, indeterminate, low-grade SIL, and high-grade SIL. The frequency of dysplasia rendered by the pathologists varied from 23% to 51%. Three of five pathologists agreed on the diagnosis in 91.9% of cases, and all five pathologists agreed in only 28% of cases. The overall interobserver agreement was poor. This study confirms the lack of reproducibility, especially in the distinction between reactive change and low-grade SIL.[136]

In cervical biopsies for cytologic diagnosis of ASCUS, after excluding CIN and normal ectocervical mucosa and squamous metaplasia, there is a heterogeneous group of reactive changes, which is termed "nondiagnostic squamous atypia" by Crum et al.[85] For purposes of this discussion, these lesions are divided into the following: (1) atypical repair/reactive change, (2) reactive squamous atypia, and (3) borderline condyloma. They occur primarily in the squamous metaplasia and less frequently in ectocervical or atrophic mucosa.

Atypical Repair/Reactive Change

Following erosion of endocervical mucosa, the re-epithelialized area is covered by three or four layers of flattened, small, immature metaplastic squamous cells. Usually a moderate acute and chronic inflammation is apparent in the underlying stroma. This change was initially designated as pseudoparakeratosis as seen in the endocervix of oral contraceptive users.[271] Subsequently, this change also was found in women who did not use oral contraceptives. These parallel layers of elongated cells have hyperchromatic nuclei, sometimes surrounded by clear space (Fig. 8–6). The cytoplasm is scant

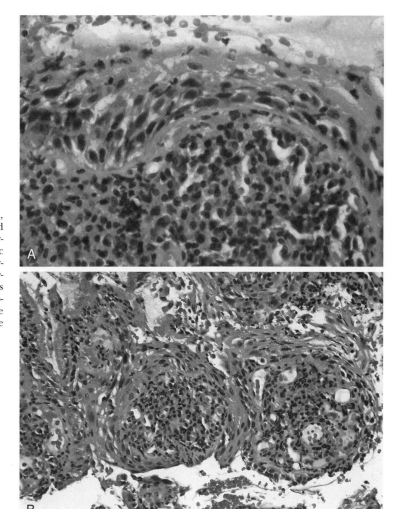

Figure 8–6. Pseudoparakeratosis. *A,* The endocervical mucosa is covered by four to five layers of flattened, parallel, small, immature metaplastic squamous cells simulating parakeratosis. The underlying stroma is heavily infiltrated by plasma cells. *B,* Cross section of endocervical papillary erosion re-epithelialized by immature metaplastic squamous cells. (See color section.)

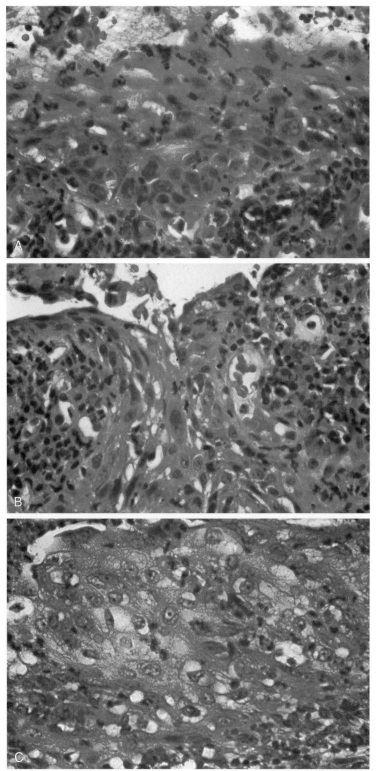

Figure 8–7. Atypical reparative change. *A, B,* and *C,* Regenerative cells with enlarged oval nuclei occur in the superficial and intermediate layers. The cytoplasm is abundant. The cells are regularly spaced without disorganization. Some nucleoli are large. (See color section.)

to moderate in amount, and the nuclear cytoplasmic ratios are increased. Spongiosis and stromal infiltration by sheets of plasma cells are prominent features.

As the metaplastic squamous cells regenerate and proliferate further, the cells have the characteristic appearance of reparative cells with enlarged nuclei and prominent nucleoli (Fig. 8–7A, B, and C). A similar change is seen in atrophic ectocervical or vaginal squamous mucosa (Fig. 8–8).

The key to differentiating these changes from CIN is the regularly spaced reactive cells with abundant cytoplasm and the enlarged regular to slightly irregular nuclei containing nucleoli. Acute or chronic inflammation, or both, is usually evident.

Reactive Squamous Atypia

The affected epithelium is slightly thickened and associated with proliferation of parabasal cells. A careful examination shows a distinct basal cell layer. No nuclear atypia or cellular disorganization is present in the parabasal layers. Mitotic activity is absent or extremely rare.

Cells in the intermediate and superficial layers contain densely eosinophilic or basophilic cytoplasm. There is a minor degree of nuclear atypia in the form of enlargement, hyperchromasia, and occasional binucleation or multinucleation. Perinuclear edema is a common finding (Figs. 8–9 and 8–10). Small nucleoli may be seen. The main distinction of reactive squamous atypia from CIN lies in the degree of nuclear changes, which are less than expected for condyloma/CIN 1.

Borderline Condyloma

Because 40% to 50% of condylomas and low-grade CINs undergo spontaneous resolution, one expects to find lesions between active HPV infection and regression in the cytologic and histologic specimens. Those changes, which have some but not all of the features of condyloma, are referred to as borderline condyloma.

Biopsies most frequently reveal normal or slightly thickened epithelium. A mild cellular proliferation is present in the parabasal layers, where mitotic figures are extremely rare or absent. No cellular disorganization is seen.

In the intermediate and superficial layers are rare, mature, slightly atypical cells with minor nuclear enlargement, hyperchromasia, and, rarely, binucleation. The nuclei remain round to oval or elongated without irregularity or a contracted popcorn appearance. Perinuclear halos are prominent. But the cell borders are not thickened (Figs. 8–11 to 8–13). Parakeratosis or atypical parakeratosis may occur on the surface.

Most important, the atypical cells do not have sufficient nuclear atypia to be classified as koilocytes. For the purpose of comparison, typical koilocytes seen in a flat condyloma are shown in Figure 8–14. The nuclei in koilocytes are enlarged, irregular in shape, and hyperchromatic. The cell borders are thickened and have a glassy appearance. This is the minimal degree of nuclear atypia required to qualify the cells koilocytes, that is, as condyloma or CIN 1 (see Fig. 8–14).

In endocervical curettage, abnormal metaplastic squamous cells meet the nuclear atypia

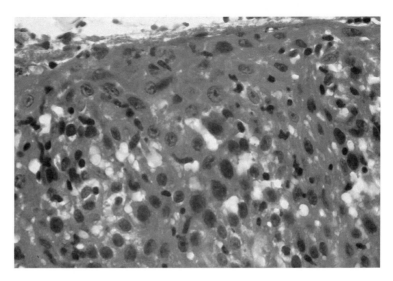

Figure 8–8. Atrophic cervicitis with atypical reparative change. The reparative cells have enlarged, regular nuclei and small nucleoli. The cells contain abundant cytoplasm and are evenly placed without altered cellular polarity. (See color section.)

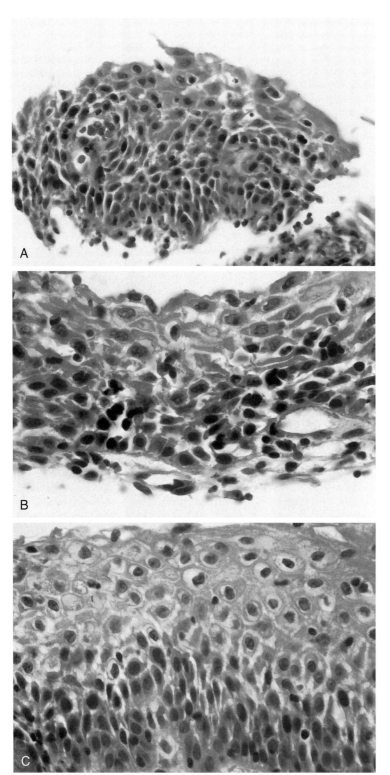

Figure 8–9. Reactive squamous atypia. *A*, *B*, and *C*, There is mild hyperplasia of parabasal cells, which maintain normal polarity, without nuclear atypia. Cells in the upper layers have minimally enlarged nuclei surrounded by clear halos. Rare binucleated cells are shown in *B*. This degree of nuclear change is insufficient for designation as koilocytes or mild squamous dysplasia. (See color section.)

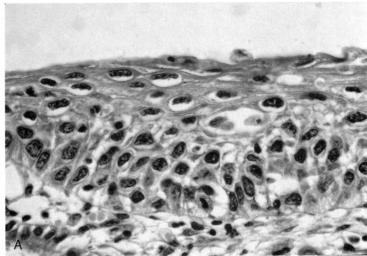

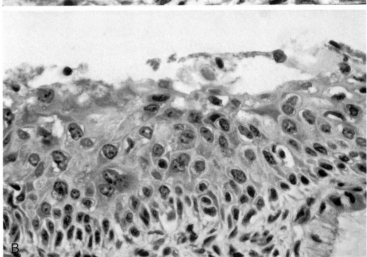

Figure 8–10. Reactive squamous atypia. Cells in the intermediate and superficial layers have slightly enlarged, irregular nuclei. A few cells are binucleated. Basal and parabasal cells maintain normal polarity without nuclear atypia or increased mitotic activity.

criteria described earlier and are classified as CIN 1 (Fig. 8–15). Inevitably some lesions are difficult to classify; in such cases, immunohistochemical stain for Ki-67 is useful. As shown in Figure 8–16, this stain demonstrates rare Ki-67 positive cells in the basal and parabasal layers. This feature favors an HPV effect.[244] Ki-67–positive cells are rarely seen in the normal ectocervical mucosa and squamous metaplasia of the basal cell layer. In addition, this stain reveals subtle cellular disorganization in the deep layers (see Fig. 8–16).

One of the common overinterpretations in cervical biopsies involves the normal glycogenated ectocervical squamous mucosa or mature squamous metaplasia, which is embedded and cut tangentially. Because of the tangential cuts, the epithelium appears to be thickened.

Closer examination reveals that the cells in the superficial layers have small nuclei without enlargement, hyperchromasia, irregularity, or binucleation. In the deep layers, no excessive proliferation of parabasal cells, increased mitotic activity, or cellular disorganization exist (Fig. 8–17). These biopsies are often taken because of a cytologic diagnosis of ASCUS. In such cases, it is always helpful to review the previous cytologic smear and to determine whether the two samples have correlated.

Atypical Immature Metaplasia (AIM) and Papillary Immature Metaplasia (PIM)

Squamous metaplasia of the cervix is basically a physiologic response to local factors, such as an

Text continued on page 291

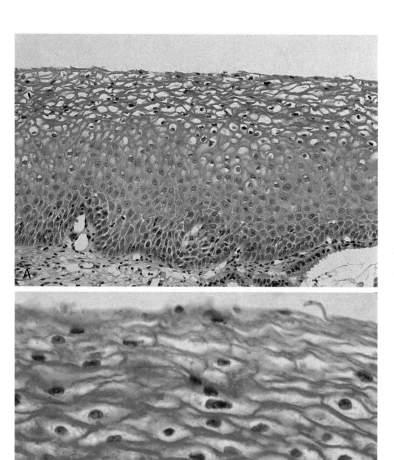

Figure 8–11. Borderline condyloma. *A* and *B,* Mature squamous mucosa with cells showing minor nuclear enlargement and prominent perinuclear halos. The cell borders are distinct without a glassy, thickened appearance.

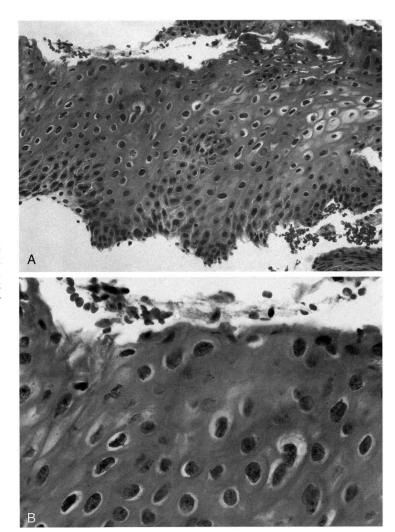

Figure 8–12. Borderline condyloma. *A* and *B*, Cells in the intermediate and superficial layers have enlarged round to oval nuclei, a few of which are binucleated. There is insufficient nuclear irregularity or hyperchromasia to be designated as koilocytes.

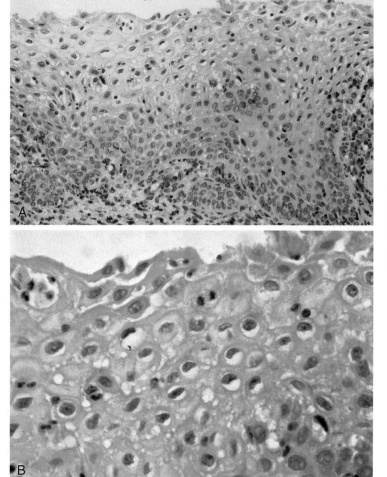

Figure 8–13. Borderline condyloma. *A* and *B,* The mature metaplastic squamous cells demonstrate a mild degree of nuclear irregularity. However, the nuclei are not enlarged in the upper layers. The cells in the deep layers are normal in appearance.

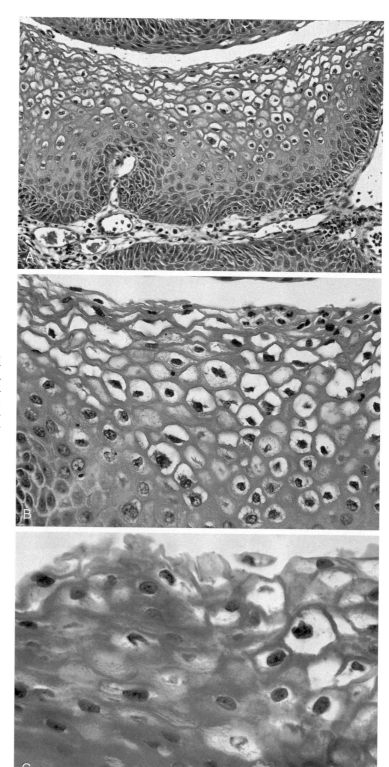

Figure 8–14. Flat condyloma/CIN 1. *A, B,* and *C,* This degree of nuclear irregularity, hyperchromasia, and enlargement is the minimal requirement for a designation as koilocytes. In addition, the cell borders are thickened and glassy/hyaline in appearance. (See color section.)

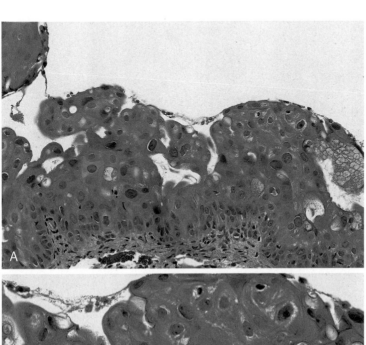

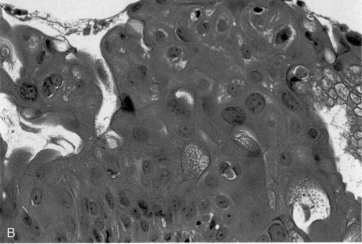

Figure 8–15. CIN 1. Endocervical curettage for cytologic diagnosis of atypical squamous cells of undetermined significance. *A* and *B*, Mature metaplastic squamous cells with nuclear enlargement, hyperchromasia, binucleation, and irregularity meet the criteria for CIN 1.

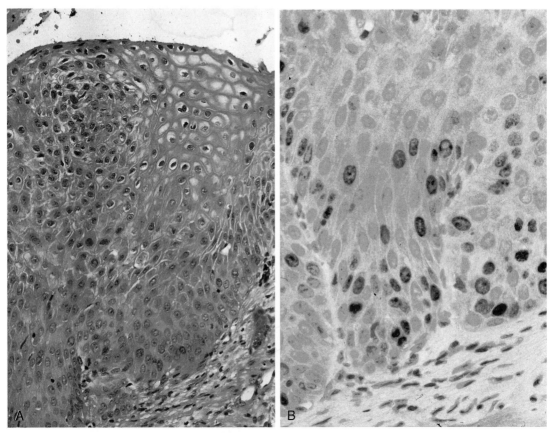

Figure 8–16. *A,* This is a borderline lesion that is difficult to classify. The upper half of the lesion does not demonstrate nuclear atypia. In the deep layers, however, cellular proliferation and overcrowded nuclei are present. *B,* Immunohistochemical stain for Ki-67 with antibody MIB-1 demonstrates an increased number of Ki-67–positive cells in the basal and parabasal layers. In addition, an irregular cellular arrangement and mild nuclear atypia become more evident in this stain and suggest condyloma/CIN 1. (See color section.)

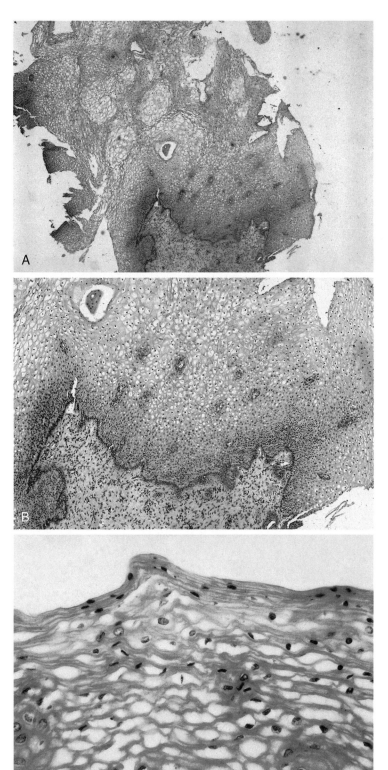

Figure 8–17. Mimicker of condyloma. *A* and *B,* Normal mature glycogenated ectocervical squamous mucosa cut tangentially results in broad sheets of cells with perinuclear halos simulating condyloma. *C,* Higher magnification of superficial and intermediate squamous cells reveals small nuclei throughout without nuclear atypia.

acidic vaginal environment following the onset of menarche, pregnancy, childbirth, or trauma. It is important to recognize that cellular response and morphologic manifestations of squamous metaplasia often differ from those of ectocervical squamous mucosa. This is especially true of response to HPV infection. Cytopathic effects of HPV require squamous differentiation. Thus, an immature squamous metaplasia, when infected by HPV, may not demonstrate koilocytosis.

AIM is found in women whose mean age is similar to that of women with cervical condyloma (27 years). They are younger than those with CIN 2 (mean 32 years) or CIN 3 (mean 37 years).[86] AIM occurs within the transformation zone or in the endocervical glands and coexists with condyloma in 34% of cases or with CIN in 16%.

Histologically, AIM consists of a monomorphic cell population with preservation of cellular polarity (Fig. 8–18). Its cellularity is slightly higher than that of immature squamous metaplasia. The monotony of cells is expressed by the uniformly round to oval nuclei, which contain prominent chromocenters and occasional small nucleoli. Mitotic activity is low to absent, and when present it is usually confined to the lower third of epithelium. Abnormal mitotic figures are absent. Occasional nuclei in the superficial layers are enlarged or multinucleated and retain uniform chromatin pattern. Koilocytosis is minimal or absent.[86]

AIM can be distinguished from CIN by its uniform cell population with minimal atypia and its low mitotic activity, usually less than one per 10 high-power fields. With the use of im-

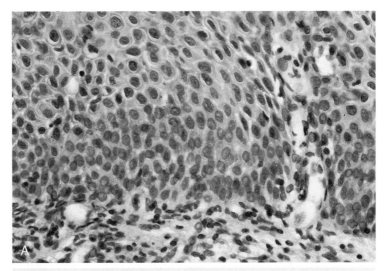

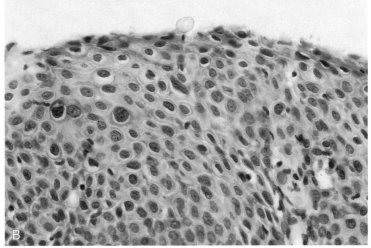

Figure 8–18. Atypical immature metaplasia. *A,* Uniform population of immature metaplastic squamous cells in most of the epithelium. No mitotic activity is seen. *B,* In the superficial layers, some of the cells have enlarged, round to oval hyperchromatic nuclei surrounded by clear halos.

munohistochemical stains, most of the cells in AIM express p63, but very few if any express Ki-67 antigen (Fig. 8–19). In CIN, scattered Ki-67–positive cells occur in relation to the severity of the lesion.

AIM sometimes is seen in endocervical curettings. The atypical metaplastic squamous cells are mixed with endocervical cells and contain large, hyperchromatic nuclei. The chromatin is finely granular, and binucleation may occur. Nucleoli, when present, are small (Fig. 8–20).

Very rarely, in the areas of immature squamous metaplasia are atypical cells with gigantic hyperchromatic nuclei that are sometimes multinucleated. Nucleoli may be seen (Fig. 8–21). Essentially, lesions demonstrating sufficient nuclear atypia or cellular disorganization are classified as CIN (see Fig. 8–21; Fig. 8–22).

Inconsistency in the diagnosis of AIM is reported by Park et al.[268] Two observers classified 44 nonpapillary atypical immature squamous proliferative lesions as (1) probably reactive, (2) not otherwise specified (NOS), and (3) SIL. The lesions were further studied for HPV by PCR technique. The interobserver reproducibility was excellent for reactive changes but poor for NOS and fair to good for SIL. The morphologic findings do not correlate strongly with HPV status. The authors concluded that AIMs exceeding the threshold of reactive change include a heterogeneous group of lesions. This view was also supported by immunohistochemical stain for Ki-67 and HPV DNA by PCR.[124]

PIM is an AIM with a papillary growth pattern (Figs. 8–23 and 8–24). In a study by Trivijitsilip et al.,[356] 11 PIMs were studied for HPV

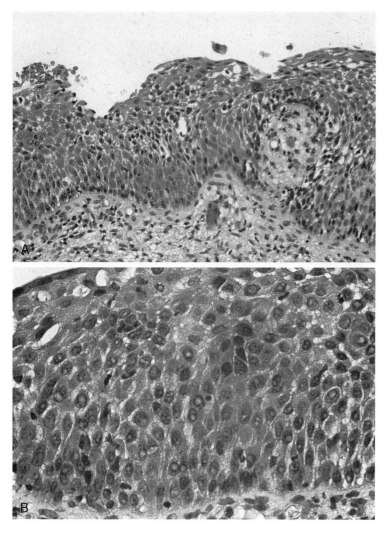

Figure 8–19. Atypical immature metaplasia. *A,* Sheet of immature metaplastic cells with rare atypical cells in the superficial layers. *B,* Higher magnification illustrates minor nuclear irregularity. No mitotic figures are present. *C,* Immunohistochemical stain for p63 reveals that immature/stem cells occupy the entire epithelium. *D,* Immunohistochemical stain for Ki-67, however, shows no positive cells, indicative of very low proliferative activity. In the case of CIN, more Ki-67–positive cells are expected. (See color section.)

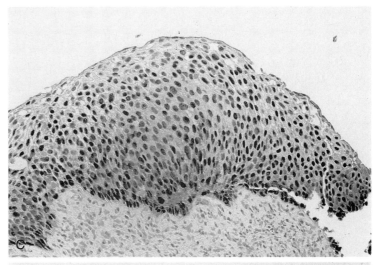

Figure 8–19. *Continued*

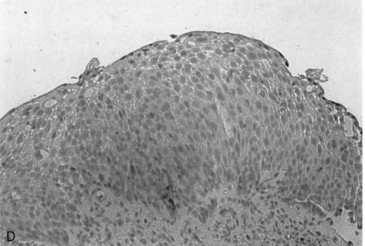

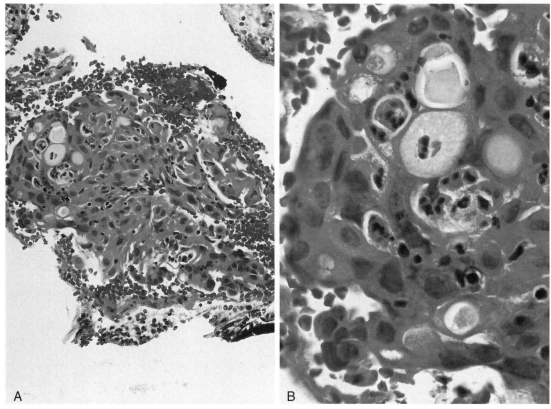

Figure 8–20 *See legend on opposite page*

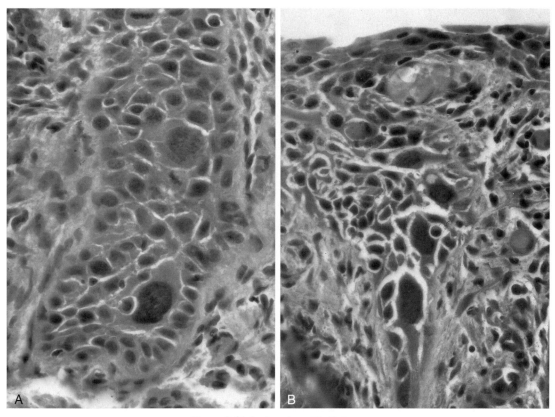

Figure 8–21 *See legend on opposite page*

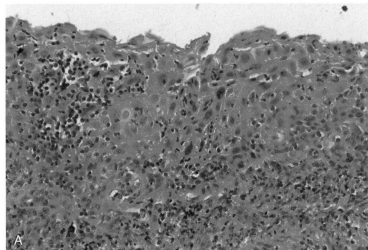

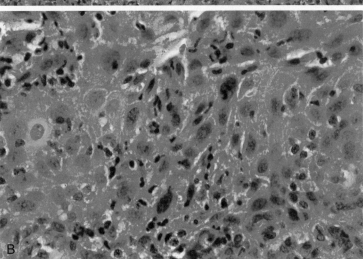

Figure 8–22. *A* and *B,* This lesion appears to be reactive; however, there are cells with enlarged, irregular hyperchromatic nuclei, best classified as at least CIN 1.

type by PCR technique. Ten (77%) of 13 PIMs were positive for HPV 6/11, and three (23%) also had areas of condyloma (see Fig. 8–24). Cone biopsy was performed in nine cases. In three of these cases, a coexisting high-grade SIL was identified that was HPV negative or other than HPV 6/11. In PIMs, Ki-67–positive cells were few in number. In contrast, all SIL and papillary squamous/squamotransitional cell carcinomas had many more Ki-67–positive cells. The authors conclude that immunohistochemical stain for Ki-67 is useful for distin-

guishing these papillary lesions.[356] When classified with strict criteria, AIM and PIM have a biologic potential comparable to that of low-grade CIN.

Cervical Intraepithelial Neoplasia (CIN)/ Squamous Intraepithelial Lesions (SIL)

Morphogenesis

Careful mapping of the lesions and their surrounding epithelia in cervical biopsies, coniza-

Figure 8–20. Atypical immature metaplasia. *A* and *B,* Endocervical curettage performed for cytologic diagnosis of atypical squamous cells of undetermined significance. Atypical metaplastic squamous cells mixed with endocervical cells. The enlarged nuclei contain small nucleoli, consistent with a reactive change.

Figure 8–21. CIN. *A* and *B,* In the background of immature squamous metaplasia are highly atypical cells with gigantic, hyperchromatic nuclei. This lesion is of uncertain nature and best classified as CIN 1.

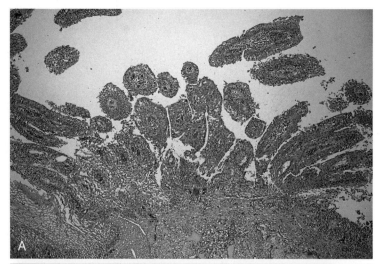

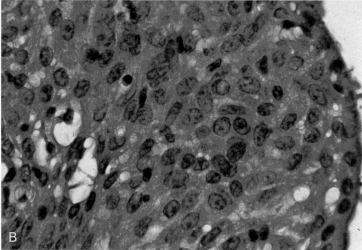

Figure 8–23. Papillary immature metaplasia. *A,* Multiple finger-like projections arising from the endocervical mucosa. *B,* Higher magnification illustrates immature metaplastic squamous cells with mild nuclear atypia. No mitotic figure is seen.

tion, or hysterectomy has confirmed that most CINs occur in the vicinity of the squamocolumnar junction, especially in relation to the squamous metaplasia and reserve cell hyperplasia.[168,287,378] Subsequent observations by colposcopy also confirm the predominant localization of CINs within the transformation zone. In a study of 319 conization specimens, using the last endocervical gland as the original squamocolumnar junction, only 3.1% of CINs were found to be localized in the ectocervix and 10% were surrounded completely by the endocervical epithelium. The remaining 87% of CINs occurred within the transformation zone.[2]

In a topographic mapping of condyloma and CIN in conization specimens by Saito et al.,[308] 94% of condylomas involved the transformation zone, usually extending distally to the last gland. Only 6% of condylomas were confined

to the ectocervix. Among the CINs, 2% were located completely in the ectocervix, 8% were predominantly distal to the last gland, and the remaining 90% were proximal to the last gland. When CINs coexist with condyloma, they are always located higher than the condyloma, suggesting that foci of CIN arise from the proximal border of condyloma[13] (Fig. 8–25). On autoradiographic in situ hybridization preparations, HPV DNA is confined to the abnormal epithelium of either condyloma and/or CIN (Fig. 8–26). This and topographic findings do not support the concept of HPV infection causing a diffuse, field change but, rather, discrete, well-defined, sometimes multiple lesions.

The topographic study by Saito et al.[308] also confirms that lower grade dysplasias occur more distally than do more advanced lesions. The CIN at the distal end extends slightly be-

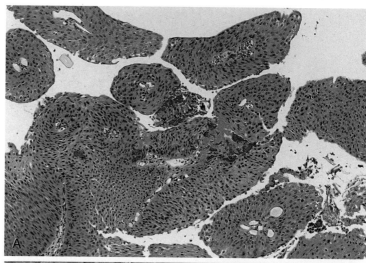

Figure 8–24. Papillary immature metaplasia. *A* and *B,* Multiple papillary fronds lined by immature metaplastic squamous cells and with atypical cells in the superficial layers. *C* and *D,* Condyloma acuminatum adjacent to lesion shown in *A* and *B. Illustration continued on following page*

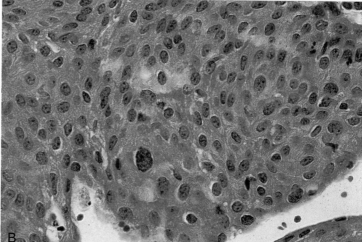

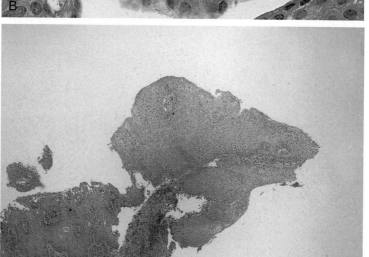

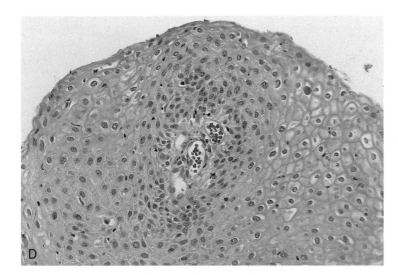

Figure 8–24. *Continued*

Figure 8–25. Topography of CIN. Low-grade CIN tends to begin from the original squamous columnar junction as indicated by the last endocervical gland (GL), and extends distally toward the ectocervix. More severe CIN is located proximally.

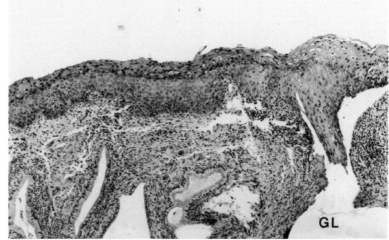

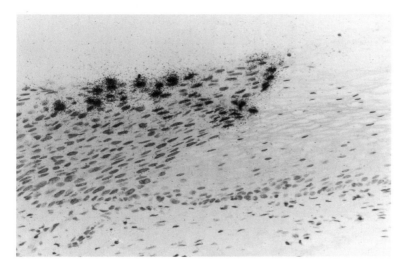

Figure 8–26. This figure illustrates the sharp border between the distal end of CIN and the ectocervical squamous mucosa (*right*). Using an autoradiographic in situ hybridization technique, HPV DNA type 16 is identified in the area of CIN as black silver grains overlying the nuclei. No HPV DNA is seen in the normal squamous mucosa. (Courtesy of Dr. J. Gupta and Dr. K. V. Shah, Johns Hopkins University, School of Public Health.)

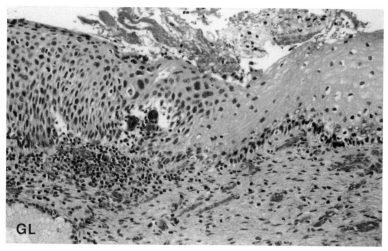

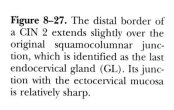

Figure 8–27. The distal border of a CIN 2 extends slightly over the original squamocolumnar junction, which is identified as the last endocervical gland (GL). Its junction with the ectocervical mucosa is relatively sharp.

yond the last gland and has a sharp border with the native squamous mucosa (Fig. 8–27). The proximal borders of CIN often appear to lift up or undermine the endocervical epithelium (Fig. 8–28).

The dimensions of CIN increase by cellular proliferation, which is strongly correlated with mitotic activity and the severity of CIN. In a study of 319 conization specimens by Abdul-Karim et al.,[2] the mean maximal length along the long axis of the cervical canal is 4.1 ± 2.8, 5.8 ± 4.1, and 7.6 ± 4.3 mm for CIN 1, 2, and 3, respectively. The mean maximal depth from the epithelial surface is 0.42 ± 0.28, 0.93 ± 0.71, and 1.35 ± 1.15 mm for CIN 1, 2, and 3, respectively. These findings also imply that to eradicate all CIN 3 le-

sions by means of local destruction, one needs to reach a depth of 4.8 mm (mean ± 3 standard deviations).

Clinical Features

Most women with CIN are asymptomatic or present with nonspecific symptoms, such as vaginal discharge, pain, or local irritation. The cervix usually appears normal, eroded, or hyperemic. Occasionally, a raised white lesion has a smooth or papillary surface. The affected areas usually fail to react with iodine solution and remain white or yellow (Schiller's test positive) (Fig. 8–29). However, similar reactions occur in nonglycogenated epithelium, such as squamous metaplasia.

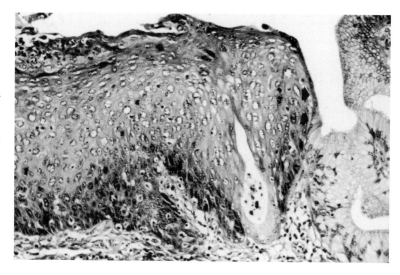

Figure 8–28. The proximal end of CIN expands by lifting up the endocervical epithelium (*arrows*). It grows downward by forming wedge-shaped processes between the base of endocervical cells and the fibrous stroma.

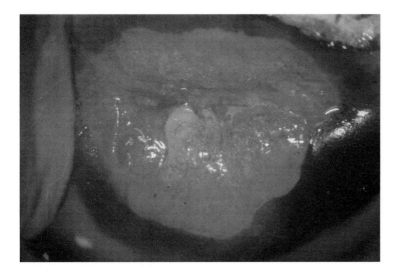

Figure 8–29. After staining with Lugol solution, the ectocervical mucosa becomes purple, while the nonstaining areas around the cervical os and carcinoma in situ remain yellow. (Courtesy of Dr. Cheng-Hsiung Roan, Taipei Medical University, Taipei, Taiwan.) (See color section.)

After the application of acetic acid, the abnormal area temporarily turns to acetowhite (Fig. 8–30). Under colposcopic examination, the dilated terminal capillary networks between the rete pegs of atypical epithelium cause a punctate pattern (see Fig. 8–30). Anastomosis of these networks produces a mosaic pattern (Fig. 8–31A). In general, increased intercapillary distance, coarse capillaries, and an irregular mosaic pattern are associated with high-grade CIN (Fig. 8–31B). Irregular, tortuous blood vessels are usually associated with invasive carcinoma (see Fig. 8–32A and B).

By colposcopic examination, CIN's boundary (complete versus incomplete visualization), extent (number of quadrants involved), and topography can be defined. These parameters, along with the findings of biopsy, endocervical curettage, and other factors, influence the therapeutic modality.

Microscopic Features

In nondiagnostic squamous atypia, AIM, and PIM, the nuclear atypia is mild. No cellular disorganization or loss of normal polarity is apparent. Mitotic activity is rare or absent. In contrast, CIN lesions demonstrate a greater degree of nuclear abnormalities and mitotic activity. With increasing severity, additional abnormalities are manifested in cellularity, differentiation, polarity, nuclear features, and mitotic activity. Once the lesion has been accepted as CIN, the next step is to determine its severity by grading further as CIN 1, CIN 2, or CIN 3.

Alternatively, the lesion is categorized as low-grade SIL (flat condyloma and CIN 1) or high-grade SIL (CIN 2 and CIN 3).

To simplify the grading of severity, it is often helpful to divide the epithelium into three zones: lower third (parabasal), middle third (intermediate), and upper third (superficial). First evaluate the type and the extent of abnormality in each zone, and then derive an overall assessment for a lesion. It is also useful to compare it with the adjacent normal epithelium zone by zone. For CIN 1 or low-grade SIL, the immature/parabasal type of abnormal cells are usually confined to the lower third of the epithelium. In contrast, in CIN 2, these immature cells reach to the middle third and in CIN 3, to the upper third.

On low-power examination, the epithelium is slightly thickened with a flat, spiky, or papillary surface (Fig. 8–33). The papillary variant of squamous CIS, although rare, deserves mention, because of the difficulty in separating it from the invasive counterpart.[191]

In most dysplasias, cells in the most superficial layers become flattened, an appearance that is suggestive of parakeratosis. In approximately 20% of dysplasias, abnormal differentiation is earmarked by hyperkeratosis, atypical parakeratosis, an excess of keratohyalin granules in the superficial layers, and dyskeratosis (see Fig. 8–33B). When prominent, these features are recognized as keratinizing dysplasia, which is readily apparent in the cytologic specimens.

The base of epithelium is flat in 20% of dysplasias, whereas the remaining 80% have the

Text continued on page 305

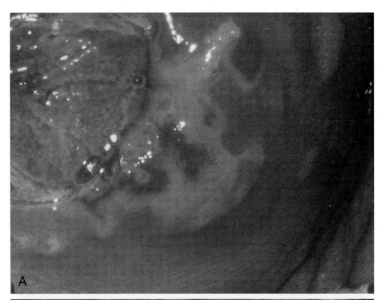

Figure 8–30. Colposcopic view after application of acetic acid. *A,* The normal endocervical epithelium has a grape-like appearance (*left field*). The outer gray-white epithelium represents squamous metaplasia. On the outer border of the transformation zone is a white thickened epithelium with mosaic pattern, consistent with mild squamous dysplasia. Two raised flat condylomas appear as white epithelium. *B,* Flat condyloma of the cervix and condyloma acuminatum in the vaginal vault. (Courtesy of Dr. Richard Reid, New Zealand.) (See color section.)

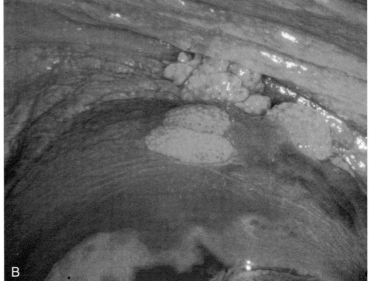

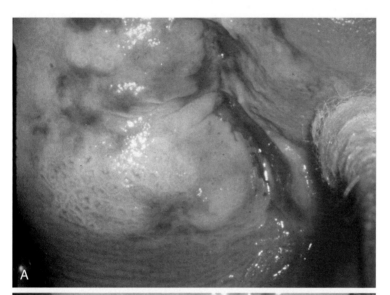

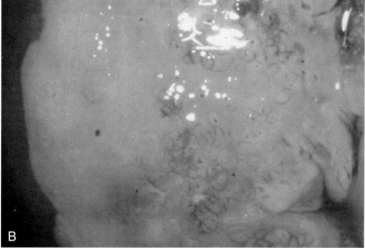

Figure 8–31. *A,* Colposcopic examination reveals a white epithelium with mosaic pattern (*left field*). A cotton swab is placed near the os. *B,* A coarse mosaicism with irregular blood vessels in a CIN 3. The thick white epithelium on the periphery was confirmed to be the result of condylomatous changes. (Courtesy of Dr. Richard Reid, New Zealand.) (See color section.)

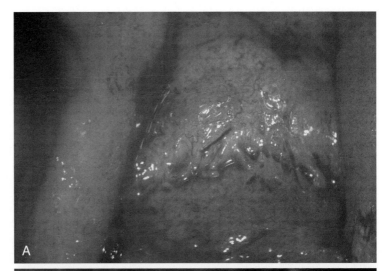

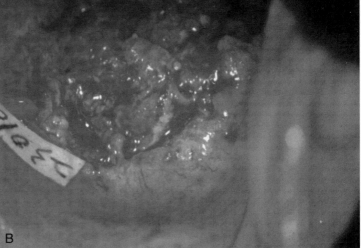

Figure 8–32. *A,* Colposcopic view of abnormal tortuous blood vessels in an invasive squamous cell carcinoma. *B,* In addition to abnormal blood vessels, the surface is ulcerated. (Courtesy of Dr. Cheng-Hsiung Roan, Taipei Medical University, Taipei, Taiwan.) (See color section.)

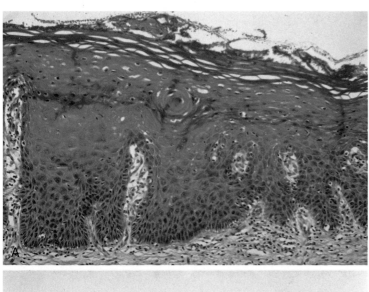

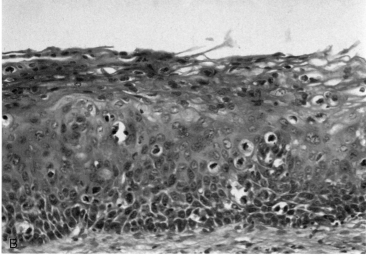

Figure 8–33. Surface and base of CIN. *A,* The surface is flat and covered by hyperkeratosis. The rete pegs are plump. *B,* The flat surface is covered by atypical parakeratosis and abnormal keratinization. The base of CIN is flat. *C,* Spiky surface with parakeratosis. *D,* Papillary fronds supported by fibrovascular cores.

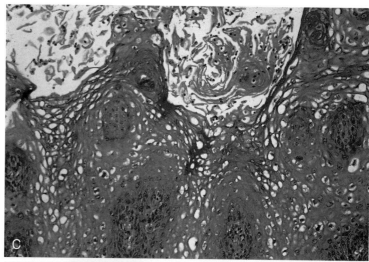

Figure 8–33. *Continued*

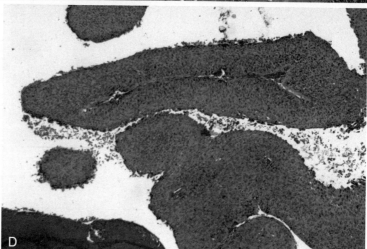

formation of rete pegs.[287] The latter generally arise from a more mature epithelium than do the former (see Fig. 8–33A). Direct extension into the underlying endocervical glands occurs regularly.

Cellular polarity refers to the architectural relationship of the neighboring cells. The normal basal cell layer consists of palisaded basal cells whose nuclei are small, uniform, and vertical to the basement membrane. This arrangement is usually maintained in condyloma and CIN 1 (Fig. 8–34A). However, in higher grade CINs, dysplastic cells replace the basal cell layer. The polarity in the superficial layers is usually horizontal in CIN 1 but becomes vertical or inconstant in high-grade CIN (see Fig. 8–34B).

Low-Grade CIN/SIL

In condyloma and mild dysplasias (CIN 1), immature cells proliferate in the lower third of the epithelium. Cells in the upper two thirds maintain squamous differentiation and horizontal polarity. A distinct basal cell layer is preserved (Figs. 8–35 and 8–36). Squamous differentiation is indicated by lower cellularity than that in the deep layers, and the cells contain a moderate amount of eosinophilic cytoplasm with distinct cell borders (see Figs. 8–35 and 8–36).

Cells in the lower third of epithelium, although enlarged, are relatively uniform with round to oval nuclei and finely granular chromatin (see Figs. 8–35 and 8–36; Fig. 8–37).

Text continued on page 309

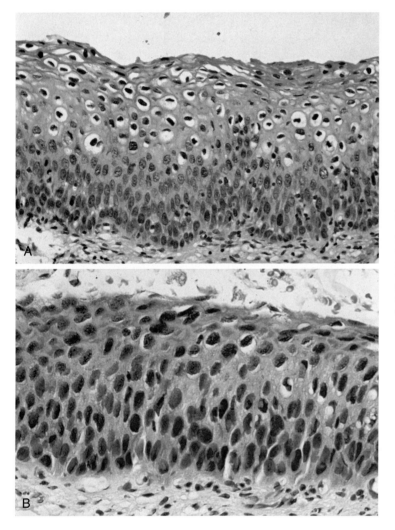

Figure 8–34. Polarity of CIN. *A,* CIN 1 with distinct basal cell layer and horizontal parallel superficial cells without loss of polarity. *B,* CIN 3 with complete replacement of normal basal cells by dysplastic cells. Disorderly arrangement of dysplastic cells is evident in the deep layers and on the surface.

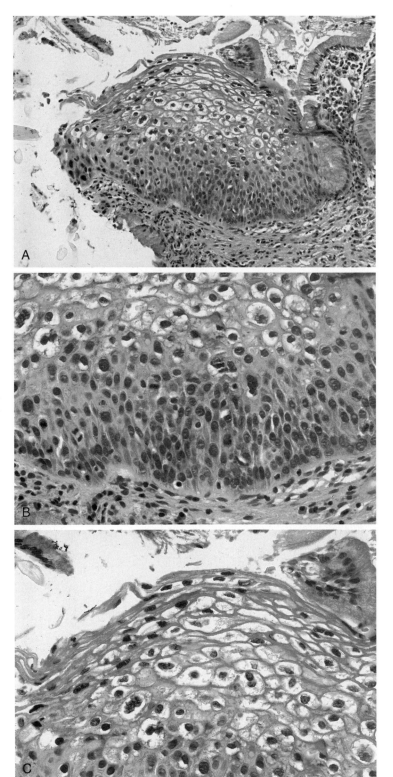

Figure 8–35. *A,* CIN 1 with koilocytosis. *B,* Proliferation of immature cells in the lower third of the epithelium with a distinct basal cell layer, mild nuclear atypia, and increased mitotic activity. *C,* Typical koilocytes occupy the upper two thirds of epithelium.

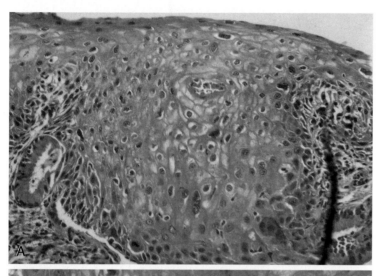

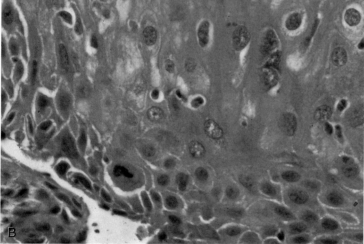

Figure 8–36. CIN 1. *A*, Koilocytes and atypical cells in the upper third of the lesion. *B*, Atypical cells with multinucleation and rare mitotic figures occur in the lower third of epithelium.

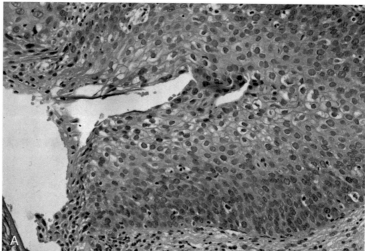

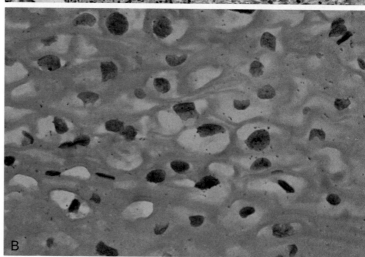

Figure 8–37. CIN 1 in immature squamous metaplasia affected by HPV type 31. *A,* Proliferation of immature cells in the lower half of epithelium and more mature cells in the upper half of the lesion. *B,* Mild nuclear atypia in koilocytes with silver grains in an in situ autoradiographic preparation.

These enlarged cells sometimes extend into the basal cell layer. Multinucleated cells may occur. The cytoplasm is diminished, and as a result nuclear cytoplasmic ratios are higher than those of normal cells at the comparable levels. Mitotic activity is rare and limited to the lower third. Abnormal forms occasionally may occur (Fig. 8–38).

In the upper layers of low-grade CIN, koilocytosis is present in most cases. By definition, koilocytes must demonstrate at least a mild degree of nuclear atypia. The nuclear abnormalities observed include enlargement, hyperchromasia, irregularity in size and shape, and chromatinic clumping. With degeneration, nuclei become pyknotic and contracted with irregular borders. Some nuclei are binucleated or multinucleated (see Figs. 8–35 to 8–37). The

nuclei are surrounded by clear halos. The cell borders are thickened. With increasing severity of CIN, the nuclei become more pleomorphic and contain coarse chromatin and chromocenters. Nucleoli are rarely seen.

In some CIN 1 lesions, the enlarged nuclei remain relatively uniformly round to oval in shape and contain finely granular chromatin with open spaces (see Fig. 8–38).

Because more than 95% of CINs are associated with HPV infection, the presence or absence of koilocytosis should not influence the determination of severity. The grading of CIN is based on cellular maturity and the nuclear and mitotic abnormalities.

Immunohistochemical stains for p63 are useful in the visualization of the level of immature cells. In condyloma and CIN 1, p63-positive

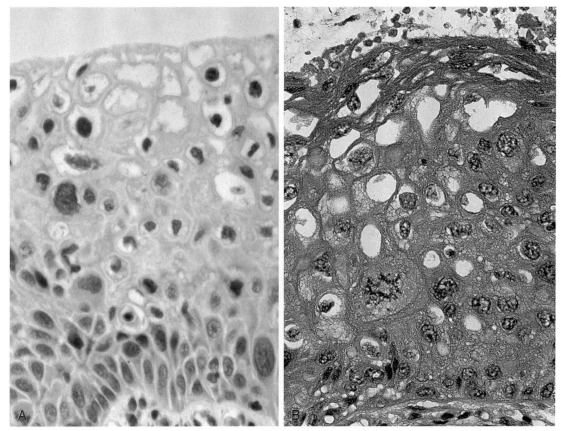

Figure 8–38. CIN 1. *A*, Large dysplastic cells occur in the lower third and middle third of the lesion. *B*, A giant mitotic figure occurs in the lower third of the lesion.

cells are localized to the lower third of the epithelium (Figs. 8–39 and 8–40). Ki-67–positive cells using MIB-1 antibody reveal rare positive cells reach to the basal and parabasal layers (see Figs. 8–39 and 8–40). In the normal ectocervical squamous mucosa, basal cells are rarely labeled by MIB-1 antibody. However, in CIN 1 lesions, some of the basal cells are positive for Ki-67.[244]

High-Grade CIN/SIL

In moderate dysplasias (CIN 2), immature cells extend from the lower third to the middle third of the epithelium. These cells demonstrate a moderate degree of nuclear irregularity in size and shape. Mitotic figures, including abnormal forms, often can be found in the middle third. Toward the surface, the abnormal cells maintain squamous maturation (Figs. 8–41 to 8–44). In lesions with koilocytosis, the nuclear atypia is much more severe than that seen in CIN 1. Immunohistochemical stains reveal p63-posi-

tive immature cells occupying the lower two thirds of epithelium, where scattered Ki-67–positive cells are present (Fig. 8–45).

In severe dysplasia and carcinoma in situ (CIN 3), almost the entire epithelium demonstrates high cellularity, immaturity, vertical orientation, and active proliferation. The polarity in the basal layer is altered. Basal cells are replaced or intermingled with abnormal cells, which have larger and irregular nuclei. In many instances, the basal cells are completely replaced by abnormal cells. In addition, the abnormal cells lose their regular parallel arrangement and become arranged in a disorderly fashion. Toward the surface, cellular disorganization is also evident, sometimes comprising entirely vertically arranged cells with elongated nuclei (Figs. 8–46 to 8–48).

The cells in CIN 3 lesions range from highly pleomorphic and heterogeneous to monotonously uniform in appearance (see Figs. 8–46 and 8–47). Individual cells have many of the cytologic hallmarks of malignancy, with coarsely

Text continued on page 319

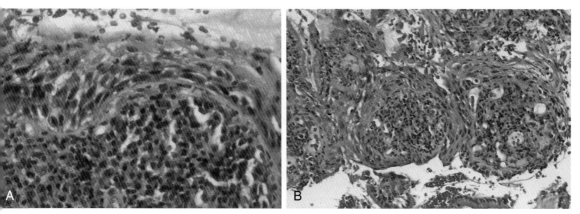

Figure 8–6. Pseudoparakeratosis. *A,* The endocervical mucosa is covered by four to five layers of flattened, parallel, small, immature metaplastic squamous cells simulating parakeratosis. The underlying stroma is heavily infiltrated by plasma cells. *B,* Cross section of endocervical papillary erosion re-epithelialized by immature metaplastic squamous cells.

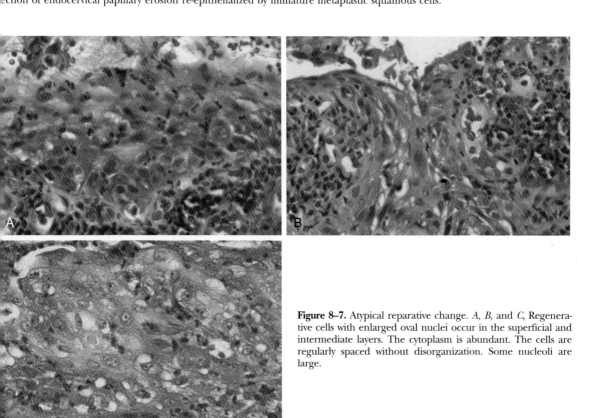

Figure 8–7. Atypical reparative change. *A, B,* and *C,* Regenerative cells with enlarged oval nuclei occur in the superficial and intermediate layers. The cytoplasm is abundant. The cells are regularly spaced without disorganization. Some nucleoli are large.

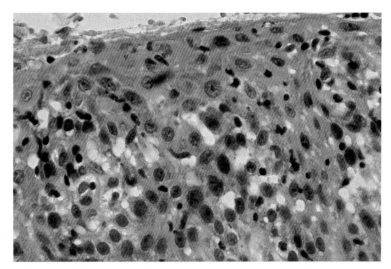

Figure 8–8. Atrophic cervicitis with atypical reparative change. The reparative cells have enlarged, regular nuclei and small nucleoli. The cells contain abundant cytoplasm and are evenly placed without altered cellular polarity.

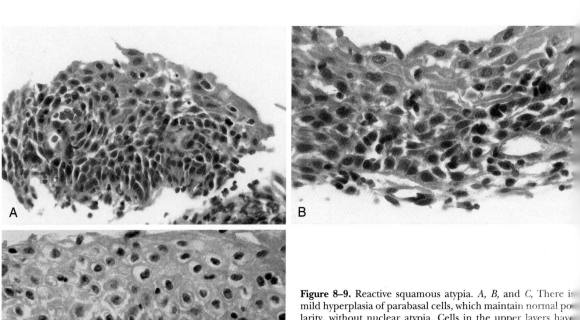

Figure 8–9. Reactive squamous atypia. *A, B,* and *C,* There is mild hyperplasia of parabasal cells, which maintain normal polarity, without nuclear atypia. Cells in the upper layers have minimally enlarged nuclei surrounded by clear halos. Rare binucleated cells are shown in *B.* This degree of nuclear change is insufficient for designation as koilocytes or mild squamous dysplasia.

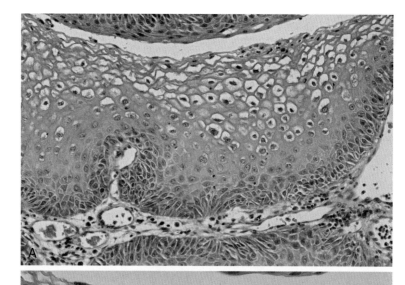

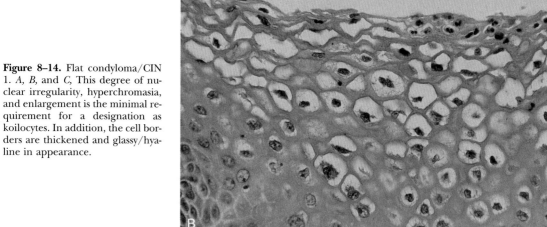

Figure 8–14. Flat condyloma/CIN 1. *A, B,* and *C,* This degree of nuclear irregularity, hyperchromasia, and enlargement is the minimal requirement for a designation as koilocytes. In addition, the cell borders are thickened and glassy/hyaline in appearance.

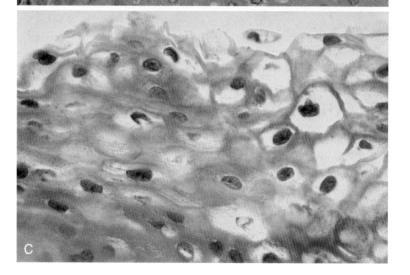

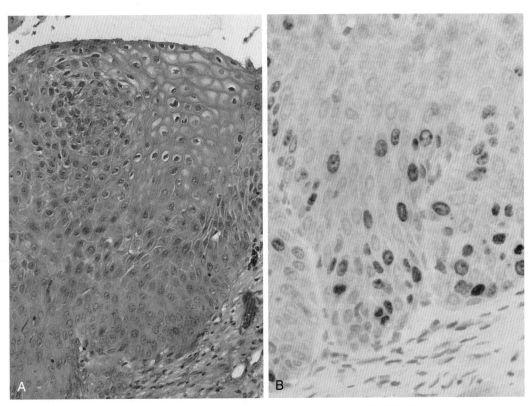

Figure 8–16. *A,* This is a borderline lesion that is difficult to classify. The upper half of the lesion does not demonstrate nuclear atypia. In the deep layers, however, cellular proliferation and overcrowded nuclei are present. *B,* Immunohistochemical stain for Ki-67 with antibody MIB-1 demonstrates an increased number of Ki-67–positive cells in the basal and parabasal layers. In addition, an irregular cellular arrangement and mild nuclear atypia become more evident in this stain and suggest condyloma/CIN 1.

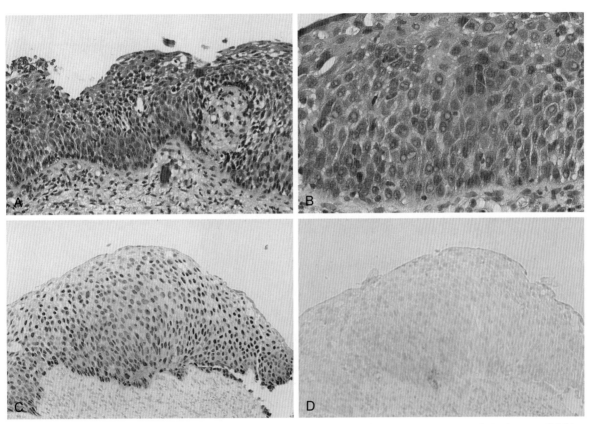

Figure 8–19. Atypical immature metaplasia. *A,* Sheet of immature metaplastic cells with rare atypical cells in the superficial layers. *B,* Higher magnification illustrates minor nuclear irregularity. No mitotic figures are present. *C,* Immunohistochemical stain for p63 reveals that immature/stem cells occupy the entire epithelium. *D,* Immunohistochemical stain for Ki-67, however, shows no positive cells, indicative of very low proliferative activity. In the case of CIN, more Ki-67–positive cells are expected.

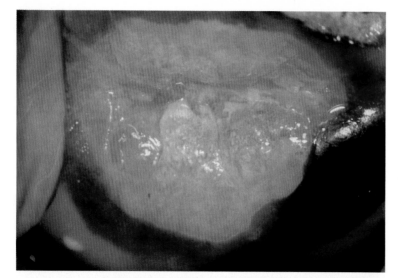

Figure 8–29. After staining with Lugol solution, the ectocervical mucosa becomes purple, while the nonstaining areas around the cervical os and carcinoma in situ remain yellow. (Courtesy of Dr. Cheng-Hsiung Roan, Taipei Medical University, Taipei, Taiwan)

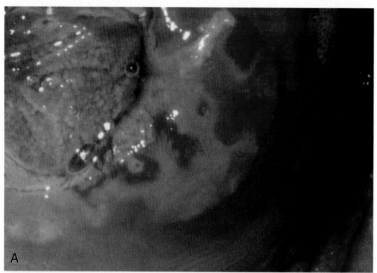

A

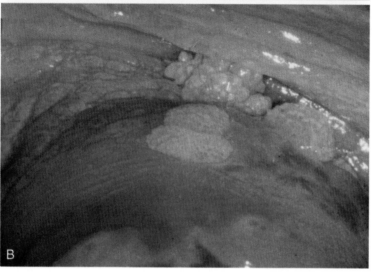

B

Figure 8–30. Colposcopic view after application of acetic acid. *A*, The normal endocervical epithelium has a grape-like appearance (*left field*). The outer gray-white epithelium represents squamous metaplasia. On the outer border of the transformation zone is a white thickened epithelium with mosaic pattern, consistent with mild squamous dysplasia. Two raised flat condylomas appear as white epithelium. *B*, Flat condyloma of the cervix and condyloma acuminatum in the vaginal vault. (Courtesy of Dr. Richard Reid, New Zealand).

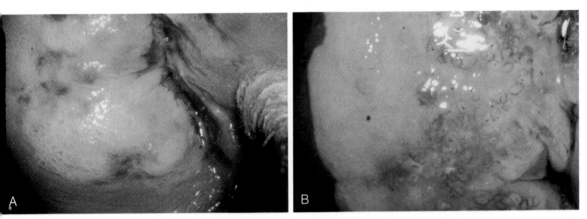

Figure 8–31. *A,* Colposcopic examination reveals a white epithelium with mosaic pattern (*left field*). A cotton swab is placed near the os. *B,* A coarse mosaicism with irregular blood vessels in a CIN 3. The thick white epithelium on the periphery was confirmed to be the result of condylomatous changes. (Courtesy of Dr. Richard Reid, New Zealand).

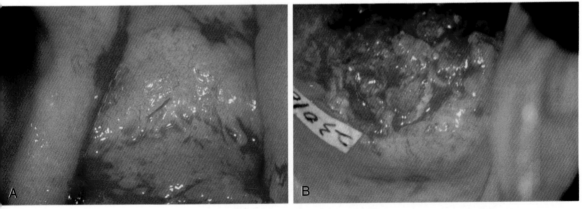

Figure 8–32. *A,* Colposcopic view of abnormal tortuous blood vessels in an invasive squamous cell carcinoma. *B,* In addition to abnormal blood vessels, the surface is ulcerated. (Courtesy of Dr. Cheng-Hsiung Roan, Taipei Medical University, Taipei, Taiwan).

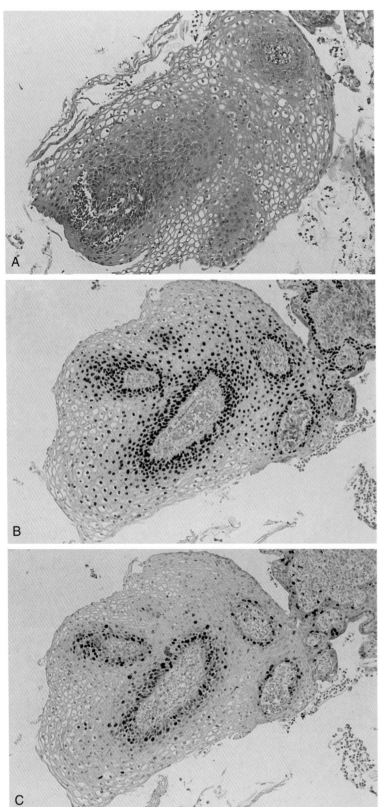

Figure 8–39. *A,* Condyloma acuminatum. *B,* Immunohistochemical stain for p63 showing immature/stem cells in the basal, parabasal, and intermediate cell layers. *C,* Ki-67–positive cells are limited to the basal and parabasal cell layers.

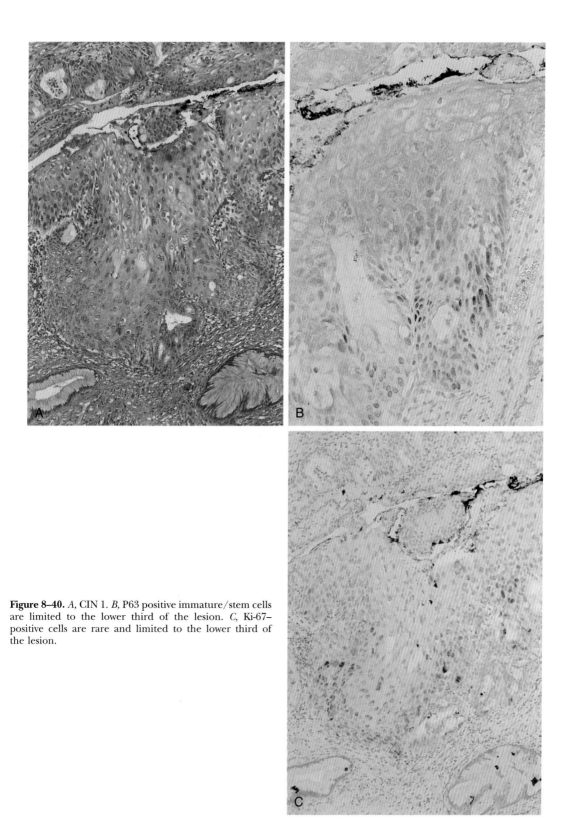

Figure 8–40. *A*, CIN 1. *B*, P63 positive immature/stem cells are limited to the lower third of the lesion. *C*, Ki-67– positive cells are rare and limited to the lower third of the lesion.

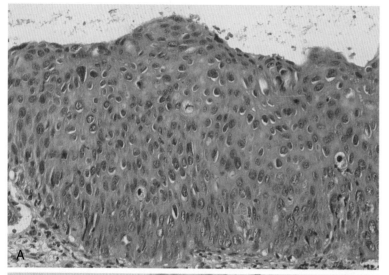

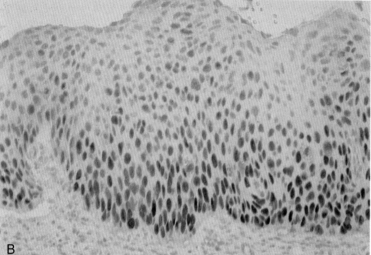

Figure 8–45. CIN 2–3. *A,* Immature cells in vertical orientation reach to the upper third in part of the lesion to support CIN 3. Atypical parakeratosis and koilocytosis occur in the superficial layers. *B,* Some p63-positive immature/stem cells occupy up to the upper third of the epithelium. *C,* Scattered Ki-67–positive cells occur mainly in the lower two thirds of the lesion.

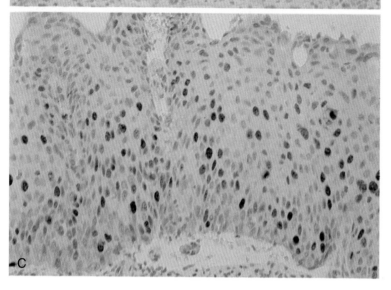

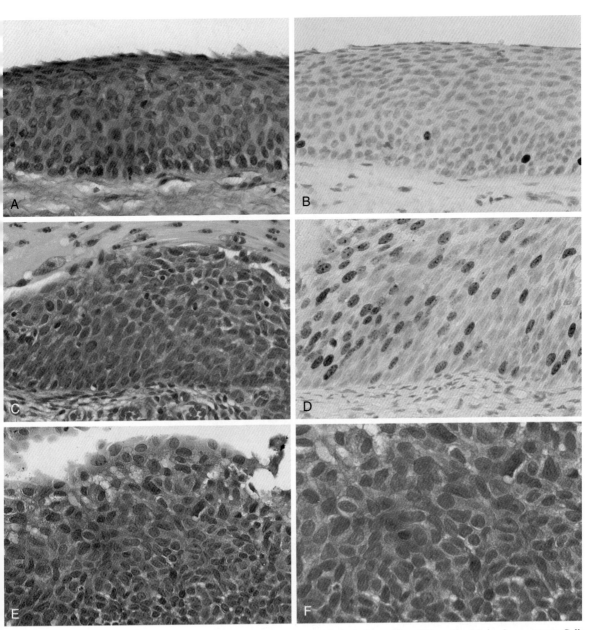

Figure 8–50. *A* and *B,* Transitional cell metaplasia. *A,* Monotonous population of transitional-like cells with nuclear grooves. Cells in the superficial layers maintain parallel arrangement. No mitotic activity is seen. *B,* Immunohistochemical stain for Ki-67 reveals very rare positive cells in the parabasal layers. *C* to *F,* High-grade CIN with transitional-like cells. *C,* Abnormal cells are arranged vertically. Cellular disorganization is seen in the superficial layers. Mitotic activity is present. *D,* Similar area as in *C.* Immunohistochemical stain for Ki-67 reveals scattered positive cells, even though mitotic figures are rare to absent. *E* and *F,* Higher magnification reveals nuclear grooves and nuclear irregularity in the upper half of the epithelium.

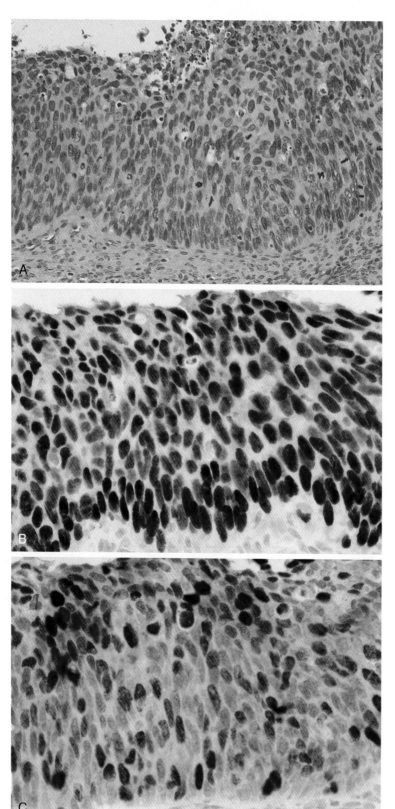

Figure 8–52. CIN 3. *A,* The entire lesion comprises vertically arranged dysplastic cells with scattered mitotic figures. *B,* P63-positive immature/stem cells occupy the entire epithelium. *C,* Ki-67–positive cells scatter over the entire epithelium, indicative of highly disordered cellular proliferation.

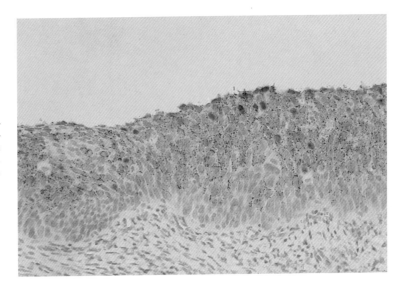

Figure 8–54. CIN 3 with neuroendocrine differentiation. Immunohistochemical stain for chromogranin is positive in the majority of cells. Same lesion as shown in Figure 8–52.

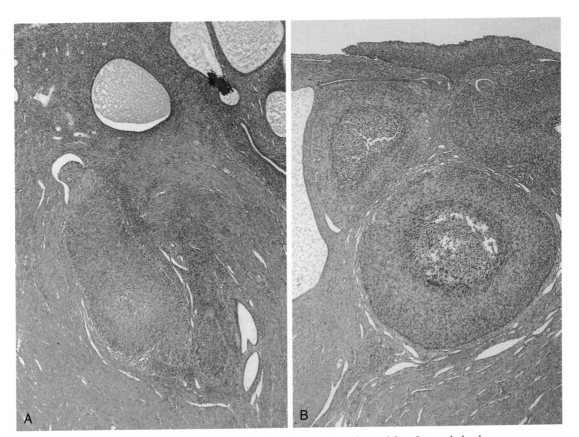

A

B

Figure 8–55. *A* and *B*, CIN 3 extends directly onto the endometrial surface and glands.

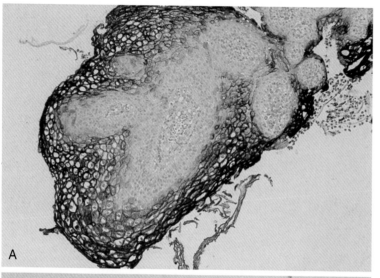

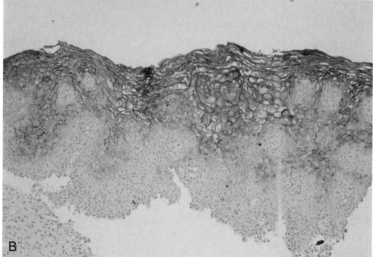

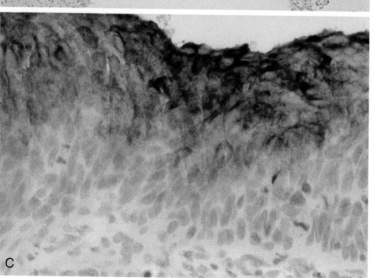

Figure 8–56. Carcinoembryonic antigen in the upper layers of condyloma (*A*), CIN 2 (*B*), and CIN 3 (*C*). Based on monoclonal antibody DAKO-CEA, AA5B7.

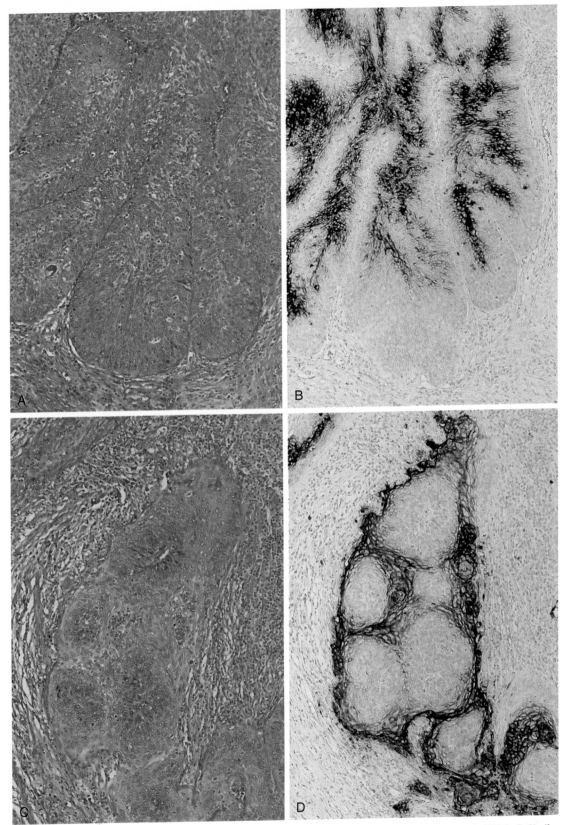

Figure 8–57. Comparison of CEA localization in CIN 3 and underlying invasive squamous carcinoma. *A*, CIN 3. *B*, Similar area as in *A*. CEA occurs in the upper half of epithelium. *C*, Underlying invasive squamous carcinoma. *D*, Similar area as in *C*. CEA is localized to the periphery of tumor nests. Based on monoclonal antibody DAKO-CEA, AA5B7.

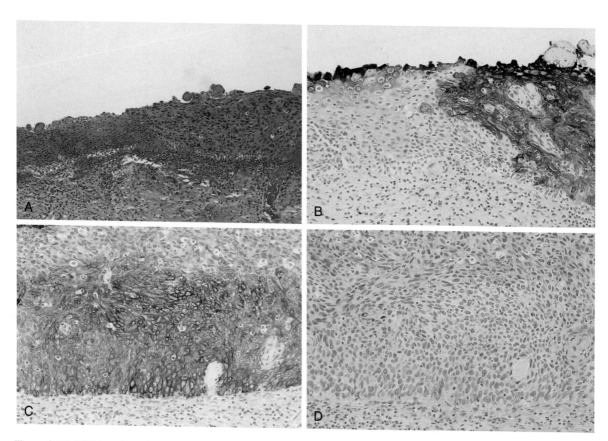

Figure 8–58. CIN 3 and cytokeratin. *A*, CIN 3 (*right*) and adjacent squamous metaplasia. *B*, CK-7 is negative in the squamous metaplasia but positive in CIN 3. *C*, CK-7 is diffusely positive, except in the superficial layers. *D*, CK-20 is negative in CIN 3 and normal squamous mucosa (not shown).

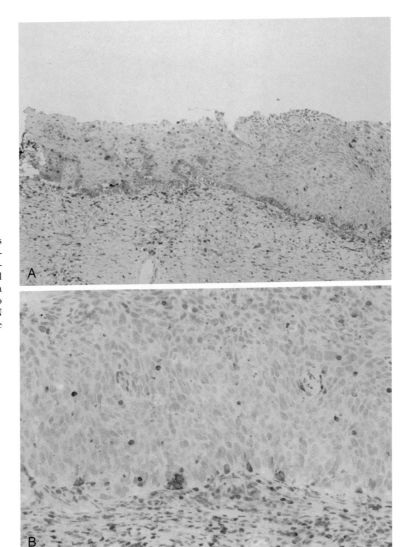

Figure 8–59. Same CIN 3 lesion as shown in Figure 8–58. Immunohistochemical stain for Bcl 2. *A,* Bcl 2–positive cells are located in the basal cell layer of squamous metaplasia and adjacent CIN 3. *B,* There is no overexpression of Bcl 2 in this CIN 3. Bcl 2–positive lymphocytes are seen in the background.

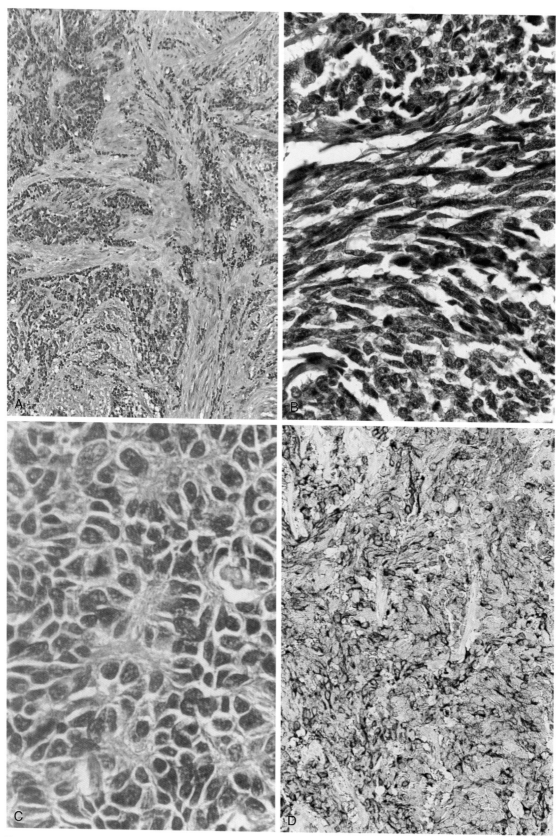

Figure 8–78. Small cell neuroendocrine carcinoma. *A,* Diffuse infiltrative pattern created by cords and nests of tumor cells in a fibrotic stroma. *B,* Small hyperchromatic nuclei are oval or elongated in shape. Cytoplasm is scant. *C,* Some tumor cells have medium-sized oval to irregular hyperchromatic nuclei and compact, coarsely granular chromatin. The nucleoli are absent or small. There is a suggestion of rosette-like arrangement. *D,* Immunohistochemical stain for chromogranin is strongly positive.

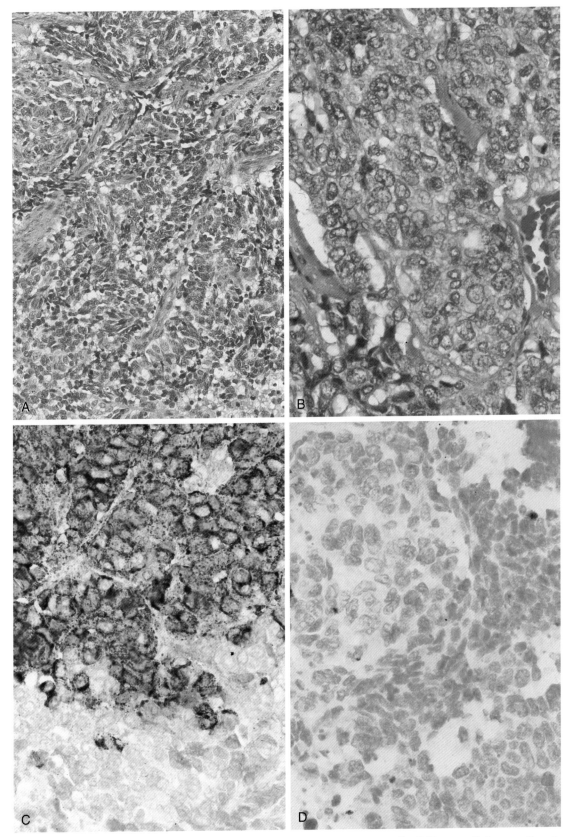

Figure 8–79. Large cell neuroendocrine carcinoma. *A,* Solid sheets of malignant cells. *B,* Tumor cells have medium to large nuclear size, open chromatin, a moderate amount of cytoplasm, and small nucleoli. *C,* Immunohistochemical stain for chromogranin is focally positive. *D,* Immunohistochemical stain for p63 is entirely negative.

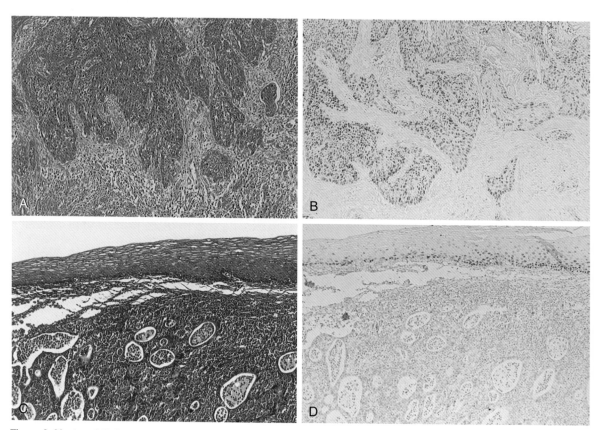

Figure 8–80. *A* and *B,* Squamous cell carcinoma. Most of the tumor cells express p63 by immunohistochemistry (*B*). *C* and *D,* Adenocarcinoma of cervix. Tumor cells are negative for p63 by immunohistochemical stain. In the overlying normal squamous mucosa, p63-positive cells are located in the deepest one to three layers. (Courtesy of Dr. Tao-Yuan Wang, Mackay Memorial Hospital, Taipei, Taiwan).

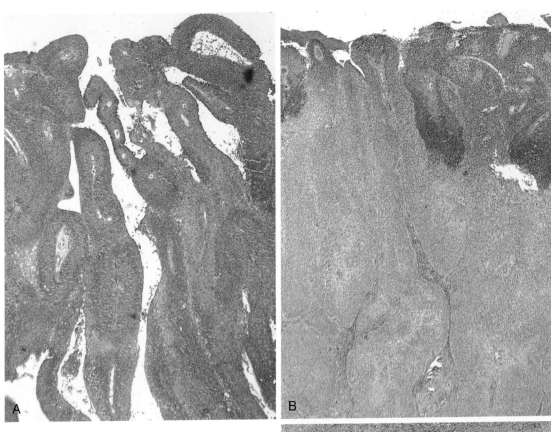

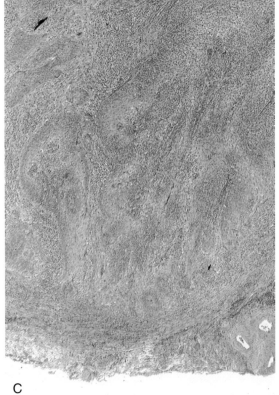

Figure 8–84. Papillary squamotransitional cell carcinoma. *A,* Initial cervical biopsy contains tumor cells in papillary fronds without stromal invasion. *B* and *C,* In the hysterectomy specimen, tumor cells grow by pushing borders and invade deeply into the stroma.

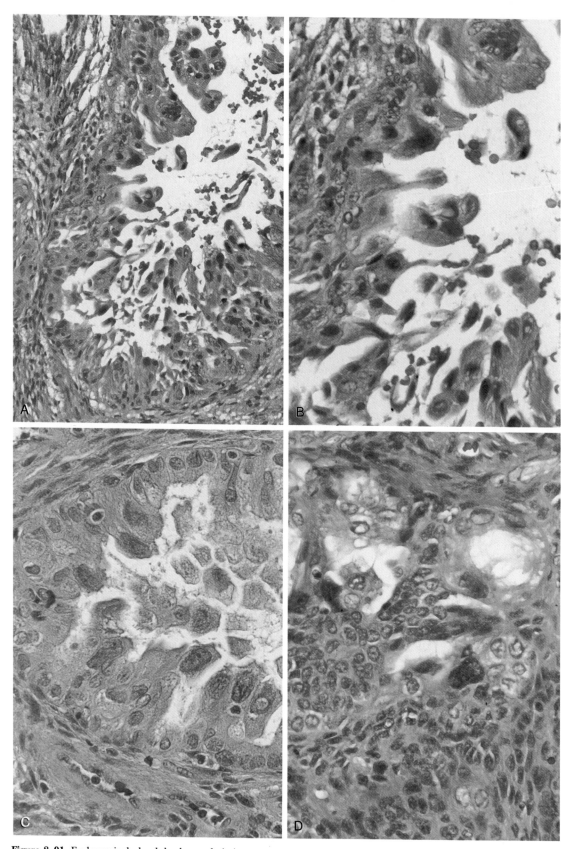

Figure 8–91. Endocervical glandular hyperplasia in a pregnant woman. *A*, Proliferating endocervical cells form papillary projections. *B*, The lining cells reveal nuclear enlargement, hyperchromasia, and irregularity. *C*, Some atypical cells have a hobnail appearance. *D*, Areas of squamous metaplasia and large atypical endocervical cells.

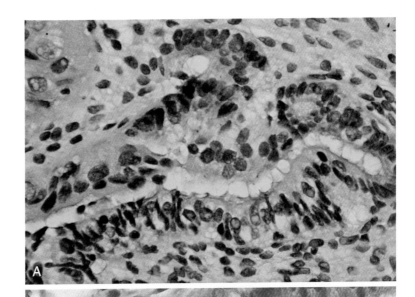

Figure 8–95. Ciliated tubal metaplasia of endocervix. *A,* Ciliated, nonciliated, and intercalated cells line the gland. In addition, there are oxyphilic metaplastic cells (*left*). *B,* A mild degree of nuclear stratification in one to two layers, and nuclear atypia is common. *C,* Squamous metaplasia in ciliated tubal glands.

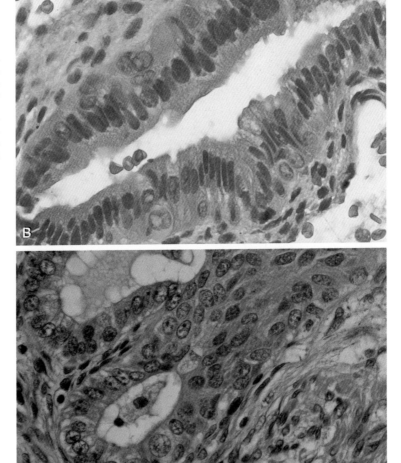

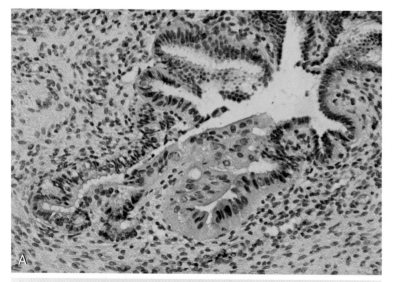

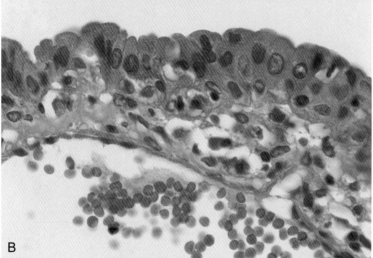

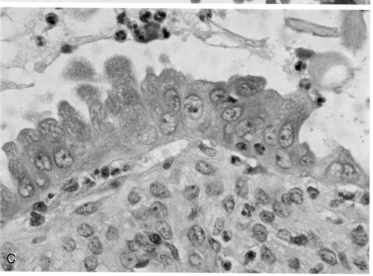

Figure 8–96. *A* and *B*, Oxyphilic cell metaplasia. *C*, Serous cell metaplasia. Serous cells contain abundant eosinophilic cytoplasm and apical cytoplasmic protrusions.

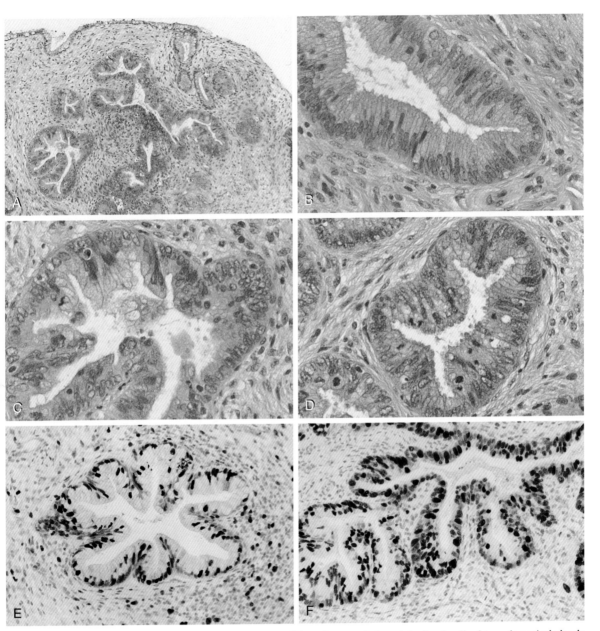

Figure 8–101. Adenocarcinoma in situ, endocervical type. *A* to *F* from the same lesion. *A*, Lesion localized to endocervical glands. *B*, Area of mild nuclear atypia and rare mitotic activity. *C*, Moderate nuclear atypia and increased mitotic activity. *D*, Moderate to severe nuclear atypia and high mitotic activity. *E* and *F*, Immunohistochemical stains for Ki-67 in low-grade atypia (*E*) and high-grade atypia (*F*). Positive cells are abundant in both areas.

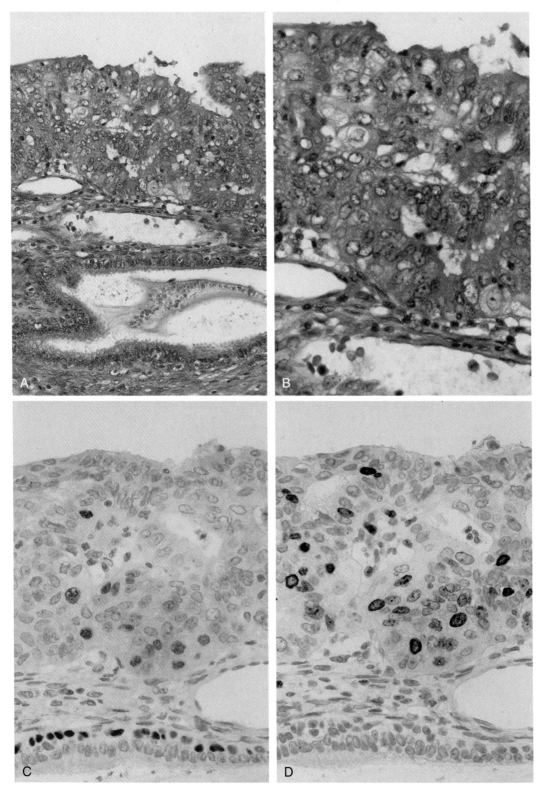

Figure 8–134. Adenosquamous carcinoma in situ. *A* and *B*, This lesion has the appearance of severe glandular dysplasia/adenocarcinoma in situ. However, there are small clusters of cells that have abundant eosinophilic to clear cytoplasm and distinct cell borders to suggest squamous cells. *C*, Immunohistochemical stain for p63 confirms the presence of p63-positive immature squamous cells corresponding to cells with eosinophilic cytoplasm. The normal endocervical gland at the lower field demonstrates the presence of p63-positive subcolumnar reserve cell. Abnormal glandular cells are negative for p63. *D*, Immunohistochemical stain for Ki-67 reveals abundant proliferative glandular and squamous cells.

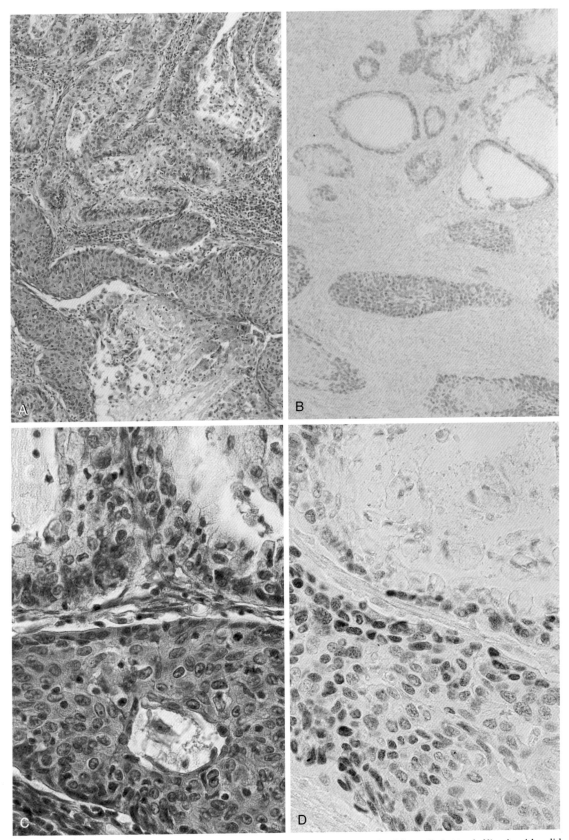

Figure 8–135. Adenosquamous carcinoma, mature type. *A,* Nests of neoplastic glandular cells (*upper half*) mix with solid nests of malignant squamous cells (*lower half*). *B,* Similar area as in *A* demonstrates p63-positive stem/immature squamous cells in the nests of glandular and squamous cells. *C,* Higher magnification demonstrates malignant glandular cells with basophilic to vacuolated mucinous cytoplasm. In contrast, squamous cells have eosinophilic cytoplasm. *D,* Similar area as in *C* reveals expression of p63 in cells beneath the glandular cells and in most of the squamous cells.

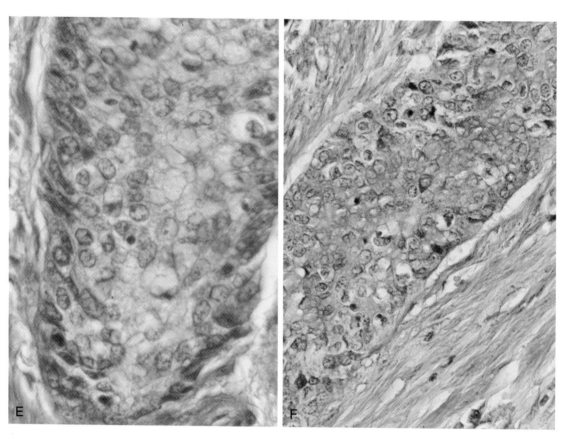

Figure 8–135. *E*, Solid nest with vacuolated tumor cells. *F*, The cytoplasm is positive for mucinous material by mucicarmine stain.

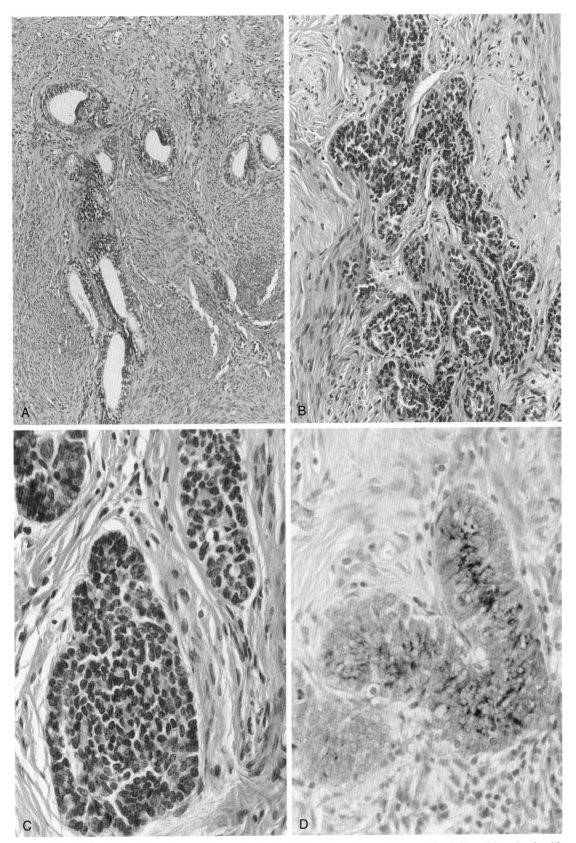

Figure 8–140. Adenoid basal carcinoma. *A,* Neoplastic glands lined by columnar tumor cells. *B,* Branching glands with basaloid cells. *C,* Solid nests of basaloid tumor cells with relatively uniform, round to oval hyperchromatic nuclei and scant cytoplasm. There is palisaded nuclear arrangement in the periphery of the solid nests. *D,* Tumor cells express carcinoembryonic antigen by immunohistochemical stain.

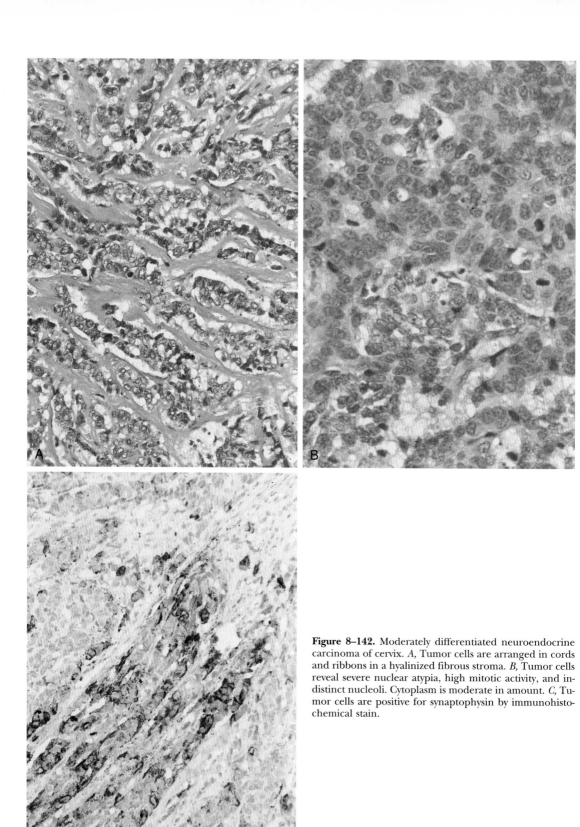

Figure 8–142. Moderately differentiated neuroendocrine carcinoma of cervix. *A,* Tumor cells are arranged in cords and ribbons in a hyalinized fibrous stroma. *B,* Tumor cells reveal severe nuclear atypia, high mitotic activity, and indistinct nucleoli. Cytoplasm is moderate in amount. *C,* Tumor cells are positive for synaptophysin by immunohistochemical stain.

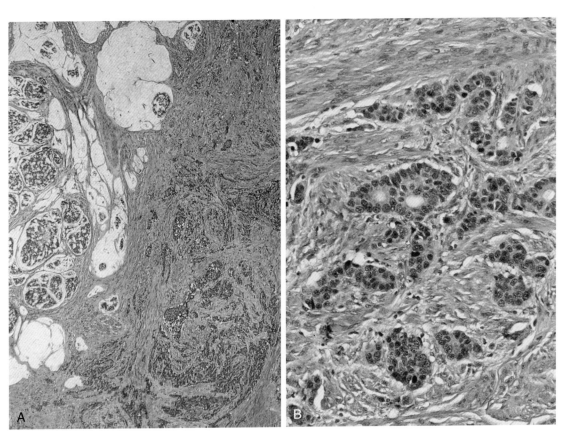

Figure 8–143. Moderately differentiated neuroendocrine carcinoma with coexisting adenocarcinoma. *A,* Low-power view of neuroendocrine carcinoma (*right field*) and mucinous adenocarcinoma (*left field*). *B,* Areas of neuroendocrine carcinoma with tumor cells forming small acini. *C,* Similar area as in *B* illustrates chromogranin-positive tumor cells by immunohistochemical stain. *D,* Areas of adenocarcinoma in situ, intestinal type. *E,* Similar areas as in *D* demonstrate chromogranin-positive cells within the neoplastic glands by immunohistochemical stain. *F,* Mucinous adenocarcinoma associated with mucinous pools. *Illustration continued on following page*

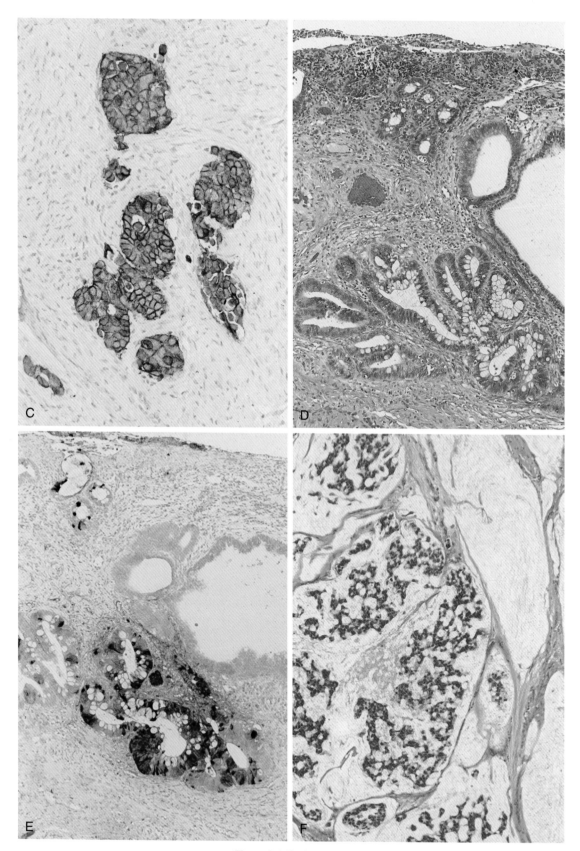

Figure 8–143. *Continued*

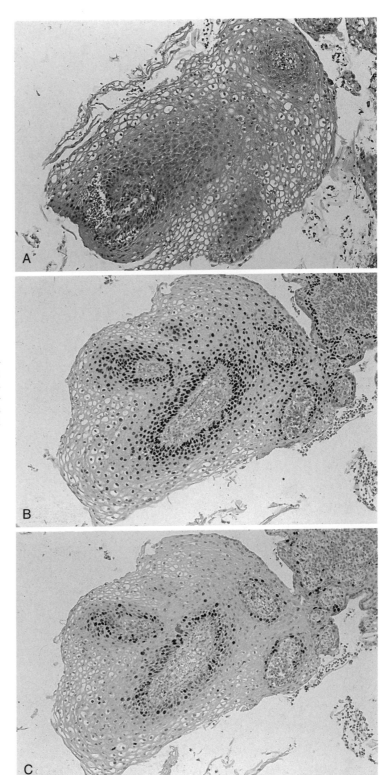

Figure 8–39. *A,* Condyloma acuminatum. *B,* Immunohistochemical stain for p63 showing immature/stem cells in the basal, parabasal, and intermediate cell layers. *C,* Ki-67–positive cells are limited to the basal and parabasal cell layers. (See color section.)

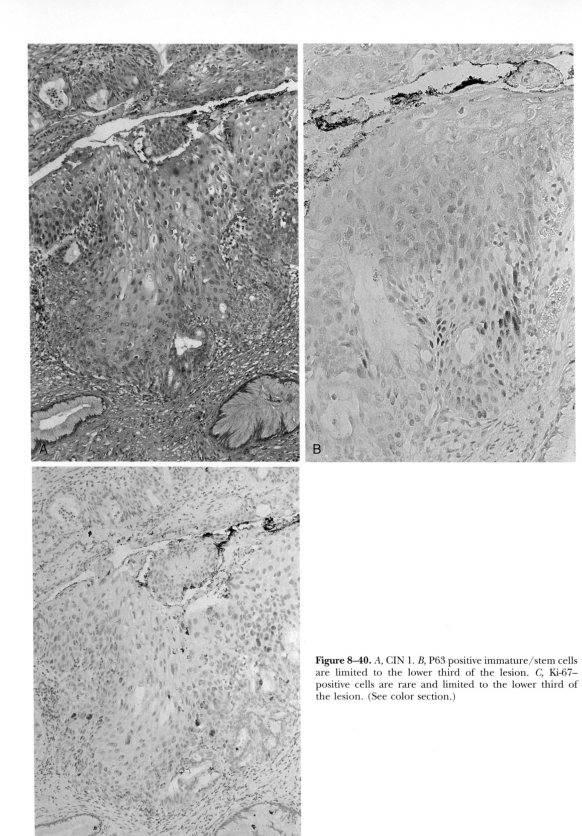

Figure 8–40. *A,* CIN 1. *B,* P63 positive immature/stem cells are limited to the lower third of the lesion. *C,* Ki-67– positive cells are rare and limited to the lower third of the lesion. (See color section.)

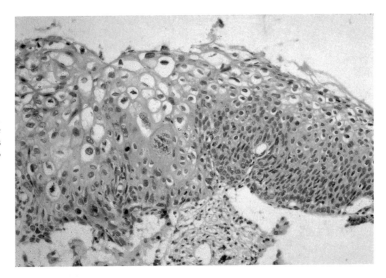

Figure 8–41. Comparison of CIN 1 (*left*) and CIN 2 (*right*). CIN 1 is more mature and less cellular and shows less nuclear atypia when compared zone to zone to CIN 2.

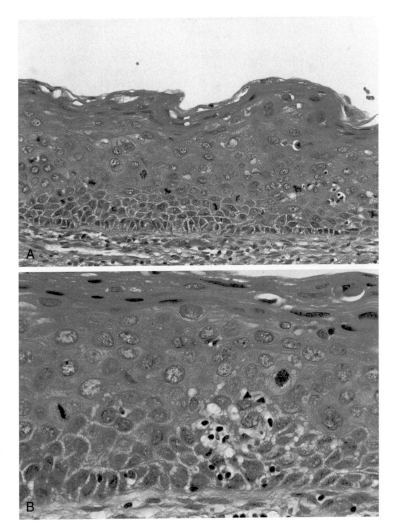

Figure 8–42. CIN 2. *A* and *B*, Although the upper half of the lesion comprises mature squamous cells, the mitotic activity and immature cells reach to the middle third of epithelium. The basal cell layer is partially replaced by dysplastic cells (*B*).

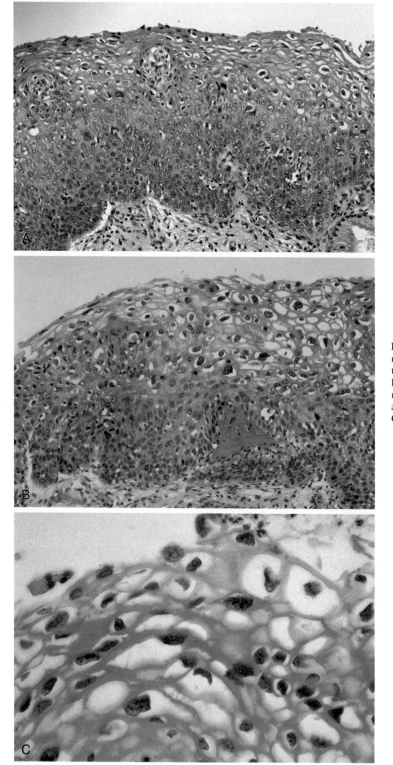

Figure 8–43. CIN 2. *A, B,* and *C,* Immature cells occupy the lower half of the lesion. Koilocytes in the upper half demonstrate a higher degree of nuclear irregularity, hyperchromasia, and enlargement than that seen in CIN 1 (see Fig. 8–35).

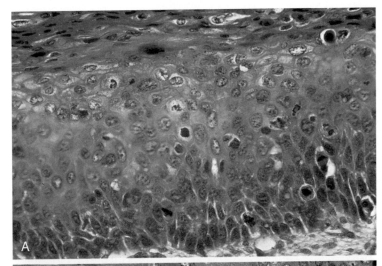

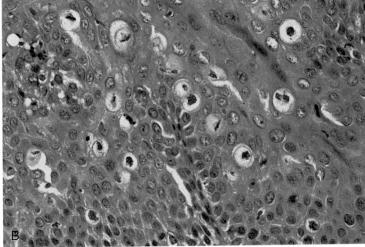

Figure 8–44. *A,* Moderate dysplasia, with immature cells proliferating in the lower half of the epithelium and abnormal keratinization on the surface. *B,* Abnormal mitotic figures occur in clusters; some are two-group metaphase.

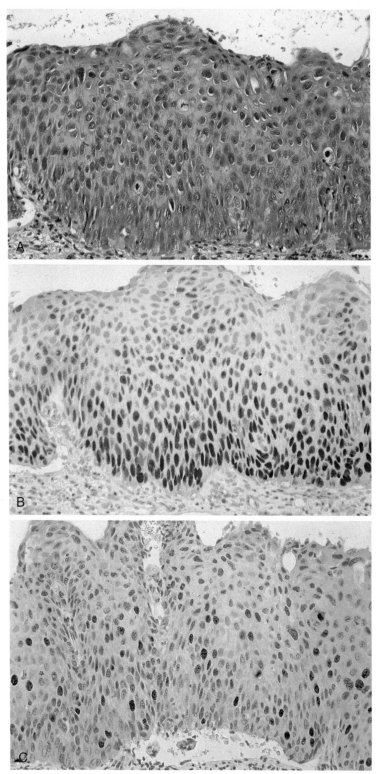

Figure 8–45. CIN 2–3. *A*, Immature cells in vertical orientation reach to the upper third in part of the lesion to support CIN 3. Atypical parakeratosis and koilocytosis occur in the superficial layers. *B*, Some p63-positive immature/stem cells occupy up to the upper third of the epithelium. *C*, Scattered Ki-67–positive cells occur mainly in the lower two thirds of the lesion. (See color section.)

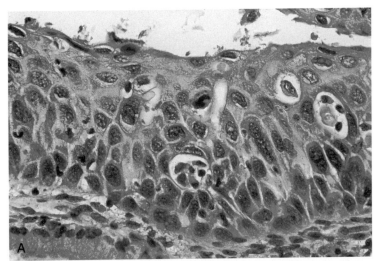

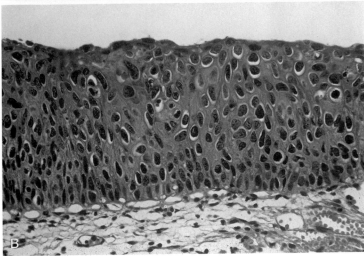

Figure 8–46. CIN 3. *A* and *B,* The entire lesion is made up of bizarre pleomorphic cells of varying sizes and shapes.

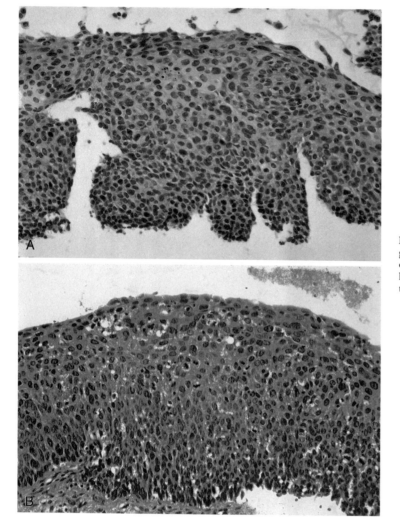

Figure 8–47. CIN 3. *A* and *B*, Homogeneous population of immature cells occupies the entire thickness of the lesion. *B*, This lesion is also referred to as metaplastic type.

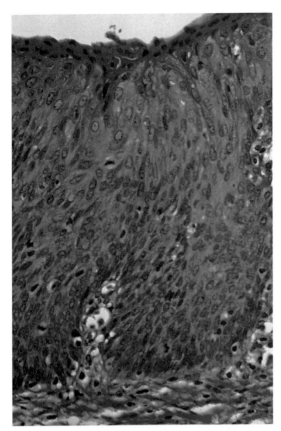

Figure 8–48. CIN 3 is made up of immature elongated cells arranged vertically throughout the lesion.

granular chromatin. The cytoplasm is scant to moderate in amount, and cell borders are ill defined. Nucleoli are rarely identified.

CINs have also been classified according to the cell type as keratinizing, nonkeratinizing, and metaplastic. On the basis of nuclear size, CINs are classified as large cell, intermediate cell, and small cell (Fig. 8–49).[271,287,288] These classifications provide useful correlation with cytologic features.

In rare CIN, transitional-like cells with nuclear grooves may predominate the lesion to simulate transitional cell metaplasia (TCM). TCM is most commonly detected in the cervix and vagina of postmenopausal women, usually as an incidental finding in hysterectomy specimens for benign conditions. On low-power view, TCM is characterized by a thick epithelium of usually more than 10 cell layers. The component cells appear immature and monotonous. In the upper layers, they become parallel to the surface. The nuclei are uniformly small, hyperchromatic, and round to oval or elongated. The chromatin is finely granular. Nuclear grooves are evident in most of the cells. Mitotic activity is absent. Some cells may have perinuclear halos and clear cytoplasm.[96] Of all the immunohistochemical stains, Ki-67 antigen is most useful. Very rare Ki-6–positive cells are seen in TCM (Fig. 8–50A, B).

In a series of 63 TCM lesions, two were described as having mild to moderate atypia with binucleation, increased nuclear to cytoplasmic ratios, and mitotic activity.[372a] In CIN with predominantly transitional-like cells, the cells reveal nuclear enlargement, irregularity, and hyperchromasia. Mitotic figures, although rare, are present. With immunohistochemical stain for Ki-67 antigen, positive cells are readily seen (see Fig. 8–50).

Mitotic abnormalities are determined by the number, the location, and the type of mitotic figures. In CIN 1, the mitotic figures are few in number, confined to the lower third of the epithelium, and normal in appearance. With increasing severity of CIN, the mitotic figures increase in number and extend to the middle third and upper third. Mitotic figures tend to occur in clusters. The abnormal forms also occur more frequently. Most of them have the appearance of abnormal metaphase with two or three uneven groups of chromosomes (Fig. 8–51). Occasionally, the mitotic figures resemble the dispersed chromosomes seen after podophyllin treatment. Other less common forms include V-shaped metaphase, ring mitosis, multipolar mitosis, giant mitosis, and other bizarre forms (see Figs. 8–50 and 8–51).

Correlations of DNA ploidy patterns and mitotic figures in punch biopsies demonstrate that 85% of CINs with aneuploid patterns contain abnormal mitoses.[117,119] Dispersed metaphase and tripolar mitoses have rarely been observed in diploid and polyploid lesions.[381] Thus, the presence of abnormal mitotic figures suggests that the lesion is likely to be aneuploid.

The morphologic differences in HPV types 6/11 and 16/18/33 were demonstrated by objective morphometric analysis. The latter had a higher proliferative activity, higher cellularity, high mitotic activity, and abnormal mitotic figures.[112] Type 6/11 lesions may occasionally contain tripolar mitosis or dispersed chromosomes. Other forms of abnormal mitoses are found mainly in lesions associated with type 16/18/33.[112]

In a study by Bergeron et al.,[35] abnormal mitotic figures were found in 16% of lower geni-

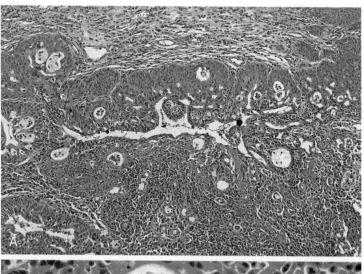

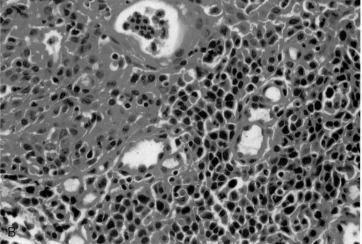

Figure 8–49. CIN 3, small cell type. *A,* Small cells permeate through the immature squamous metaplasia. *B,* Small immature cells have scant cytoplasm and hyperchromatic nuclei. The nuclear size is similar to that of the adjacent immature metaplastic squamous cells.

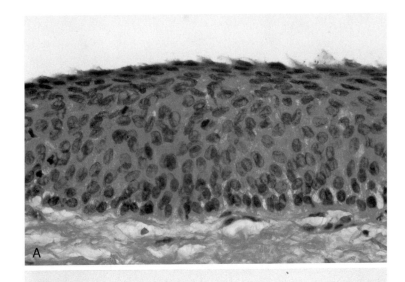

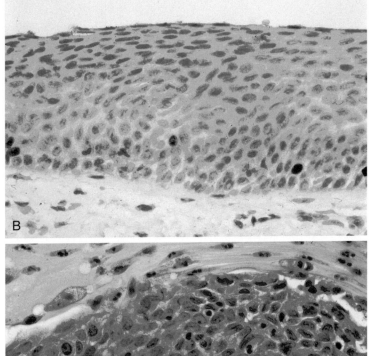

Figure 8–50. *A* and *B*, Transitional cell metaplasia. *A*, Monotonous population of transitional-like cells with nuclear grooves. Cells in the superficial layers maintain parallel arrangement. No mitotic activity is seen. *B*, Immunohistochemical stain for Ki-67 reveals very rare positive cells in the parabasal layers. *C* to *F*, High-grade CIN with transitional-like cells. *C*, Abnormal cells are arranged vertically. Cellular disorganization is seen in the superficial layers. Mitotic activity is present. (See color section.)
Illustration continued on following page

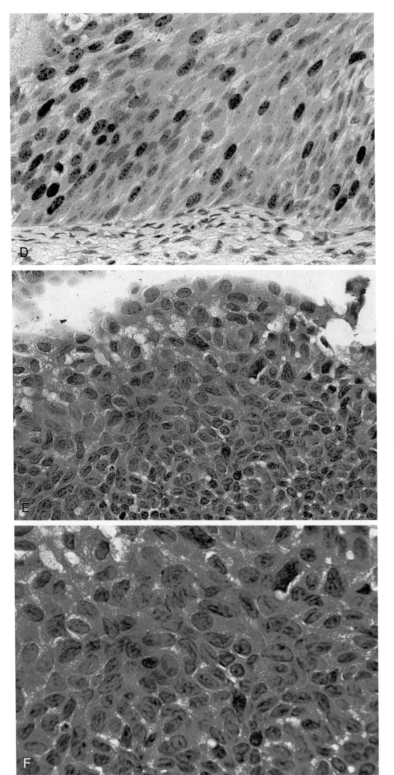

Figure 8–50. *Continued D,* Similar area as in *C.* Immunohistochemical stain for Ki-67 reveals scattered positive cells, even though mitotic figures are rare to absent. *E* and *F,* Higher magnification reveals nuclear grooves and nuclear irregularity in the upper half of the epithelium. (See color section.)

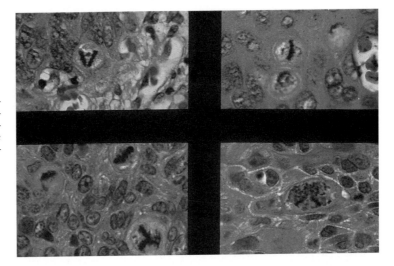

Figure 8–51. Different types of abnormal mitotic figures. V-shape metaphase (*upper left*); three-group metaphase (*upper right*); normal metaphase and multipolar mitosis (*lower left*); giant mitosis (*lower right*).

tal squamous dysplasias associated with type 6/11, in 87% of type 16 lesions, and in 75% of changes with mixed infection. These qualitative and quantitative differences support a higher oncogenic potential for type 16/18/33 than for type 6/11.[112]

Mittal et al.[245] studied cervical condylomas and low-grade dysplasias with different types of HPV. Their study included eight condylomas with HPV 6/11, eight with HPV 31/33/35, and nine with HPV 16/18. The HPV typing was determined with the use of biotinylated probes. Proliferative cell fraction was based on staining with antibody MIB-1. One of the most distinct findings was the more frequent MIB-1 staining of basal cells in association with HPV type 16 than with other types (35 ± 19.3% versus 18 ± 8.3%, $P = 0.013$). There was no difference in the number of proliferative cells in the parabasal layers of different HPV types. The mitotic index for HPV 6/11 was 6.5 ± 4.6%, as compared with 7.9 ± 6.8% for other HPV types ($P = 0.6$). Abnormal mitotic figures were high in lesions with HPV 16/18/31/33/35. The mitotic index was 1.7 ± 1.6% versus 0.5 ± 1.4% for condylomas with HPV 6/11 ($P = 0.049$). One of eight HPV 6/11 lesions contained abnormal mitotic figures, as compared with 12/17 associated with other HPV types ($P = 0.02$). Thus, in diagnosing low-grade CIN, the presence of abnormal mitotic figures is likely to indicate high-risk HPV lesions.

By immunohistochemical stains, p63-positive immature cells occupy the entire thickness of CIN 3 lesion. In addition, many Ki-67–positive cells occur throughout the lesion (Fig. 8–52).

Some rare CINs are made up of largely abundant clear vacuolated cytoplasm. These clear cells contain abundant glycogen with PAS stain (Fig. 8–53). No mucinous material is seen by mucicarmine stain. Such clear cells may be seen in rare papillary squamotransitional cell carcinomas.[191] High-grade CIN with mucin-positive cells is classified as adenosquamous carcinoma in situ, which is discussed in the section on adenosquamous carcinoma. Rare CIN may also contain cells that are positive for neuroendocrine markers, such as chromogranin and synaptophysin (Fig. 8–54).

Cervical squamous carcinomas that spread into the endometrium and fallopian tube are usually invasive carcinoma and verrucous carcinoma and rarely in situ carcinoma (Fig. 8–55). These carcinomas cover the mucosa of the upper genital tract without stromal invasion. Pins et al.[276] reported an unusual case of a 55-year-old woman who had squamous cell carcinoma in situ of the cervix that spread diffusely into the endometrium, fallopian tube, and ovaries. In the tubes and ovaries, the tumor cells become invasive. HPV DNA type 16 was demonstrated in the tumor cells by PCR technique.[276]

Differential Diagnosis

Based on the criteria described in the foregoing section, the distinction between atypical, reactive changes and CIN can be made in the majority of cases. Essentially, CIN lesion must meet the minimal degree of nuclear atypia for koilocytes and mild dysplasia. Any lesion without suf-

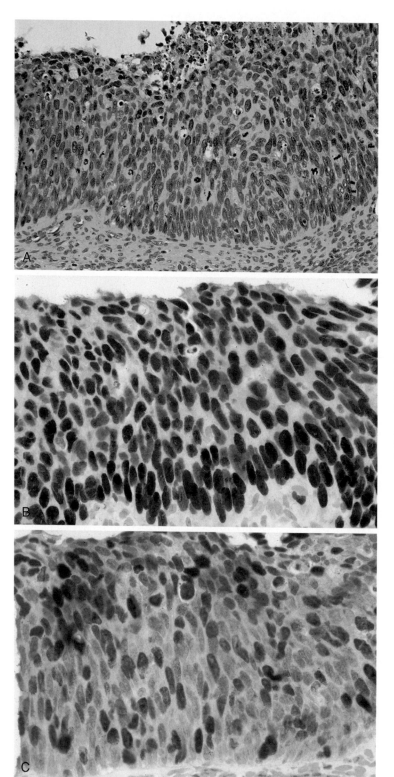

Figure 8–52. CIN 3. *A*, The entire lesion comprises vertically arranged dysplastic cells with scattered mitotic figures. *B*, P63-positive immature/stem cells occupy the entire epithelium. *C*, Ki-67–positive cells scatter over the entire epithelium, indicative of highly disordered cellular proliferation. (See color section.)

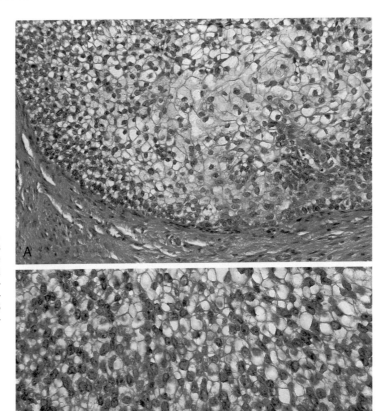

Figure 8–53. CIN 3, clear cell variant. *A* and *B,* Most of the abnormal cells contain clear cytoplasm. Some have eosinophilic cytoplasm and distinct cell borders, indicative of squamous differentiation (*A*). Clear cytoplasm corresponds to abundant glycogen by PAS stains, and is negative for mucin by mucicarmine stain.

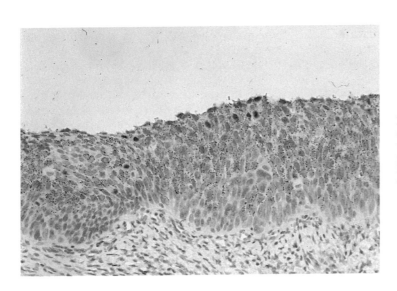

Figure 8–54. CIN 3 with neuroendocrine differentiation. Immunohistochemical stain for chromogranin is positive in the majority of cells. Same lesion as shown in Figure 8–52. (See color section.)

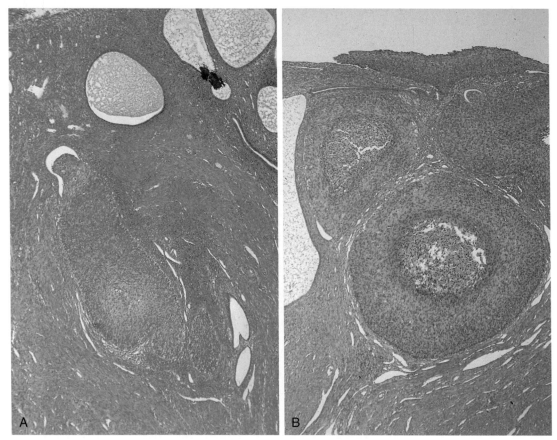

Figure 8–55. *A* and *B*, CIN 3 extends directly onto the endometrial surface and glands. (See color section.)

ficient nuclear atypia is placed in the nondiagnostic squamous atypia category. HPV testing of cervicovaginal cells is reported by some as useful. If HPV DNA is negative by hybrid capture II assay, the chance of the patient having CIN is very small.[333] If the assay results are positive, more than 30% of women have no colposcopically and pathologically identifiable CIN lesion.[333] Studies by specialized technique may be helpful.

Studies with the Use of Special Techniques

Tumor Markers

Several tumor markers have been studied in an effort to improve diagnostic and prognostic accuracy. Carcinoembryonic antigen (CEA) is one of the most extensively tested tumor markers. Using immunoperoxidase technique, CEA was detected in 25% of mild dysplasias, 37% of severe dysplasias, and 60% of CIS lesions (Fig. 8–56).[212] However, the presence or absence of

CEA was not useful in distinguishing between immature squamous metaplasia and CIN, because 60% of control samples with squamous metaplasia were positive.[24] Epithelial membrane antigen, although frequently positive in CIN and invasive carcinoma, was positive in 19% of benign samples with cervicitis and squamous metaplasia.[24]

The localization of CEA may aid in differentiating CIN from invasive squamous neoplasm. In the former, CEA was found in the superficial layers or in the entire thickness of the epithelium, whereas in invasive carcinoma CEA was located at the periphery of invasive nests (Fig. 8–57).[64]

In a more recent study, by Tendler et al.,[350] CEA was determined by immunohistochemical stain using monoclonal antibody COL-1. The percentage of moderate immunoreactivity or higher for CEA is 0% in the normal cervix, 0% in CIN 1, 11.1% in CIN 2, 58.3% in CIN 3, 90% in invasive squamous cell carcinomas, and 14.3% in cervical adenocarcinomas. The au-

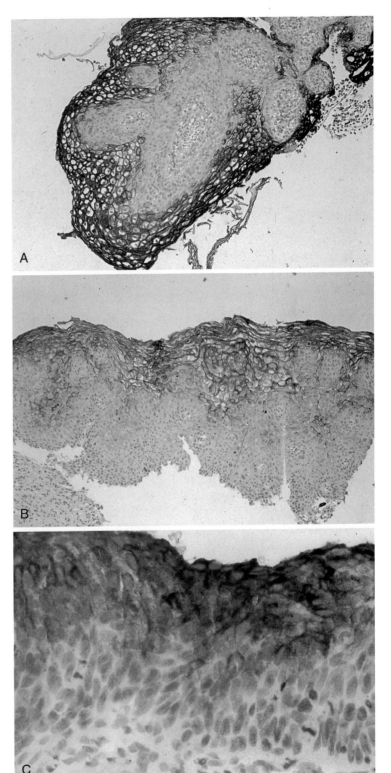

Figure 8–56. Carcinoembryonic antigen in the upper layers of condyloma (*A*), CIN 2 (*B*), and CIN 3 (*C*). Based on monoclonal antibody DAKO-CEA, AA5B7. (See color section.)

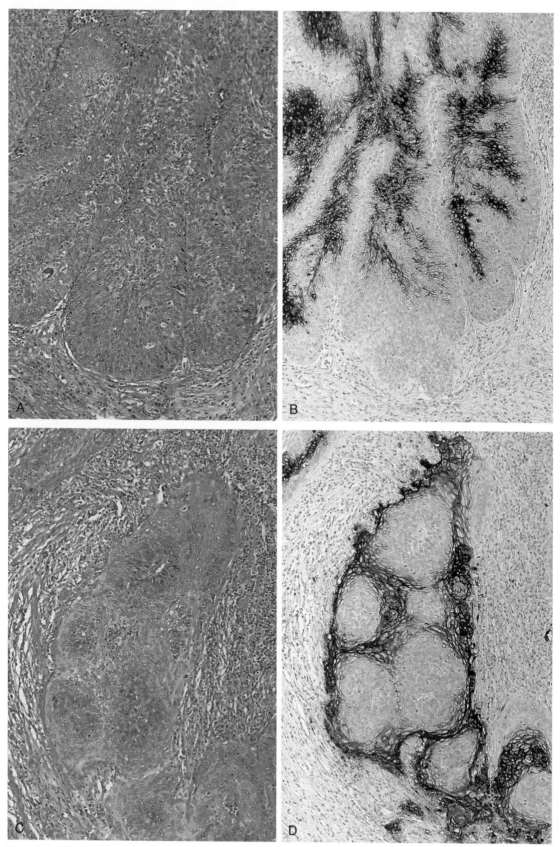

Figure 8–57. Comparison of CEA localization in CIN 3 and underlying invasive squamous carcinoma. *A,* CIN 3. *B,* Similar area as in *A.* CEA occurs in the upper half of epithelium. *C,* Underlying invasive squamous carcinoma. *D,* Similar area as in *C.* CEA is localized to the periphery of tumor nests. Based on monoclonal antibody DAKO-CEA, AA5B7. (See color section.)

thors conclude that CEA expression may be a useful diagnostic tool and marker of progressive CIN.[350]

Intermediate Filaments

Staining for intermediate filaments, such as different molecular weights (MW) of cytokeratin, may be useful in the grading of CIN. Normal ectocervical squamous cells express CK 4 (MW 59 KD), CK 6 (MW 56 KD), CK 13 (MW 53–54 KD), and CK 14 (MW 50 KD). In CIN 1 and CIN 2, the majority of abnormal cells are positive for CK 4 (MW 59 KD), CK 5 (MW 58 KD), CK 13 (MW 53–54 KD), CK 14 (MW 50 KD), and CK 19 (MW 40 KD). In CIN 3, the component cells express CK 4 (MW 59 KD), CK 5 (MW 58 KD), CK 13 (MW 53–54 KD), CK 14 (MW 50 KD), CK 17 (MW 46 KD), CK 18 (MW

45 KD), and CK 19 (MW 40 KD).[331] In the majority of high-grade CIN and invasive squamous cell carcinoma, the component cells are positive for CK 7 (MW 54 KD) and negative for CK 20 (MW 46 KD) (Fig. 8–58).

In a study by Smedts et al.,[331] CK 17 was detected in only a small number of CIN 1 and CIN 2 lesions but was found in 50% of CIN 3 lesions and in almost all invasive squamous cell carcinomas. The authors suggest that CIN lesions expressing CK 17 are progressive.[331]

Proliferative Cell and Cell Cycle Markers

A study by Mittal et al.[243] included 20 samples of normal ectocervix, 11 of metaplastic squamous epithelium, five of condylomas, three of mild dysplasias, three of moderate dysplasias, nine of severe dysplasias, and six of atrophic

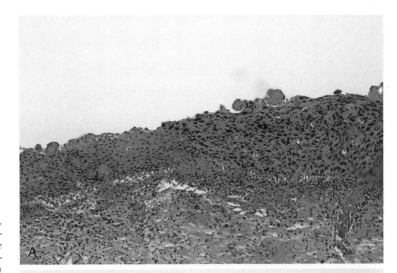

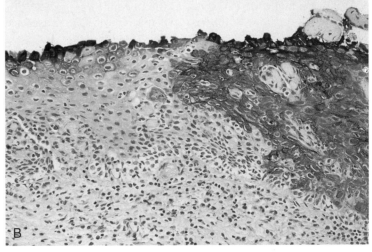

Figure 8–58. CIN 3 and cytokeratin. *A,* CIN 3 (*right*) and adjacent squamous metaplasia. *B,* CK-7 is negative in the squamous metaplasia but positive in CIN 3. (See color section.) *Illustration continued on following page*

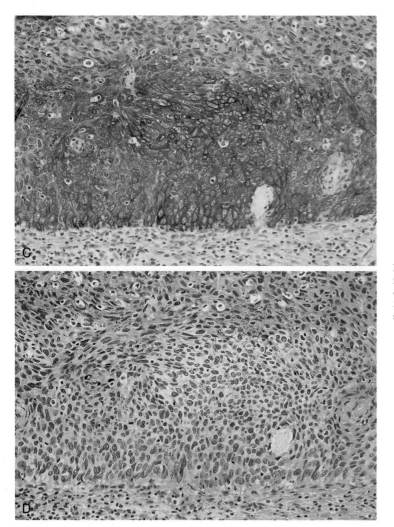

Figure 8–58. *Continued C,* CK-7 is diffusely positive, except in the superficial layers. *D,* CK-20 is negative in CIN 3 and normal squamous mucosa (not shown). (See color section.)

changes. Immunohistochemical stain was performed for proliferating cell nuclear antigen (PCNA). As might be expected, in the normal ectocervical squamous mucosa positive cells were found only in the parabasal layers and ever fewer cells in the basal cell layer. In the atrophic mucosa, only one of six samples stained cells in the lower third of the epithelium. In the squamous metaplasia, the staining was usually confined to the lower third but sometimes extended to the middle third.[243]

In a subsequent study, antibody MIB-1 was used to compare cervical condyloma, squamous metaplasia, and cervicitis. The mean mitotic activity was 7.6 in cervical condyloma, 1.4 in squamous metaplasia, 1.6 in cervicitis, and 1.5 in normal ectocervix per 10 high-power fields. MIB-1–positive cells were also more likely to occur in the basal cells of condyloma than in

squamous metaplasia, cervicitis, and normal ectocervix.[244]

In CIN, the number of PCNA-positive cells increased with severity of the lesion.[243] By using antibody MIB-1, there was also a progressive increase of Ki-67–positive cells from normal to CIN-1, CIN-2, and CIN-3. In the case of CIN-3, the labeled cells were scattered throughout the epithelium. A similar distribution is seen in invasive squamous cell carcinoma.[230,281]

In another study, Ki-67–positive cells were found in the upper two thirds of 71.4% of low-grade SIL lesions and in 94.7% of high-grade SILs. This immunoreactivity was found in 7.7% (2 of 29) of squamous metaplasias ($P < 0.001$).[184a] Ki-67 was found to be particularly useful in differentiating atrophy from SIL. In atrophy, Ki-67 is entirely absent.[184a]

Cho et al.[69] investigated normal cervix, CIN, squamous cell carcinoma, and adenocarcinoma for cyclin D1 and cyclin E. In addition, PCR technique was used to detect HPV DNA. Cyclin D1 was detected in the normal basal and parabasal cells but was decreased in CIN and squamous cell carcinoma. In contrast, cyclin E was absent in the normal ectocervical squamous cells but increased in CIN and squamous cell carcinoma. The expression of cyclin E was significantly higher in HPV-positive lesions. These findings suggest that cyclin E is responsible for the neoplastic transformation, whereas cyclin D1 is decreased when HPV infection is present.[69] This observation is supported by Quade et al.,[281] who found a moderate or strong immunohistochemical expression of cyclin E in 5% of nondiagnostic squamous atypia, 92.3% of low-grade SIL, 51.6% of high-grade SIL, and 50% of invasive squamous cell carcinomas.[281]

Cyclin E was most frequently seen in the intermediate layers and koilocytes of CIN. Superficial squamous cells were occasionally positive.[281] Binding of high-risk HPV E7 with retinoblastoma gene product is believed to decrease E2 transcription factor, to increase cyclin E gene, or to decrease degradation of cyclin E to result in cellular proliferation. In the initial study, the index of cyclin E expression was higher in low-grade SIL than in high-grade SIL. In a subsequent report from the same investigators, this difference was less apparent, perhaps because different antibodies were used in the two studies.[184a] Both studies confirm that cyclin E expression is a marker of HPV-related lesions.[184a,281]

P16[INK4,] also known as CDK inhibitor 2 (CDKN2), antagonizes the functions of CDK 4 and CDK 6, which are activated by binding with cyclin D1. Interestingly, p16 is upregulated in HPV-related lesions. Immunohistochemical stains for cyclin E and p16 demonstrate moderate or strong immunoreactivity in nearly 90% of low-grade and high-grade SILs, with a positive predictive value of 88.7%.[184a] The authors conclude that these stains are particularly useful in separating SIL from reactive changes.[184a]

Apoptosis Markers and Oncogenes

The BCL-2 gene was initially identified in human follicular lymphoma and later in the immature and stem cells of adult tissues. Its property is believed to extend cell survival. In the immunohistochemical stain, BCL-2 is localized in the basal cell layer of normal ectocervical squamous mucosa and squamous metaplasia, supporting the concept that stem cells in the basal cell layer maintain proliferative capability with a prolonged life span through the inhibition of programmed cell death.[77]

In the cervical reserve cell hyperplasia, about 1% to 20% of cells expressed Ki-67, whereas almost all the reserve cells contained BCL-2. In immature squamous metaplasia, about 5% of cells were positive for Ki-67, whereas the number of cells containing BCL-2 was variable. In CINs and invasive squamous cell carcinomas, cells expressing both Ki-67 and BCL-2 were reported to increase with severity by some authors.[146,147,305] These authors also suggest that CIN with overexpression of both Ki-67 and BCL-2 is likely to progress.[146,147]

On the other hand, Cooper et al.,[77] found no difference in BCL-2 expression between low-grade and high-grade CIN lesions. In addition, there was no difference in the BCL-2 expression with or without HPV DNA. These authors concluded that BCL-2 does not play a major role in CIN lesions.[77]

In this author's opinion, BCL-2 in CIN lesions is variable and unpredictable from lesion to lesion and from area to area (Fig. 8–59).

Kurvinen et al.[200] found that progression of HPV-positive CIN was associated with a low percentage of p53-positive cells and BCL-2 overexpression in the upper layers of CIN. However, overexpression of BCL-2 alone was not predictive of the clinical outcome of HPV lesions.[200]

Overexpression of BCL-2 implies that cells of CIN lesions are protected from programmed cell death, thus maintaining the ability for continuous proliferation. BCL-2 overexpression may induce genetic instability.

Dellas et al.[93] investigated the relationship of Ki-67 by antibody MIB-1, BCL-2, and C-myc in CIN. There was a gradual increase in the number of Ki-67 and C-myc from normal to low-grade CIN and to high-grade CIN. In low-grade CIN, the number of BCL-2–labeled cells was found to correlate with HPV status. There also was a higher labeling of BCL-2 in the absence of HPV DNA than in HPV positive lesions. The highest labeling of BCL-2 was found in high-grade CIN. Similarly, C-myc expression is associated with high-grade CIN and high-risk HPV types. Based on these stains, the authors found correlation between C-myc and BCL-2 overexpression.[93]

Ras genes are involved in the normal cell receptor signal transduction pathways. Golijow et

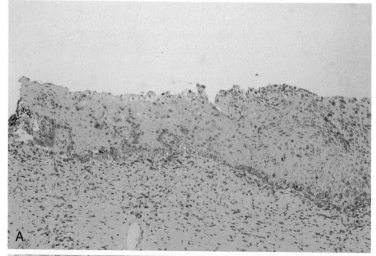

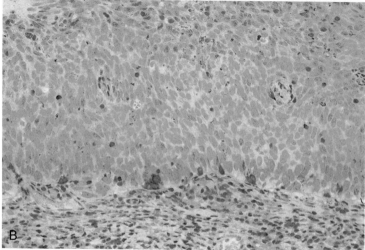

Figure 8–59. Same CIN 3 lesion as shown in Figure 8–58. Immunohistochemical stain for Bcl 2. *A,* Bcl 2–positive cells are located in the basal cell layer of squamous metaplasia and adjacent CIN 3. *B,* There is no overexpression of Bcl 2 in this CIN 3. Bcl 2–positive lymphocytes are seen in the background. (See color section.)

al.[132] studied 155 cytologic samples for HPV DNA and K-ras codon 12 mutation by PCR. K-ras codon 12 mutation was detected in 15% (8 of 53) of HPV 16–positive lesions, 23% (8 of 38) of HPV 18–related lesions, and 1.6% (1/64) of HPV 6–positive lesions ($P < 0.01$). The authors suggest that Ras mutation occurred after HPV E6 and E7 binding to p53 and retinoblastoma gene protein.[132]

Wisman et al.[382] analyzed telomerase in the normal cervix, in CIN, and in invasive cervical carcinoma by in situ hybridization technique. Human telomerase RNA was not identified in the normal cervix but was found in 7% (1 of 14) of CIN 1 lesions, 54% (15 of 28) of CIN 2, 70% (21 of 30) of CIN 3, and 89% (16 of 18) of invasive carcinomas. Increased telomerase

activity was also correlated with the presence of HPV types 16 and 18.[382]

Immune Response

The number of Langerhans' cells in CIN was quantified by S100 protein–positive cells by immunohistochemistry. The mean number of Langerhans' cells in the normal cervical squamous mucosa was 16.7 per mm, as compared with 8.6 cells per mm in low-grade CIN, and 6.0 cells per mm in high-grade CIN ($P = 0.04$).[76] In the HPV-positive CIN, the mean number of Langerhans' cells was 5.9 per mm. In the HPV negative CIN, it was increased to 12.9 cells per mm. It is interesting to note that in the presence of acute inflammation, Langerhans' cells were even higher, up to 15.9 ± 3.5 cells per mm versus 6.9 ± 1.4 cells per mm, in the absence of acute cervicitis. The authors concluded that HPV has an immunosuppressive effect.[76]

Majeed et al.[220] used PCR to analyze interleukin-1beta (IL-1beta) +5887 C to E mutation in 147 CIN lesions of varying grades. Eighty low-grade CINs demonstrated a high frequency of IL-1beta phenotype. This was higher than in CIN 2 or CIN 3 ($P = 0.039$) lesions. These findings suggest a host immune reaction, perhaps through the production of interleukin-2 lymphocytes and interferon. It is also possible that cytolytic T lymphocytes, natural killer cells, and monocytes are stimulated to result in host immune response.[220]

Angiogenesis

In a study by Davidson et al.,[89] immunohistochemical stains were used to assess the number of blood vessels in the subepithelial stroma of normal cervix, CIN, and invasive carcinoma. The normal cervix contained about six blood vessels per 10 high-power fields ($\times 400$), whereas in CIN and invasive carcinoma the average number of blood vessels was in the range of 15. Most of the vascular spaces were blood vessels, and not lymphatics. There was no correlation between the number of blood vessel counts and the types of HPV.

Ultrastructure

The ultrastructural features of CIN correspond closely to the cellular maturation and metabolic activity. Tonofilaments are abundant in mature squamous cells and low-grade CIN. Golgi complexes, rough endoplasmic reticulum, and glycogen particles appear occasionally. The desmosomal junctions, although fewer than normal cells at the comparable level, are readily identified. With increasing immaturity of cells, most of the cytoplasmic organelles are scanty, except for free ribosomes, which are abundant. The cell membranes demonstrate numerous microvillous projections, which are wavy and lack the compact microfilaments seen in the microvilli of glandular cells. Pseudopodia and hemidesmosomes on the basal cell membrane, as well as desmosomal junctions, are markedly diminished.[99,206] These abnormalities contributed to a decrease in mutual cohesiveness and contact inhibition. With the use of scanning electron microscopy, the micro ridges normally seen on the surface of superficial cells

are replaced by microvillous processes. This phenomenon further diminishes the horizontal stability of the cells.

The nuclear abnormalities are demonstrated by irregular configuration, coarse chromatin aggregates, and thickened chromatinic membrane. In some CIS, the basal lamina is reported to be absent focally. Whether this represents an incipient invasion remains to be confirmed.

In frankly invasive squamous cells, the number of tonofilaments and desmosomes is closely related to the degree of differentiation. In general, the desmosomes are fewer in number, poorly developed, or defective. Basal lamina appears only focally.

Factors Related to the Outcome of CIN

In the past 4 decades, many investigators have attempted to determine the natural history of cervical dysplasia and CIS. Women with CIN were followed by cytology alone or with biopsy without treatment for certain periods of time. Many studies had inherent limitations, such as including women with biopsy, which may alter the outcome by removing a small lesion. The length of follow-up is another limiting factor. Despite these drawbacks, Ostor[261] provided a comprehensive review of the literature to demonstrate a general trend for the regression, persistence, and progression in relation to severity of CIN (Table 8–1).

Among women with CIN 1, the lesion regressed in 57%, persisted in 32%, progressed to CIN 3 in 11%, and progressed to invasive carcinoma in less than 1%. Among women with CIN 2, lesions regressed in 43%, persisted in 35%, progressed to CIN 3 in 22%, and progressed to invasive carcinoma in 5%. CIN 3 lesions regressed in 32%, persisted in less than 56%, and progressed to invasive carcinoma in more than 12% (see Table 8–1). It is impossi-

Table 8–1. Outcome of CIN Based on Ostor's Literature Review

Outcome	CIN I	CIN 2	CIN 3
Regress	57%	43%	32%
Persist	32%	35%	<56%
Progress to CIS	11%	22%	—
Progress to invasive	<1%	5%	>12%

From Ostor AG. Natural history of cervical intraepithelial neoplasia: A critical review. Int J Gynecol Pathol 12:186, 1993.

ble to predict the outcome of an individual patient with CIN.

DNA ploidy patterns are closely related to the outcome of the lesion.[117,118] Included in this retrospective study were 120 women who had histologically confirmed dysplasia or CIS but did not receive therapy for at least 1 year. Of the 47 lesions that returned to normal, as confirmed by negative cervical smears or histologic sample, 40 (85%) had a diploid or polyploid DNA pattern and the remaining 7 (15%) had an aneuploid distribution. Regression of the latter cases may not be spontaneous because of the use of biopsy. The disease-free period was 1 to 13 years (mean 4.9 years). Among lesions that persisted for 1 to 14 years (mean 3.2 years), 60 (92%) had an aneuploid pattern and 5 (8%) had a diploid or polyploid pattern.[118] All initial dysplasias from 8 women who developed invasive carcinoma 1 to 18 years (mean 7.2 years) later had an aneuploid distribution.[118] The majority of diploid and polyploid lesions are low-grade CIN, including condyloma, mild dysplasia, and atypical immature metaplasia. In contrast, aneuploid lesions were predominantly CIN 2 and higher and were likely to persist or progress to invasive carcinoma.[117,118] Although no HPV typing was available at the time of these studies, it is likely that those regressed lesions are associated with low-risk HPV. As shown by recent studies, the persistence and the progression of CIN are strongly influenced by HPV types and their persistent infection.[157,267,370]

The impact of pregnancy on CIN was investigated by Yost et al.,[386] who followed 82 pregnant women with CIN 2 for at least 6 weeks postpartum with cytology or colposcopically directed biopsies. In 68% of women, the lesions regressed, 7% progressed to CIN 3, and 25% remained the same. Among 71 women with CIN 3, 70% of lesions regressed or became less severe postpartum (including 37% that returned to normal, 18% to CIN 1, and 15% to CIN 2). The lesions remained the same as CIN 3 in 30% of the women. None of the lesions progressed to invasive carcinoma. The method of delivery, whether vaginal or by caesarean section, makes no difference. It is interesting that the regression rates for CIN 2 and CIN 3 appear to be higher than those in the literature review by Ostor.[261] Because regression is unrelated to the mode of delivery, immunosuppression during pregnancy and subsequent return to the normal state postpartum may be a reasonable explanation for regression.

The risk of progression from CIN to invasive carcinoma is more difficult to assess. In the McIndoe et al. series,[232] less than 5% (7 of 131) of CIS cases resolved, 69% (90 of 131) persisted as CIS, 4% (5 of 131) persisted as dysplasia, and 22% (29 of 131) progressed to invasive carcinoma. Of the 25 women with CIS who received only punch and/or wedge biopsy, 15 (60%) had normal cytology following biopsy. Their lesions were presumably removed by biopsy. One of these 15 women developed invasive carcinoma 4 years later. Of the 10 women with persistent abnormal cytology, 9 (90%) subsequently developed invasive carcinoma 1 to 9 years (median 4 years) after the initial biopsy. Overall, 10 of 25 (40%) women with CIS who received diagnostic biopsies developed invasive carcinoma. If only cases with persistent abnormal cytology are considered, 90% of women with CIS eventuated in invasive carcinoma.

If CIS is eradicated by conization and/or hysterectomy as indicated by negative follow-up smears, only 1.4% (11 of 802) of patients developed invasive carcinoma of the cervix or vagina. These carcinomas most likely represent a new squamous neoplasm.[232]

Treatment and Prognosis

The treatment modalities for CIN include cryotherapy, laser therapy, local excision, loop electrocautery excision procedure (LEEP), cervical conization, and hysterectomy. Treatment failure is generally related to incomplete eradication of CIN owing to its large size, depth, or position high in the cervical canal. In some instances, invasive carcinoma was not detected before cryotherapy. The importance of strict adherence to the protocol with adequate sampling of the cervical canal, acquisition of representative tissue for histologic diagnosis, and accurate interpretation of colposcopic findings cannot be overemphasized.[355]

The surgical margins of conization specimens should be investigated for completeness of the excision. When the margins were free of abnormal epithelium, 9%[3] to 15%[63] of hysterectomy specimens were found to contain residual disease, usually CIN 1 or CIN 2. This is in contrast to the persistence of CIN in 41%[63] to 55%[3] of hysterectomy specimens. It should be emphasized that a positive margin for CIN is also a risk for coexisting or subsequent development of invasive squamous carcinoma. The lack of residual disease in hysterectomy specimens can be explained by the false-positive margins (usually caused by oblique or inadequate sectioning of true margins or lack of proper inking) and tissue necrosis secondary to surgical procedures.

Cervical smears performed between the period of conization and subsequent hysterectomy are useful in determining persistent disease. When the cervical smears are normal, none of the hysterectomy specimens have residual disease.[63] In the presence of abnormal cells, 57% of women have residual disease in the hysterectomy specimens. The reason that no disease is found in the remaining 43% of women may be explained by false-positive smears owing to overdiagnosis of reparative epithelial changes as CIN following conization.[63]

INVASIVE SQUAMOUS CELL CARCINOMA

Clinical Staging

To assess the extent of cervical neoplasm, the International Federation of Obstetricians and Gynecologists (FIGO) has established a clinical staging system based on the findings of pelvic examination, radiology, and endoscopy, such as sigmoidoscopy, cystoscopy, chest and skeletal x-rays, and intravenous pyelogram. The cri-

teria are summarized in Table 8–2. Briefly, Stage 0 is an in situ carcinoma. An invasive tumor confined to the cervix is Stage I. Early tumors less than 5 mm in depth and up to 7 mm in width are classified as Stage IA, or microinvasive carcinoma. Stage I tumors exceeding this limit are designated IB. Tumors up to 4.0 cm in size are State IB1, and those greater than 4.0 cm are Stage IB2. Stage IB2 tumors have a worse prognosis than Stage IB1 tumors and a small IIA neoplasm with minimal vaginal extension.[80] Cervical tumors that extend beyond the cervix but do not affect the lower third of the vagina or do not affect the pelvic wall are Stage II. Stage III tumors extend to the pelvic wall or lower third of the vagina. Invasion of the urinary bladder or rectum or metastasis to distant sites is Stage IV disease.

This staging system allows comparison of the treatment results with different modalities from various centers. Although it does not govern the method of treatment, it proves to be one of the most important prognostic indicators. For example, the 4-year cancer-free probability of American women with Stage I, II, and III disease following treatment is 87%, 66%, and 28%, respectively.[143] In patients treated with radiotherapy, Reddy et al.[289] report that the 5-year survival rates are 92% for Stage IA, 88%

Table 8–2. Definition of FIGO Clinical Staging for Cervical Cancer

Stage 0	Carcinoma in situ, intraepithelial carcinoma
Stage I	Carcinoma is strictly confined to the cervix (extension to the corpus should be disregarded)
Stage IA	Invasive cancer, identified only microscopically. Invasion is limited to measured stromal invasion with maximum depth of 5 mm and no wider than 7 mm. (The depth of invasion should not be more than 5 mm taken from the base of the epithelium, either surface or glandular, from which it originates. Vascular space involvement, either venous or lymphatic, should not alter the staging.)
Stage IA1	Measured invasion of stroma no greater than 3 mm in depth and no wider than 7 mm.
Stage IA2	Measured invasion of stroma greater than 3 mm and no greater than 5 mm and no wider than 7 mm.
Stage IB	Clinical lesions confined to the cervix or preclinical lesions greater than stage IA.
Stage IB1	Clinical lesions no greater than 4 cm in size.
Stage IB2	Clinical lesions no greater than 4 cm in size.
Stage II	The carcinoma extends beyond the cervix but has not extended to the pelvic wall. The carcinoma involves the vagina but not as far as the lower third of the vagina.
Stage IIA	No obvious parametrial involvement.
Stage IIB	Obvious parametrial involvement.
Stage III	The carcinoma has extended to the pelvic wall. On rectal examination, there is no cancer-free space between the tumor and the pelvic wall. The tumor involves the lower third of the vagina. All cases with a hydronephrosis or nonfunctioning kidney are included unless they are known to be the result of other causes.
Stage IIIA	No extension to the pelvic wall.
Stage IIIB	Extension to the pelvic wall and/or hydronephrosis or nonfunctioning kidney.
Stage IV	The carcinoma has extended beyond the true pelvis or has clinically involved the mucosa of the bladder or rectum. A bullous edema as such does not permit a case to be allotted to Stage IV.
Stage IVA	Spread of the growth to adjacent organs.
Stage IVB	Spread to distant organs.

From Creasman WT. New gynecologic cancer staging. Gynecol Oncol 58:157, 1995.

for IB, 74% for IIA, 58% for IIB, 60% for IIIA, 65% for IIIB, and 25% for IV, with an overall survival rate of 74%.

There is a tendency to underestimate the disease clinically. When compared with surgical findings, 15%[228] to 25%[202] of Stage IB and 50%[202,228] of Stage II and III cancers are understaged. Overall, the disease is underestimated in 36% of women with cervical cancer.[202] The risk of both pelvic and para-aortic nodal metastasis as well as distant metastasis increases with advancing clinical stage.

FIGO Stage IA Microinvasive Squamous Cell Carcinoma

The concept of a prognostically favorable, early cervical cancer was credited to Mestwerdt,[237] who defined "microcarcinoma" as a lesion that invades less than 5 mm into the cervical stroma measured from the basement membrane. In the current FIGO Stage IA1 tumor, the stromal invasion is up to 3.0 mm and in Stage IA2, between 3.0 to 5.0 mm. The linear extent for both conditions is up to 7.0 mm. The presence of vascular lymphatic space invasion does not exclude the tumor from Stage IA by FIGO definition. In contrast, the Society of Gynecologic Oncologists (SGO) limits the microinvasive squamous carcinoma to up to 3 mm in depth without vascular lymphatic space invasion.

Most microinvasive carcinomas are seen in asymptomatic women, are detected initially by cytologic smears, and are confirmed subsequently by excision, conization, or hysterectomy specimens.[57,58] Thus, the frequency is closely related to a cervical cancer screening program. Over a period of 2 decades, the relative frequency of microinvasive cancers increased from 1.2% in the 1940s to 20.9% of all cervical cancers in the 1960s, an increase attributed to effective cytologic detection.[254] In regions with an established screening program, about 15% of all invasive cervical cancers are Stage IA, 35% are Stage IB, and the remaining 50% are Stage II and higher.[246] At the beginning of cytologic screening, microinvasive carcinomas made up 7% of all cervical cancers in 1970. In contrast, in 1990 microinvasive carcinomas were 19% of all cervical cancers.[246]

Microscopic Features

In the earliest development of recognizable microinvasion, a nidus of a few tumor cells is found to have more abundant eosinophilic cytoplasm than do adjacent cells. The nuclei also appear different, with more irregularity, open chromatin, and prominent nucleoli (Fig. 8–60). These cells form one or more small protrusions at the point of invasion (see Fig. 8–60). With increasing size, tongue-like processes project into the underlying stroma (Fig. 8–61). Tumor cells penetrate throughout the basement membrane to form isolated cells and small aggregates in the stroma, which undergo chronic inflammation and fibrosis (Fig. 8–62). Progressively, multiple foci of invasion arise from the mucosa and the periphery of endocervical glands involved by CIN. (Fig. 8–63).

The tumor dimensions increase vertically and laterally. This process is accompanied by further genetic alterations and stem cell evolution.[107,120] The stroma reacts to invasion through a band-like lymphoplasmacytic infiltration, proliferation of fibrous tissue, and the formation of granulomas to the necrotic tumor cells and keratin debris. The tumor processes are surrounded by clear spaces resulting from shrinkage artifact of the stroma and simulate vascular lymphatic space invasion (Fig. 8–64). True vascular space invasion also occurs.

Among the microinvasive cervical cancers that measure 5 mm or less in depth, 56% involve the anterior lip, 33% involve both the anterior and posterior lips, and 11% involve the posterior lip alone.[254] The invasive foci are mostly multicentric (92%). The epithelia overlying the invasive carcinoma resemble CIS in 68% of cases and dysplasia in 5%, are indeterminate in 14%, are normal in 2%, and are ulcerated in the remainder. Islands of well-differentiated squamous cells occur in 60% of intraepithelial neoplasms.[254] Such features are also found at the point of invasion in 85% of microinvasive carcinomas of 5 mm or less in depth.[315]

Microinvasive cervical cancers grow in different patterns. Some infiltrate in finger-like processes (Fig. 8–65A) or form networks of invasive cords with confluence (see Fig. 8–65B). Infrequently, the tumors invade diffusely in small clusters or infiltrate as bulky solid sheets. The confluent pattern is generally defined as a lesion in which anastomosing tongues of tumor with pushing borders are present.[254,317,365] Other investigators define confluent pattern in terms of tumor area of at least 1 square mm.[81]

There is evidence to support that the confluent pattern is a covariable of the depth of invasion. When the studies by Sedlis et al.[315] and

Text continued on page 341

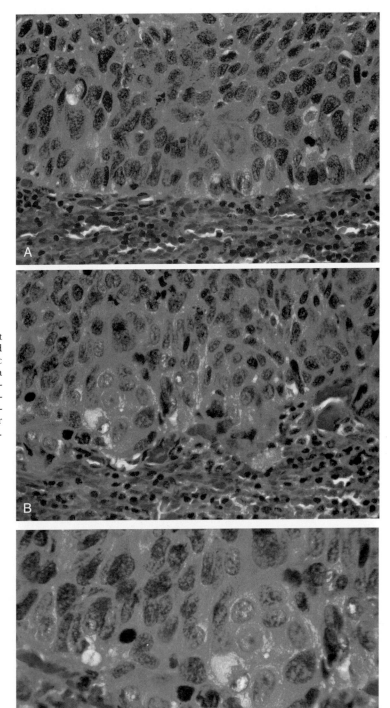

Figure 8–60. Serial sections of earliest stage of microinvasion characterized by *A*, the development of anaplastic cells, and *B* to *D*, the formation of a nidus made up of tumor cells with nuclear anaplasia and prominent nucleoli. The abundant eosinophilic cytoplasm gives the impression of better differentiation than in the adjacent cells. *Illustration continued on following page*

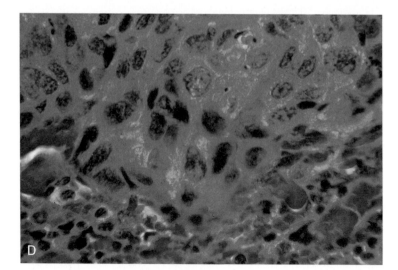

Figure 8–60. *Continued*

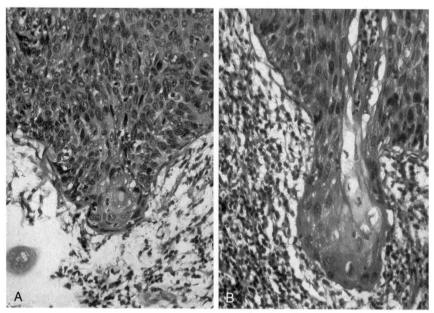

Figure 8–61. Very early stage of microinvasion. *A* and *B*, Tumor cells form tongue-like protrusion surrounded by intact basement membrane.

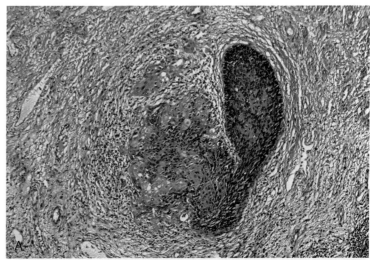

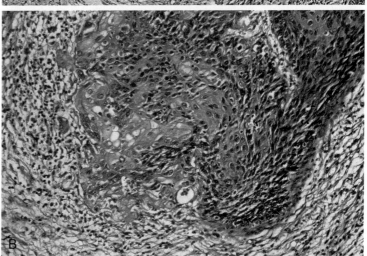

Figure 8–62. Early stage of microinvasion. *A* and *B,* Tumor cells break through the basement membrane at the point of invasion to form isolated tumor nests. Invasive tumor cells have more eosinophilic cytoplasm than the noninvasive tumor cells.

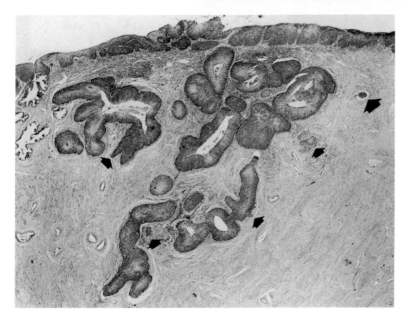

Figure 8–63. Multiple foci of microinvasion originating from the endocervical glands involved by CIN. Irregular and sometimes pointed invasive processes alter the normally smooth borders of endocervical glands (*arrows*). Areas of periglandular fibrosis and a capillary-lymphatic invasion (*right upper corner*) are noted. In such tumor with multifocal stromal invasion, the depth of stromal invasion is measured from the base of overlying CIN to the deepest tumor.

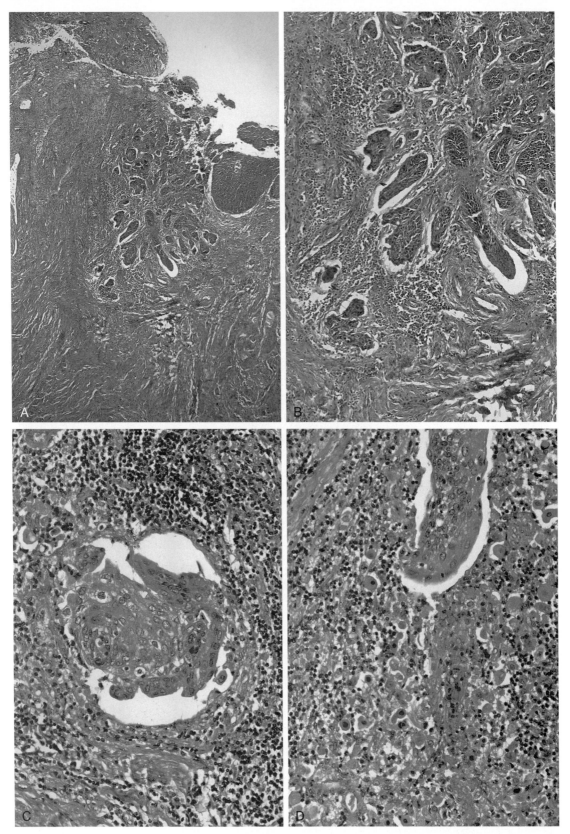

Figure 8–64. Microinvasive squamous cell carcinoma and pseudovascular lymphatic space invasion. *A* and *B,* Close to the base of the tumor, the tumor nests are surrounded by clear spaces without endothelial lining. *C,* Some of the pseudovascular lymphatic space invasions occur in areas with histiocytic reaction. Note tumor cells and adjacent multinucleated giant cells. *D,* Tumor nest surrounded by a clear space and histiocytes mixed with degenerated tumor cells.

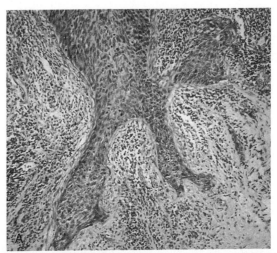

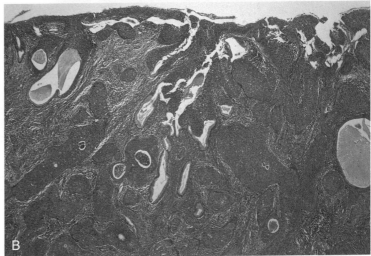

Figure 8–65. Microinvasive squamous cell carcinoma. *A,* Tongue-like infiltrative pattern. *B,* Confluent pattern.

Creasman et al.[81] are combined, the confluent pattern is associated with 3% (2 of 75) of tumors less than 1 mm in depth, 27% (30 of 111) of neoplasms between 1 and 3 mm, and 43% (18 of 42) of tumors between 3 and 5 mm in depth ($P = 0.0001$). Confluent pattern does not increase local recurrence or pelvic lymph node metastasis.[78]

The histologic cell type of early invasive carcinomas is large cell nonkeratinizing type in 76% to 88%, whereas 9% to 18% are of the keratinizing type, and 3 to 6% are of the small cell type.[204,365]

Tumor cells gain access to the vascular lymphatic channels early in their invasion. Because a distinction between capillary and lymphatic spaces is impossible in routine histologic preparations, invasion of such spaces is generally considered together as capillary-lymphatic (C-L) invasion. The reported frequency of C-L invasion varies from 8%[254] to 57%.[298] Such divergent results among studies can be explained by the different morphologic criteria used, variable types of histologic preparations, and the depth of invasion.

In H&E-stained histologic sections, it is common to find clear spaces around the tumor cells, which is caused by shrinkage of fibrous stroma after fixation (see Fig. 8–64). These artifacts can be mistaken for vascular invasion. True vascular invasion should be lined by clearly recognizable endothelial cells. The involved vessel is generally small. The presence of fibrin thrombi further confirms the vascular nature (Fig. 8–66A). It would be helpful to confirm the vascular channel by finding other ves-

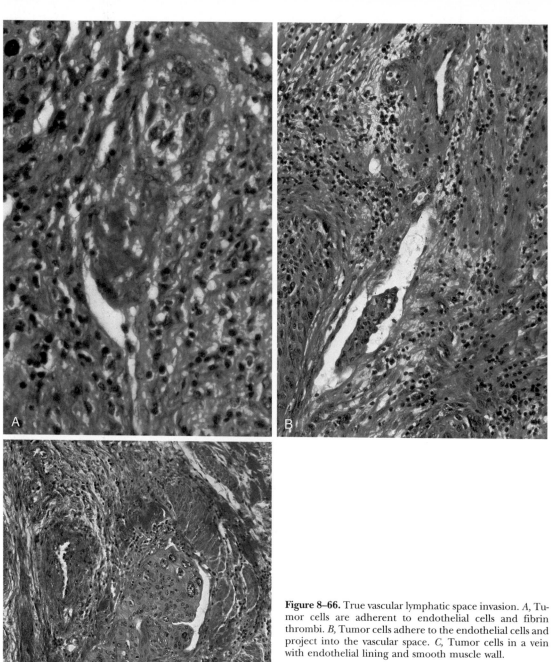

Figure 8–66. True vascular lymphatic space invasion. *A,* Tumor cells are adherent to endothelial cells and fibrin thrombi. *B,* Tumor cells adhere to the endothelial cells and project into the vascular space. *C,* Tumor cells in a vein with endothelial lining and smooth muscle wall.

sels in the vicinity, because capillaries, lymphatics, arterioles, and venules often travel together (see Fig. 8–66B). Smooth muscular wall is evident when blood vessels are involved (see Fig. 8–66C). Using these criteria, it should be possible to correctly identify vascular invasion. Immunohistochemical stains for endothelial markers do not appear to improve diagnostic accuracy. Endothelial cells lining the lymphatic spaces may not express endothelial cell markers.

Roche and Norris[298] demonstrated that, by step section of conization specimens, the frequency of C-L invasion is increased from 30% to 57%. Finally, C-L invasion and the depth of invasion are closely related. By combining the series of Sedlis et al.[315] and Creasman et al.,[81] C-L invasion occurs in 8% (6 of 75) of tumors less than 1 mm, 22% (24 of 111) of neoplasms between 1 and 3 mm, and 38% of tumors between 3 and 5 mm in depth ($P = 0.0004$). In the study by Orlandi et al.,[260a] the frequency of C-L invasion is 0%, 10%, and 47.3% with stromal invasion of up to 1.0 mm., 1.0 to 3.0 mm, and 3.0 to 5.0 mm, respectively. Similar results have been reported by others.[78,223]

Depth of Invasion

The current FIGO staging method recommends that measurement be made from the base of epithelium from which invasion occurs to the deepest point of tumor in a vertical line (Fig. 8–67). In the majority of microinvasive squamous carcinomas, invasion occurs either from the base of the surface mucosa or originates from both the mucosa and endocervical glands simultaneously. In such cases, measurement should be made from the base of mucosa involved by CIN (see Fig. 8–63). In only a small number of cases is invasion limited to the periphery of a few endocervical glands without surface involvement. In such instances, measurement is made from the base of the gland to the deepest tumor (Fig. 8–68).

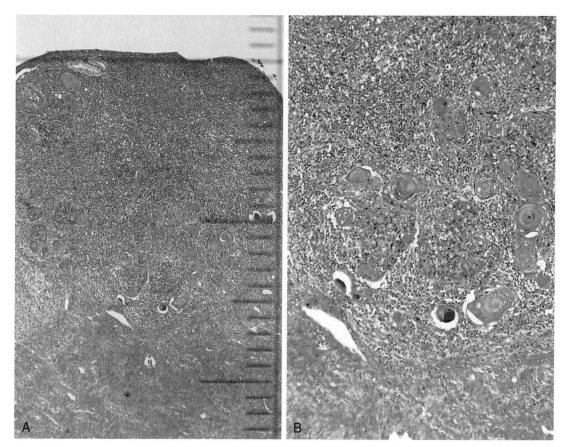

Figure 8–67. Measurement of the depth of stromal invasion. *A,* This tumor originates from the base of CIN and invades to a depth 1.5 mm. *B,* Higher magnification demonstrates keratinizing type of squamous carcinoma and pseudovascular space invasion at the base of tumor.

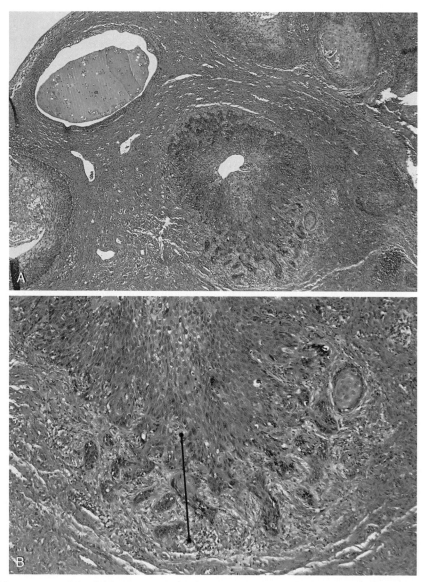

Figure 8–68. Measurement of the depth of stromal invasion. *A,* In this case, the area of stromal invasion is limited to this endocervical gland involved by CIN 3. *B,* The depth of stromal invasion is measured from the point of invasion or pre-existing basement membrane of endocervical gland to the deepest tumor (*solid line*). Multiple tongue-like protrusions are associated with desmoplastic stroma. In this case, the depth of invasion is less than 1 mm without vascular-lymphatic space invasion.

When the series of Sedlis et al.[315] and Hasumi et al.[149] are combined, 41% of the tumors measure 1 mm or less, 40% are between 1.1 and 3.0 mm, and 19% are between 3.1 and 5.0 mm.

Diagnostic Problems

In a study by Sedlis et al.,[315] 37% (99 of 265) of specimens initially submitted by the participating pathologists of the Gynecologic Oncology Group as microinvasive carcinoma were judged to be noninvasive neoplasms. Overdiagnosis of invasive carcinoma is most frequently caused by misinterpretation of tangential cuts of glandular extension by CIN (Figs. 8–69 and 8–70). Solid nests of dysplastic cells appear to extend into the stroma, but the periphery of tumor nests is smooth (see Fig. 8–69).

Sometimes irregular, tongue-like processes with surrounding fibrosis seem to invade the stroma. In such cases, deeper cuts usually confirm glandular extension (see Fig. 8–70). In the

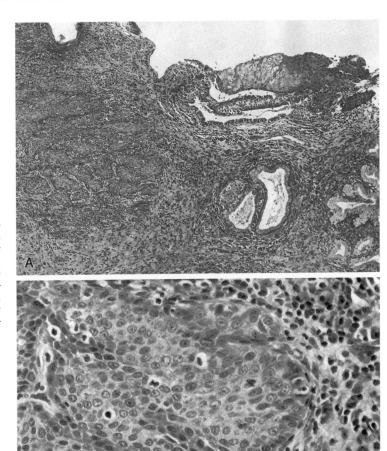

Figure 8–69. Mimicker of microinvasive squamous carcinoma. *A,* A focus of endocervical glands involved by CIN. Owing to the tangential cut, multiple bud-like protrusions resemble early invasion. *B,* On higher magnification, the solid cell nests maintain smooth borders. Although the cells are dysplastic with increased mitotic activity, no nuclear anaplasia is seen.

case of true stromal invasion, isolated single tumor cells or irregular tumor nests can be found in the stroma.

Edema and chronic inflammatory reaction beneath the benign mucosa or CIN often obscures the basement membrane and simulates early invasion (Fig. 8–71). Examination for the presence or absence of basement membrane on routine H&E slide or PAS stain seldom yields conclusive information. At the site of true early invasion, cellular anaplasia and stromal fibrosis are expected. It is useful to recall that only 2% of microinvasive carcinomas originate from the base of normal-appearing epithelium.[254]

Finally, entrapped atypical cells in the stroma may result from previous procedures, such as biopsy and conization. Inquiry about recent

medical intervention may offer important clues as to the cause of artifacts.

Although early invasive carcinoma can be seen in punch biopsies, the depth of invasion may not represent the maximal depth. Therefore, the diagnosis of microinvasive cancer requires a comprehensive histologic examination of the entire cervix, that is, study of specimens obtained with LEEP, conization, trachelectomy, or hysterectomy. It is important to handle the conization specimens appropriately, allowing for accurate assessment of the depth of invasion and the surgical margins. We prefer the method of sectioning along the long axis of the cervical canal and around the clock following adequate fixation. Tangentially cut sections invariably result in inaccurate measure-

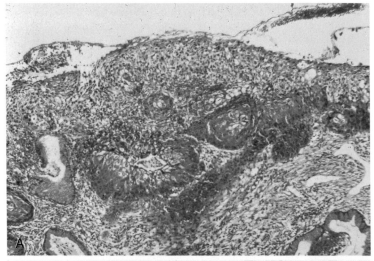

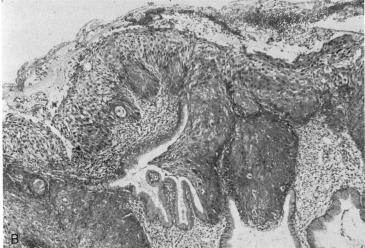

Figure 8–70. Mimicker of microinvasive squamous carcinoma. *A,* Multiple irregular tongue-like protrusions from the base of CIN suggest early stromal invasion. *B,* Deeper cut of area shown in *A* reveals endocervical extension by overlying CIN.

ments, and excessive manipulations of the specimen cause denudation and crush artifacts, impeding optimal evaluation. As indicated in Chapter 1, in fragmented LEEP specimens with early cancer it is difficult to assess the tumor dimension and completeness of the excision.

According to a study by Creasman et al.,[81] if the surgical margins of conization specimens were clear of microinvasive carcinoma, the chance of finding residual invasive carcinoma in the subsequent hysterectomy specimens was 4% (2 of 45; both were less than 0.5 mm in depth). If the surgical margins were involved by invasive carcinoma, 77% (10 of 13) of hysterectomy specimens contained residual invasive carcinoma.[81] More important, the depth of invasion in 8 of 12 hysterectomy specimens ex-

ceeded that of conization specimens.[315] Thus, invasive carcinomas that extend to the surgical margins of the conization specimen should be excluded from the FIGO clinical Stage IA. Larsson et al.[204] found that surgical margins involving only dysplasia or CIS were a significant risk factor for tumor recurrence.

Factors Affecting Pelvic Lymph Node Metastasis and Tumor Recurrence

In their critical review of literature, Benson and Norris[32] found that most of the previous studies are biased in assessment of pelvic nodal status. In some studies, the depth of invasion was not confirmed histologically or was based on inadequate cone or punch biopsies. The latter

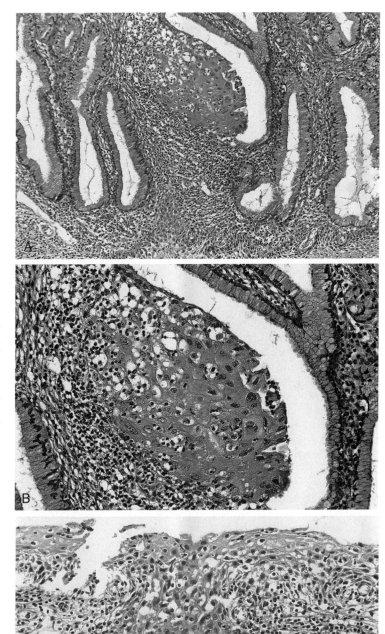

Figure 8–71. Mimicker of microinvasive squamous carcinoma. *A* and *B,* Mild squamous dysplasia in an endocervical gland. The base of dysplasia undergoes inflammatory change with irregular borders to simulate invasion. Note the lack of nuclear anaplasia as expected at the point of invasion. *C,* Atypical cells extend from the mucosa, suggestive of early invasion.
Illustration continued on following page

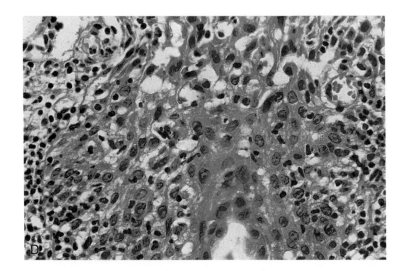

Figure 8–71. *Continued D,* Higher magnification of *C* reveals reactive metaplastic squamous cells with uniform nuclei and small nucleoli. Note that the chronic inflammatory cells obliterate the basement membrane.

often underestimate the true depth and are biased toward a higher frequency of pelvic nodal metastasis. Some studies included cases with questionable invasion or excluded those having capillary-lymphatic invasion or confluent pattern, thus favoring a lower rate of pelvic nodal metastasis. Treatment modality, such as selection of more advanced tumor for lymphadenectomy and radiotherapy given before lymphadenectomy, might have influenced the frequency of pelvic nodal status. Using the same criteria as those of Benson and Norris,[32] additional series are listed (Tables 8–3 to 8–5). Only patients treated with radical hysterectomy and pelvic lymphadenectomy are included.

If the depth of invasion is 1 mm or less, the risk of having pelvic nodal metastasis is 0.2% (1 of 427) and that of tumor recurrence is 0% (see Table 8–3). The only metastasis occurred in a tumor of 0.7 mm in depth without C-L invasion.

Table 8–3. Cervical Squamous
Carcinoma up to 1 mm in Depth

Authors	No. Pts.	LN+	Rec/DOD
Averette et al.[17]	162	0	0/0
Seski et al.[317]	14	0	0/0
Hasumi et al.[150]	61	1*	NA
Sevin et al.[319]	166	0	0/0
Maiman et al.[223]	24	0	0/0
Total	427	1 (0.2%)	0/0 (0%/0%)

*0.7 mm in depth, no evidence of vascular lymphatic space invasion.

LN+, lymph node metastasis present; NA, not available; Rec/DOD, recurrence/dead of disease.

In patients whose invasive tumor measures 0.1 to 3.0 mm, 1% (5 of 494) had pelvic lymph node metastasis. Two of these women developed tumor recurrence and died, representing an overall risk of 0.4% (see Table 8–4).

Of the 198 tumors between 3.1 and 5.0 mm in depth, 7.6% metastasized to the pelvic lymph nodes. Tumor recurred in 3.5% (seven) of women and 3% (six) women died of tumor (see Table 8–5).

In two large series, the treatment modalities included conization, simple to radical hysterectomy, and radiotherapy.[78,192] The recurrent rates were 1.6% for tumors up to 1 mm in depth, 3.5% for tumors 1.1 to 3.0 mm in depth, and 3.9% for tumors between 3 and 5 mm in depth (Table 8–6). The mortality rates were 0%, 0.4%, and 1.3% for tumors less than 1 mm, 1 to 3 mm, and 3 to 5 mm, respectively.

The significance of capillary-lymphatic space invasion and its relationship to pelvic lymph node metastasis and tumor recurrence is controversial. In a review of the literature, Copeland et al.[78] found that C-L space invasion in tumors 1 to 3 mm in depth correlated with increased pelvic nodal metastasis and tumor recurrence. The frequency of nodal involvement without C-L space invasion was 0.3% (1/339), but with C-L space invasion frequency increased to 2.6% (1/63). Tumor recurrence without and with C-L space invasion was 0.9% (4/453) and 4% (4/99), respectively. These differences are not statistically significant, however.

For tumors 3 to 5 mm in depth, 9.1% (3/33) of tumors with C-L space invasion recurred, as compared with 0% (0/88) without invasion

Table 8–4. Cervical Squamous Carcinoma 0.1 to 3.0 mm

Authors	No. Pts.	LN+	Rec/DOD
Foushee et al.[105]	16	0	0/0
Roche and Norris[298]	9	0	0/0
Leman et al.[210]	32	0	0/0
Bohm et al.[40]	56	4	2/2
Seski et al.[317]	37	0	0/0
Hasumi et al.[150]	106	1	NA
Van Nagle et al.[365]	52	0	0/0
Creasman et al.[81]	24	0	0/0
Simon et al.[329]	43	0	0/0
Sevin et al.*[319]	54	0	0/0
Maiman et al.[223]	65	0	0/0
Total	494	5 (1%)	2/2 (0.4% /0.4%)

*Excluding tumor with vascular-lymphatic space invasion.
LN+, lymph node metastasis present; NA, not available; Rec/DOD, recurrence/ dead of disease.

Table 8–5. Cervical Squamous Carcinoma 3.1 to 5.0 mm

Authors	No. Pts.	LN+	Rec/DOD
Foushee et al.[105]	13	1	0/0
Roche and Norris et al.[298]	21	0	0/0
Leman et al.[210]	3	0	0/0
Hasumi et al.[150]	29	4	NA
van Nagle et al.[365]	32	3	3/2
Creasman et al.[81]	8	0	0/0
Simon et al.[329]	26	1	0/0
Sevin et al.[319]	36	2	4/4
Maiman et al.[223]	30	4	0/0
Total	198	15 (7.6%)	7/6 (3.5% /3.0%)

LN+, lymph node metastasis present; NA, not available; Rec/DOD, recurrence/ dead of disease.

Table 8–6. Tumor Recurrence and Dead of Disease of FIGO Stage IA Tumor*

Authors	Stromal Invasion	Recurrence	Dead of Disease
Kolstad[192]	≤ 1 mm	3/232	0/232
Copeland et al.[78]	≤ 1 mm	1/24	0/24
Total		4/256 (1.6%)	0/256 (0%)
Kolstad[192]	1.1–2.9 mm	8/224	1/224
Copeland et al.[78]	1.1–3.0 mm	2/59	0/59
Total		10/283 (3.5%)	1/283 (0.4%)
Koldstad[192]	3.0–5.0 mm	8/187	3/187
Copeland et al.[78]	3.1–5.0 mm	1/42	0/42
Total		9/229 (3.9%)	3/229 (1.3%)

*Treatment modalities include conization, simple to radical hysterectomy, and radiotherapy.

$(P < 0.05)$.[78] There was no correlation between C-L space invasion and nodal metastasis. Nodal metastasis occurred in 6.6% (7/106) of tumors without C-L space invasion, as compared with 3.9% (2/51) with such invasion. Thus, C-L space invasion increases local recurrence in tumors 3 to 5 mm in depth.[78]

The confluent pattern, cell type, and amount of lymphoplasmacytic stromal response have no apparent impact on pelvic nodal metastasis or tumor recurrence.[210,298,317,365]

FIGO Stage IB and Higher Frankly Invasive Squamous Cell Carcinoma

Clinical and Gross Features

In the early stage, cervical squamous cell carcinoma presents as a poorly defined, hyperemic, granular, eroded lesion, which bleeds on contact (Fig. 8–72A). With the aid of colposcopy, tortuous abnormal blood vessels become evident. With progression, a localized, nodular lesion develops. The center becomes ulcerated (see Fig. 8–72B). Patients with more advanced carcinomas present with exophytic, papillary, verrucous, or polypoid masses projecting from the ectocervix (see Fig. 8–72C). The endophytic variants tend to occur within the cervical canal and infiltrate into the stroma, causing diffuse enlargement and hardening of the cervix (see Fig. 8–72D). These are typified by a barrel-shaped cervix[216] or the spray cancer described by Schiller et al.[311] In 25% to 30% of patients, the cervix appears normal in size and shape and is covered by smooth, intact mucosa. Unless adequate cytologic and histologic samples are taken from the endocervix, the tumor may go undetected.

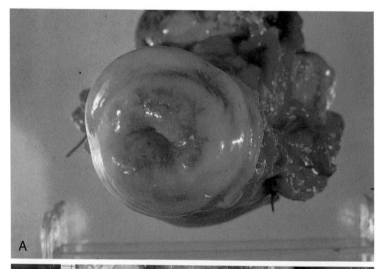

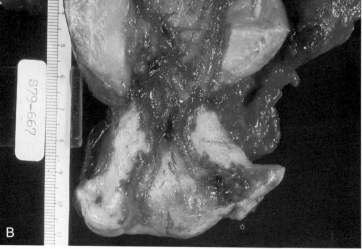

Figure 8–72. Gross features of invasive squamous carcinoma. *A,* In the early stage, it has a granular, hyperemic appearance without induration. *B,* A nodular, ulcerated lesion. *C,* A fungating, exophytic mass on the ectocervix. *D,* A large, bulky, ulcerating mass.

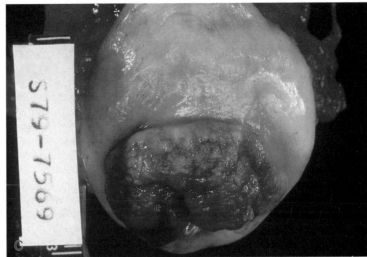

Figure 8–72. *Continued*

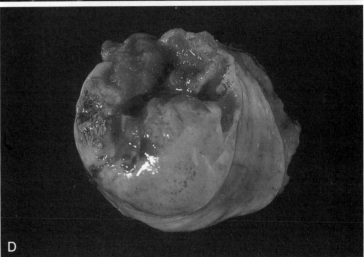

Locally, the tumors spread downward to involve the vagina and upward to the endometrium. Rarely, invasive carcinoma spreads superficially to involve the endometrium and fallopian tube in a manner similar to that of in situ carcinoma.[180,276] Infiltrations through the cervical stroma eventually reach to the parametrium and further extend anteriorly to the base of urinary bladder and the ureteral tissue and posteriorly to the rectum. Necrosis, ulceration, and fistula ultimately develop. In addition to the local spread, some tumors metastasize to the pelvic lymph nodes in the early stage. Involvement of the external and iliac lymph nodes is most commonly identified in lymphadenectomy specimens. Metastasis to the sacral, parametrial, paracervical, and common iliac lymph nodes is less common. Tumor emboli may follow efferent lymphatic channels of pelvic lymph node to para-aortic node to the cisterna chyli and the thoracic duct and then to the scalene node.[187]

Tumor Volume

Tumor volume can be estimated by clinical size or by reconstruction of giant tissue sections prepared from conization or hysterectomy specimens. In a study of Stage IB and IIA tumors by van Nagell et al.,[363] pelvic lymph node metastasis occurred in 9% of tumors less than 2 cm in size, but this figure increased to 31% when the tumor was greater than 2 cm. Following radical hysterectomy, tumor recurred in

9% and 44% of women whose tumor was less than and greater than 2 cm, respectively.

Among the clinical Stage IB tumors of less than 3 cm, the risk of pelvic nodal metastasis was 21% but increased to 35% when tumor was greater than 3 cm. The corresponding 5-year survival rates were 90% and 66% for women whose tumors were less than and greater than 3 cm, respectively.[277]

For patients with Stage IIA disease, metastasis to the pelvic lymph node occurred in 21% and 42% of tumors less than and greater than 3 cm, respectively. The 5-year survival rates were 72% to 81.8% if the tumor was less than 3 cm, and 38% to 41.6% if it was greater than 3 cm.[277] Thus, tumor size as determined by pelvic examination provides important prognostic information. In women receiving radiotherapy for Stage IB to IIB cervical cancer, bulky tumor, which is defined as tumor equal to or greater than 6 cm in size, has the highest frequency of recurrence.[236]

Baltzer and Koepcke[22] estimated the tumor volume by a meticulous sectioning of 684 hysterectomy specimens using giant histologic sections. The tumor volume was calculated by $(pi/6) \times TH \times TL \times TB$. TH represents the distance between the anterior and posterior margins of tumor or tumor height (tumor thickness in both anterior and posterior lips). TL, tumor length, is the vertical distance from the upper (proximal) to the lower (distal) borders. TB, tumor breadth, is the horizontal distance of the tumor borders. When the tumor volume was 500 to 1500 cubic mm, 17% of tumors had pelvic lymph node metastasis; when tumor volume was 6500 to 10,000 cubic mm, the figure was 46%; and when tumor volume was greater than 20,000 cubic mm, it was 55%. The respective 5-year survival rates were 84%, 75%, and 60%. This and other studies document the importance of tumor volume in relation to pelvic lymph node metastasis, tumor recurrence, and survival.

Depth of Invasion

The depth of stromal invasion adds critical information about survival rates and the risk for pelvic nodal metastasis and tumor recurrence (Tables 8–7 and 8–8). In ulcerated tumor, the adjacent intact mucosal base is used as a reference point for measurement. Stromal invasion is also expressed by dividing the cervical wall into thirds. In a study of Stages IB, IIA, and IIB squamous cell carcinomas, pelvic lymph node

Table 8–7. Five-Year Survival Rates in Surgically Treated Cases

Parameter	Kamura et al.[179]		Sevin et al.[318]	
No. cases	211 IB and II		370 I and II	
Cell type	Squamous CA	91.1%	Squamous CA	
	Adenocarcinoma	70.1%	vs. adenocarcinoma	
	P value significant		Not significant	
Tumor size	<2 cm	97.6%	<1 cm	93%
	2–4 cm	85.6%	1.1–2.0 cm	76%
	>4 cm	80.1%	2.1–3.0 cm	64%
			>3.0 cm	60%
Stromal invasion	<3 mm	95.7%	<5 mm	92%
	3–5 mm	91.7%	6–10 mm	74%
	5–10 mm	83%	>10 mm	60%
	>10 mm	81.8%		
Cervical wall	<1/3	94.8%		
Invasion	middle 1/3	88.1%		
	outer 1/3	79.9%		
LVSI	Absent	91.5%	Absent	85%
	Present	82.4%	Present	62%
Parametrial disease	Absent	90.3%		
	Present	77.3%		
Lymph node metastasis	Negative	90.8%	Negative	77%
	1+	96.7%	1–2 +	55%
	2+	44.3%	>2 +	39%
	3+	36%		
Histologic grade	Not evaluated		Not significant	

LVSI, lymphatic vascular space invasion.
From Fu YS. Pathology of cervical carcinoma. In Sciarra JJ, ed. Gynecology and Obstetrics. Philadelphia, Lippincott Williams & Wilkins, 2000.

Table 8–8. Frequency of Lymph Node Metastasis
in Surgically Treated Cases

	Delgado et al.[92]		Fuller et al.[121]	
Study population	745 Stage I squamous CA, >3 mm in depth		431 IB and IIA squamous CA, adenocarcinoma, and others	
FIGO stage	I	15.5%	IB	15%
			IIA	22%
Cervical wall invasion			<1/3	0%
			middle 1/3	12%
			outer 1/3	24%
Stromal invasion	3–5 mm	3.4%		
	6–10 mm	15.1%		
	11–15 mm	22.2%		
	16–20 mm	38.8%		
	≥21 mm	22.6%		
LVSI	Absent	8.2%	Absent	14%
	Present	25.4%	Lymphatic	36%
			Vascular	56%
Parametrial disease	Absent	13.5%	Not evaluated	
	Present	25%		
Tumor size	Occult	8.9%		
	Gross	20.9%		
Histologic grade	Grade 1	9.7%	Grade 1	9%
	Grade 2	13.9%	Grade 2	16%
	Grade 3	21.8%	Grade 3	25%
Cell type	LCK	17.2%	Squamous	18%
	LCNK	17.2%	Adenocarcinoma	18%
	Small cell		Adenosquamous CA	17%
	and others	17.6%		
	Not significant		Not significant	

LCK, large cell keratinizing type; LCNK, large cell non-keratinizing type; LVSI, lymphatic vascular space invasion.

From Fu YS. Pathology of cervical carcinoma. In Sciarra JJ, ed. Gynecology and Obstetrics. Philadelphia, Lippincott Williams & Wilkins, 2000.

metastasis was found in none of 62 tumors involving the inner one third, in 16 of 130 (12%) tumors invading up to the middle third, and in 55 of 226 (24%) tumors extending into outer third.[121]

Viewed from a different perspective, Kishi et al.[190] measured the thickness of uninvolved cervical stroma from the deepest tumor to the external cervical wall in 287 of Stage IB, IIA, or IIB cervical squamous cancer. The pelvic nodal metastatic and 5-year cancer death rates were 7% and 8%, respectively, when the uninvolved stroma measured greater than 3 mm. Corresponding figures were 37% and 26% when the uninvolved stroma measured less than 3 mm. The authors felt that the uninvolved stroma acts as a barrier to cancer spread and that therefore its width is a more important measurement than the depth of tumor invasion.[190]

The depth of invasion in Stage I tumors clearly influences the pelvic lymph node metastasis and prognosis. When the tumor is less than 5 mm, 5% of the tumors had pelvic lymph node involvement, and only 1 (2.5%) of 41 women died. This was in contrast to an incidence of 23% nodal metastasis and 19% mortality when the tumor was deeper than 5 mm. Similarly, in patients with Stage IB, IIA, or IIB cervical squamous carcinoma, the depth of invasion correlated strongly with pelvic lymph node metastasis, parametrial extension, and survival.[162]

Cell Type

In 1959 Wentz and Reagan[376] divided cervical squamous cell carcinomas into three types: large cell keratinizing, large cell nonkeratinizing, and small cell. With the advent of electron microscopy and immunohistochemistry, it has become apparent that the original small cell "squamous" carcinoma really includes a heterogeneous group of tumors, such as small cell squamous carcinoma, small cell undifferentiated carcinoma, and small cell "neuroendocrine" carcinoma. In the WHO Histological Typing of Female Genital Tract Tumors, published in 1994,[314a] the conventional squamous cell carcinoma includes keratinizing and nonkeratinizing types. Small cell carcinomas with individual cell keratinization are classified as the nonkeratinizing type. Small cell carcinomas that resemble small cell anaplastic carcinoma of the lung are separately designated as "small cell carcinoma."[314a] Furthermore, a newly proposed classification has expanded the spectrum of neuroendocrine carcinoma to include both small cell and large cell types.[7]

For the purpose of comparison with squamous cell carcinoma, small cell and large cell neuroendocrine carcinomas are discussed here. Well and moderately differentiated neuroendocrine carcinomas are discussed in the section on neuroendocrine carcinoma.

Keratinizing squamous carcinoma is characterized by sheets and nests of cells with abundant cytoplasm, large pleomorphic nuclei, and inconspicuous nucleoli. Keratin pearls and intercellular bridges are evident (Fig. 8–73). Mitotic figures are noted occasionally, and the growth pattern is largely infiltrative.[286]

Nonkeratinizing large cell squamous carcinoma comprises predominantly cells containing a moderate or abundant amount of eosinophilic to amphophilic cytoplasm. Some cells reveal individual cell keratinization with distinct cell borders (Figs. 8–74A and B). Less differentiated cells have indistinct cell borders in a syncytial pattern (see Fig. 8–74C). By definition, keratin pearl formation should be absent. Nucleoli are prominent and mitotic figures are common. The invasive nests often have a smooth periphery.[286]

Nonkeratinizing small cell squamous carcinoma is characterized by broad, solid sheets of tumor cells associated with desmoplastic stroma (Fig. 8–75). Crush artifact and nuclear smudging are not prominent. Small to medium-sized tumor cells have hyperchromatic nuclei, scant cytoplasm, and small nucleoli. Keratinization is minimal or absent, and mitotic figures are abundant (Fig. 8–76). The nuclear chromatin is finely to coarsely granular, and small nucleoli are often evident.[113] The nuclear cytoplasmic ratio is lower than that for small cell anaplastic carcinoma, and the cell borders are more distinct.[113] The overlying mucosa may contain coexisting squamous dysplasia or carcinoma in situ.

The category of small cell carcinoma is reserved for cervical tumors that resemble small cell or intermediate cell anaplastic carcinoma of the lung.[72,125,137,326,369] In some tumors, diffuse sheets of small round cells infiltrate the stroma without reaction in a way similar to that of malignant lymphoma (Fig. 8–77A). In others, tumor cells infiltrate by irregular cords and nests in a delicate fibrovascular stroma (Fig. 8–78A). Desmoplastic reaction of the stroma is minimal or absent. At the lesion's periphery, an infiltrative pattern and vascular space invasion are invariably present.

On closer examination, some tumor cells have small round to oval hyperchromatic nuclei and scant cytoplasm resembling those seen in oat cell carcinoma of the lung (see Fig. 8–78B). In others, the tumor cells are arranged in rosettes, an organoid pattern, or trabeculae (see Fig. 8–78C). The nuclei range from oval

Text continued on page 360

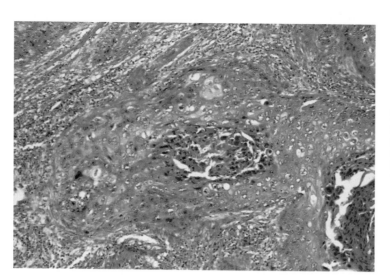

Figure 8–73. Keratinizing type of squamous cell carcinoma. Tumor cells reveal individual cell keratinization and keratin pearls with concentric arrangement of hyperkeratotic cells in the center of tumor nests.

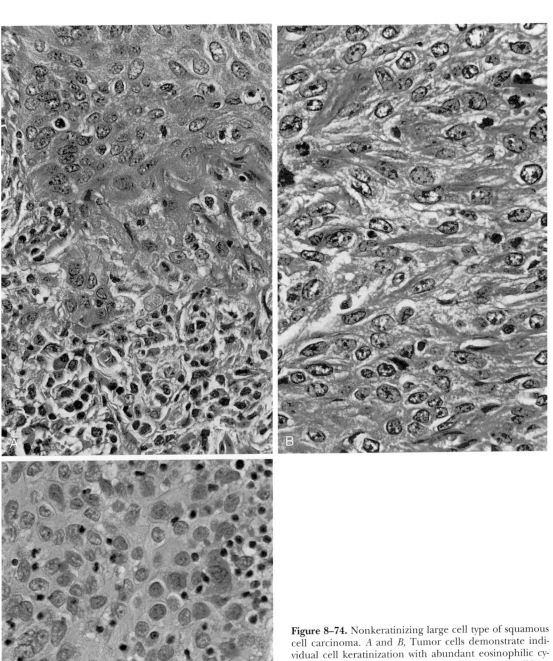

Figure 8–74. Nonkeratinizing large cell type of squamous cell carcinoma. *A* and *B,* Tumor cells demonstrate individual cell keratinization with abundant eosinophilic cytoplasm. The cell borders are well defined. *C,* The cell borders become indistinct with a syncytial appearance. The nuclei contain finely to coarsely granular chromatin and small to large nucleoli.

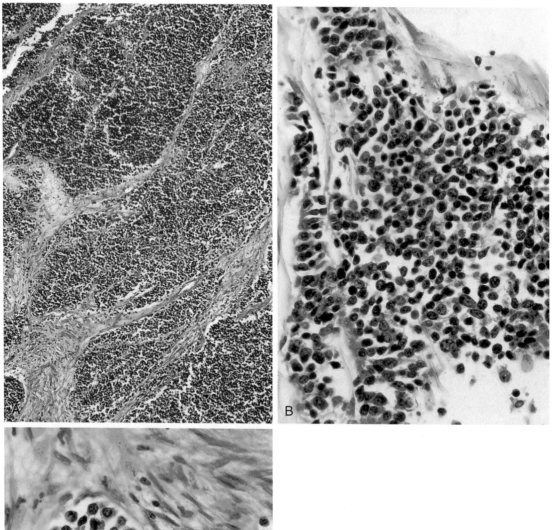

Figure 8–77. Small cell (anaplastic) carcinoma. *A,* Diffuse sheets of malignant small, round cells resembling malignant lymphoma. No desmoplastic stromal reaction is seen. *B,* Higher magnification reveals small, round to oval nuclei with coarsely granular chromatin, indistinct nucleoli, and scant cytoplasm. *C,* Rare columnar tumor forms a rosette-like arrangement. Tumor cells are positive for keratin but negative for neuroendocrine markers (not shown).

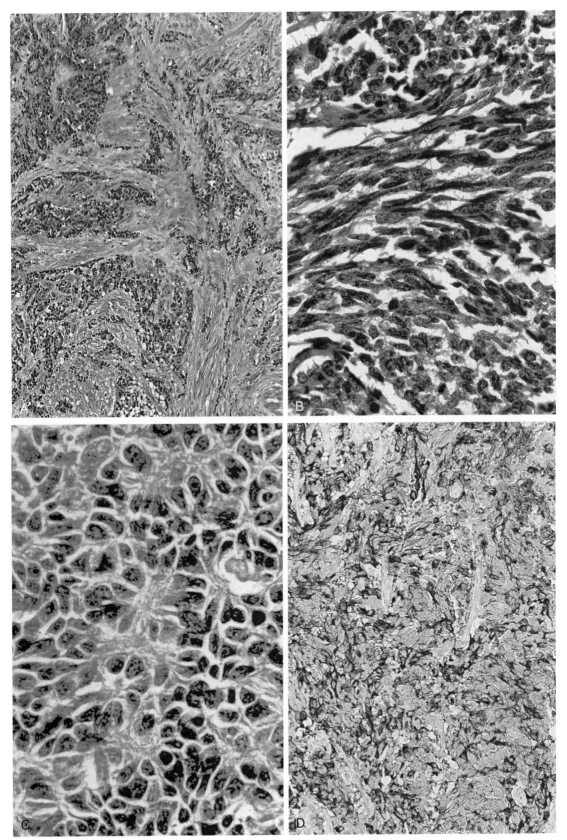

Figure 8–78. Small cell neuroendocrine carcinoma. *A,* Diffuse infiltrative pattern created by cords and nests of tumor cells in a fibrotic stroma. *B,* Small hyperchromatic nuclei are oval or elongated in shape. Cytoplasm is scant. *C,* Some tumor cells have medium-sized oval to irregular hyperchromatic nuclei and compact, coarsely granular chromatin. The nucleoli are absent or small. There is a suggestion of rosette-like arrangement. *D,* Immunohistochemical stain for chromogranin is strongly positive. (See color section.)

to elongated and are small to intermediate in size. The nuclear chromatin ranges from coarsely granular to dark and smudged (see Fig. 8–78B and C). Nucleoli are inconspicuous and mitotic figures are frequent. The cytoplasm in the majority of tumor cells is scant, resulting in nuclear molding and a high nuclear cytoplasmic ratio. A minority of tumor cells have a moderate amount of eosinophilic cytoplasm. Necrosis and crush artifact are common features. Evidence of neuroendocrine differentiation can be visualized with immunohistochemical stain by chromogranin, synaptophysin, or neuron specific enolase (see Fig. 8–78D).

In the case of large cell neuroendocrine carcinoma, the tumor cells also grow in diffuse infiltrative patterns. The tumor cells present with medium to large nuclear size and are round to oval or elongated in shape. Some cells have punctate coarsely chromatin and indistinct nucleoli, suggestive of neuroendocrine cells. However, many others have small to even large nucleoli and a moderate amount of cytoplasm. Overall, they resemble large cells of poorly differentiated carcinoma. Neuroendocrine markers are positive by immunohistochemistry (Fig. 8–79C).

Gilks et al.[127] reported on 12 patients with large cell neuroendocrine carcinoma, who ranged from 21 to 62 (mean 34) years of age. Two tumors were Stage IA2, nine were Stage IB, and one was Stage IIA. The predominant growth patterns included insular, trabecular, glandular, and solid. The tumor cells contained a moderate amount of eosinophilic cytoplasm and large nucleoli. In addition, eight tumors had coexisting adenocarcinoma in situ and three had adenocarcinomas. The mitotic activity in all tumors exceeded 10 mitotic figures per 10 high-power fields. By immunohistochemical stain, all 12 tumors expressed chromogranin. A poor prognosis was indicated by 7 of 10 patients dying of disease with more than a year of follow-up. Tumor recurred in the pelvis and lung in three women and in the liver in four others.[127] Three patients had no evidence of disease at 2.5, 3, and 3 years following treatment. Two had follow-up of less than a year.

Gilks et al.[127] also reviewed the literature for cases known as non–small cell neuroendocrine carcinomas and identified 20 of 31 (65%) of patients who died of disease, usually within the first 3 years after diagnosis. Among 21 women with Stage I disease, 12 (57%) died of disease, with a median survival of 16 months. It appears that the survival rates for small cell and large cell neuroendocrine carcinomas are comparable.[127]

In view of these findings, poorly differentiated small cell and large cell carcinomas with features of neuroendocrine differentiation should be studied by immunohistochemistry. With the use of routine hematoxylin and eosin–stained slides, these tumor cells demonstrate some of the characteristics common to neuroendocrine carcinoma, such as coarsely granular chromatin. Nucleoli in large cell neuroendocrine carcinoma vary from indistinct to large in size. In addition to the diffuse infiltrative pattern, tumor cells are also arranged in trabeculae, ribbons, and rosettes in close association with capillaries—the so-called organoid pattern.

The distinction of squamous cell carcinoma and other poorly differentiated carcinoma can be facilitated by immunohistochemical stain for p63, a homologue of p53. P63 is expressed in the immature squamous epithelium and reserve cells of the normal uterine cervix (see Chapter 2). In a survey of 250 cervical invasive carcinomas of all histologic types, a strong p63 expression (greater than 70% of tumor cells) was found in 97% of squamous cell carcinomas, including 100% of large cell keratinizing and nonkeratinizing types and 91% of small cell nonkeratinizing squamous carcinomas (Fig. 8–80A and B). None of the adenocarcinomas were positive for p63 (see Fig. 8–80C and D). Of the 11 neuroendocrine carcinomas, eight (73%) were positive for chromogranin, but all were negative or showed low expression (less than 30%) for p63 (see Fig. 8–79D).[370a] In the case of mixed adenosquamous carcinoma, p63 was positive in areas with squamous cell differentiation but negative in the glandular cells. One major advantage of this stain is its nuclear localization, which facilitates interpretation.

Small cell anaplastic/neuroendocrine carcinomas are believed to derive from multipotential cells or argyrophilic cells in the basal cell layer of the endocervical mucosa.[103] These tumors have the propensity to occur in young women (mean age 36 years versus 50 years in patients with small cell squamous carcinoma),[12] strong association with HPV type 18,[125,341] and aggressive behavior. When treated with radical hysterectomy and pelvic nodal dissection, four of six patients (67%)

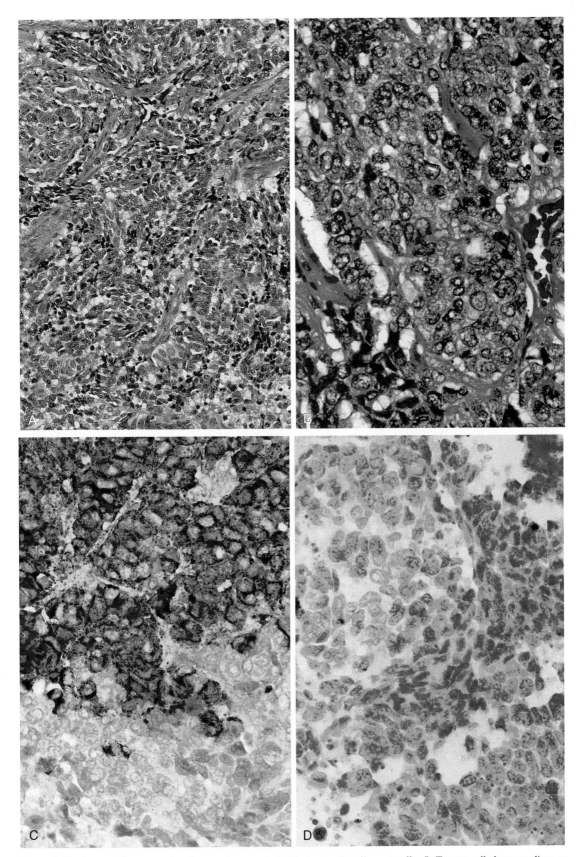

Figure 8–79. Large cell neuroendocrine carcinoma. *A,* Solid sheets of malignant cells. *B,* Tumor cells have medium to large nuclear size, open chromatin, a moderate amount of cytoplasm, and small nucleoli. *C,* Immunohistochemical stain for chromogranin is focally positive. *D,* Immunohistochemical stain for p63 is entirely negative. (See color section.)

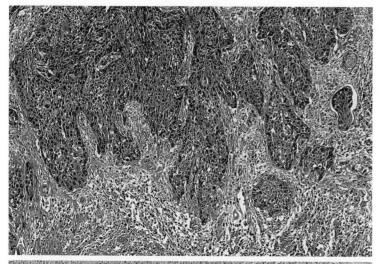

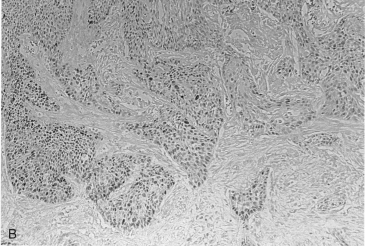

Figure 8–80. *A* and *B,* Squamous cell carcinoma. Most of the tumor cells express p63 by immunohistochemistry (*B*). *C* and *D,* Adenocarcinoma of cervix. Tumor cells are negative for p63 by immunohistochemical stain. In the overlying normal squamous mucosa, p63-positive cells are located in the deepest one to three layers. (Courtesy of Dr. Tao-Yuan Wang, Mackay Memorial Hospital, Taipei, Taiwan.) (See color section.)

with small cell carcinoma had pelvic nodal metastasis and five of eight women (63%) developed tumor recurrence, as compared with 18% nodal metastasis and 9% tumor recurrence in women with small cell squamous carcinoma.[12] Spread beyond the uterus and pelvis is common even for Stage I tumors. Small cell anaplastic/neuroendocrine carcinoma is recognized as one of the most aggressive types of cervical cancer, with a 5-year survival rate of 14% in one study.[4]

Sevin et al.[318] reported on 12 women with small cell carcinoma, including one Stage IA, 10 Stage IB, and one Stage II. When compared with Stage IB and II cervical squamous carcinoma and adenocarcinoma combined, small cell carcinoma had a higher frequency of vascular lymphatic space invasion (82% versus 62%), more frequent lymph node metastasis (45.5% versus 18.9%), and lower 5-year survival rate (36.4% versus 71.6%). Only 42% (5 of 12) of patients were disease free at the time of the report. In view of these findings, a combined therapy of surgery, radiotherapy, and cytotoxic chemotherapy is recommended.[318]

The value of separating squamous carcinoma by cell type was evaluated using the data of the Gynecologic Oncology Group (GOG). Among women with Stage I squamous cell carcinoma treated surgically, the cell type was not predictive of pelvic nodal metastasis and outcome.[392]

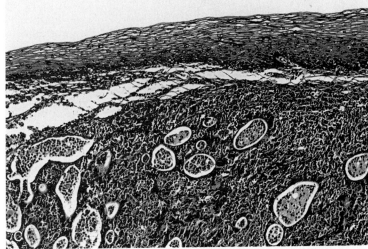

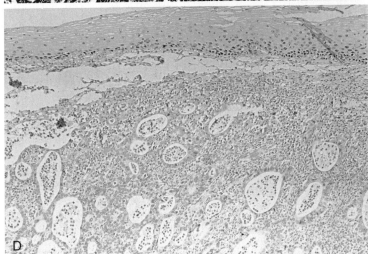

Figure 8–80. *Continued*

The progression-free rate at 5 years was 84% for large cell keratinizing and 74% for large cell nonkeratinizing (P = not significant) and 75% for grade 1, 82% for grade 2, and 78% for grade 3 (P = not significant).[392]

In the GOG study of women with Stage IIB to IVA squamous carcinoma treated by radiation therapy, the classification of keratinizing or nonkeratinizing type by the original criteria did not correlate with prognosis. However, when tumors with individual cell keratinization were reclassified in the keratinizing category, this group of tumors had a significantly higher recurrence/death rate than the nonkeratinizing type (65.8% versus 53.5%, P = 0.0074).[340]

Histologic Grade

The histologic grade reflects the degree of differentiation of the tumor cells. The most commonly used grading system for squamous carcinoma is a modification of the original Broders' system consisting of three grades based on the amount of keratin, the degree of nuclear atypia, and the mitotic activity. Grade 1, well-differentiated lesions exhibit abundant intercellular bridging, cytoplasmic keratinization, and keratin pearls. The cells are relatively uniform with minimal nuclear pleomorphism. The mitotic rate should be less than 2 per high-power field.[113] Grade 2, moderately differentiated lesions show primarily individual cell keratinization, moderate nuclear pleomorphism, and up to four mitotic figures per high-power field.[113] Grade 3, poorly differentiated lesions show little evidence of squamous differentiation. The tumor cells are immature, with marked nuclear pleomorphism, scant cytoplasm, and greater than four mitotic figures per high-power field.[113]

The histologic grade of Stage I and II cervical carcinomas (including squamous carcinoma and adenocarcinoma) did not affect survival rates in a study by Sevin et al.[318] Others have found poorly differentiated tumor to have a higher pelvic nodal metastasis (Table 8–8).[91,121] The degree of differentiation in adenocarcinoma is closely related to prognosis and pelvic nodal metastasis. In Stage I and II adenocarcinomas, pelvic nodal metastases were found in 5% of grade 1, 11% of grade 2, and 50% of grade 3 tumors.[34]

In surgically treated patients with Stage I and II squamous cell carcinomas, some studies have found histologic grade to influence prognosis and pelvic nodal metastasis.[91] In a GOG study of Stage I squamous carcinoma, the histologic grade was correlated to the frequency of pelvic nodal metastasis. Pelvic nodal metastasis occurred in 9.7%, 13.9%, and 21.8% of grade 1, grade 2, and grade 3 tumors, respectively.[91] Fuller et al. reported a comparable result (see Table 8–8).[121] Some investigators of Stage IB and IIA carcinomas have found that grade 3 tumors were larger and had a higher incidence of lymph node metastasis than did lower grade lesions.[121] Fuller et al.[121] found that 25% of grade 3 tumors had pelvic lymph node metastases, compared with 9% and 16% in grades 1 and 2 tumors, respectively.

Among 445 patients with Stage IIB through IVA squamous cell carcinoma treated by radiation therapy following GOG protocols, the histologic grade had no impact on prognosis.[340] Similar findings were reported by others.[82,285]

In the early 1980s, an alternative malignancy grading system (MGS) was proposed.[337] In the MGS system, eight morphologic parameters of a tumor, consisting of four characteristics of the tumor cell population (structure [i.e., papillary versus solid], degree of cell differentiation, nuclear pleomorphism, and mitotic activity) and four characteristics of the tumor-host relationship (mode of invasion, stage of invasion, extent of vascular invasion, and degree of host inflammatory response [lymphoplasmacytic]) were evaluated and scored on a scale of 1 to 3 points, with minimum score of 8 and a maximum score of 24.[338] When this grading system was applied to 445 Stage IIB to IVA squamous carcinoma patients treated by radiation therapy, the recurrence/death rates were 32.9% for women whose tumors scored up to 12 points, 57.3% for tumors rated 14 to 16 points, and 64.8% for neoplasms over 18 points ($P = 0.004$).[340]

Vascular Lymphatic Space Invasion

Shrinkage artifact after formalin fixation often results in clear empty spaces in the periphery of tumor nests, simulating vascular space. These artifacts do not have well-defined endothelial cells. In true vascular invasion, the tumor cells are partially adherent to the endothelial cells, which should be clearly identifiable. In addition, blood and sometime fibrin thrombi are present in the vascular lumen. The frequency of lymphatic-vascular space invasion is closely related to the depth of stromal invasion.[48] Vascular invasion is associated with increased pelvic nodal metastasis, higher tumor recurrence, and decreased survival in Stage I and II squamous carcinoma and adenocarcinoma (see Tables 8–7 and 8–8).[48,91,121,179,377]

Some studies have reported a significant difference in progression of Stage I tumors with lymphatic or blood vessel invasion. In women treated with surgery alone (hysterectomy and pelvic lymphadenectomy), 5-year survival was 69% in the presence of lymphatic invasion compared with 30% in women with blood vessel invasion.[23] The comparable rate was 90% in the absence of any vascular or lymphatic space invasion. Pelvic lymph node metastasis is higher when blood vessel invasion occurs.[34]

A positive association between vascular invasion and disease recurrence is not evident in Stage II and higher neoplasms. In fact, several studies of Stage II and III cervical squamous carcinomas found that vascular invasion had no bearing on long-term survival.[36]

A study by Sakuragi et al.[309] included 189 women with squamous cell carcinomas and 50 with adenocarcinomas and adenosquamous carcinomas, all of whom were treated by radical hysterectomy. Their clinical stage was 94 tumors in Stage IB, 15 in Stage IIA, 93 in Stage IIB, and 37 in Stage IIIB. The lymphatic space invasion was defined as the presence of tumor in a space lined by flattened endothelial cells, with or without lymphocytes. In contrast, blood vessel invasion is determined by the presence of flattened endothelial lining cells and red blood cells in the lumen.[309]

Using these criteria, the parameters related to increased risk for the development of pelvic lymph node metastasis by logistic regression model included invasion of the uterus, parametrial invasion, lymphatic space invasion, and blood vessel invasion. By multivariate analysis, only parametrial invasion and lymphatic space invasion were significant for the development of nodal metastasis.[309] There was no difference in the frequency of lymphatic space invasion between squamous cell carcinoma (52.9%) and adenocarcinoma and adenosquamous carcinoma (66%). However, there was a statistically significant difference for blood vessel invasion: 18% for squamous cell carcinoma and 34% for adenocarcinoma and adenosquamous carcinomas had blood vessel involvement ($P < 0.05$). There were also strong correlations among depth of stromal invasion, FIGO stage, and the frequency of lymphatic space invasion and blood vessel invasion.[309] Based on these findings, it appears that it is important to distinguish between lymphatic and blood vessel invasion. The question remains as to whether the authors' criteria are reliable in separating lymphatic and blood vessel invasions.

Growth Patterns and Stromal Response

A variety of growth patterns and stromal reactions have been described in cervical squamous cell carcinoma, but none are prognostically useful. Similarly, the results of vascular density counts are conflicting in relation to radiosensitivity of the tumor and prognosis.[303]

Parametrial Extension

The parametrial tissue surrounding the uterine cervix contains major blood vessels, lymphatics, and occasionally lymph nodes. Involvement of parametrium usually results from direct extension of locally advanced tumor and less frequently by lymphatic or vascular spread (Fig. 8–81A and B). Parametrial invasion is defined as tumor extension beyond the deepest portion of cervical smooth muscle layer (see Fig. 8–81A and B). In the presence of parametrial invasion, tumor cells occur in the fibroadipose tissue outside the muscular layer (see Fig. 8–81C).

Histologic documentation of parametrial spread is critical prognostically. A positive finding correlates strongly with (1) vascular invasion, (2) presence of tumor cells close to or at the surgical margins, (3) pelvic nodal metastasis, (4) tumor recurrence, and (5) death from disease.[59,325] Of women with Stage I cervical cancer who were treated surgically, 50% with parametrial extension died of disease. This is in contrast to 8% of those without parametrial spread.[325]

Bemedetto-Panici et al.,[29] studied 69 radical hysterectomy specimens removed for Stage IB and IIA cervical carcinomas by giant sections. Ninety-three percent of women had lymph nodes in the parametrium. Parametrial involvement was found in 31% of Stage IB1 tumors, 63% of Stage IB2 tumors, and 58% of Stage IIA tumors. Thirty-six percent of women had pelvic lymph node metastasis or had involvement of parametrium. The overall 5-year survival rate for this group of patients was 91%. In the absence of parametrial disease and lymph node metastasis, the 5-year survival rate was 100%, as compared with 78% with parametrial or lymph node involvement. This study emphasizes the importance of detecting parametrial involvement. In many cases, parametrial extension was not clinically suspected.[29]

In a study by Kamura et al.,[179] the 5-year survival rates for Stage IB and II patients treated by radical surgery were 90.3% and 77.3% without and with parametrial involvement, respectively (see Table 8–7).[179]

Tumor extension into the parametrium, a highly vascular site, occurs by contiguous spread and less often by lymphatic or vascular invasion. When present, parametrial invasion is associated with a higher incidence of vascular invasion, positive lymph nodes, tumor recurrence, and death (see Table 8–8).[59,91]

Lymph Node Metastasis

The frequency of pelvic lymph node metastasis is influenced by parameters such as FIGO stage, tumor size, depth of stromal invasion, lymphatic-vascular space invasion, and histologic grade (see Table 8–8).[91,121,126,294,275] In some series, 15% of clinical Stage I and 26% to 35% of Stage II cervical carcinomas have positive lymph nodes at the time of diagnosis.[121,228,354] The pelvic lymph nodes most frequently involved are the paracervical, obturator, and external iliac chains.[211] The likelihood of recurrence and death increases in the presence of pelvic lymph node metastases and is related to the number of positive

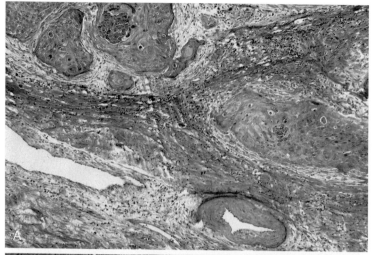

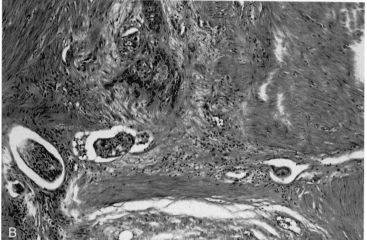

Figure 8–81. *A,* Deeply invasive squamous carcinoma still within the outermost layer of smooth muscle cells. Parametrium is not invaded by tumor. *B,* Vascular invasion in the deep cervical stromal. *C,* Tumor extension into the parametrial fibroadipose tissue. The resection margin, although close to tumor, is not involved by tumor.

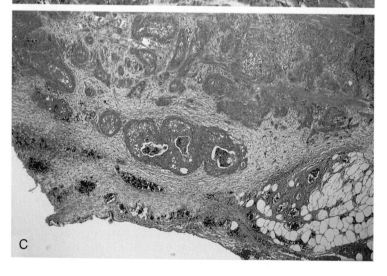

nodes.[126,275] In a series of 97 patients with Stage IB to IIB carcinoma, one third of patients with one positive lymph node and two thirds with three or more positive nodes had tumor recurrence within 5 years. In another study of Stage I and II carcinomas, the survival rate was 59% with unilateral and 20% with bilateral lymph node metastases.[275]

From the iliac lymph nodes, tumor cells may spread to the para-aortic lymph nodes and then to the scalene and other nodes.[302] Tumor involvement of these sites is associated with disseminated disease in more than 75% of patients.[50] Para-aortic lymph node involvement is present in 6% of Stage IB carcinoma and 30% of Stage II and III disease. When all series are combined, the overall incidence of scalene lymph node metastasis from all cervical carcinomas is about 15%.[366] When para-aortic lymph nodes are involved, the frequency of an occult scalene metastasis ranges from 0% to 50% (mean 28%).[366] Identification of such patients through scalene biopsy may result in more accurate staging.

In women with Stage I or II cervical adenocarcinoma treated surgically, lymph node metastases in the pelvic or para-aortic region occurred in 15% of Stage I and 40% of Stage II tumors. In the presence of pelvic lymph node metastasis, the 5-year survival rate decreased from 92% to 10%.[34]

Kim et al.[189] investigated 43 women with para-aortic lymph node metastasis from Stage IB to IVB. The overall 5-year survival rate was 24%, with a median survival of 18 months. Of women without gross residual disease in the para-aortic lymph nodes following surgical staging, 31% were alive and free of disease, as compared with only 6% when gross residual disease remained.[189]

These data were confirmed by more recent studies. For women with Stage IB and II carcinoma, the 3-year survival rate was 94% without any lymph node metastasis, 64% with pelvic lymph node metastasis, and 35% with para-aortic lymph node involvement. When metastasis was limited to unilateral pelvic lymph nodes, the 3-year survival rate was 74%, as compared with 37% for those with bilateral disease. If para-aortic lymph nodes were not involved, the 3-year survival rate was 88%; when they were involved, the rate dropped to 35%.[247] With up to two positive pelvic lymph nodes, the 3-year survival rate was 65%; in contrast, 3-year survival dropped to 40% when more than two

nodes were involved. The presence of extracapsular spread further worsened the prognosis.[247]

Ovarian Metastasis

Cervical cancer rarely metastasizes to the ovary.[276] In a study of 318 women with Stage IA cervical squamous cell carcinoma treated by simple hysterectomy with ovarian preservation, no ovarian disease was noted in any of the patients with long-term follow-up.[346] In a separate study of 105 women with Stage I cervical squamous cell carcinoma, no ovarian metastasis was found in the removed ovaries.[267] In a series of 770 women with Stage IB cervical squamous cell carcinoma treated by radical hysterectomy, only 4 women (0.5%) were found to have ovarian metastasis.[345]

The risk of ovarian metastasis in a study with the use of a logistic regression model was associated with cell type (squamous cell carcinoma versus adenocarcinoma), corpus invasion, parametrial invasion, and lymphatic-vascular invasion. Adenocarcinomas and adenosquamous carcinomas caused more metastasis than did squamous cell carcinoma. There was no metastasis in Stage IB or IIA tumors. The rate of metastisis increased to 5.4% for Stage IIB tumors and 13.5% for Stage III disease, however. Ovarian metastasis was significantly associated with blood vessel invasion.[309]

Cervical Cancer in Pregnant Women

Hacker et al.[139] reviewed the literature on the occurrence of cervical in situ and invasive carcinoma detected during pregnancy or in the first 12 months postpartum. The incidence of squamous carcinoma in situ was 1.3 per 1000 pregnancies, or 1 per 770 pregnancies. Invasive carcinoma occurred in 1 per 2205 pregnancies, or 0.45 per 1000 pregnancies. This suggests that one in 34 cervical cancer patients is pregnant.

Pregnant women with cervical cancer are generally younger than are nonpregnant women with cervical cancer. The mean age of pregnant women with carcinoma in situ is 29.9 years (versus 35 years for nonpregnant women); the mean age for women with invasive carcinoma is 33.8 years (versus 48 years for nonpregnant women).[139]

Cervical cancer is generally detected at an earlier stage in pregnant women, with 42% in Stage IB, 33% in Stage II, and 25% in Stage III or IV.[139] When the disease is detected late in pregnancy or postpartum, however, it tends to be more advanced. Overall, 50% of invasive carcinomas in this population are detected postpartum. Histologically, 93% of women have squamous carcinoma, 3% adenocarcinoma, 3% anaplastic carcinoma, 1% adenosquamous carcinoma, and 0.1% each adenoacanthoma and sarcoma. The survival rates for Stage I cancer are similar in pregnant and in nonpregnant women.[11,139,209] In more advanced disease, survival is adversely affected by pregnancy.[139,209]

Cervical Cancer in Young Women

Stanhope et al.[334] found a lower survival rate for cervical cancer patients younger than 35 years. When compared stage by stage, the survival rates in women younger than 35 years were 10% lower for Stage IB disease and 32% lower for Stage II disease, when compared with older population. The treatment failure was particularly high in young women with Stage IIB disease, primarily owing to distant metastasis. A subsequent study showed a similar trend. Among women aged 23 and 39 years who received radiotherapy for cervical cancer, 5-year survival rates were 70%, 54%, 17%, and 0%, respectively, for Stage I to IV disease.[279] These findings are best explained by an unusual number of distant metastases (26% in Stage I and 42% in Stage II) and poorly differentiated carcinoma that occurred in this population.

In a study by Morice et al.[247] among women with Stage IB and II disease, those younger than 30 years were found to have a higher rate of pelvic lymph node metastasis than older patients.

Carcinoma of the Cervical Stump

Following subtotal hysterectomy, the retained cervix may be affected by an in situ or invasive carcinoma, mostly of the squamous type. In one study, carcinoma was detected in 18% of the resected cervical stumps, including 15% in situ and 3% invasive carcinomas.[278] The reported frequency of invasive carcinoma in the cervical stump is in the range of 1% to 2%. This occurrence is expected to decline further, because subtotal hysterectomy is currently performed only under special circumstances. The outcome for women with carcinoma of the stump diagnosed more than 2 years after subtotal hysterectomy is generally comparable to that of women with an intact uterus. Lower survival is noted, however, among women whose carci-

noma was detected within 2 years of subtotal hysterectomy. Presumably, the carcinoma in these women was present but not identified at the time of surgery.

Prognosis

Several large series have applied statistical models to identify prognostic parameters of cervical carcinoma among women treated by radical surgery and radiation therapy. In a study by Sevin et al.,[318] 370 women with Stage I or II carcinomas were treated by radical hysterectomy and pelvic lymphadenectomy. By univariate analysis, the disease-free survival rates were closely related to the depth of stromal invasion, tumor size, presence or absence of lymphatic-vascular space invasion, pelvic lymph node status, tumor volume, and clinical stage.[318]

Kamura et al.[179] studied 211 women with Stage IB or II cervical carcinoma treated by radical hysterectomy and pelvic lymphadenectomy. By univariate analysis, the 5-year survival rates were correlated with lymph node status, cell type (squamous carcinoma versus adenocarcinoma), tumor dimension, depth of stromal invasion, lymphatic-vascular space invasion, and parametrial invasion.[179]

Fuller et al.[121] studied 431 women with Stage IB or IIA carcinoma treated by radical hysterectomy, including 85% squamous carcinomas, 9% adenocarcinomas, 3% adenosquamous carcinomas, 2% small cell carcinomas, and 1% clear cell carcinomas. A decreased survival was strongly related to the presence of pelvic lymph node metastasis.[121] Among cases with no lymph node metastisis, the adenocarcinoma cell type, increasing tumor size, deeper stromal invasion, and poor histologic grade were associated with decreased survival.[121] Increasing tumor size and depth of invasion and histologic grade were covariable and predictors of both lymph node metastasis and recurrence.[121] In this study, poorly differentiated tumors were larger.[121]

Most authors thus agree that for surgically treated Stage IB and II cervical carcinomas, the depth of stromal invasion, tumor dimension, the presence or absence of lymphatic-vascular space invasion, and pelvic lymph node status are the most important prognosticators. The value of classification by cell type and histologic grade continues to be controversial.[27,362]

With a multivariate stepwise regression model, it is possible to use several parameters to subdivide tumors into different risk groups.

Kamura et al.[179] developed such a scheme based on lymph node status, cell type, and tumor dimension. Sevin et al.[320] identified three risk groups on the basis of depth of stromal invasion, lymphatic-vascular space invasion, age, and lymph node status.

In the series of Barillot et al.,[25] 1875 women were treated by radiotherapy, including Stage IA to IB, 25.5%; Stage IIA, 12%; Stage IIB, 29%; Stage IIIA, 5%; Stage IIIB, 25%; and Stage IV, 3.5%. By univariate analysis of Stage I to II cases, FIGO stage, tumor diameter, and lymph nodal status were significant parameters. The 5-year survival rates were 83.5% for Stage IB, 81% for Stage IIA, 71% for Stage IIB, 65% for Stage IIIA, and 59% for Stage IIIB.[25] The 5-year survival rates were 86% for tumors less than 3 cm, 76% for tumors 3 to 5 cm, and 61.5% for tumors greater than 5 cm. The survival rates was 90% in the case of negative lymphangiogram, as compared to 65% if positive. Women younger than 30 years had better survival rates than older women (91% versus 75%). Women with adenocarcinoma had a 10% lower 5-year survival rate than those with squamous cell carcinoma.[25]

By multivariate analysis, FIGO stage and nodal involvement remained significant for all stages. For Stage I to II tumors, those greater than 5 cm and adenocarcinoma were notably poor prognosticators.[25]

Tumor Recurrence

Tumor recurrences are divided into three categories: central (involving vaginal cuff, bladder, or rectum), pelvic sidewall, and distant or extrapelvic. By combining multiple studies, tumor recurrence is reported to be central in 14% to 28% of cases, sidewall or sidewall and central in 37% to 59%, and distant in 35% to 42%.[196,203,213] In a large study, 40 of 303 (13%) women with Stage IB to IIB cervical cancers developed recurrence following radical hysterectomy and pelvic lymphadenectomy.[196] In a literature review, tumor recurrence develops within 12 months of initial treatment in 45% to 58% of cases and within 3 years in 70% to 90% of cases.[196] Pelvic recurrence may be asymptomatic and detected only on physical examination, or it may be suspected by nonspecific symptoms such as vaginal bleeding or discharge. Pelvic sidewall recurrence may produce pain in the lower abdomen, back, hip, or leg. Patients with distant metastasis may present with pain or a mass lesion.

Usual sites of distant metastasis in cervical carcinoma include the periureteral, abdominal, hepatic, and para-aortic regions. Spread to scalene node occurs through the thoracic duct. Unusual sites of recurrence, such as cutaneous lymphatic dissemination, are occasionally reported.[20]

Survival statistics following tumor recurrence are discouraging. In one study, 36% of women with central recurrence died within 1 year, compared with 65% with sidewall or distant metastases. Only 13% of patients had no evidence of disease 5 years following tumor recurrence.[196]

Successful treatment of pelvic recurrence by radiation therapy has been reported. In a study by Larson et al.,[203] eight of 15 (53%) patients with pelvic recurrence who were treated with irradiation were free of disease 10 to 126 (median 48) months after recurrence. In a literature review, 80% of patients with recurrent disease failed to be controlled.[203]

Autopsy studies reveal that the cause of death in cervical cancer has changed over the years. Although the incidence of ureteral blockage has remained unchanged, subsequent death from uremia has decreased in incidence from 28% between the years 1935 and 1964 to 6.7% in the years 1965 to 1979. This difference is attributed to the benefits of radiotherapy. The most frequent terminal events are pulmonary embolus, myocardial infarct, bronchopneumonia, and cachexia.[184]

Variants of Squamous Cell Carcinoma

Verrucous Squamous Carcinoma

Verrucous squamous carcinoma of the cervix, like that of other sites, represents a well-differentiated form of squamous cell carcinoma. Grossly, these tumors appear exophytic and warty and may simulate a condyloma acuminatum. Histologically, the cells in this variant show orderly maturation and lack of cytologic atypia. The tumor grows by expansion with smooth pushing margins, as opposed to the infiltrating pattern of conventional squamous cell carcinoma (Fig. 8–82).

To differentiate verrucous squamous carcinoma from condyloma, pseudoepitheliomatous hyperplasia, or conventional squamous carcinoma, full-thickness biopsies are necessary. Some squamous carcinomas have a verrucous appearance but show severe nuclear atypia and foci of invasion by nests of single cells. These tumors behave like conventional squamous carcinoma and should be identified as such. Condyloma

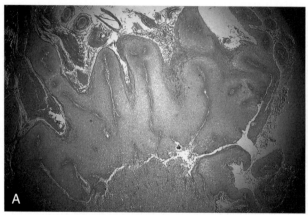
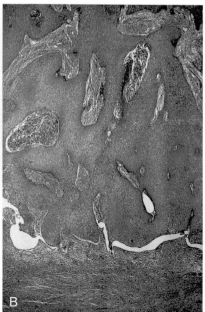
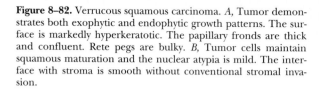

Figure 8–82. Verrucous squamous carcinoma. *A,* Tumor demonstrates both exophytic and endophytic growth patterns. The surface is markedly hyperkeratotic. The papillary fronds are thick and confluent. Rete pegs are bulky. *B,* Tumor cells maintain squamous maturation and the nuclear atypia is mild. The interface with stroma is smooth without conventional stromal invasion.

acuminatum has prominent koilocytosis and delicate fibrovascular cores, as opposed to the compressed cores and confluent epithelial growth pattern seen in verrucous squamous carcinoma. Condylomas also lack the expansile, endophytic extension into the stroma seen in verrucous squamous carcinomas.

According to Tiltman and Atad,[353] although none of the reported cervical verrucous squamous carcinomas metastasized to the lymph node, direct local extension to the adjacent organ, including the vagina and endometrium, is common. Some of these extensions appear as carcinoma in situ. Incomplete excision or resistance to radiotherapy led to local tumor recurrence in 40% to 50% of cases.[31]

Papillary Squamous (Squamotransitional) Cell Carcinoma

Randall et al.[283] initially reported nine squamous cell carcinomas of the cervix having a papillary, fungating, wart-like appearance. In recent years, terms such as *papillary squamotransitional cell carcinoma* and *transitional cell carcinoma* were used.[10,191]

In contrast to verrucous carcinoma, a moderate to severe degree of nuclear atypism occurs. Fibrovascular cores in a papillary pattern support solid sheets of dysplastic cells. In superficial biopsies, stromal invasion is generally

not demonstrable (Figs. 8–83 and 8–84). Similar to the diagnosis of verrucous carcinoma, deep biopsies or an excisional specimen is required to distinguish between an in situ and an invasive carcinoma (see Figs. 8–83 and 8–84).

In a series of 32 women, aged 22 to 93 (mean 50) years, they presented with abnormal bleeding or abnormal cervical smears.[191] Tumor size ranged from 0.7 to 6.0 (mean 3.0) cm. The diagnostic problems are indicated by the fact that only 63% (20 of 32) of specimens were considered adequate. The remaining 37% were too superficial to determine in situ or invasive carcinoma. Of those with suitable specimens, 90% (18 of 20) had stromal invasion.[191] Full-thickness biopsies, to include the underlying stroma, are necessary to distinguish in situ from invasive lesions.

Histologically, most of the tumor cells resemble large cell nonkeratinizing squamous cells with moderate to severe nuclear atypia and high mitotic activity. Some of the tumor cells have convoluted nuclei with nuclear grooves and resemble urothelial cells (see Fig. 8–83C). By immunostain, only 9.5% (2 of 21) of tumors expressed cytokeratin 20, a marker of urothelial cells. Their immunoreactivity is similar to conventional squamous cell carcinomas manifesting almost exclusively cytokeratin 7.[191]

In a series of nine cases, one tumor was an in situ carcinoma, whereas the remaining eight

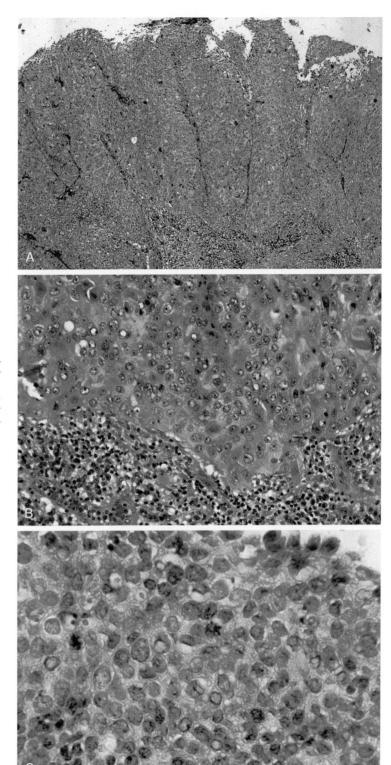

Figure 8–83. Papillary squamotransitional cell carcinoma. *A,* Papillary growth pattern on low-power view. *B,* At the interface with stroma, there is minimal stromal invasion. *C,* Tumor cells reveal severe nuclear atypia, vesicular nuclei, and nuclear grooves.

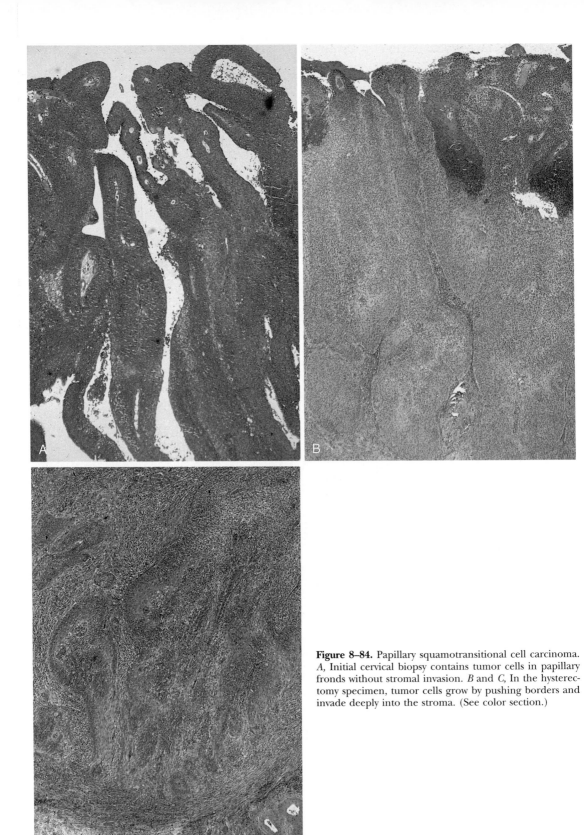

Figure 8–84. Papillary squamotransitional cell carcinoma. *A,* Initial cervical biopsy contains tumor cells in papillary fronds without stromal invasion. *B* and *C,* In the hysterectomy specimen, tumor cells grow by pushing borders and invade deeply into the stroma. (See color section.)

cases ranged from Stage I to Stage IV invasive carcinoma.[283] In another study, the FIGO stage was known in 11 women, including two Stage 0, three Stage IA, two Stage IB, one Stage IIA, one Stage IIB, and two Stage IIIB.[191] In this series, only 12 women had follow-up information, and all three patients with Stage IIB or higher died, with a mean survival of 13 months after diagnosis.[191] One patient developed ovarian metastasis, one had vaginal recurrence 12 years later, and in the third patient adenosquamous carcinoma of the endometrium occurred. Five women were alive and well, and three died of other causes. Late recurrence and metastasis were known to occur many years following treatment.[283]

Circumscribed Carcinoma, Lymphoepithelioma-like Carcinoma

Hasumi et al.,[148] in 1977, reported on 39 cervical carcinomas, which were characterized grossly by a well-circumscribed, expansile mass with a bulging, homogeneous cut surface and superficial ulceration. Microscopically, tumor cells were uniform in size and shape and were arranged in solid cords with minimal squamous differentiation. The large nuclei revealed one or two prominent nucleoli and numerous mitotic figures (Fig. 8–85). The cytoplasm appeared clear, slightly eosinophilic, or finely granular. The loose fibrillary stroma was infiltrated by numerous lymphocytes and eosinophils. All 39 carcinomas were more than 5.0 mm in depth but were confined to the cervix. When compared with conventional squamous carcinoma of comparable clinical stage, this variant has a favorable outcome, with a 5-year survival rate of 97% (versus 79% for squamous carcinoma, $P < 0.05$) and low pelvic lymph node metastasis (5% versus 18% for squamous carcinoma, $P < 0.05$).[148]

This group of tumors may be similar to those described by Bostrom and Hart,[46] Kapp and

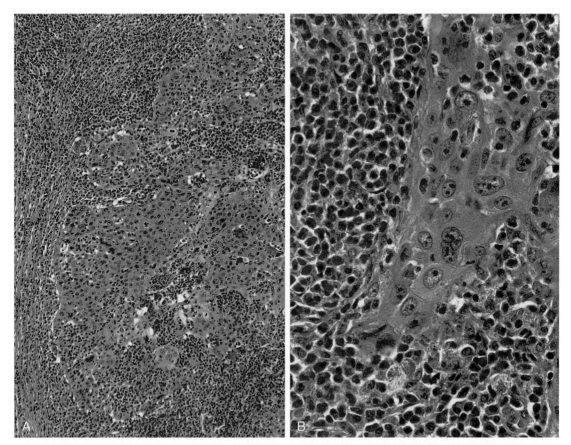

Figure 8–85. Circumscribed carcinoma, lymphoepithelioma-like carcinoma. *A,* Solid tumor nests are surrounded by abscess-like infiltration of eosinophils. *B,* Tumor cells have large, irregular nuclei; prominent nucleoli; and syncytial-like arrangement with ill-defined cell borders. Eosinophils are abundant in the stroma.

LiVolsi,[181] and Mills et al.[242] The latter authors used the term *lymphoepithelioma-like carcinoma.* The tumor bears some resemblance to undifferentiated nasopharyngeal carcinoma and malignant lymphoepithelial lesion of the salivary gland.[140,142,250] The malignant cells had abundant eosinophilic cytoplasm, round to oval nuclei, and prominent nucleoli. Some of the nuclei are bizarre and multinucleated (Fig. 8–86). The stroma was infiltrated by abundant lymphocytes, eosinophils, and plasma cells and might be confused with that seen in lymphoproliferative disorder.

In a study by Tseng et al.,[357] 15 such tumors were compared with conventional squamous cell carcinomas. With the use of PCR, Epstein-Barr viral gene sequences were found in 73% (11 of 15) of tumors, as compared to 27% (4 of 15) of the usual squamous cell carcinomas ($P = 0.001$). Interestingly, HPV types 16 and 18 were also detected in 20% (3 of 15) of these tumors, as compared with 80% (12 of 15) of the usual squamous cell carcinomas ($P = 0.001$).[357]

Although the total number of cases in the literature is too small for complete understanding of these neoplasms, they appear to have a better prognosis than conventional squamous cell carcinoma. After radical hysterectomy, all 15 patients were alive and well.[357]

Spindle Cell Squamous Carcinoma

Spindle cell squamous carcinoma is a rare variant of poorly differentiated carcinoma and may be confused with either melanoma or sarcoma. This tumor comprises cells with large, spindle-shaped or oblong nuclei arranged in fascicles (Figs. 8–87 and 8–88). A portion of the tumor sometimes contains cells with individual cell keratinization that is diagnostic for squamous cell origin. However, in many instances the entire tumor is made up of poorly differentiated spindle cells in a fibromyxoid stroma. The spindle cells may be arranged in interlacing bundles that simulate fibrosarcoma and leiomyosarcoma. When tumor cells are arranged in a

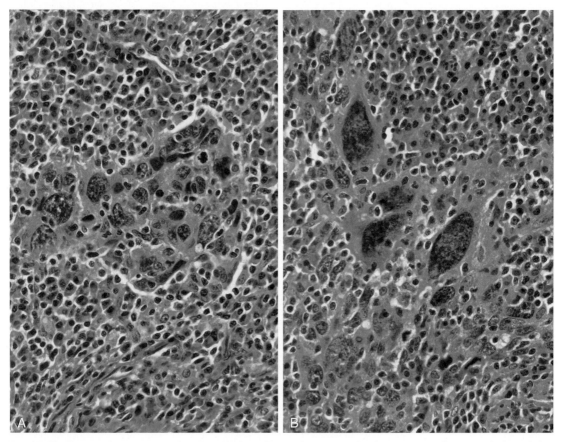

Figure 8–86. Circumscribed carcinoma, lymphoepithelioma-like carcinoma. *A* and *B,* Some tumor cells are anaplastic and pleomorphic in appearance.

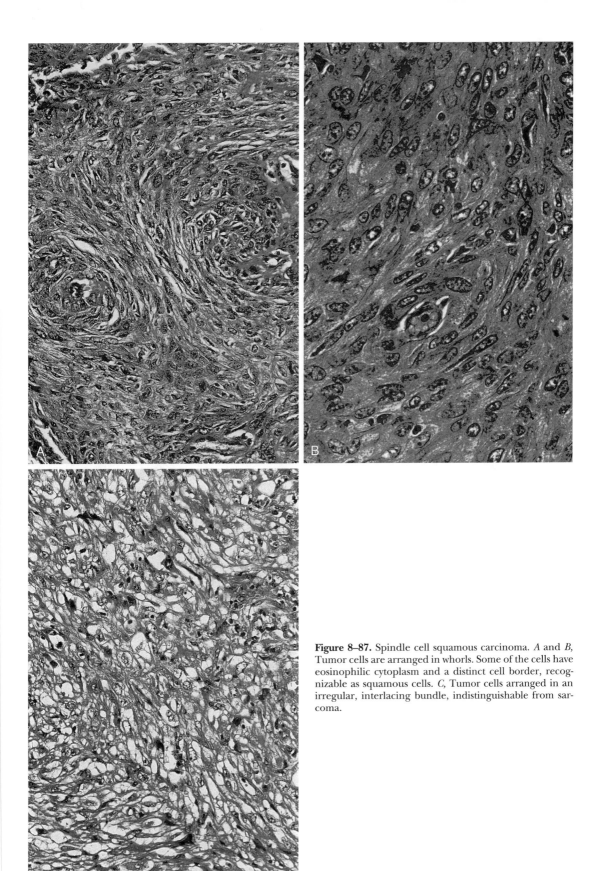

Figure 8–87. Spindle cell squamous carcinoma. *A* and *B,* Tumor cells are arranged in whorls. Some of the cells have eosinophilic cytoplasm and a distinct cell border, recognizable as squamous cells. *C,* Tumor cells arranged in an irregular, interlacing bundle, indistinguishable from sarcoma.

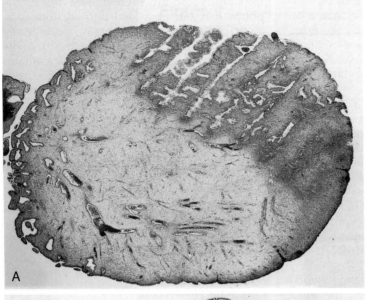

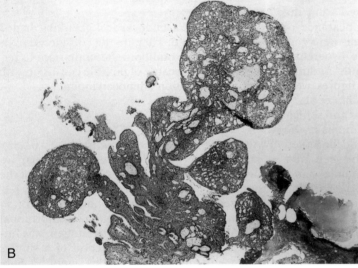

Figure 8–89. Endocervical polyp with predominantly fibrous stroma (*A*) and adenomatous tissue (*B*). Blood vessels are prominent in the base and the stalks of the polyp. Focal necrosis is noted in *A*.

During pregnancy, Arias-Stella change occurs in the microglandular hyperplasia and other endocervical glands. Hobnail cells present with large, irregular, hyperchromasial nuclei that project into the apical cytoplasm (Fig. 8–91A to D). Mitotic figures are generally absent or rare. Unlike those seen in clear cell carcinoma, most of the cells lack prominent nucleoli. Reserve cell hyperplasia, squamous metaplasia, stromal edema, and chronic inflammation are common findings (see Fig. 8–91D). Microglandular hyperplasia is a benign proliferation without malignant potential.

Young and Scully[390] described atypical features seen in microglandular hyperplasia of the cervix, including solid epithelial proliferation, signet-ring cells, hobnail cells, moderate nuclear atypia, stromal hyalinization, and myxoid change. Some of these changes suggest infiltrating adenocarcinoma. Awareness of the focal nature of these atypical features helps to minimize overdiagnosis.

Conversely, about 20% of well-differentiated adenocarcinomas of the endometrium have extensive areas of endocervical metaplasia with malignant cells arranged in a microglandular pattern. Helpful features in favor of this diagnosis include the presence of endometrial hyperplasia or conventional endometrial adenocarcinoma, moderate nuclear atypia in glan-

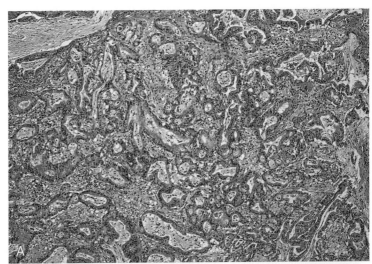

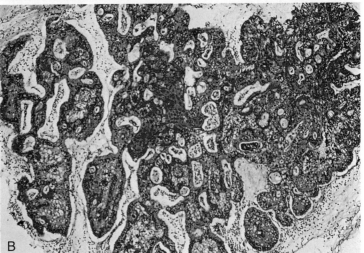

Figure 8–90. Microglandular hyperplasia of endocervix. *A* and *B*, Complex branching glands and clusters of closely apposed small glands. Areas of squamous metaplasia are seen in *B*.

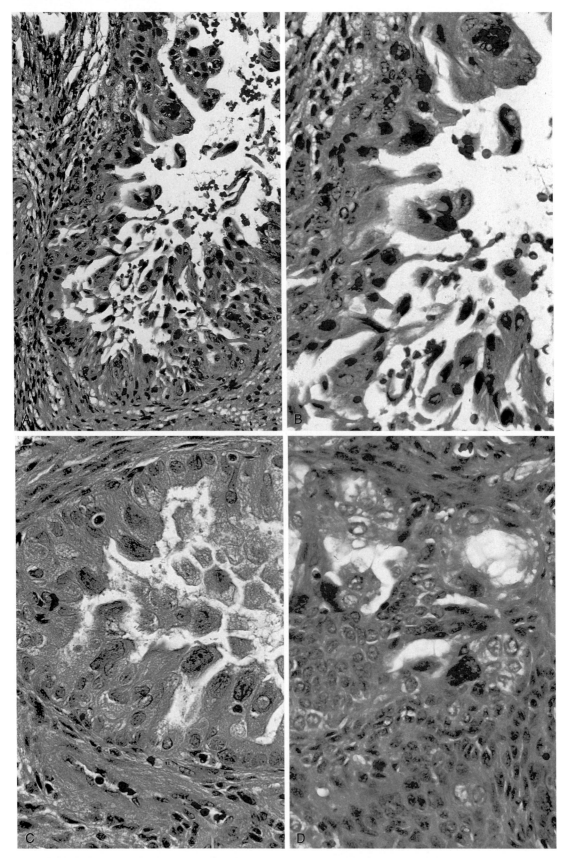

Figure 8–91. Endocervical glandular hyperplasia in a pregnant woman. *A*, Proliferating endocervical cells form papillary projections. *B*, The lining cells reveal nuclear enlargement, hyperchromasia, and irregularity. *C*, Some atypical cells have a hobnail appearance. *D*, Areas of squamous metaplasia and large atypical endocervical cells. (See color section.)

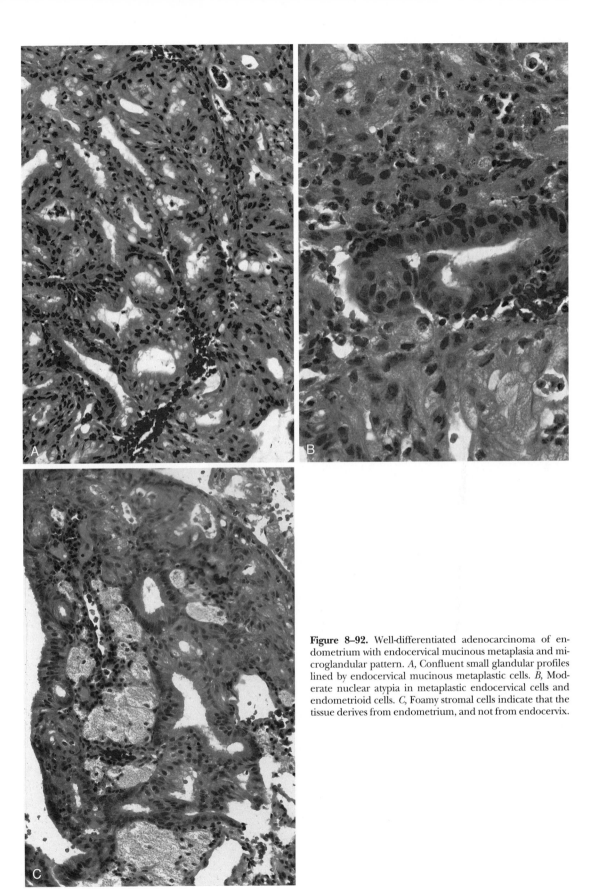

Figure 8–92. Well-differentiated adenocarcinoma of endometrium with endocervical mucinous metaplasia and microglandular pattern. *A,* Confluent small glandular profiles lined by endocervical mucinous metaplastic cells. *B,* Moderate nuclear atypia in metaplastic endocervical cells and endometrioid cells. *C,* Foamy stromal cells indicate that the tissue derives from endometrium, and not from endocervix.

dular cells, and foamy histiocytes in the stroma (Fig. 8–92).

Cystic and Noncystic Endocervical Tunnel Clusters

In a study of 29 cases of cystic tunnel clusters, the age of patients varied from 33 to 72 (mean 55) years. The clusters were identified in 5.9% of consecutive hysterectomy specimens and 9.7% of consecutive cervical conization specimens. Ninety-seven percent of women were multigravidas. The size of the tunnel clusters varied from 0.5 to 18.8 mm, with a mean of 2.4 mm. They were multifocal in 83% of the specimens. The deepest cluster was 9.0 mm from the endocervical mucosa. Nabothian cysts were usually present.[316]

The most distinctive feature is the arrangement in lobules. The majority of the glands are dilated and cystic with branching and budding patterns (Fig. 8–93A and B). In the lumen, abundant inspissated mucinous material is usually present. The lining cells vary from low cuboidal to columnar in shape. The nuclei are basally located, and the cytoplasm is abundant and has a mucinous character. The nuclear atypia is minimal or absent (see Fig. 8–93B). Branching tubular glands less frequently are the predominant component. The borders of the clusters are smooth (see Fig. 8–93A). Immunohistochemical stain for carcinoembryonic antigen is negative in all the tunnel clusters.[316]

Noncystic (type A) tunnel clusters, as compared with cystic variants, tended to occur in younger women, with a mean age of 44.8 (32–54) years.[171] They varied from 2.5 to 7 (mean 3.5) mm in size and usually coexisted with type B cystic variant. The characteristic fea-

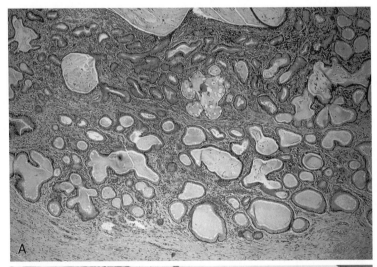

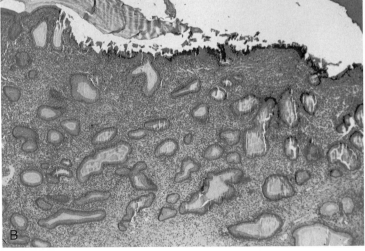

Figure 8–93. Cystic tunnel clusters. *A,* Many of the crowded cystic endocervical glands are lined by flattened cells. The outer border of the cluster is smooth. *B,* Dilated glands are lined by benign endocervical cells.

tures are lobules of branching, budding, and overcrowded small glands close to back-to-back pattern. Central dilated glands and papillary glands are sometimes present (Fig. 8–94A and B). These glandular profiles may become irregular and associated with stromal fibrosis and chronic inflammation, but a lobular arrangement is maintained (see Fig. 8–94A).[171]

The lining cells are columnar to cuboidal in shape and contain basophilic or amphophilic mucinous cytoplasm. Nuclear enlargement, irregularity, hyperchromasia, and prominent nucleoli are present. Mitotic figures are generally absent. The nuclei are round to oval in shape with minimal nuclear stratification. In the case of severe glandular dysplasia and adenocarcinoma in situ, nuclear stratification, hyperchromasia, elongation, and increased mitotic activity are readily appreciated.[171] Similarly, in the

microcystic variant of adenocarcinoma, moderate to severe nuclear atypia is evident, at least focally.[347]

Nucci et al.[258] reported a variant of lobular hyperplasia in which the borders of lobular hyperplasia are not very well demarcated and glands are present deep in the stroma to simulate adenoma malignum. These hyperplasias are made up of small to medium-sized glands, which are generally lined by a layer of tall columnar cells with benign-appearing nuclei and abundant mucinous cytoplasm. However, reactive nuclear atypia and rare mitotic figures were seen. The immunohistochemical stain for carcinoembryonic antigen was negative in two specimens studied. In lesions with poorly demarcated borders, these glands were not associated with desmoplastic stroma. The 13 women in this report varied from 37 to 71

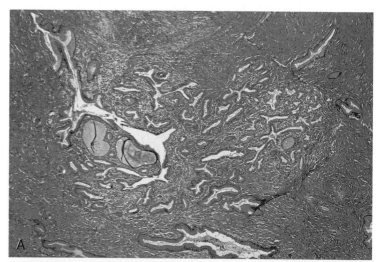

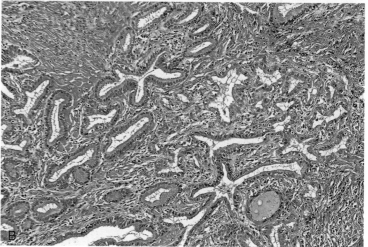

Figure 8–94. Noncystic tunnel clusters. *A* and *B,* Lobular hyperplasia. Branching, budding glands maintain a lobular pattern. A few cystic glands are present in the center of the lobule. *Illustration continued on following page*

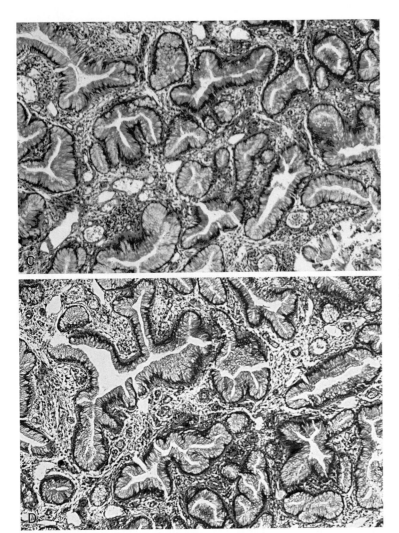

Figure 8–94. *Continued C* and *D*, Diffuse laminar hyperplasia. Tall columnar endocervical cells form complex outpouchings without lobular pattern. The nuclei are small and basally located without atypia or mitosis.

(mean 45) years of age. The majority of lesions were incidental findings in hysterectomy specimens, but a few women presented with increased vaginal discharge or a cervical mass.

A diffuse laminar form of endocervical glandular hyperplasia was reported by Jones et al.[172] This lesion was an incidental finding in hysterectomy specimens removed for uterine bleeding or leiomyoma. The age of the patients varied from 20 to 48 (mean 37) years. Five were multigravida; one was a user of oral contraceptive pills.[172]

Histologically, in contrast to tunnel clusters, there is no lobular architecture. The proliferative endocervical glands form closely apposed medium-sized glands mixed with cystic glands. Branching and outpouching patterns are prominent (see Fig. 8–94C and D).[172] These glands are lined by a layer of tall columnar cells with abundant mucinous cytoplasm and basally located nuclei. In five cases, nuclear atypia was associated with nuclear enlargement, chromatinic vacuolization, and prominent nucleoli. All five specimens had heavy chronic inflammatory infiltrates in the stroma. Acute and chronic inflammatory cells also occur in the glandular lumens. Periglandular fibrosis sometimes occurs and simulate desmoplastic reaction. However, these glands maintain a smooth configuration without an angulated appearance or tongue-like protrusions (see Fig. 8–94D). The main differential diagnosis for diffuse hyperplasia is well-differentiated adenocarcinoma. In the latter, a greater degree of nuclear atypia is expected.[171]

Daya and Young[90] described two hysterectomy specimens removed for benign conditions, in which florid glandular hyperplasia was deeply seated up to 10 mm and 13 mm in depth. One of the two cases was diagnosed as adenoma malignum, and the patient received radiation therapy. Immunohistochemical stain for carcinoembryonic antigen was negative in both cases.[90]

Glandular Metaplasia

Several types of glandular metaplasia can occur in the endocervix. Tubal metaplasia is typically found high in the cervical canal and uterine isthmus. It is commonly found in the endocervical end of LEEP and conization specimens. Following local excision or conization for CIN, these glands can be found near the squamocolumnar junction. The tubal metaplastic glands are lined by ciliated and nonciliated cells and intercalated cells (Fig. 8–95). These cells are arranged in 1 to 2 stratified layers. The nuclei of ciliated cells tend to be slightly enlarged and irregular, giving the impression of mild nuclear atypia (see Fig. 8–95A and B). Chromocenters and small nucleoli are often present. Rare mitotic figures may be found. Squamous metaplasia sometimes occurs (see Fig. 8–95C). In the case of significant glandular dysplasia and adenocarcinoma, the degree of nuclear atypia, mitotic activity, and nuclear stratification is more pronounced. In addition, the architecture of the glands is complex.

Suh and Silverberg[343] reported on 11 cases of ciliated metaplasia of the endocervix and called attention to the misinterpretation of tubal metaplasia as glandular dysplasia or adenocarcinoma in situ. In a subsequent study by Johannessen et al.,[167] 31% of the cone biopsies and hysterectomy specimens demonstrated ciliated tubal metaplasia. The mean age of this group of women was 41 years.

Oliva et al.[260] described 25 cases of tubal or tubo-endometrioid metaplasia of the cervix among women 21 to 51 (mean 39) years. They reported certain unusual features, such as overcrowded, back-to-back glands that simulated adenocarcinoma. Some of the cystic glands are deeply seated and raise the question of adenoma malignum. In others, the stroma undergoes myxoid change and hypercellular zone, simulating endometriotic stroma. Some of the glands contain very few ciliated cells, to justify the designation of tubo-endometrioid metaplasia.[260]

In a study by Umezaki et al.,[360] epidermal growth factor receptor and epithelial specific antigen were described in tubal metaplasia and adenocarcinoma of the cervix. These findings led the authors to consider whether tubal metaplasia may have neoplastic character.

Endometrial glands found in the cervix most likely represent endometriosis, especially when accompanied by endometrial stroma. Isolated endometrial glands without endometrial stroma are probably derived by metaplasia. These glands may simulate adenocarcinoma in situ because of their nuclear stratification and occasional mitotic figures. However, nuclear atypia is absent.

Oncocytic, oxyphilic cell metaplasia occurs within the tubal metaplasia or on the endocervical mucosa (Fig. 8–96A and B). Oxyphilic cells accumulate abundant eosinophilic granular cytoplasm. Rare examples of serous cell metaplasia are also noted (see Fig. 8–96C). Intestinal metaplasia is usually part of glandular dysplasia and adenocarcinoma.

ADENOCARCINOMA AND POTENTIAL PRECURSORS

Malignant glandular neoplasms of the cervix generally arise from the glandular tissue of the endocervix. For this reason, the adjective *endocervical* is often used to indicate their origin from the cervical canal. However, the neoplasms of this site are not limited to the endocervical epithelium. All types of müllerianderived epithelial cells, as well as cells of mesonephric ducts, are potential progenitors. In this chapter, the word *endocervical* refers specifically to the mucus-secreting endocervical cells. In addition to pure adenocarcinoma, about 50% of adenocarcinomas contain additional squamous elements, the adenosquamous carcinoma. This group of tumors is discussed separately from pure glandular neoplasms.

Epidemiology

Although cervical cancer screening programs have contributed to a significant reduction in squamous cancer, no comparable reduction has occurred for adenocarcinoma. As a result, the relative frequency of adenocarcinoma among the cervical cancers has increased in recent years.[122,286] Several authors reported as many as 23% to 34% of cervical cancers comprised of glandular neoplasms.[229,344]

In the Los Angeles County population between 1972 and 1982, an increase of cervical ade-

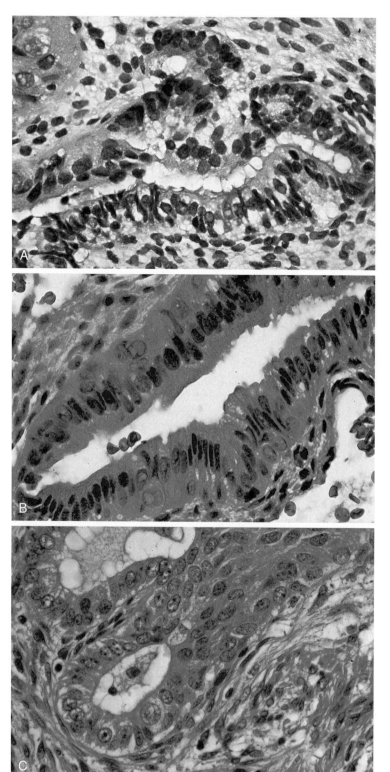

Figure 8–95. Ciliated tubal metaplasia of endocervix. *A,* Ciliated, nonciliated, and intercalated cells line the gland. In addition, there are oxyphilic metaplastic cells (*left*). *B,* A mild degree of nuclear stratification in one to two layers, and nuclear atypia is common. *C,* Squamous metaplasia in ciliated tubal glands. (See color section.)

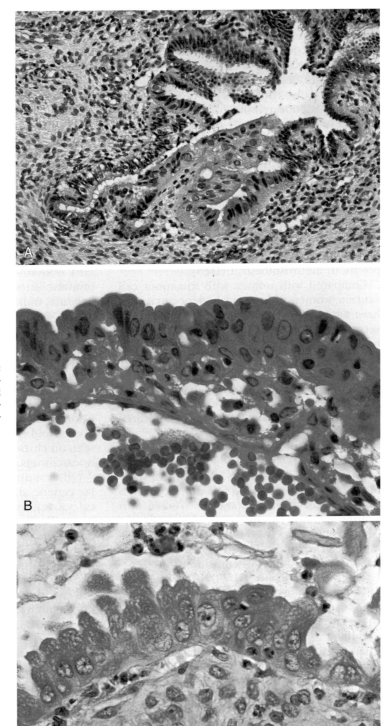

Figure 8–96. *A* and *B*, Oxyphilic cell metaplasia. *C*, Serous cell metaplasia. Serous cells contain abundant eosinophilic cytoplasm and apical cytoplasmic protrusions. (See color section.)

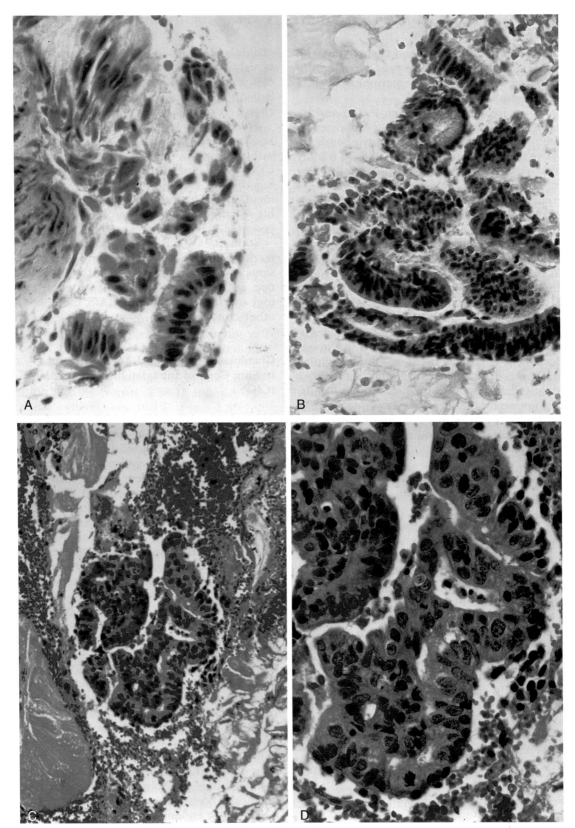

Figure 8–97. Atypical glandular cells in endocervical curettage preceding the diagnosis of in situ or invasive adenocarcinoma. They can be overlooked on low-power view without careful survey of nuclear features. *A,* Strips of benign-appearing endocervical cells with nuclear stratification in one to two layers and nuclear hyperchromasia. *B,* Atypical endocervical cells in ribbons and honeycomb sheets with nuclear hyperchromasia, elongation, and stratification. *C,* Small glands lined by eosinophilic cells. *D,* Higher magnification of cells in *C* reveals nuclear stratification, moderate nuclear atypia, and mitotic figures.

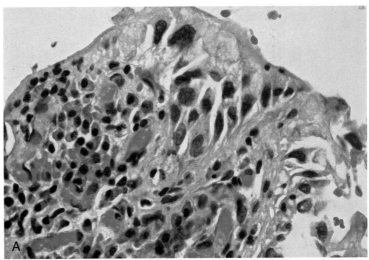

Figure 8–98. Reactive glandular atypia. *A,* Atypical endocervical cells present with large, irregular hyperchromatic nuclei associated with chronic endocervicitis. *B,* Endocervical gland lined by a layer of markedly atypical endocervical cells with nuclear enlargement, hyperchromasia, and irregularity. No mitotic activity is seen. *C,* An atypical cell with a gigantic hyperchromatic nucleus.
Illustration continued on following page

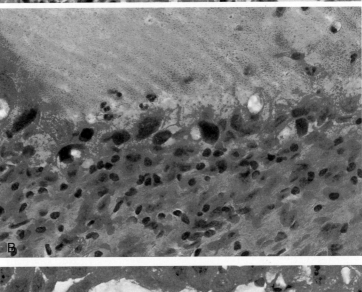

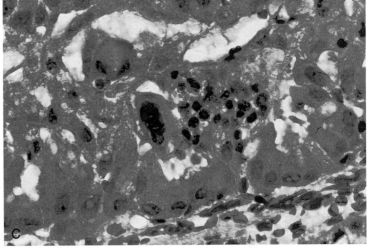

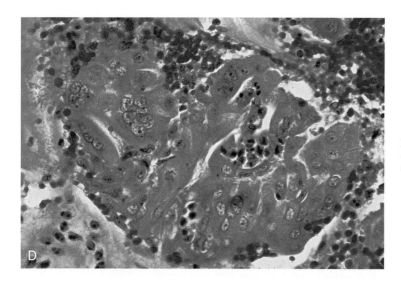

Figure 8–98. *Continued D,* Atypical endocervical cells with multinucleation and small nucleoli.

ognize benign cellular change or glandular atypia as a precursor of AIS.[131]

Lee et al.[207] studied 117 consecutive cone biopsies and hysterectomy specimens that were removed for in situ or invasive adenocarcinoma. The morphologic changes less severe than those of AIS were classified into low-grade atypia and high-grade atypia. These atypias were further dissected for HPV testing by PCR. Immunohistochemical stains were performed for Ki-67 using MIB-1 antibody. Eight specimens (6.8%) had glandular atypia. An additional 20 cases of high-grade and low-grade atypias were included in this study with a total of 27 lesions.[207]

Lee et al.[207] defined:

A. low-grade atypia as having (1) low mitotic activity (two or fewer mitotic figures per five high-power fields) and moderate nuclear atypia or (2) higher mitotic rate and mild nuclear atypia;

B. high-grade atypia as having (1) a low mitotic rate and severe nuclear atypia, or (2) a high mitotic rate and moderate nuclear atypia; and

C. AIS as having both a high mitotic rate and severe nuclear atypia.

Six of nine high-grade atypias and one of six low-grade lesions had HPV DNA. In a group of 13 isolated atypias without associated high-grade glandular or squamous lesions, only two had HPV DNA.[207]

In contrast, Higgins et al.[155] found a high frequency of HPV RNA in all grades of glandular dysplasia by in situ hybridization with [125]iodine labeled–riboprobes. HPV RNA was detected in 95.2% of 42 biopsies of CIGN from grade 1 to grade 3. HPV 16 RNA was found in 12, HPV 18 in 27, and both in 1 specimen. Of the 16 specimens with coexisting CIN 3, all had HPV RNA, including 31% for type 16, 63% for type 18, and 6% for type 31. The authors conclude that their findings support progression of CIGN from low grade to high grade in a manner similar to that of CIN and invasive squamous carcinoma.[155]

In terms of proliferative rate with MIB-1 antibody, all 10 AIS had greater than 25% MIB-1–positive cells. Six of eight high-grade lesions had more than 25% MIB-1–positive cells. None of five low-grade lesions had more than 25% MIB-1–positive cells. In the isolated atypias, three of 13 lesions had MIB-1–positive cells exceeding 25%.[207] Based on a low frequency (6.8%) of low-grade atypia found in in situ and invasive adenocarcinomas and infrequent association with HPV DNA, the authors question the malignant potential of low-grade atypia. High-grade atypias associated with AIS or CIN 2 or CIN 3 may be precursors of AIS.[207] The authors recommend that, if 25% or more MIB-1 cells are present, the lesion is acceptable as AIS.[207]

Low-grade atypia, as defined by Lee et al.,[207] exists alone (Fig. 8–99) or coexists with high-grade dysplasia or AIS (Figs. 8–100 to 8–106). Low-grade glandular atypia in cervical smears

Text continued on page 405

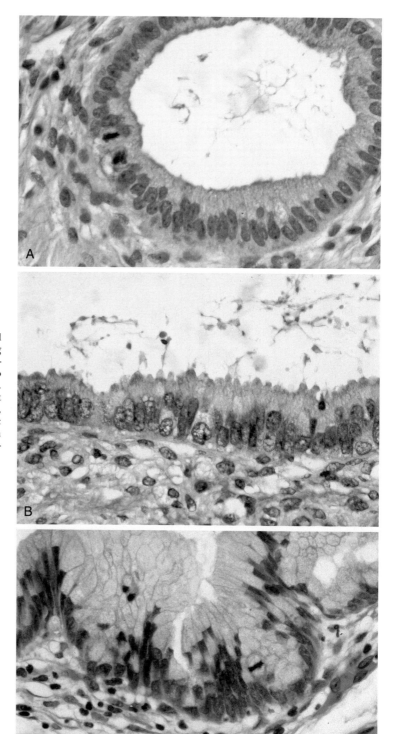

Figure 8–99. Low-grade endocervical glandular atypia without coexisting adenocarcinoma in situ. *A,* Mild nuclear atypia and stratification in one to two layers with rare mitotic figures. *B,* Moderate nuclear atypia without mitotic activity. *C,* Mild nuclear atypia, nuclear stratification, and rare mitotic figure. (Courtesy of Dr. Shu-Yuan Liao, St. Joseph Medical Center, Orange, California.)

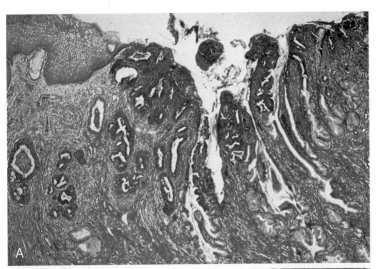

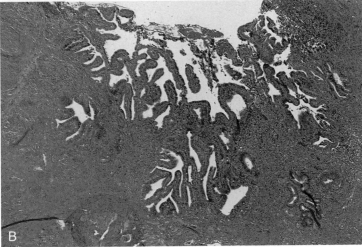

Figure 8–100. Adenocarcinoma in situ. *A,* The lesion starts from the squamocolumnar junction and extends proximally. It involves the endocervical mucosa and underlying glands. *B,* The involved surface is papillary, resembling villoglandular adenocarcinoma. *C,* Clusters of endocervical glands involved by adenocarcinoma in situ retain their original branching pattern. *D,* The lesion extends to the deep margin of conization specimen.

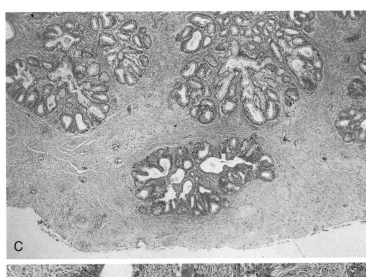

Figure 8–100. *Continued*

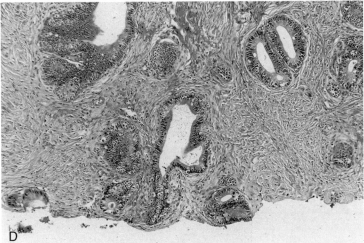

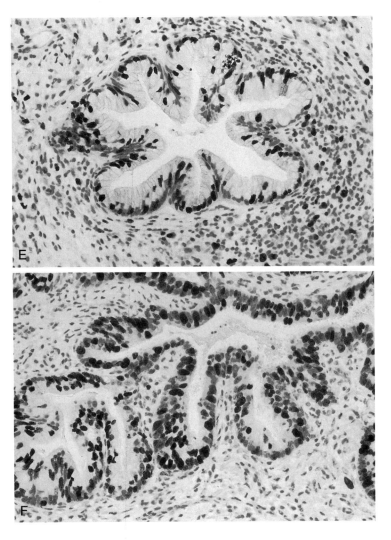

Figure 8–101. *Continued E* and *F,* Immunohistochemical stains for Ki-67 in low-grade atypia (*E*) and high-grade atypia (*F*). Proliferative cells are abundant in both areas. (See color section.)

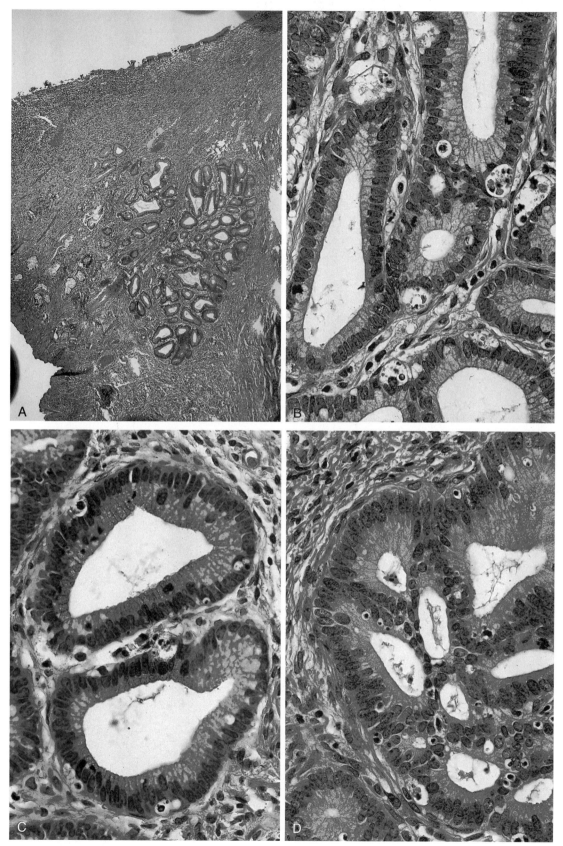

Figure 8–102. Adenocarcinoma in situ, endocervical type. *A* to *D*, from the same lesion. *A*, Low-magnification view of the lesion, involving multiple endocervical glands. *B*, Low-grade nuclear atypia with rare mitotic activity. *C*, Moderate nuclear atypia with rare mitotic activity. *D*, Moderate nuclear atypia with increased mitotic activity.

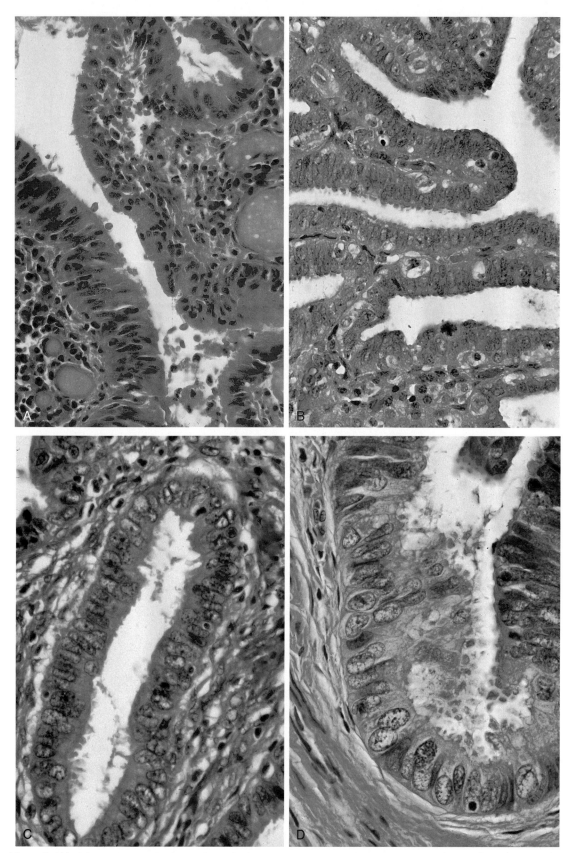

Figure 8–103. Adenocarcinoma in situ, endometrioid type. *A,* Nuclear stratification, mild nuclear atypia, and rare mitotic activity. *B,* Mild nuclear atypia and rare mitotic activity. *C,* Moderate nuclear atypia and rare mitotic activity. *D,* Severe nuclear atypia and high mitotic activity.

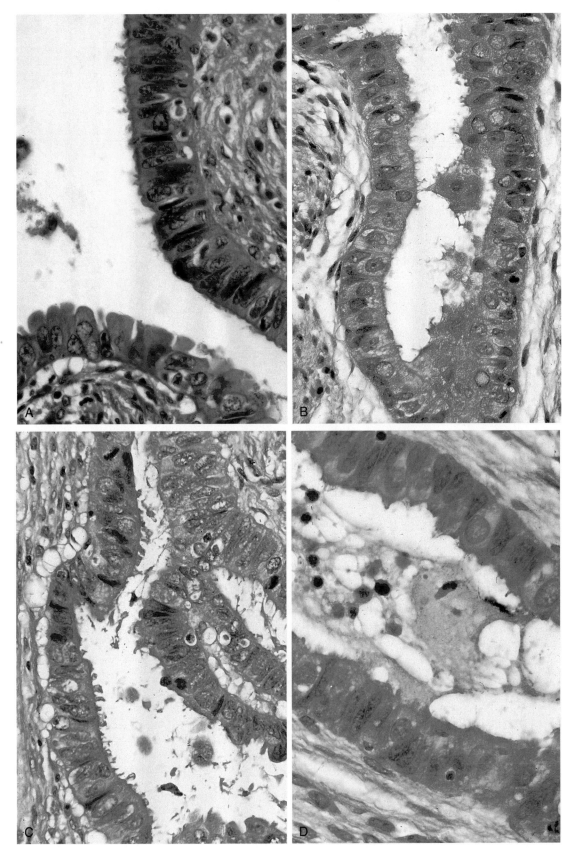

Figure 8–104. Adenocarcinoma in situ, ciliated tubal type. *A*, Moderate nuclear atypia and rare mitotic activity. *B*, Moderate nuclear atypia and rare mitotic activity. *C*, Severe nuclear atypia and increased mitotic activity. *D*, Severe nuclear atypia.

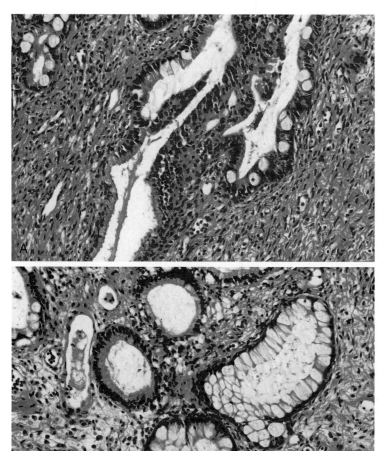

Figure 8–105. Glandular dysplasia adjacent to adenocarcinoma in situ, intestinal type. Same specimen as shown in Figure 8–106. *A,* Intestinal type cells with absorptive cells and goblet cells. The junction with the normal endocervical cells is sharp (*low center field*). *B,* Tall columnar cells with basally located nuclei and without nuclear stratification or atypia. *C,* Mild nuclear atypia and rare mitotic activity. *D,* Moderate nuclear atypia and rare mitotic activity.

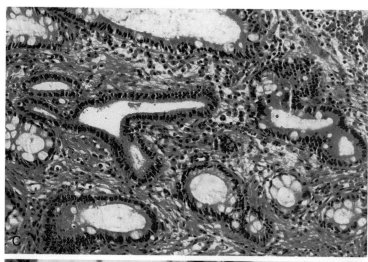

Figure 8–105. *Continued*

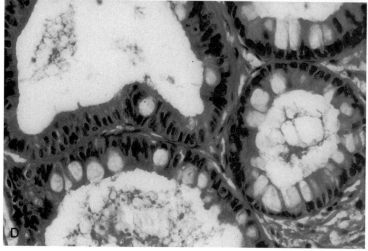

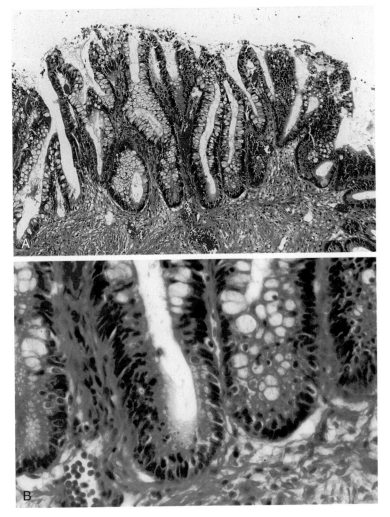

Figure 8–106. Adenocarcinoma in situ, intestinal type. *A* to *D* from same lesion. *A*, A villous growth pattern resembling villous adenoma of the colon. *B*, Moderate to severe nuclear atypia with increased mitotic activity. *C*, Squamous cell carcinoma in situ and overlying adenocarcinoma in situ. *D*, High-magnification view of squamous carcinoma in situ consisting of small cells.

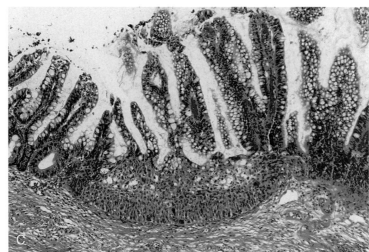

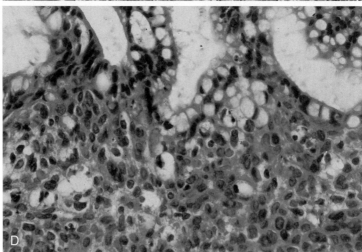

Figure 8–106. *Continued*

is difficult to recognize and usually is reported as normal, benign, or AGUS. In the latter case, cervical biopsy or endocervical curettage may be performed. In such specimens, the chance of finding the lesion is small without a more comprehensive survey of the entire cervix, such as through LEEP or conization specimen. Studies based on specimens removed for CIN, in situ and invasive adenocarcinomas[131,207] are biased for high-grade dysplasia and worse lesions.

In my opinion, endocervical cells with the following features meet the criteria for a low-grade glandular dysplasia:

1. Nuclear stratification in two to three layers
2. Mild nuclear atypia, enlargement, irregularity
3. Rare mitotic figures

4. Presence of Ki-67–positive cells by immunohistochemical stain

High-grade glandular dysplasia, as described by Lee et al.,[207] is difficult to distinguish from AIS, especially in cervical biopsy and endocervical curettage. In this author's experience, a spectrum of glandular dysplasia is found within AIS (see Figs. 8–101 to 8–106). For this reason, when a high-grade glandular dysplasia is seen in cervical smears, endocervical curettage, or cervical biopsies, additional studies are required to exclude in situ or invasive adenocarcinoma. In some instances, the area of glandular dysplasia/AIS is small and can be identified only by careful examination of LEEP or conization specimen and sometimes only by multiple levels of sections. Thus, for practical purposes, high-grade glandular dysplasias should be recognized as potential precursor lesions of in situ and invasive adenocarcinoma of the uterine cervix. In this monograph, high-grade glandular dysplasia and AIS of the cervix are considered together as one entity under the term AIS.

Most AIS begin in the region of the squamocolumnar junction and spread proximally (see Fig. 8–100). With few exceptions, both the endocervical mucosal surface and the underlying glands are involved. The affected surface may be flat or papillary (see Fig. 8–100). The neoplastic glands form budding and crowded back-to-back glands. Excessive proliferation within large glands sometimes results in a cribriform pattern. The most characteristic features are the preservation of normal branching patterns, the smooth configuration of the glandular profiles, and normal fibromuscular stroma without desmoplasia (see Fig. 8–100).

Over 80% of cervical AIS is composed exclusively or predominantly of mucus-secreting endocervical cells.[114] Endometrial cells, ciliated tubal cells, intestinal cells, and clear cells occur in the remaining 20%. These different cell types with distinct cytoplasmic characters allow separation. However, many lesions contain more than one cell type and not otherwise specified (NOS).

Morphologic features of high-grade glandular dysplasia and AIS of all cell types share most of the following characteristics:

1. An architecture of branching, budding, or cribriform glandular pattern
2. Nuclear features of stratification, enlargement, hyperchromasia, elongation, and irregularity
3. Chromatin pattern of fine to coarse granularity with even or uneven distribution
4. Increased mitotic activity
5. Indistinct to prominent nucleoli
6. A sharp transition with normal endocervical cells

In addition, in a study of 43 AIS, apoptotic cells were found in all cases. These cells have densely eosinophilic or clear cytoplasm. The apoptotic bodies are characterized by masses of compact, sharply defined, fragmented and pyknotic chromatin.[38]

Normally, endocervical cells are arranged in a single layer and have basally located small nuclei. Nucleoli and mitotic figures are absent or rarely observed. Cells occasionally are arranged in 2 to 3 stratified layers especially in tangential sections. In the endocervical type of AIS, the tumor cells maintain a tall, columnar shape and basophilic to clear cytoplasm. A wide range of nuclear atypia and mitotic activity is seen within the lesion (see Figs. 8–101 to 8–102). In the most advanced areas, severe nuclear atypia and increased mitotic activity are evident. By immunohistochemical stains for Ki-67, a high proliferative index is seen in both low-grade and high-grade areas (see Fig. 8–101E and F).

In the endometrioid type of AIS, the cells have densely eosinophilic cytoplasm, which is less abundant than in the endocervical type (see Fig. 8–103).

In the tubal type of AIS, ciliated, nonciliated, and intercalated cells with nuclear atypia and increased mitotic activity are seen. The number of ciliated cells may be few; in such cases, tubal AIS is difficult to separate from the endometrioid type. Schlesinger and Silverberg[312] found atypical tubal metaplasia associated with the tubal type of AIS. Of the 10 ciliated glandular atypias (three high grade and seven low grade) reported by Lee et al., all were HPV negative.[207]

The intestinal type of glandular dysplasia and AIS consist of absorptive cells with brush borders and goblet cells with discrete vacuoles (see Figs. 8–105 and 8–106). Some authors proposed that all atypical intestinal metaplasia be classified as AIS.[207]

In some NOS types of AIS lesion, the tumor cells have pleomorphic nuclei and large nucleoli (Fig. 8–107).

Squamous cell dysplasias and carcinomas in situ coexist with 35% to 71% of AIS.[70,129,383] Rarely has microinvasive squamous carcinoma been recorded.[129] The squamous and glandular elements often merge into one lesion.

Although the diagnosis of AIS may be made on the basis of cytologic and biopsy specimens, it is difficult to separate in situ from well-differentiated invasive adenocarcinoma. Because both lesions may occur concurrently, cervical conization is usually performed to reach a definitive diagnosis.

Figure 8–107. Adenocarcinoma in situ and nuclear abnormalities. *A,* Severe nuclear atypia with uneven, finely granular chromatin. *B,* Severe nuclear atypia with finely granular chromatin, small nucleoli, and mitotic figures. *C,* Severe nuclear atypia and large nucleoli. *D,* Pleomorphic nuclei and prominent nucleoli.

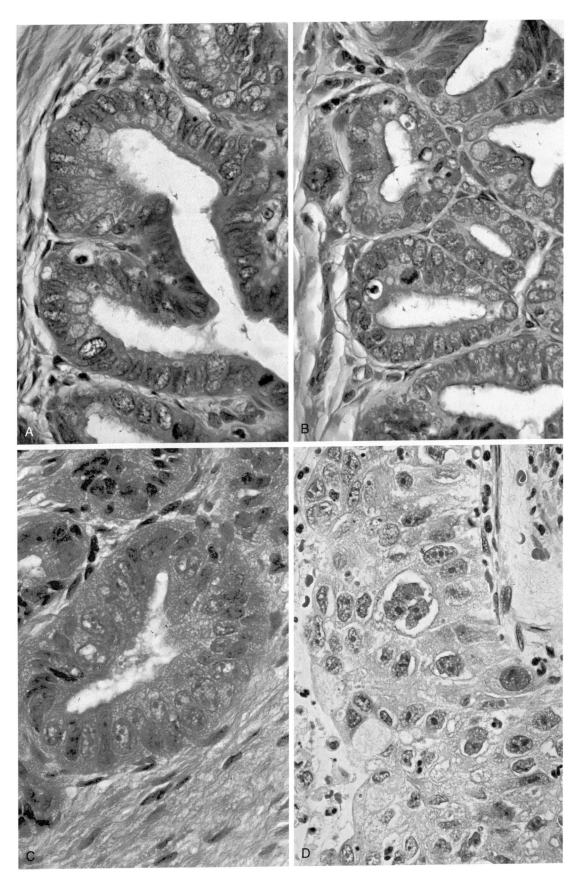

Figure 8–107 *See legend on opposite page*

Estimates based on conization and hysterectomy specimens have found AIS extending as deep as 3 to 5 mm from the mucosal surface. The linear extent along the cervical canal varies from 0.5 to 25 mm (mean 12 mm).[264] If measured from the external os, these lesions may extend to 30 mm.[36] This implies the need for deep conization to encompass the entire lesion. Young women, who prefer to retain the uterus, may be treated by conization alone and followed regularly by endocervical aspiration or curettage.[264] However, even when the surgical margins of the conization specimen appear uninvolved, residual tumor may exist. A possible explanation is that this is a multifocal disease, which is estimated to be 15%.[264]

Wolf et al.[383] studied 61 women (mean age 35.9 years) with AIS. Of the 55 women who underwent cone biopsies, 50 had known status of cone margins and 44 had subsequent hysterectomy. The conization margins were positive in 23 of 50 (46%) women, and 19 of these had hysterectomy. Residual tumor was found in 53% (10 of 19) of hysterectomy specimens, including AIS in four, invasive adenocarcinoma in five, and glandular atypia in one.[383] Three of four women who received no further treatment were well 2 to 9 years later. The fourth woman was lost to follow-up.[383]

The conization margins were negative in 27 of 50 patients (54%), and 21 had hysterectomy. Residual tumor was found in 7 of 21 cases (33%), including invasive adenocarcinoma in three (two neoplasms 2 mm or less, one tumor 5 mm in size), AIS in three, and glandular atypia in one.[383] Of six women who refused hysterectomy after cone biopsy, two were lost to follow-up, one developed 5 mm deep invasive adenocarcinoma 2 years after the cone biopsy, one developed glandular atypia that was treated by cone biopsy, and the remaining two have no evidence of disease.[383]

Azodi et al.[18] studied 40 women with AIS; all had cone biopsy. The mean age of the patients was 37 years. Ninety-eight percent of women had abnormal Pap smears. In the initial biopsy of the cervix, 70% of patients had glandular dysplasia or AIS, 5% had squamous dysplasia, 5% had chronic cervicitis, and 5% were normal. The other 7.5% were nondiagnostic, and 7.5% had no biopsy. The endocervical margin was positive in 24% of cold-knife cones, 75% of LEEP specimens, and 57% of laser cones. The ectocervical margin was positive in 8% of cold-knife cones, 13% of LEEP specimens, and 57% of laser cones.[18]

When the margins were clear, residual disease was found in 31% of second cone or hysterectomy specimens (one AIS, one mild glandular dysplasia, and three glandular atypias).[18] When the margin was involved, 56% had residual disease (two invasive adenocarcinomas, four AIS, one severe glandular dysplasia, one moderate glandular dysplasia, and one mild glandular dysplasia).[18] These findings provide sufficient evidence of the malignant and multifocal nature of AIS to justify hysterectomy. When such lesions are treated by conization alone, a close follow-up with endocervical samples is recommended.

FIGO Stage IA Microinvasive Adenocarcinoma

Microinvasive adenocarcinomas were initially described as tongue-like protrusions arising from the base of AIS (Fig. 8–108) or from the periphery of endocervical glands replaced by AIS (Figs. 8–109 and 8–110).[280] Since then, investigators have attempted to define the criteria for microinvasive adenocarcinoma. Teshima et al.[351] defined early adenocarcinoma as less than 5 mm of stromal invasion as measured from the mucosal surface. All 30 patients in this study were treated by hysterectomy, and one woman developed tumor recurrence. This patient had a 3 mm deep tumor, which did not involve the capillary-lymphatic spaces or pelvic lymph node, but tumor recurred in the vaginal cuff.[351]

Buscema and Woodruff[62] also reported a 3 mm deep adenosquamous carcinoma that metastasized widely. Among women with Stage I or II cervical adenocarcinoma up to 5 mm in depth, Berek et al.[34] found that 2 of 24 women (8%) had pelvic lymph node metastasis, and the overall 5-year survival rate was 92%. Thus, adenocarcinomas as superficial as 5 mm have a small risk of nodal metastasis.

In a study of 77 early invasive adenocarcinomas by Ostor et al.,[263] microinvasive adenocarcinoma was defined as less than 5 mm in depth. The invasive tumor was measured from the mucosal surface to the deepest point of tumor. This type of measurement is referred to as "tumor thickness" by other authors. The tumor thickness was 0.1 to 1.0 mm in 12 (15.5%) tumors, 1.1 to 2.0 mm in 12 (15.5%), 2.1 to 3.0 mm in 19 (24.7%), 3.1 to 4.0 mm in 22 (28.8%), and 4.1 to 5.0 mm in 12 (15.5%). The histologic type of these tumors is heterogeneous, including AIS with early stromal inva-

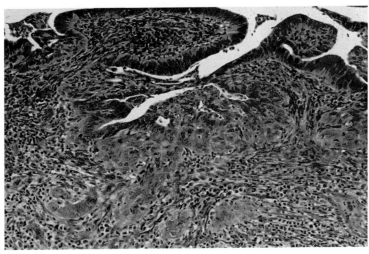

Figure 8–108. Microinvasive adenocarcinoma of cervix. Stromal invasion originates from the endocervical mucosa replaced by adenocarcinoma in situ. Invasive tumor cells form several bud-like protrusions from the base of adenocarcinoma in situ. Invasive cells have more abundant eosinophilic cytoplasm than do the noninvasive cells.

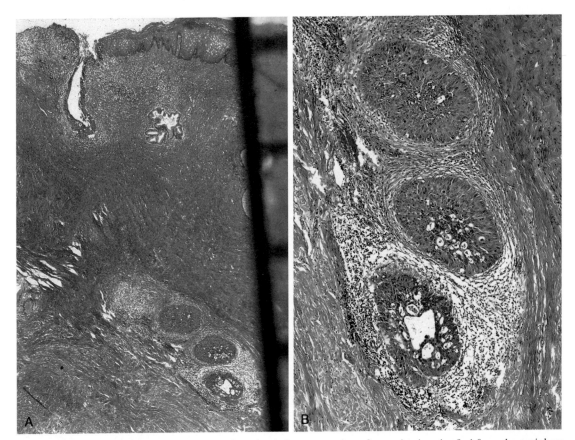

Figure 8–109. Microinvasive adenocarcinoma of cervix. *A,* Low-power view of two microinvasive foci from the periphery of endocervical gland involved by adenocarcinoma in situ. One occurs at the 1 mm mark and the other at 3 mm. *B,* Higher magnification of early invasion at 3 mm demonstrates tongue-like extension associated with peri-glandular fibrosis, edema, and chronic inflammation.

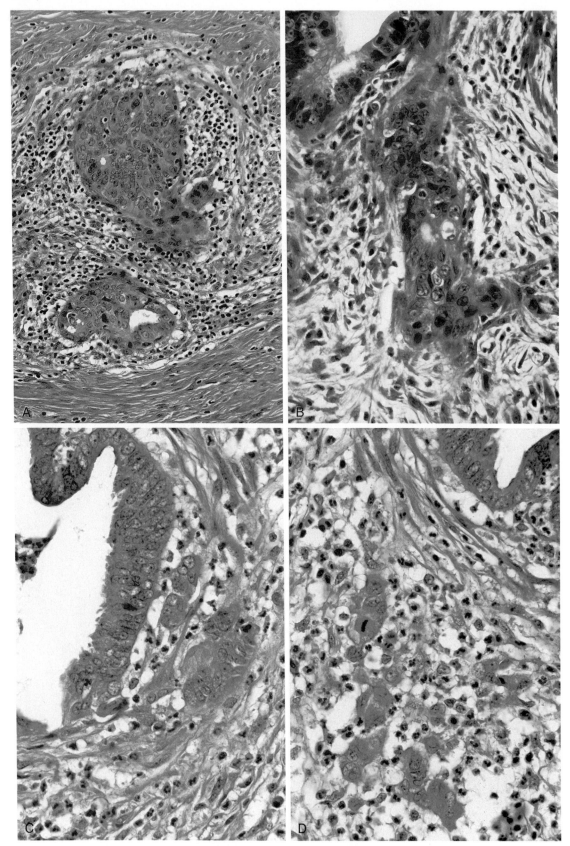

Figure 8–110. Microinvasive adenocarcinoma of cervix. *A,* Formation of small protrusion at the point of invasion. *B,* Expansion of cords of malignant cells with desmoplastic reaction. Severe nuclear atypia is evident. *C,* Two tumor nests separate from the point of origin. *D,* Isolated groups of tumor cells invade further into the stroma.

sion, well-differentiated adenocarcinoma, and papillary villoglandular adenocarcinoma. Seven (9%) tumors had vascular lymphatic space invasion, and 21 (27%) neoplasms had multifocal lesion involving both cervical lips. Other findings included 66% of women had abnormal glandular cells in Pap smear, 38% had abnormal colposcopic findings, and 53% had used oral contraceptive pills.[263]

The study by Ostor et al.[263] provides an alternative approach to express the extent of stromal invasion by measuring from the surface of the lesion to the deepest point of tumor in the form of tumor thickness. However, not all early invasive adenocarcinomas arise from the mucosal surface (see Fig. 8–108). Some microinvasive adenocarcinomas have several foci of invasion simultaneously arising from the periphery of endocervical glands involved by adenocarcinoma in situ (see Fig. 8–109). In others, invasive neoplastic glands predominate the early adenocarcinoma, and the degree of differentiation varies (Fig. 8–111).

Treatment modalities in a study by Ostor et al.[263] included cold-knife conization and simple to radical hysterectomy. There was no parametrial involvement in any of the 26 radical hysterectomy specimens. Pelvic lymph nodes in 48 women undergoing nodal sampling were all negative. Twenty-three women had one or both ovaries removed, and all were free of tumor.[263] Two women had tumor recurrence. The original tumor of one 62-year-old woman was 3.2 mm in depth, 21 mm in length, and 670 cubic mm in volume. Five years after total abdominal hysterectomy, bilateral salpingo-oophorectomy, and external pelvic irradiation, she developed recurrent tumor in the vaginal vault, which was excised. Four years later, tumor recurred in the vault, which was treated by upper vaginectomy. The patient died postoperatively. In a second woman, the original tumor was 5 mm in depth, 10 mm in length, and 450 cubic mm in volume. Nine years following total abdominal hysterectomy, a squamous carcinoma was found in the vaginal vault.[263]

In a series of 200 women with cervical adenocarcinoma of Stage IIA or earlier, 21 tumors met the criteria of FIGO Stage IA1, which is less than 3 mm in depth and 7 mm in length. In this study, microinvasion was defined as "small buds of malignant glandular cells protruding into the stroma from glands with AIS." The depth of invasion was measured from "the surface of the tumor or overlying benign epithelium to the deepest point using a calibrated 40× magnification field." The linear extent of the tumor was based on the maximal horizontal extension of the tumor.[313]

The mean age of 21 women with FIGO Stage IA1 disease was 38 (24–75) years. Three (14%) women were younger than 30 years, and 14 (67%) were younger than 40 years of age, including eight who were nulliparous.[313]

The histologic type includes 18 adenocarcinomas, two adenosquamous carcinomas, and one clear cell carcinoma. Sixteen tumors were grade 1, and five were grade 2. No grade 3 tu-

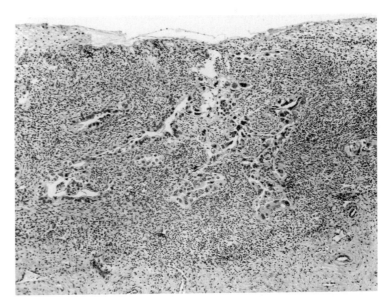

Figure 8–111. Early invasive adenocarcinoma. Complex neoplastic glands lined by pleomorphic cells invade into the stroma to a depth of 3 mm. Using Ostor's criteria, this tumor is acceptable as microinvasive adenocarcinoma.

mor or vascular lymphatic space invasion was seen. Eight patients had less than 1 mm of invasion, nine patients had 1.1 to 2.0 mm invasion, and four patients had 2.1 to 3.0 mm invasion. The invasive foci occurred predominantly close to the endocervical mucosal surface at or within 5.0 mm of the squamocolumnar junction. Four tumors had multifocal invasion.[313] All patients except one were treated by simple or radical hysterectomy. One woman was treated by LEEP alone; she remained disease free at 45 months. Of the 16 women who underwent type II or type III radical hysterectomy and pelvic lymph node dissection, including two patients who had paraaortic lymph node dissection, all were free of parametrial extension or lymph node metastasis.[313]

In a study by Kaku et al.,[176] of 21 women with 3.0 mm or less of stromal invasion, none had extension beyond the cervix and none developed tumor recurrence.

In a review of the literature, Ostor et al.[262] found no evidence of tumor recurrence or extension beyond the cervix in 43 women with disease up to 3.0 mm in depth.

Kaspar et al.[182] reported two cases with tumor recurrence among 36 women with 3.0 mm or less of stromal invasion. Both women with recurrence had disease exceeding 7.0 mm in length and thus should be classified as FIGO stage IB1.

Lee and Flynn[208] reported on 40 cases of early invasive adenocarcinoma of the cervix with stromal invasion of 5.0 mm or less. The mean age of the patients was 40.9 (25–63) years. The histologic type included 32 endocervical type, three mixed endometrioid and endocervical type, and three adenosquamous type. The histologic grade was grade 1 in 33 tumors, grade 2 in five, and grade 3 in two. The maximal tumor length was 0.3 to 20 mm (mean 5.8 mm). The depth of stromal invasion was 0.1 to 5.0 mm (mean 2.3 mm). The invasive foci were located beneath the transformation zone or adjacent to the squamocolumnar junction in 78% of the cases. Four (10%) cases had more than one focus of invasion. Eighty-five percent of the cases had AIS, and 33% had coexisting AIS and CIN. No follow-up information was available.[208]

Ostor[262] reviewed the literature and identified 436 cases of early invasive adenocarcinoma of the cervix with stromal invasion up to 5.0 mm. One hundred twenty-six women were treated by radical hysterectomy, and none had parametrial involvement. Of the 155 women

who had one or both ovaries removed, no tumor was identified. Of the 219 women with pelvic lymph node dissection, five (2%) had metastasis. Fifteen (3.4%) women had tumor recurrence, and there were six (1.4%) tumor-related deaths among 436 patients. Twenty-one patients were treated only by conization, and none had developed recurrence. In Ostor's opinion, cold-knife conization is acceptable when the margins are free and when fertility is desired. Loop excision often obscures the depth of invasion and excision margins and is not acceptable for diagnosis or for therapy.[262]

FIGO Stage IB and Higher Frankly Invasive Adenocarcinoma

In dealing with glandular neoplasm of the cervix, one should keep in mind the possibility of a secondary carcinoma arising from the endometrium, ovary, breast, colon, or other site. To assist in distinguishing primary from secondary carcinoma, certain criteria have been suggested.

Diagnostic Criteria and Procedure

Maier and Norris[221] suggested the following criteria for primary cervical adenocarcinoma:

1. a demonstrable transition from normal endocervical glands to neoplasm in the specimen
2. normal endometrium present in curettage or hysterectomy specimen
3. adenocarcinoma present in a cervical stump 5 or more years after removal of the corpus
4. gross tumors located on the cervix with a normal-sized uterus and absence of gross tumor in the endometrial cavity

These guidelines are useful. In some instances, the decision can be difficult, and other factors must be included in the determination of an individual case.

When an obvious tumor is detected in the cervix, the diagnosis can be established by the presence of an invasive carcinoma in the cervical biopsy and benign endometrial sample. When neoplastic glandular cells are detected in the cervical smears and no visible lesion is present on the cervix, a fractional curettage often is obtained, first from the endocervix and then from the endometrium. These procedures were performed in 29 patients with confirmed cervical adenocarcinoma, and the tumor was confined to the endocervical curettings in 11 cases (38%). In the remaining 62%, the tumor was present in the corporal fraction, giving an equivocal result.[193] This false-positive finding results from contamination of the endometrial sample as the curette passed through the cervical canal. Another problem is that abnormal tissue present in the endocervical sample is often fragmented and superficial in nature, precluding the determination of stromal invasion.

When the fractional curettage fails to determine the primary source or the extent of disease (in situ versus invasive), cervical conization followed by dilatation and curettage is the recommended procedure. From the amount of tumor in the two samples, it should be possible to determine the exact primary site. In the case of cervical primary adenocarcinoma, the tumor should be confined largely to the conization specimen. The endometrium in the curettage should be free of tumor or only minimally involved. If the tumor involves only the endometrial curettings or both the conization and endometrial samples, a primary endometrial tumor is favored. Based on the primary site of origin, patients are staged with the FIGO system.

Clinical and Gross Features

Endocervical carcinomas usually present as polypoid, nodular, exophytic, papillary, or ulcerated growths. Less frequently, the cervix is diffusely enlarged and indurated, having a barrel-shaped configuration. In one study, the cervix appeared normal by clinical examination in 29% of patients.[193] Cross-sections of tumors produce a cystic, mucoid, or solid appearance (Fig. 8–112).

In a series by Greer[135] et al. of 55 women with Stage IB adenocarcinoma, 44% had no symptoms and 58% had no gross lesions. The diagnosis was suspected on the basis of abnormal cervical smears in 16 women (29%). Of these, 15 required conization for diagnosis.[135]

Miller et al.[241] studied 124 women from the Memphis, Tennessee, area who had invasive glandular neoplasms treated between 1964 and 1988. During this study period, the relative ratio of glandular neoplasm increased from 9% to 25%. In addition, the ratio of women younger than 36 years increased from 16% in 1964 to 24% in 1988. In women younger than 35 years, the tumor in 74% was first detected by cytopathology, as compared with 27% from those older than 35 years. Thirty-one percent of women were asymptomatic. Those who were symptomatic included 53% with vaginal bleeding, 6% with vaginal discharge, and 6% with pain.[241]

This study demonstrates the importance of cytologic screening for the detection of cervical adenocarcinoma.[241] The histologic type of the glandular neoplasms include 56% adenocarcinoma, 14% adenosquamous carcinoma, 11% adenoid cystic carcinoma, 10% papillary adenocarcinoma, and 9% clear cell, mucoid, and mixed type. The median age of the patients was 49 years for adenocarcinoma, 39 years for adenosquamous carcinoma, and over 60 years for adenoid cystic carcinoma and papillary carcinoma. The breakdown from Stage

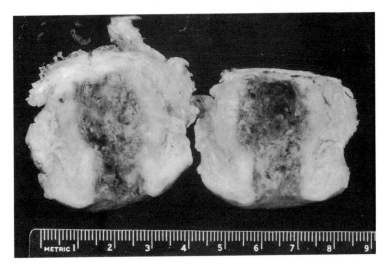

Figure 8–112. Adenocarcinoma in a cervical stump. A cystic, partially hemorrhagic, necrotic mass fills the cervical canal. With this amount of tumor tissue, it would not be surprising to find fragments of tumor in both the endometrial and endocervical curettings.

I to Stage IV was 57%, 16%, 9%, and 8%, respectively.

Endocervical Adenocarcinoma

The endocervical type of adenocarcinomas is composed of cells that resemble endocervical or, less frequently, intestinal cells. The predominant growth pattern may be glandular, mucinous (colloid), papillary, solid, or mixed. The degree of nuclear atypia also varies from case to case. Evaluation of the degree of differentiation may be based on the nuclear features alone or a combination of growth pattern and nuclear atypia. Tumors with a glandular pattern and mild to moderate nuclear atypia are graded as well differentiated, whereas those with a solid pattern and marked nuclear anaplasia are classified as poorly differentiated. Moderately differentiated tumors refer to those whose characteristics fall between these two.

Among the well-differentiated tumors with a predominantly glandular pattern, the glands are small and closely packed in back-to-back pattern (Fig. 8–113). Moderately differentiated neoplasms contain glandular, cystic structures and solid nests (Fig. 8–114). The lining cells are tall and columnar and have eosinophilic or finely vacuolated, pale-staining cytoplasm resembling that of normal endocervical cells. Some tumors closely resemble intestinal carcinoma, with tumor cells forming abundant intracellular and extracellular mucin (Fig. 8–115).

In poorly differentiated mucinous carcinoma, the malignant cells form cords, nests, or solid sheets with few glandular spaces. Most of the cells exhibit a high degree of nuclear anaplasia, and some have the appearance of signet-ring cells (Fig. 8–116). Mucicarmine and PAS stains are helpful in confirming their glandular differentiation.

A complex papillary pattern predominates in a small number of tumors. Those with exophytic papillary architecture are discussed under the section on well-differentiated villoglandular adenocarcinoma. In tumors with endophytic papillary growth, the lining cells are tall, columnar, and well-differentiated (Fig. 8–117).

Tambouret et al.[347] described eight cases of microcystic variant of endocervical adenocarcinomas. The eight women ranged from 34 to 78 (mean 46) years of age. Four women presented with abnormal cervical smears, and three had vaginal bleeding.[347] Gross appearance was recorded for three women, including a 3.0 cm polypoid mass, an endocervical hemorrhagic lesion, and multiple cystic lesions. These tumors, on low-power view, strongly simulate benign cystic tunnel clusters with predominantly cystic glands and lobular architecture. These cystic glands were usually lined by flattened epithelium, suggesting deeply seated Nabothian cysts or endocervical glandular hyperplasia (Fig. 8–118). Some of the tubules and glands contained eosinophilic material in the glandular lumens, resembling mesonephric hyperplasia.

On closer examination, these glands were lined by cells with nuclear stratification and hyperchromasia. All tumors had an infiltrative pattern of conventional endocervical adenocarcinoma, and mitotic figures were present in all tumors (see Fig. 8–118; Fig. 8–119). Only two tumors had desmoplastic stroma. The remaining tumors showed no stromal reaction. Six tumors were endocervical type (see Fig. 8–118), and two were intestinal type (see Fig. 8–119) with focal goblet cells and Paneth cells. All tumors had coexisting AIS. Three were well differentiated, and five were moderately differentiated. The depth of stromal invasion varied from 3.0 to 13.0 mm. The tumor dimension varied from 1.0 to 8.0 mm.[347]

The authors recommend careful survey of the cytologic and histologic features to avoid underdiagnosis of this variant of adenocarcinoma as benign glandular hyperplasia or benign cyst. Areas of neoplastic glands with nuclear atypia can be limited and focal.[347] Of the three women with follow-up, two were alive and well at 1 and 6.5 years after diagnosis. The third woman died of pelvic recurrence 2 years after initial diagnosis.[347]

Minimal Deviation Adenocarcinoma (Adenoma Malignum)

The term *adenoma malignum of the cervix* was used by McKelvey and Goodlin[233] to refer to a group of extremely well-differentiated mucinous adenocarcinomas that demonstrated minimal nuclear atypia and retained the branching pattern of normal endocervical glands. The desmoplastic stromal response may be minimal or absent. This term was chosen to express the lesion's deceptively benign appearance. Silverberg and Hurt[328] prefer the term *minimal deviation adenocarcinoma* (MDA), which has recently been extended to well-differentiated endometrioid, clear cell, and mesonephric carcinomas, which maintain regular glandular profiles.[177,351]

Text continued on page 422

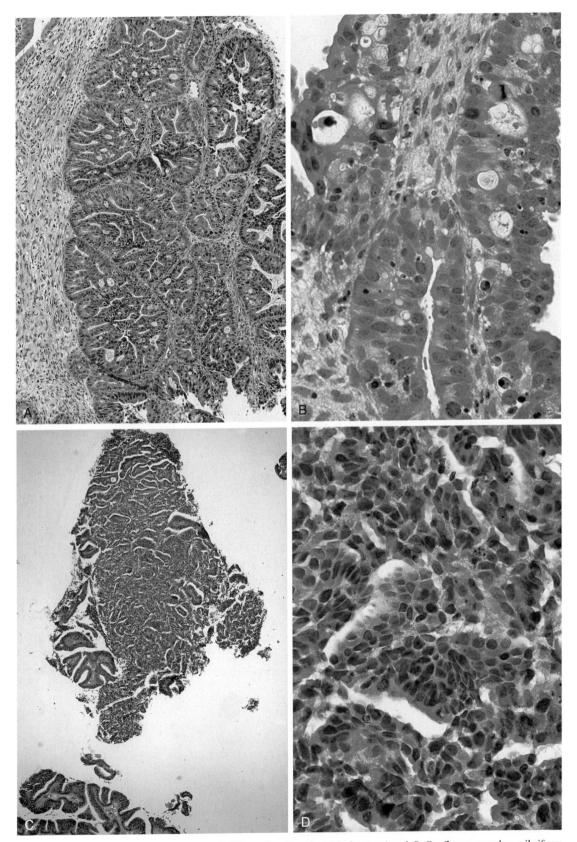

Figure 8–113. Adenocarcinoma of cervix, well-differentiated, endocervical type. *A* and *B,* Confluent complex cribriform glands with loss of the normal branching pattern of endocervix, indicative of stromal invasion. Moderate nuclear and high mitotic activity in the tumor cells. *C* and *D,* Papillary and compact glands with moderate nuclear atypia and increased mitotic activity.

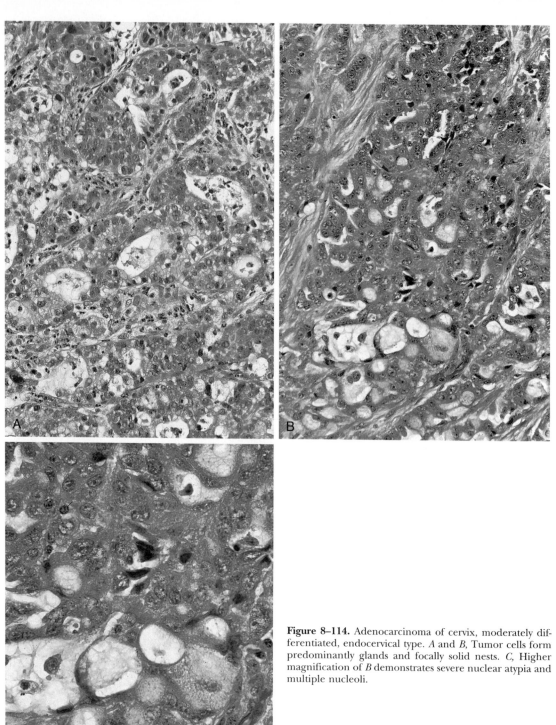

Figure 8–114. Adenocarcinoma of cervix, moderately differentiated, endocervical type. *A* and *B,* Tumor cells form predominantly glands and focally solid nests. *C,* Higher magnification of *B* demonstrates severe nuclear atypia and multiple nucleoli.

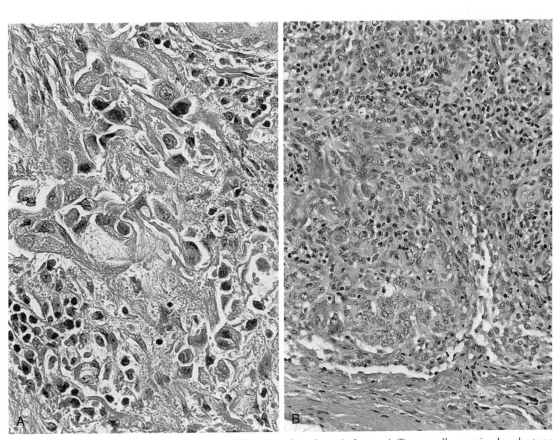

Figure 8–115. Mucinous adenocarcinoma with abundant extracellular mucin. The tumor cells have the appearance of intestinal type.

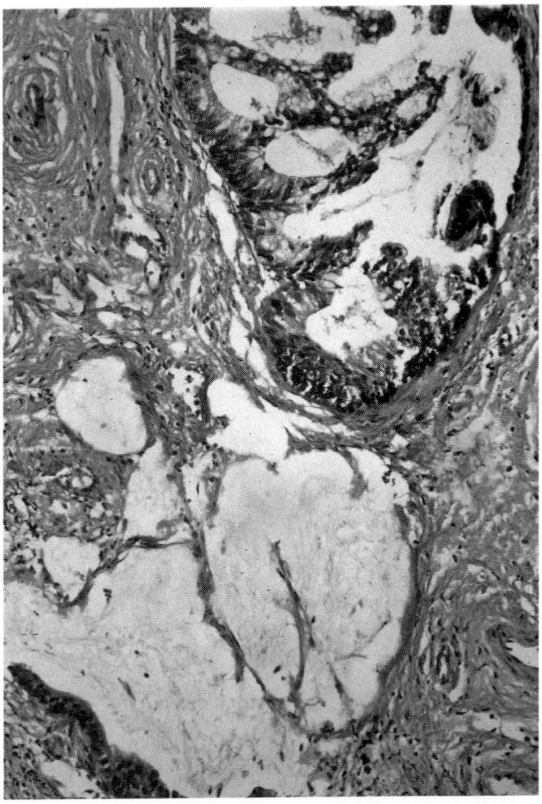

Figure 8–116. Adenocarcinoma of cervix, poorly differentiated, endocervical type. *A,* Tumor cells contain abundant vacuolated cytoplasm and pleomorphic nuclei. *B,* Metastasis in the pelvic lymph node. Tumor cells are predominantly solid.

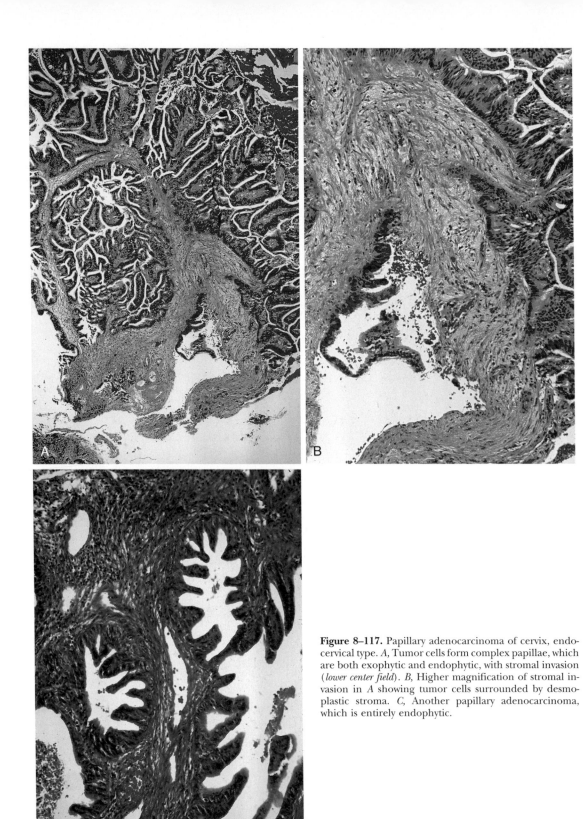

Figure 8–117. Papillary adenocarcinoma of cervix, endocervical type. *A,* Tumor cells form complex papillae, which are both exophytic and endophytic, with stromal invasion (*lower center field*). *B,* Higher magnification of stromal invasion in *A* showing tumor cells surrounded by desmoplastic stroma. *C,* Another papillary adenocarcinoma, which is entirely endophytic.

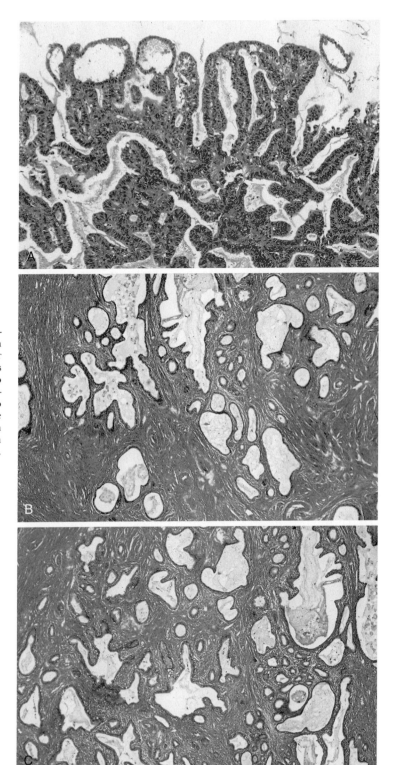

Figure 8–118. Microcystic endocervical adenocarcinoma of cervix. *A,* In the initial cervical biopsy, the tumor cells form complex papillary glands and reveal moderate nuclear atypia to justify the diagnosis of a well-differentiated adenocarcinoma of cervix. *B* to *D,* In the hysterectomy specimen, the tumor cells maintain a lobular pattern resembling cystic tunnel clusters. *C,* In other areas, the lobular pattern is lost. *Illustration continued on following page*

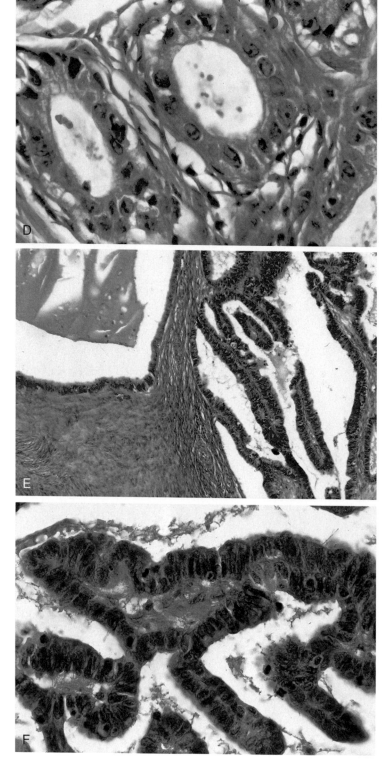

Figure 8–118. *Continued D,* Higher magnification of tumor cells reveals moderate nuclear atypia and medium-sized nucleoli. This tumor measures 5 mm in depth and 10 mm in width. *E* and *F,* Ovarian metastasis showing tumor cells forming complex papillary glands and moderate nuclear and increased mitotic activity. (Courtesy of Dr. B.F. Chen, Mackay Memorial Hospital, Taipei, Taiwan.)

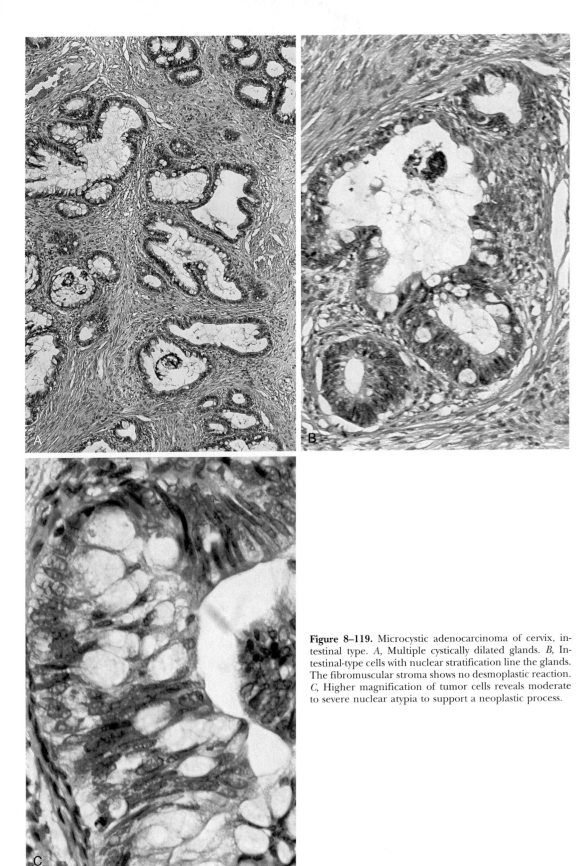

Figure 8–119. Microcystic adenocarcinoma of cervix, intestinal type. *A,* Multiple cystically dilated glands. *B,* Intestinal-type cells with nuclear stratification line the glands. The fibromuscular stroma shows no desmoplastic reaction. *C,* Higher magnification of tumor cells reveals moderate to severe nuclear atypia to support a neoplastic process.

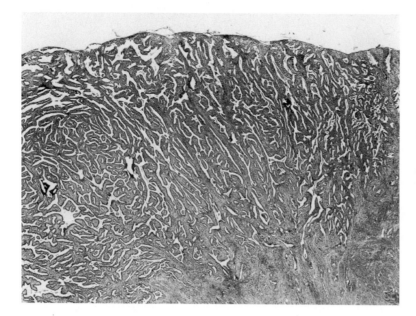

Figure 8–120. Minimal deviation adenocarcinoma of cervix, endocervical type. Irregular, complex, slit-like glandular spaces extend deeply into the cervical stroma.

Microscopic Features

The surface of the tumor is usually covered by normal squamous or endocervical epithelium. Less frequently, tumor cells proliferate on the mucosal surface, resembling well-differentiated villoglandular adenocarcinoma or villous adenoma of the colon.[239] Despite the regular branching patterns of the neoplastic glands, they differ from the normal endocervical glands in several ways. They tend to be more complex and more irregular in size and shape. Under low-power examination, the appearance of complex convoluted glands and slit-like glands with pointed ends is an important clue as to the neoplastic nature (Figs. 8–120 to 8–122).[175,238] Encroachment of the blood vessels and nerve fibers is an additional sign of stromal invasion. The lining cells, while retaining a single layer without nuclear stratification, may reveal focal papillary infoldings and nuclear atypia with enlargement and chromatin clumping. Nucleoli may be prominent.

Another helpful feature is the presence of large mucous pools or an inflammatory response similar to that of the mucocele of the oral cavity or Bartholin's gland (Fig. 8–123).

Within the granulation tissue, mucin-containing macrophages are mixed with lymphocytes and plasma cells. This type of tissue reaction also can be seen following stromal invasion with leakage of mucinous content, and therefore it is important to search for signet-ring cells to rule out a malignant disease. In essence, when features are suggestive of but not diagnostic for MDA, more tissue with adequate depth should be requested.

With immunoperoxidase stain, cytoplasmic CEA was demonstrable in all five MDAs. However, one of five benign, histologically atypical endocervical lesions was also positive.[238]

In MDA of the endometrioid type, the lining cells have the appearance of proliferative or hyperplastic endometrium (Fig. 8–124). Although mild nuclear stratification may be seen, atypia is minimal. In the clear cell variant, clear cells and hobnail cells line the small, round to oval, regular, and isolated glands. Mitotic activity in mucinous and clear cell variants of MDA is, on average, one to three mitoses per 10 high-power fields, but it is higher in the endometrioid type. All cases of MDA were deeply invasive, with the most superficial one having a depth of 7 mm.[177]

McGowan et al.[231] reported two cases of Peutz-

Figure 8–121. Minimal deviation adenocarcinoma of cervix, endocervical type. *A,* Branching and budding endocervical glands resembling normal endocervix. In small biopsies, it is impossible to know the depth of lesion. *B,* Lining cells in many areas have small, basally located nuclei without nuclear atypia, identical to normal endocervical cells. *C,* In other areas, low-grade nuclear atypia appear in some of the tumor cells. *D,* Rarely the tumor cells form papillary architecture and reveal moderate nuclear atypia to indicate a neoplastic process.

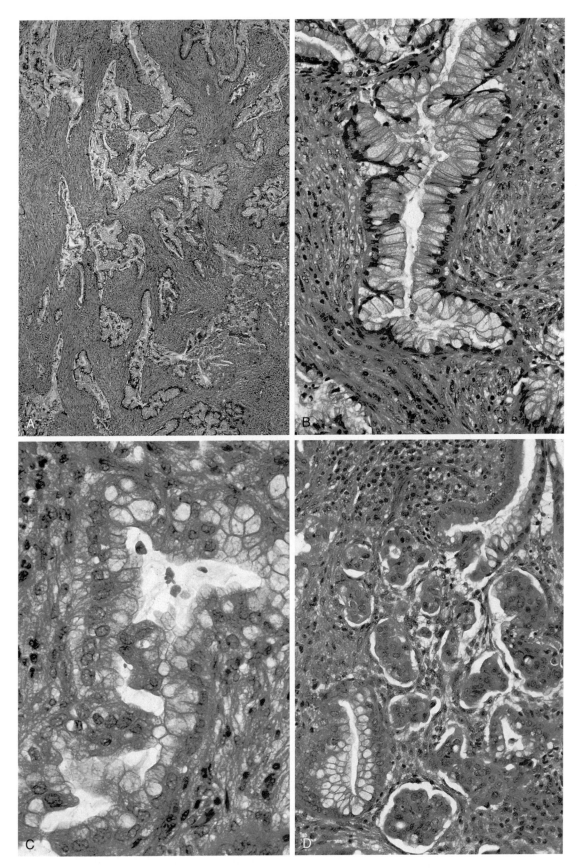

Figure 8–121 *See legend on opposite page*

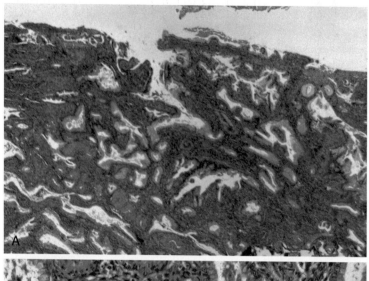

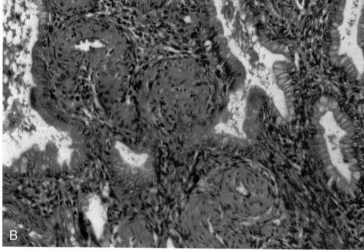

Figure 8–122. Minimal deviation adenocarcinoma of cervix, endocervical type. *A,* Branching glands are more complex than expected in normal endocervix. *B,* Lining cells with tall columnar configuration and abundant amphophilic cytoplasm. Nuclear atypia is minimal, but the close relationship with the arterioles is unusual for benign endocervical glands.

Jeghers syndrome associated with hamartomatous intestinal polyps, mucocutaneous melanin pigmentation, and mucinous MDA. In addition, one woman had bilateral ovarian sex-cord tumors with annular tubules, whereas the other women had bilateral ovarian mucinous cystadenoma of borderline malignancy. Both patients died of cervical MDA. A review of the literature indicates that cervical adenocarcinoma is relatively common in women with Peutz-Jeghers syndrome and its detection warrants careful examination of the genital tract.[231]

Differential Diagnosis

Misdiagnosis of MDA as benign lesions has received considerable emphasis. Correct diagno-

sis begins from recognition of subtle abnormal cells in the cervical smears. They reveal mild nuclear enlargement, irregularity, and uneven chromatin. Nucleoli may be evident. The cytoplasm has a vacuolated appearance. The smear has a mucinous or watery background. The subtle irregularity in the size and shape of glandular cells and encroachment of the blood vessels and nerve fibers support stromal invasion (see Fig. 8–124C).

It is equally important, however, not to overdiagnose tunnel clusters of endocervical gland, hyperplastic mesonephric ducts, and endometriosis as MDA. Michael et al.[238] reported additional benign conditions that are difficult to distinguish from MDA. These include (1) hyperplastic endocervical glands and reserve cell

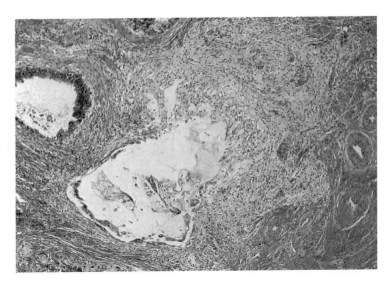

Figure 8–123. Mucoceles with histiocytic reaction following rupture of a neoplastic gland.

hyperplasia arranged in a cribriform pattern, (2) highly reactive endocervical glands secondary to inflammation, and (3) slit-like distortion of endocervical glands caused by fixation and mechanical artifacts. In addition, rupture of mucus-filled glands, which results in extravasated mucin and entrapped cells in the stroma, can simulate mucinous carcinoma.[238] These benign changes might reveal nuclear enlargement and hyperchromasia resulting from poor fixation, mechanical distortion, and cellular degeneration. Mitotic activity is low to absent. Immunoperoxidase stain for CEA may be useful.[238]

Prognosis

Patients with MDA are reported initially to have a dismal outcome by some investigators[175,233] but more favorable survival rates by others.[156,177,328] A closer examination of the extent of disease reveals that the survival rates in patients with Stage I or II neoplasm without pelvic lymph node metastasis are favorable after radical hysterectomy. Most patients with clinical Stage III or IV disease died. In some advanced cases, a delay in diagnosis was attributed to failure to recognize abnormal cells evident in earlier cytologic or histologic samples.

Well-Differentiated Villoglandular Adenocarcinoma

Young and Scully[388] initially reported on a series of 13 villoglandular papillary adenocarci-

nomas of the uterine cervix. This tumor tends to occur in young women (mean age 33 years). The lesions are described clinically as polypoid, condylomatous, eroded, nodular, white, friable, or fungating. Microscopically, the superficial portion of the tumor consists of complex papillae lined by well-differentiated endocervical cells. In the deeper portion of the tumors, tumor cells form branching tubular glands surrounded by a fibrous stroma (Figs. 8–125 and 8–126). The tumor was confined to the superficial one third of the cervical wall in six women, whereas deep invasion occurred in two women. After hysterectomy, no tumor recurrence was noted in 10 women followed for 2 to 14 years.[388]

In a subsequent study of 24 cases by Jones et al.,[174] the mean age was 37 years (range 27 to 54 years), and 50% were in their third decade of life. There was a history of oral contraceptive use in 63% of women, which was higher than the 28% among women with other types of cervical adenocarcinoma (*P* = 0.02). Grossly, the tumor had an exophytic polypoid appearance. Microscopically, the predominant cell type was endocervical in 50%, endometrioid in 33%, and intestinal in 17%. Coexisting squamous dysplasia or carcinoma in situ was present in 33%. Five (21%) tumors were entirely in situ without stromal invasion; 75% (18) were superficial and confined to inner third of the cervical wall; and 4% (1) invaded 75% of the cervical wall.[174]

Treatment modalities included local excision or cone biopsy in five, simple hysterectomy in four, and radical hysterectomy in 15 women.[174]

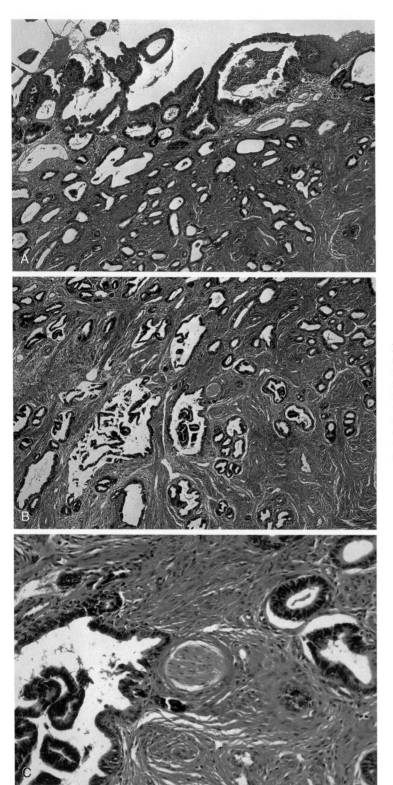

Figure 8–124. Minimal deviation adenocarcinoma of cervix, endometrioid type, removed by conization. *A,* Adenocarcinoma in situ and underlying invasive adenocarcinoma. In the latter, the tumor cells form small and cystic glands. *B,* The tumor cells are deeply invasive. *C,* Well-differentiated tumor cells come close to perineural space.

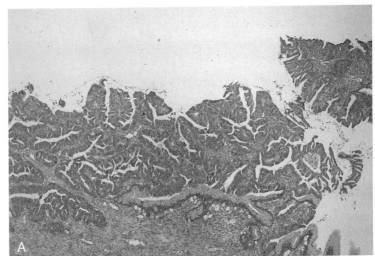

Figure 8–125. Well-differentiated villoglandular adenocarcinoma of cervix. *A,* Exophytic papillary growth on the surface. No evidence of stromal invasion appears in the conization specimen. *B,* Moderate nuclear atypia of tumor cells. This is an example of villoglandular adenocarcinoma in situ.

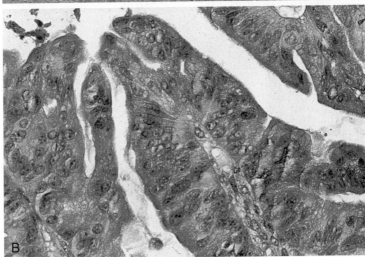

All tumors were confined to the cervix without pelvic lymph node metastasis. All women were alive and well 7 to 77 (mean 36) months later. In view of the distinct clinical and pathologic features, these tumors are separated from other cervical adenocarcinomas. A conservative treatment is considered to be justified, especially in young women who want to retain fertility.[174]

The term *villoglandular papillary adenocarcinoma* should be reserved for only those tumors that meet the strict morphologic criteria. The degree of nuclear atypia should be no worse than moderate. The tumor borders should be smooth, and clear cells and serous cells are excluded (see Figs. 8–125 and 8–126). In the cervical biopsies and endocervical curettage are fragments of tumor with a villous pattern; however, in subsequently excised specimens, some of these tumors prove to have poorly differentiated elements (Fig. 8–127). Thus, the diagnosis of well-differentiated villoglandular papillary adenocarcinoma should be made on the basis of the completely excised neoplasm.

Endometrioid Adenocarcinoma

This group of tumors has the appearance of grade 1 or grade 2 adenocarcinoma of the endometrium. The predominant growth pattern is glandular or, less commonly, papillary. The lining cells are tall and columnar, and have densely basophilic or eosinophilic cytoplasm (Fig. 8–128). Mature metaplastic squamous cells sometimes occur within the neoplastic glands.[110,115] The diagnosis is justified only if

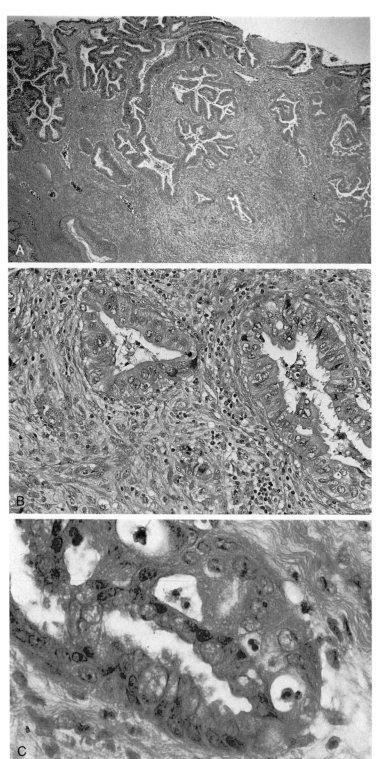

Figure 8–126. Well-differentiated villoglandular adenocarcinoma of cervix. *A,* Exophytic papillary growth and limited stromal invasion on conization specimen. *B,* Invasive neoplastic glands surrounded by desmoplastic stroma. *C,* Moderate nuclear atypia.

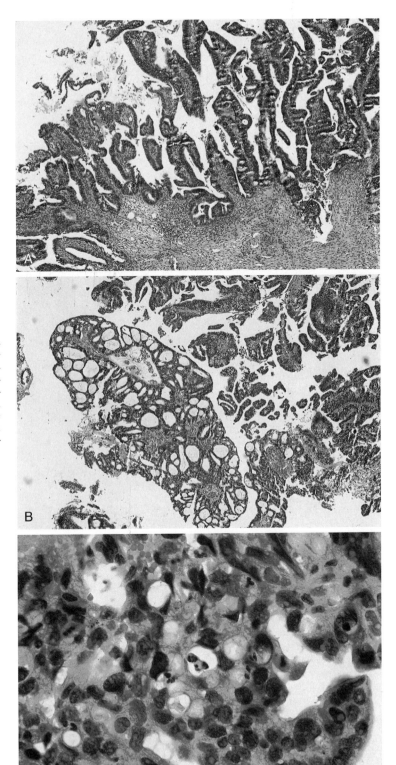

Figure 8–127. Mimicker of villoglandular adenocarcinoma with poorly differentiated elements. *A,* In the cervical biopsy, the tumor has the appearance of villoglandular adenocarcinoma. *B* and *C,* However, a small portion of exophytic tumor is made up of tumor cells forming cribriform glands. These cells demonstrate severe nuclear atypia.

Illustration continued on following page

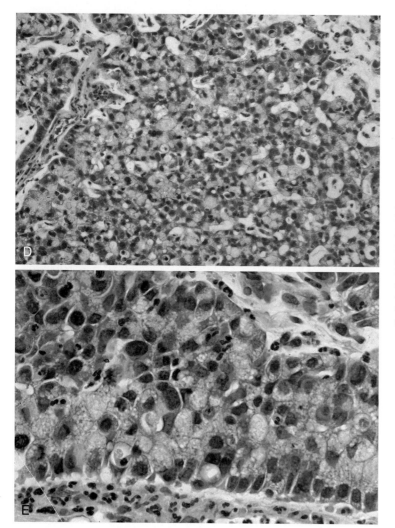

Figure 8–127. *Continued D* and *E,* In the hysterectomy specimen, part of the invasive adenocarcinoma is poorly differentiated and tumor cells have a signet-ring appearance. This case illustrates the importance of complete excision of the tumor for histologic examination before the tumor can be accepted as well-differentiated villoglandular adenocarcinoma.

the endometrium is normal after careful sampling for histologic examination.

Differential Diagnosis of Primary and Secondary Cervical Adenocarcinomas

Although the true frequency of secondary malignancies of the cervix is unknown, there is no question that the majority result from direct extensions of endometrial carcinoma, and especially those of the adenosquamous type. This poses a significant problem in the pathologic diagnosis and management of patients. It is highly desirable to distinguish between primary endometrial and endocervical carcinomas because of the differences in prognosis and treatment plans for the two diseases. Special stains using histochemical and immunoperoxidase techniques are useful to an extent.

More than 90% of endocervical adenocarcinomas, irrespective of their differentiation, have demonstrable mucin and PAS diastase-resistant material in the cytoplasm of malignant cells.[74] In endometrial adenocarcinomas, many cells contain glycogen particles, which are digested by diastase. Mucin and PAS diastase-resistant material, although frequently present in the lumen and the apical cell borders, is rarely found in the cytoplasm. When present, it is usually found in tumor cells with endocervical mucinous metaplasia.

With the use of the immunoperoxidase technique, carcinoembryonic antigen (CEA) was reported by Wahlstrom et al.[368] as being useful for differentiating between endocervical and endometrial adenocarcinomas. Of 107 endocervical adenocarcinomas, 80% were positive for CEA, whereas none of 122 endometrial ade-

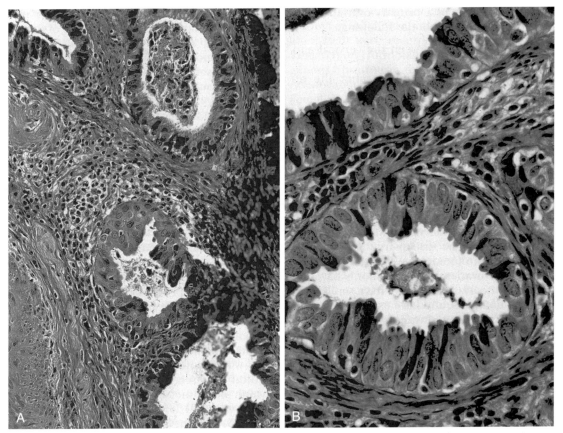

Figure 8–128. Adenocarcinoma of cervix, endometrioid type. *A,* Irregular infiltrative glands. There is focal squamous metaplasia. *B,* Tumor cells show moderate nuclear atypia.

nocarcinomas were positive. Clear cell carcinomas of the cervix and endometrium were consistently negative for CEA. Most adenosquamous carcinomas of the cervix and endometrium were positive for CEA.[368] A study by Cohen et al.[74] confirmed that all endocervical adenocarcinomas were positive for CEA, with the majority having strong staining, including 77% cytoplasmic and 77% diffuse. The immunostaining for CEA in endometrial adenocarcinomas was mostly weak (82%), located on the cell surface (82%) and focal (64%). However, 52% of endometrial adenocarcinomas contained CEA, including 19% in the cytoplasm.[74] In a study by Dabbs et al.,[87] CEA was demonstrated in 87% of endocervical adenocarcinomas (47% predominantly luminal, 40% cytoplasmic) and in 72% of endometrial adenocarcinomas (55% predominantly luminal, 17% cytoplasmic).

Antivimentin turns out to be useful because endocervical adenocarcinomas are consistently nonreactive, whereas 65% of endometrial adenocarcinomas are reactive to antivimentin.[87] Its localization corresponds to the intermediate filaments present in the perinuclear region. Although quantitative and topographic differences for CEA and vimentin exist between endocervical and endometrial adenocarcinomas, the sensitivity and specificity remain to be improved.

Young and Scully[389] reported 16 cases of mucinous tumor involving ovaries and cervix. The women ranged in age from 25 to 70 (mean 44) years. Two had evidence of Peutz-Jeghers syndrome. The ovarian tumors had the appearance of cystic mucinous adenocarcinoma. The cervical tumors resembled adenoma malignum in 10 cases and moderately to poorly differentiated adenocarcinoma in six cases. In this group of 16 cases, 10 ovarian tumors were considered to be independent primaries, three neoplasms metastatic from the cervix, and in three cases the ovaries contained both primary and metastatic tumors.[389]

Of the seven women with Stage IB disease, six were free of disease from 1.5 to 8.3 years. The seventh woman died of disease at 6.2 years, with mediastinal and pleural metastases. Two women with Stage IIB and Stage IVB tumor were dead of pelvic recurrence.[327a]

MIXED ADENOSQUAMOUS CARCINOMA

Histologic Classification and Diagnostic Problems

Approximately 50% of cervical adenocarcinomas contain malignant squamous cells. Of these, adenoid cystic carcinoma and adenoid basal carcinoma are sufficiently distinct to be recognized as separate entities. The remaining neoplasms have been designated as mixed carcinoma, adenosquamous carcinoma, adenoepidermoid carcinoma, mucoepidermoid carcinoma, adenoacanthoma, reserve cell carcinoma, double primary carcinoma, collision carcinoma, and squamous carcinoma with mucin secretion.[5,109,116,123,130] This monograph accepts the term *adenosquamous carcinoma* and its variants as originally proposed by Glucksmann and Cherry.[130] The precursor lesion is designated as adenosquamous carcinoma in situ.

The relative frequency of adenosquamous carcinoma among all cervical cancers is highly variable owing to a lack of uniform criteria used by the investigators. Most authors accept the designation of adenosquamous carcinoma when squamous cell carcinoma and adenocarcinoma are clearly identifiable on regular H&E-stained section. However, in some adenosquamous carcinomas, histochemical stains are required to define glandular differentiation. In a study by Benda et al.[30] of 69 consecutive Stage IB cervical cancers, the original histologic classification included 55 (80%) squamous cell carcinomas, 12 (17%) adenocarcinomas, and two (3%) undifferentiated carcinomas. With the use of mucicarmine and PAS staining, 18 of 55 (33%) squamous carcinomas contained mucinous material in the cytoplasm. If this finding is accepted as evidence of glandular differentiation, and thus mixed carcinoma, only 54%[37] of tumors remain as squamous type (35% keratinizing, 16% nonkeratinizing, 3% small cell), and the frequency of mixed carcinoma is increased to 26%. As is discussed in a later section, this group of tumors should be recognized as a variant of adenosquamous carcinoma and should be differentiated from ordinary squamous carcinoma.

Adenosquamous Carcinoma In Situ

Two types of precursors of adenosquamous carcinoma have been recognized. The first group includes adenocarcinomas in situ with coexisting squamous carcinoma in situ (see Fig. 8–106C and D). Their invasive counterparts resemble the mature type of adenosquamous carcinoma, in which glandular and squamous elements are readily recognized.

The second type of adenosquamous CIS was first described by Steiner and Friedell,[336] who reported the presence of mucin-producing signet-ring cells within the squamous cell CIS as revealed by PAS stain. This change was noted in 5 of 13 (38%) pregnant women, in contrast to only 2 of 45 (4%) nonpregnant women. This lesion was considered to be the precursor of the signet-ring variant of mixed carcinoma.

Histologically, the second type of adenosquamous CIS consists of intermingled dysplastic glandular cells and squamous cells (Fig. 8–132). This change may involve the endocervical surface or the underlying glands, or both. Without the aid of PAS or mucicarmine stain, the lesion is most often classified as squamous SIL. The cytoplasm, however, has a distinct vacuolated or basophilic quality (Fig. 8–133). Mucin-producing cells can be identified in small groups or in isolated forms scattered throughout the squamous epithelium. Qilzibash[280] found only one such case in a total of 14 in situ and microinvasive adenocarcinomas. This change was recently named "stratified mucin-producing intraepithelial lesions" and is considered to be a poorly differentiated or stratified variant of adenocarcinoma in situ.[269]

The proliferating cells had highly atypical, large, irregular nuclei, many of which were elongated in shape. Mitotic figures were abundant. Many cells had vacuolated or basophilic cytoplasm, containing mucinous material as demonstrated by PAS or mucicarmine stain. However, the mucinous differentiation was inapparent in some lesions, even with special stains. The age of 18 patients ranged from 23 to 57 years. The mean age of women without invasive carcinoma was 34.5 years, as compared to 41.8 years for those with invasive carcinoma. Other coexisting lesions included CIN 2 or CIN 3 in 14 (78%) cases, adenocarcinoma in situ in 11 (61%) cases, invasive adenocarcinoma in

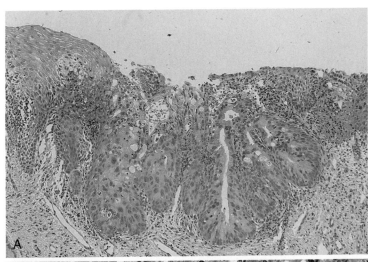

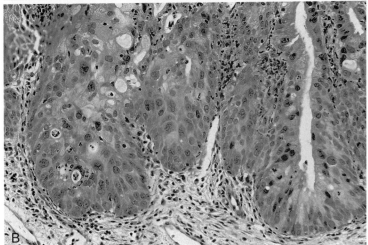

Figure 8–132. *A* and *B*, Coexisting squamous dysplasia and gladular dysplasia.

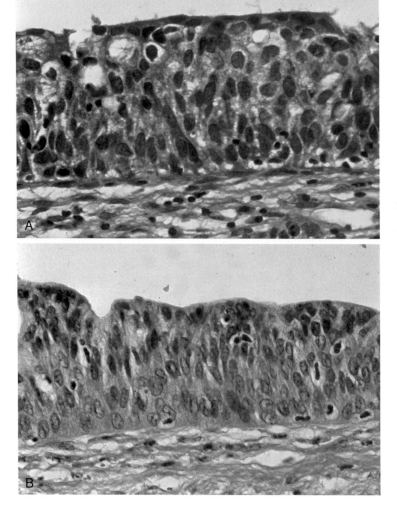

Figure 8–133. Adenosquamous carcinoma in situ. *A* and *B*, Multiple layers of vertically arranged, elongated dysplastic cells on endocervical mucosa resembling CIN 3. Some cells have vacuolated cytoplasm that contains mucicarminophilic material (not shown).

four (22%) cases, separate squamous carcinoma and adenocarcinoma in one (5.5%) case, adenosquamous carcinoma in five (25%) cases, and papillary squamous neoplasm in two (11%) cases.

Immunohistochemical stain for Ki-67 with MIB-1 antibody disclosed a high index of cell proliferation in all cases.[269] All lesions were negative for cytokeratin 14. The stain for P63 was variable. P63-positive squamous cells were confined to the basal layer of the lesion and were not seen in areas of columnar cell differentiation. Immunohistochemical stain for p63 is helpful to visualize neoplastic squamous cells in a background of glandular cells (Fig. 8–134).

Invasive Mixed Adenosquamous Carcinoma

Microscopic Features

Glucksmann and Cherry[130] subdivided adenosquamous carcinomas into mature, well-differentiated type (35%) and immature, poorly differentiated type. The latter is divided into signet-ring (44%) and glassy cell (21%) types and is estimated to make up 2% of all cervical cancers and 13% of glandular neoplasms.[130] Maier and Norris[222] recorded only 2% of 389 primary cervical adenocarcinomas as glassy cell type.

In the mature type of adenosquamous carcinoma, the glandular and squamous elements are readily recognized (Fig. 8–135). The majority of squamous carcinomas have the appearance of the large cell nonkeratinizing type. Keratinizing and small cell types are less common. The squamous cells contain abundant eosinophilic cytoplasm and evidence of individual cell keratinization (see Fig. 8–135). Sometimes, the predominant cells have clear cytoplasm with abundant glycogen.

The glandular elements are well to moderately differentiated. Most of the tumor cells contain vacuolated cytoplasm, which is mucicarminophilic. With the use of immunohistochemical stain for p63, most of the malignant squamous cells are positive for p63. Even in the areas of neoplastic glands, p63-positive tumor cells are present in the outermost layers, indicative of the presence of squamous cells (see Fig. 8–135).

In the signet-ring type, the tumor cells grow in solid nests and sheets closely resembling nonkeratinizing squamous cell carcinoma. However, some cells have basophilic, vacuolated, or clear cytoplasm, and many have the appearance of signet-ring cells (Fig. 8–136). With mucicarmine staining, mucous secretion can be confirmed. Some of the tumors reported as "mucoepidermoid carcinoma" and "squamous cell carcinoma with mucin secretion" by Benda et al.[30] and Ireland et al.[163] fall into this category.

In glassy cell carcinoma, the tumor cells are separated into small nests by fibrous stroma, which is heavily infiltrated by eosinophils and plasma cells. The individual cells have abundant eosinophilic, granular, and ground-glass–appearing cytoplasm as well as distinct cell borders (Fig. 8–137). The uniformly round to oval nuclei contain prominent nucleoli. Mitotic figures are abundant. In the original cases of Glucksmann and Cherry,[130] no mucinous secretion was noted. Maier and Norris[222] found intracellular mucin in seven of eight tumors studied with mucicarmine stain. Three of eight neoplasms contained glandular lumens, and three others had squamous differentiation. One tumor had both glandular and squamous foci. These findings tend to support dual differentiation of these neoplasms.

Ultrastructural studies of glassy cell carcinoma similarly support the presence of glandular cells with intracytoplasmic lumens and additional cells, which are rich in tonofilaments, suggesting squamous differentiation.[272,358,391] In addition, cells that retain prominent microvilli but accumulate abundant tonofilaments have been observed. These cells may represent an intermediate stage of development from glandular to squamous differentiation.

Prognosis

The clinical and pathologic parameters in relation to the prognosis of adenosquamous carcinoma are conflicting owing to the inconsistent morphologic criteria and different treatment modalities used by investigators. Shingleton et al.[323] did not find differences in the 3-year survival rates among patients with adenocarcinoma, adenosquamous carcinoma, or squamous carcinoma. Others have found that the outcome of patients with adenosquamous carcinoma is significantly worse than for those with pure adenocarcinoma.[61,116,123,306]

Text continued on page 447

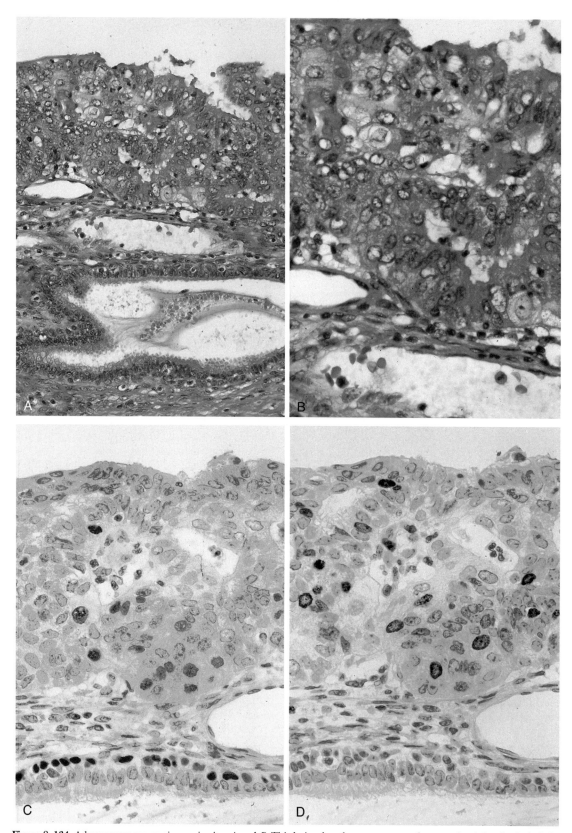

Figure 8–134. Adenosquamous carcinoma in situ. *A* and *B,* This lesion has the appearance of severe glandular dysplasia/adenocarcinoma in situ. However, there are small clusters of cells that have abundant eosinophilic to clear cytoplasm and distinct cell borders to suggest squamous cells. *C,* Immunohistochemical stain for p63 confirms the presence of p63-positive immature squamous cells corresponding to cells with eosinophilic cytoplasm. The normal endocervical gland at the lower field demonstrates the presence of p63-positive subcolumnar reserve cell. Abnormal glandular cells are negative for p63. *D,* Immunohistochemical stain for Ki-67 reveals abundant proliferative glandular and squamous cells. (See color section.)

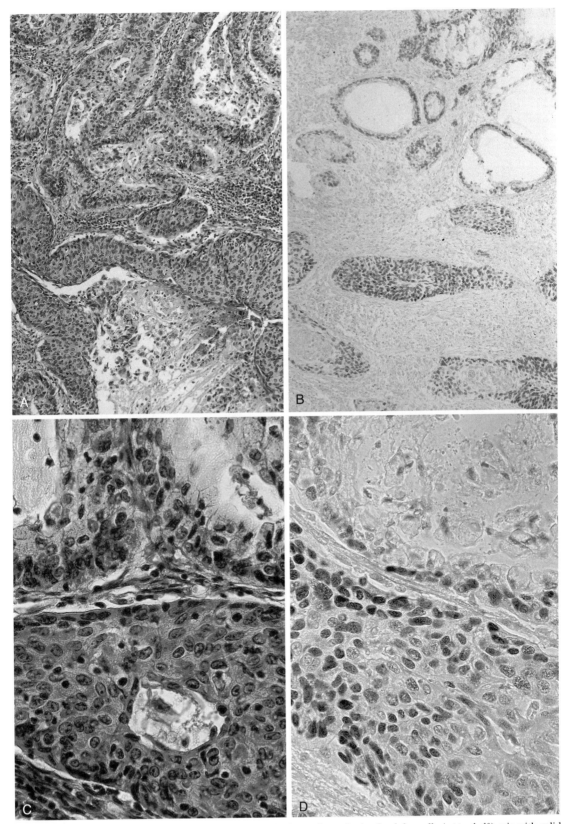

Figure 8–135. Adenosquamous carcinoma, mature type. *A,* Nests of neoplastic glandular cells (*upper half*) mix with solid nests of malignant squamous cells (*lower half*). *B,* Similar area as in *A* demonstrates p63-positive stem/immature squamous cells in the nests of glandular and squamous cells. *C,* Higher magnification demonstrates malignant glandular cells with basophilic to vacuolated mucinous cytoplasm. In contrast, squamous cells have eosinophilic cytoplasm. *D,* Similar area as in *C* reveals expression of p63 in cells beneath the glandular cells and in most of the squamous cells. (See color section.)

Illustration continued on following page

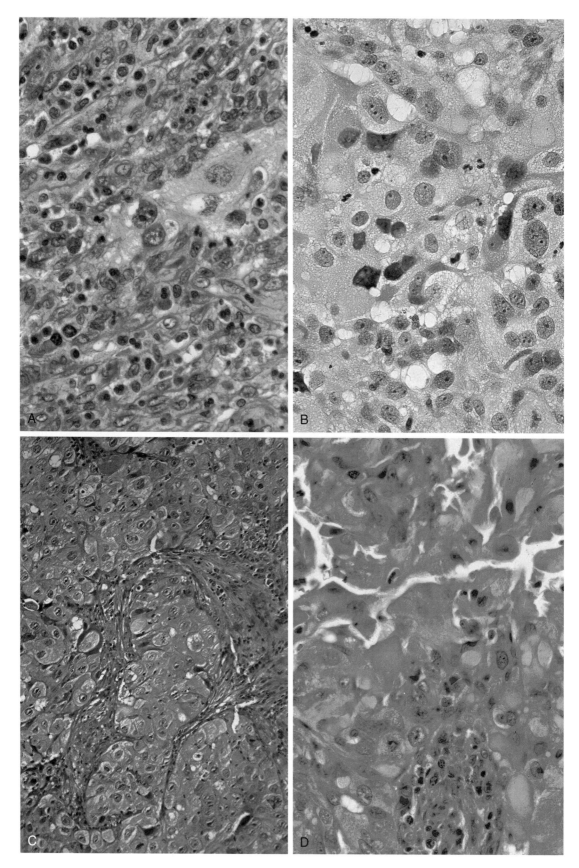

Figure 8–137 *See legend on opposite page*

In a study of Stage IB carcinoma by Gallup et al.,[123] the survival rate for women with adenosquamous carcinoma was 27%, compared with 91% for those with squamous carcinoma and 83% for those with adenocarcinoma. The frequency of tumor recurrence following radical hysterectomy for Stage IB cervical cancer was 9.2% for squamous cell carcinoma and 17.4% for both adenocarcinoma and adenosquamous carcinoma.[61] In our series of patients with adenosquamous carcinoma, the poor prognosis can be attributed to a high frequency of vascular lymphatic invasion (50%), persistence of tumor following preoperative radiotherapy (86%), and metastasis to distant site (25%).[116]

Reports of glassy cell carcinoma have shown a high frequency of pelvic and extrapelvic spread and poor response to surgery and/or radiotherapy, with 5-year survival rates in the range of 31% to 33%.[212a,265] This poor outcome was attributed to radioresistance and understaging of the tumor.[265] When compared according to surgical staging, the proportion of patients with Stage III disease increased from 23% to 60%, and those with Stage IV cancer increased from 0% to 20%.[265]

A study by Bethwaite et al.[37] included 165 cases of cervical cancer of Stage IB or higher. Representative paraffin blocks were stained for PAS with and without diastase and alcian blue at pH 2.6 to identify mucinous material. Based on the results of these stains for mucin, the relative frequency of squamous cell carcinoma decreased from 85.7% to 64%. Frequency of adenocarcinoma remains similar from 7.5% to 6.9%. On the other hand, adenosquamous carcinoma increased from 3.1% to 24.2%. Only 49% of adenosquamous carcinomas were Stage IB (49%), in contrast to 60% for squamous cell carcinoma ($P = 0.004$). The overall 5-year survival rate for patients with squamous cell carcinoma was 75%, as compared with 52% for those with adenosquamous carcinoma ($P = 0.006$).

A high frequency of lymph node metastasis also contributed to a poor outcome in the signet-ring variant. In a study by Benda et al.[30] of Stage IB cervical carcinoma, six of 18 (33%) women with squamous carcinomas and mucin production had pelvic lymph node metastasis. This is in contrast to only two of 37 (5%) squamous carcinomas without mucin ($P = 0.01$). In a series of 23 squamous cell carcinomas studied by PAS and alcian blue stains for mucin, only two of eight (25%) women whose tumors demonstrated cytoplasmic mucin were alive after 3 years. Among 15 women whose tumors did not contain mucin, 13 (87%) survived ($P < 0.01$).[163] These studies indicate that squamous cell carcinoma with mucin production represents a distinct entity that should be differentiated from conventional squamous carcinoma.

In another study, 12 Stage I "mucoepidermoid" carcinomas were compared with 265 Stage IB squamous cell carcinomas.[352] In this study, *mucoepidermoid carcinoma* is defined as the presence of mucin in what appears to be squamous cell carcinoma without any glandular formation but having demonstrable intracellular mucin as shown by mucicarmine staining. Ten of 12 tumors had focal mucin secretion. The remaining two had more than 40% to 50% mucus-secreting cells. The frequency of pelvic lymph node metastasis was 33% in mucoepidermoid carcinoma, as compared with 14% for squamous cell carcinoma. Capillary-lymphatic space invasion occurred in 50% of tumors.[352]

In a study by Costa et al.[79] that included 35 pure adenocarcinomas, 26 adenosquamous carcinomas (4 glassy cell carcinoma), and 4 villoglandular papillary adenocarcinomas, 21 (38%) patients had tumor recurrence, including three local, 10 distant, and eight both. Thirty-five (62%) women were disease free. Tumors with adenosquamous or serous differentiation were the only histological types that developed tumor recurrence.[79] Other risk factors for recurrence included vascular space invasion, deep invasion, high nuclear grade, large tumor on clinical or pathologic examination, and lymph node metastasis at surgery. There was no difference in prognosis among mucinous, endometrioid, or clear cell tumors. All patients with villoglandular adenocarcinoma were alive and well.[79]

Adenoid Cystic Carcinoma

Adenoid cystic carcinoma of the female lower genital tract occurs most commonly in the

---

Figure 8–137. Adenosquamous carcinoma, glassy cell type. *A,* Tumor cells are surrounded by abundant eosinophils, lymphocytes, and plasma cells. *B,* Tumor cells have abundant granular eosinophilic cytoplasm. *C,* Nests of tumor cells have opaque, eosinophilic, ground glass cytoplasm. *D,* Typical glassy cells with densely eosinophilic cytoplasm, prominent nucleoli, and distinct cell borders.

Bartholin's gland, followed by the uterine cervix. Most women with adenoid cystic carcinoma of the cervix are postmenopausal and in their seventh decade of life, which is about 20 years later than those with squamous cell carcinoma.[324] The histologic features are similar to those that occur in the salivary gland. It is suggested that multipotential reserve cells in the endocervical glands acquire myoepithelial differentiation, which is not normally seen in the cervix.

Histologically, basaloid cells are typically arranged in cribriform glands with hyaline or mucinous material in the microcystic spaces (Fig. 8–138). Tubules and solid nests are less common. Tumors with a predominantly solid growth pattern may metastasize early. The individual cells have scanty cytoplasm and small, uniform, hyperchromatic nuclei. Mitotic figures are variable, depending on the degree of differentiation.[101]

In about 50% of cases, squamous differentiation is apparent. In such cases, squamous cells replace the glandular lumens partially or completely and invade the adjacent stroma, resembling squamous cell carcinoma (Fig. 8–139). When squamous elements predominate, adenoid cystic carcinoma may not be recognized in a small biopsy sample. Adenoid cystic carcinoma may also be associated with squamous carcinoma in situ; because of this, some cases are detected initially by abnormal cervical smears. Other types of adenocarcinoma, undifferentiated carcinoma, or sarcoma may sometimes coexist with adenoid cystic carcinoma.[101,205]

In one study, the 3- to 5-year survival rate for patients with Stage I adenoid cystic carcinoma was 56%, compared with 27% for Stage II. None of the patients with Stage III or IV disease survived.[279] Most of the treatment failures were caused by distant and/or local pelvic recurrence. Metastases occurred most frequently in the lung (44%) and less commonly in the bone, liver, and brain. With only 32% of patients free of disease at last follow-up, the overall prognosis of adenoid cystic carcinoma is worse than that of squamous carcinoma or pure adenocarcinoma of the cervix.[279] In one review, the authors suggested that bulky early stage tumors are best treated with combined surgery and postoperative radiation therapy and chemotherapy by cisplatin.[95]

Adenoid Basal Carcinoma

This rare tumor was initially described by Baggish and Woodruff.[21] Most women with this tumor were in their fourth to seventh decades of life and had abnormal cervical smears that were suggestive of squamous CIS. In all patients, disease was confined to the cervix (Stage I).[101]

Histologically, the round to oval-shaped invasive nests seem to drop off from the overlying squamous cell CIS. Individual cells have the appearance of basaloid cells, with uniform and hyperchromatic nuclei, scanty cytoplasm, and distinct peripheral palisading (Fig. 8–140). Under lower power magnification, there is a resemblance to basal cell carcinoma of the skin. Mitotic activity is low, usually none to one mitotic figure per nest.[101] Occasional cells may contain eosinophilic cytoplasm, suggesting individual cell keratinization. The stroma elicits minimal desmoplasia. Vascular lymphatic invasion was not seen in any of the cases.[101] Approximately 50% of tumors also coexist with in situ or invasive adenocarcinoma with mucous secretion.[21,88] The depth of invasion tends to be superficial.

Most adenoid basal carcinomas have coexisting squamous severe dysplasia or squamous carcinoma in situ. Microinvasive squamous carcinoma may evolve from the periphery of solid nests replaced by neoplastic squamous cells. All reported cases were Stage IA or IB. The prognosis is excellent following hysterectomy. In a review of 26 cases reported in the literature, 85% of patients were alive without tumor recurrence. Three women (12%) died of other causes. Only one patient is known to have died of disease with metastasis in the lung.[49]

In a study of five cases of adenoid basal carcinoma by Jones et al.,[173] HPV DNA type 16 was detected in all the tumors studied by PCR. No K-ras-2 point mutation was detected. One tumor had a point mutation of p53; four others had weak reaction of p53 and two of these expressed WAF-1 (an effector protein induced by wild type p53). Grayson et al.[134] studied nine tumors by non-isotopic in situ hybridization and PCR using E6 consensus primers to HPV. HPV DNA type 16 was detected in four tumors (44%) and HPV 33 in two cases (27%) by in situ method, and three tumors were positive by PCR. HPV DNA was thought to be integrated based on punctate and combined punctate and diffuse signals. It is postulated that HPV integration leads to E2 disruption and loss of suppressive effects on E6 and E7 by binding to p53 and Rb gene product.[134]

The differential diagnosis includes adenoid basal hyperplasia, which occurs in the superficial endocervical glands. Adenoid cystic carcinoma presents with infiltrative cribriform glands

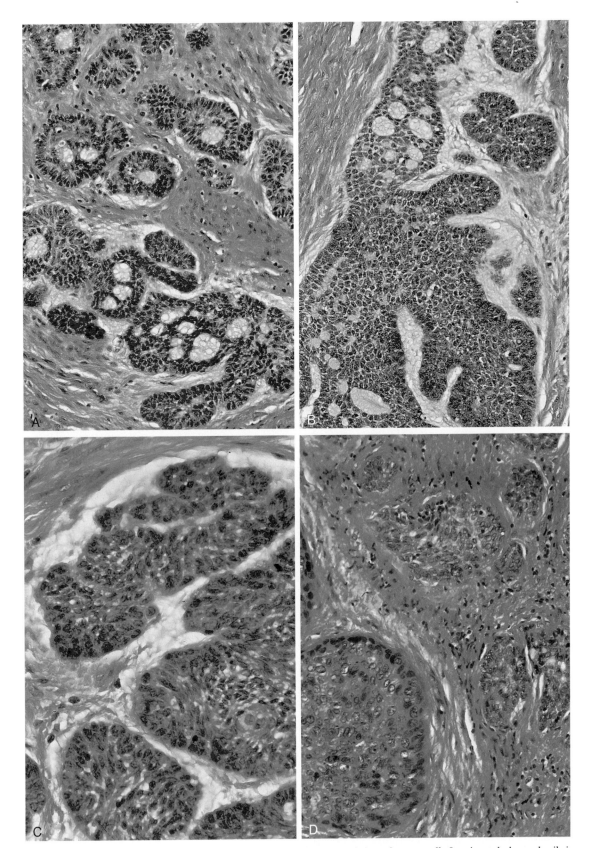

Figure 8–138. Adenoid cystic carcinoma. *A*, Well-differentiated area consisting of tumor cells forming tubules and cribriform glands. *B*, Moderately differentiated area containing cribriform glands and solid nests. Mucinous material is seen in the cribriform spaces. *C*, Higher magnification reveals basaloid tumor cells with hyperchromatic nuclei and scant cytoplasm. *D*, Solid nests in poorly differentiated tumor with basaloid appearance and nuclear pleomorphism (*left lower field*).

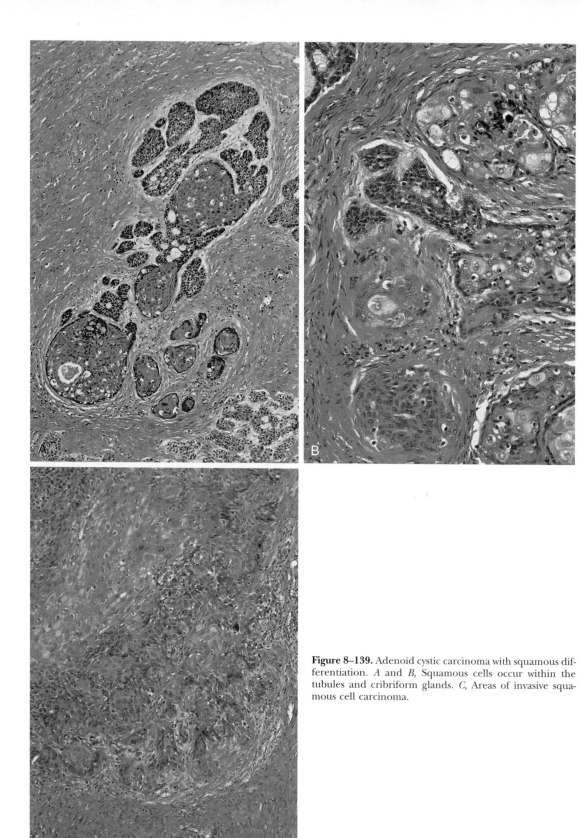

Figure 8–139. Adenoid cystic carcinoma with squamous differentiation. *A* and *B*, Squamous cells occur within the tubules and cribriform glands. *C*, Areas of invasive squamous cell carcinoma.

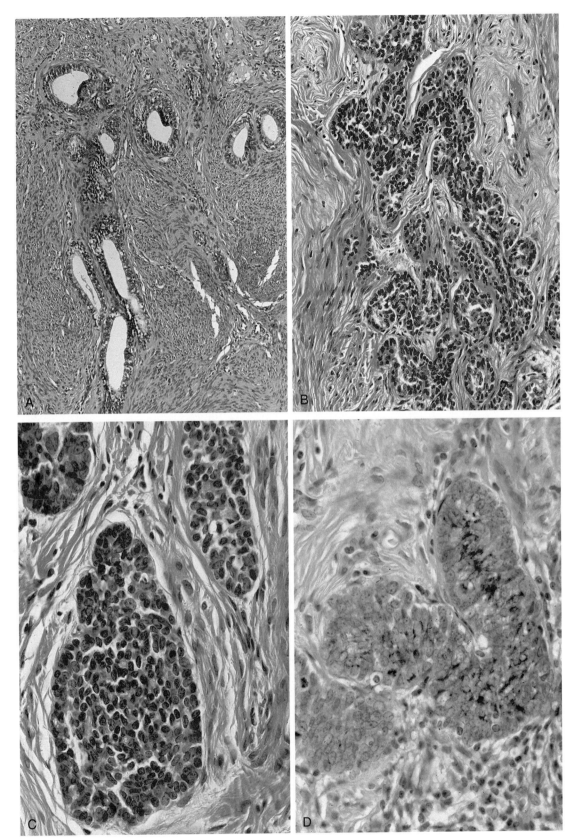

Figure 8–140. Adenoid basal carcinoma. *A,* Neoplastic glands lined by columnar tumor cells. *B,* Branching glands with basaloid cells. *C,* Solid nests of basaloid tumor cells with relatively uniform, round to oval hyperchromatic nuclei and scant cytoplasm. There is palisaded nuclear arrangement in the periphery of the solid nests. *D,* Tumor cells express carcinoembryonic antigen by immunohistochemical stain. (See color section.)

associated with extracellular mucinous material or hyaline cylinders. Cytologic atypia is evident in the tumor cells. In the case of rare basaloid squamous carcinoma, the tumor cells are cytologically malignant and mitotically active. The infiltrative tumor nests are surrounded by desmoplastic stroma that is sometimes hyalinized and resembles hyaline cylinders.

The solid nests in adenoid basal carcinoma have a distinct peripheral palisading. The tumor cells have low mitotic activity and do not invade vascular or lymphatic channels. In contrast to adenoid cystic carcinoma, adenoid basal carcinoma rarely demonstrates cribriform pattern. Unlike small cell carcinoma, the mitotic activity is low. Histochemical and immunohistochemical stains fail to reveal neuroendocrine differentiation.

OTHER MALIGNANT NEOPLASMS

Carcinoid Tumor and Neuroendocrine Carcinoma

Neuroendocrine neoplasms of the cervix are uncommon and have a wide morphologic spectrum, ranging from well-differentiated tumors that resemble carcinoid tumor of the lung and gastrointestinal tract to poorly differentiated neuroendocrine carcinomas, which are indistinguishable from small cell and large cell neuroendocrine carcinoma of the lung. These tumors are discussed in the earlier section on squamous cell carcinoma.

Between the two extremes are atypical carcinoid tumors. Some authors have adopted the terminology and morphologic criteria of lung tumors for cervical tumors.[127]

In the typical carcinoid tumor, mitotic activity is rare, nuclear atypia is mild, and no necrosis is seen (Fig. 8–141). Atypical carcinoid tumor has increased mitotic activity of up to 10 mitotic figures per high-power field, mild to moderate nuclear atypia, and focal necrosis (Fig. 8–142). Large cell neuroendocrine carcinoma has more than 10 mitotic figures per high-power field, moderate to severe nuclear atypia, and geographic necrosis. This diagnostic scheme simplifies the diagnosis and eliminates old terms

used in the past, such as argyrophil cell carcinoma,[227,248] endocrine cell carcinoma,[169,327] neuroendocrine carcinoma,[273] oat cell carcinoma,[165] small cell nonkeratinizing carcinoma,[170] small cell tumor,[218] and others.

The frequency of cervical cancer with neuroendocrine differentiation by immunohistochemistry is unknown. Neuroendocrine differentiation by argyrophilic stain or electron microscopy was described in a variety of cervical neoplasms, including CIN,[167,335,371] invasive squamous carcinoma,[371] small cell carcinoma,[26] adenocarcinoma,[26,227,248,249] and adenosquamous carcinoma.[26]

Clinical Features

The age of patients with neuroendocrine tumor varies from the fourth to eighth decade, with the majority being in their fourth and fifth decades. The clinical presentations are not different from those of other cervical malignancies. Vaginal bleeding, especially postcoital spotting, and vaginal discharge are the most common complaints. On physical examination, the tumor has an exophytic, polypoid, infiltrative, or ulcerated appearance. Endocrinologic manifestations include Cushing's syndrome[170,227] and hypoglycemia.[188] Carcinoid syndrome and symptoms related to vasoactive polypeptides have not been documented.[8,9]

Gross and Microscopic Features

The tumor ranges in size from 0.8 cm[227] to greater than 5 cm[9] and has a firm, white to yellow cut surface. Invasion of the adjacent structures is common, and the tumor borders are well demarcated. Although the microscopic growth patterns vary, the most distinct pattern is the organoid arrangement, characterized by delicate fibrovascular septae surrounding ribbons, clusters, cords, nests, or solid sheets of cells (see Figs. 8–141 and 8–142). Within the nests, rosettes and glands containing mucinous material are sometimes present. Less commonly, the cells are arranged radially around the blood vessels in so-called pseudorosettes. Hyaline material, calcification, and amyloid may be seen in the stroma.

Figure 8–141. Well-differentiated neuroendocrine carcinoma of cervix. *A* and *B,* Tumor cells are arranged in ribbons and sheets closely associated with blood vessels, the so-called organoid pattern. *C* and *D,* Tumor cells have relatively uniform, round to oval hyperchromatic nuclei with low mitotic activity. No tumor necrosis is seen.

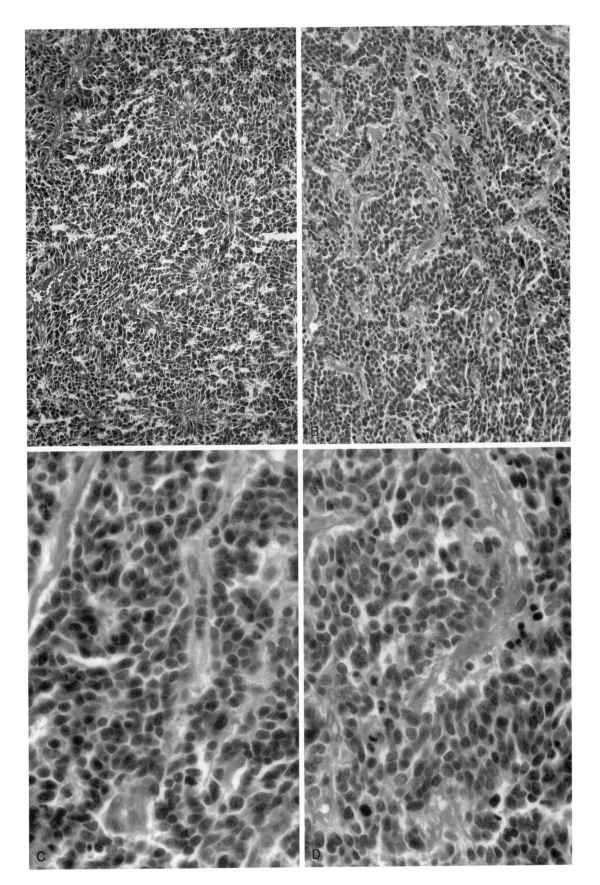

Figure 8–141 *See legend on opposite page*

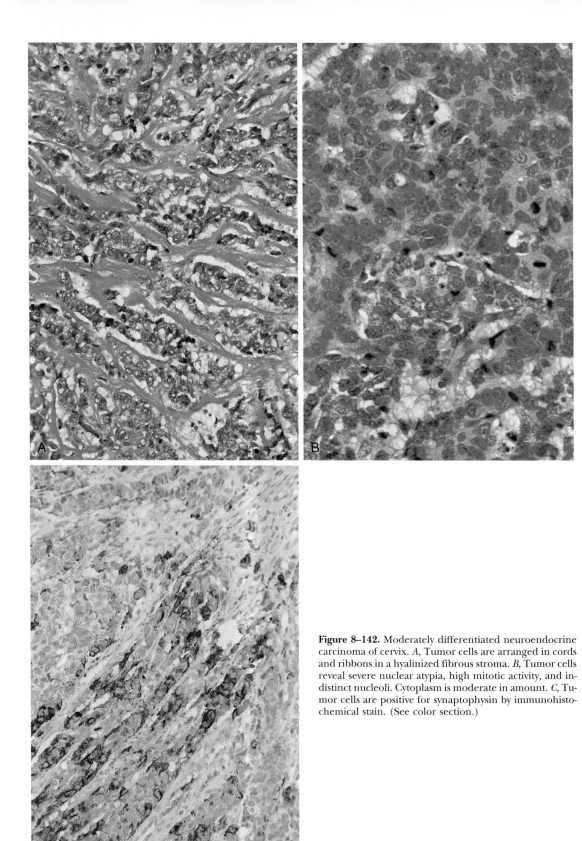

Figure 8–142. Moderately differentiated neuroendocrine carcinoma of cervix. *A,* Tumor cells are arranged in cords and ribbons in a hyalinized fibrous stroma. *B,* Tumor cells reveal severe nuclear atypia, high mitotic activity, and indistinct nucleoli. Cytoplasm is moderate in amount. *C,* Tumor cells are positive for synaptophysin by immunohistochemical stain. (See color section.)

The separation of well-differentiated (see Fig. 8–141) and moderately differentiated (see Fig. 8–142) neuroendocrine carcinomas is based on the degree of nuclear atypia, mitotic activity, and necrosis as outlined in the beginning of this section. In situ and invasive adenocarcinomas sometimes coexist with neuroendocrine carcinoma (Fig. 8–143).

With immunohistochemical staining, depending on the degree of differentiation, tumor cells usually express keratin, CEA, neuron-specific enolase, chromogranin, and synaptophysin. Serotonin, intestinal polypeptide, and somatostatin are variable.[327,359] By ultrastructure, neurosecretory granules are easily found in well-differentiated tumors. Extensive search and multiple sections are sometimes required for poorly differentiated neoplasms.

The prognosis of this group of tumors is related to the extent of the disease and the degree of differentiation. In a series of Albores-Saavedra et al.,[8] three of six women with well-differentiated tumors developed pelvic lymph node metastasis. A fourth woman had vaginal and pelvic recurrences. Only two of the women were known to be asymptomatic 2 years following surgery. Of the 13 patients with poorly differentiated neoplasms, four had local recurrence, and seven had proven lymph node metastasis. At the time of the report, six women had died from tumor, and only two were living and well 2 and 3 years following treatment.[8] The overall survival rates are lower than those for additional squamous cell carcinoma or adenocarcinoma.[327]

Other authors have confirmed the aggressive behavior of cervical neuroendocrine tumor, especially the poorly differentiated variants. The majority of patients developed metastasis and responded poorly to treatment.[218,227,273,335]

Wilms' Tumor

Although extrarenal Wilms' tumor has been reported to occur in the retroperitoneum, inguinal regions, mediastinum, chest wall, and testis, its occurrence in the female genital tract is unusual. Bittencourt et al.[39] reported on a Wilms' tumor involving the endometrium, left mesosalpinx, and pouch of Douglas in a 14-year-old female. Bell et al.[28] reported on a 13-year-old female who presented with a 12 × 12 cm, pedunculated mass connected to the cervical canal. It was removed by local excision. Histologically, the tumor is indistinguishable from

Wilms' tumor. It contains tubules of columnar epithelial cells, well-formed glomeruloid bodies, and spindle-shaped stromal cells with foci of smooth muscle, skeletal muscle, and cartilage. No residual tumor was found in the hysterectomy specimen. The kidneys were reported as normal by intravenous pyelogram and palpation at the time of laparotomy. The patient has remained free of disease 9.6 years after surgery. It is postulated that the tumor was derived from metanephros, which were misplaced in the müllerian duct during embryonic development.[28]

Babin et al.[19] described a 13 year-old female who presented with vaginal spotting for 2 months. Physical examination revealed a 6.5 × 4.5 × 2.5 cm pedunculated mass from the anterior cervix. The initial treatment included cervical polypectomy and LEEP conization of the polyp base. A local recurrence developed 8 months later with a 2.0 × 1.0 cm mass in the cervical os. Radical vaginal hysterectomy with pelvic and periaortic lymph node dissection was subsequently performed. The patient also received chemotherapy for Wilms' tumor including vincristine, actinomycin D, and Adriamycin. The patient was alive and well without disease 5 years after the radical surgery. Pathologically, this tumor met the criteria of extrarenal Wilms' tumor, consisting of tubular epithelial elements, glomeruloid structures, and primitive mesenchymal tissue resembling renal blastema elements.[19] In a review of the literature, Babin et al.[19] identified four cases of extrarenal Wilms' tumor occurring in the uterus.

The differential diagnosis includes immature teratoma, embryonal rhabdomyosarcoma, and malignant mixed mesodermal sarcoma. To qualify for the diagnosis of extrarenal Wilms' tumor, the following criteria are suggested: (1) no associated renal tumor; (2) no teratomatous elements, (3) no anaplastic features, (4) prominent epithelial elements with tubular and glomeruloid structures, and (5) the presence of primitive blastomatous spindle cell stroma. Wilms' tumor in the uterus may have derived from a primitive or undifferentiated remnant of metanephric or mesonephric tissue.[19]

SPECIALIZED TECHNIQUES FOR INVASIVE CARCINOMA

Tumor Markers

A variety of tumor antigens have been identified in cervical carcinoma with the use of im-

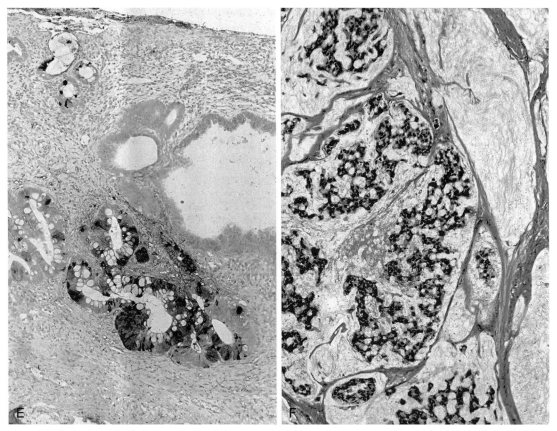

Figure 8–143. *Continued E,* Similar areas as in *D* demonstrate chromogranin-positive cells within the neoplastic glands by immunohistochemical stain. *F,* Mucinous adenocarcinoma associated with mucinous pools. (See color section.)

trogen and progesterone receptor status and survival. Among those alive, 36% had positive estrogen receptor protein and 44% were positive for progesterone receptor protein. Among those dead of disease, only 6% were positive for estrogen or progesterone receptor proteins.[226] There was no correlation between the FIGO stage and receptor status.

DNA Ploidy Pattern and S-Phase Fractions

Many investigators have carried out flow cytometric analysis of cervical squamous carcinoma. In his review of the literature, Strang[342] summarized the data on DNA ploidy patterns and S-phase fractions. Aneuploidy was found in the majority of cervical tumors, with only 20% to 40% of cases studied being peridiploid. A higher proportion of tumors with aneuploidy and high S-phase rates were found in Stage III and IV cancers compared with lower stage tumors, possibly reflecting successive changes in karyotype with

tumor progression. Increasing age and postmenopausal status were also associated with aneuploidy and high S-phase rates ($P < 0.01$). Correlations were found between aneuploidy and aggressive histopathologic features, such as infiltrative growth pattern, vascular invasion, and sparse lymphoplasmacytic infiltrate.[342]

Results have been conflicting concerning the prognostic significance of DNA ploidy in cervical squamous cell carcinoma. It appears that the prognosis for diploid and aneuploid tumors is similar. This may be because aneuploid tumors are more radiosensitive than are diploid tumors. High S-phase rates, on the other hand, were correlated with early recurrence and decreased survival in many studies. In a study of 133 patients, 17 of 81 (21%) cervical tumors with an S-phase rate of less than 20% presented with early relapses, compared to 25 of 52 (48%) tumors with S-phase rates greater than 20% ($P < 0.01$).[342]

Connor et al.[75] studied 53 IB cervical carcinomas by flow cytometry. Of these, 25 (47%)

tumors were aneuploid, with a mean DNA index of 1.52 ± 0.4. The mean S phase was $7.6 \pm 0.4\%$ for diploid tumors and $9.2 \pm 0.4\%$ for aneuploid neoplasms. Only the depth of invasion was correlated with recurrence or survival following radical hysterectomy and pelvic lymphadenectomy. DNA index and S-phase cells did not correlate with recurrence or survival.[75] A similar finding was reported for Stage I to IIA cervical carcinomas.[197]

Studies of nuclear DNA by static cytometry and morphometric measurements found increased tumor recurrence for Stage I and II adenocarcinomas when DNA ploidy level was greater than 3N, and mean nuclear areas were greater than 53 square microns.[111,115]

A study by Magitbay et al.[219] included 66 Stage IB and IIA mucinous endocervical adenocarcinomas. The DNA ploidy patterns by flow cytometric analysis were 27% diploid, 12% tetraploid, and 47% aneuploid. The remaining 14% were undetermined. The authors correlated the age, maximal tumor dimension, stage, histologic grade, and pelvic lymph node status with ploidy patterns. Tumor recurred in 20% of the patients. There was no correlation between the DNA ploidy pattern and tumor recurrence. By multivariate analysis, positive pelvic lymph node metastasis was highly associated with tumor recurrence. In eight of nine women with positive lymph nodes, tumor recurred. In the node negative group, a high proliferative index of S and G2M cells exceeding 20%, was the only significant factor for increased tumor recurrence. The authors conclude that in the absence of nodal metastasis a combined S and G2M cells of greater than 20% indicated high risk for tumor recurrence ($P = 0.002$).[219]

Oncogenes

Mutations and overexpression of C-myc and ras oncogenes have been demonstrated in cervical carcinoma.[6,84,296,307] Some studies have correlated the degree of abnormal expression with prognosis. In one study, overexpression of C-myc was found in 25 of 72 Stage I and II cervical carcinomas. There was an eightfold increase of early relapse in patients with C-myc overexpression.[296]

Mandai et al.[224] used immunohistochemical stains for the expression of nm23-H1 and c-erB-2 proteins. The nm23-H1 gene was originally cloned from the murine melanoma cell lines

with low and high metastatic potential. It was identified later in human genes. Expression of nm23-H1 is associated with a better prognosis and a lower level of lymph node metastasis in breast ductal carcinoma, hepatocellular carcinoma, and gastric carcinoma patients.[127] A member of epidermal growth factor receptor family, c-erB-2, is associated with poor prognosis in breast carcinoma when overexpressed nm23-H1 was expressed in 46% of adenocarcinomas and 36% of squamous carcinomas.[224] In 49% of adenocarcinomas and 38% of squamous carcinomas, c-erb-2 was overexpressed. Negative nm23-H1 and overexpressed c-erb-2 were associated with increased lymph node metastasis and poor prognosis in adenocarcinoma. These findings were not applicable to squamous carcinoma.[224]

Other Markers

Oka et al.[259] studied 59 women with Stage I to Stage IV adenocarcinoma of the cervix that was treated by radiation alone. The authors stained tumor cells for S-100 protein and vimentin by immunohistochemistry. They found that the presence of Langerhans' cells by S-100 protein was a significant prognostic factor for women with Stage III tumors. S-100 protein–positive dendritic cells were found adjacent to the malignant cells and in the fibrous stroma around the tumor nests. The disease-free survival rate with expression of S-100 protein in Stage III disease was 42%, as compared with 10% without S-100 protein expression. The presence of vimentin in tumor cells is a poor prognostic indicator. The disease-free 5-year survival rate with negative vimentin expression is 38% as compared with 0% with vimentin expression. These immunohistochemical stains are not of prognostic significance in Stage II tumors. It is interesting to note that vimentin positive cells were found in 25% of adenosquamous carcinomas as compared with 6% in adenocarcinoma ($P < 0.05$).[259] It is unclear whether there is any quantitative relationship between the S-100 protein–positive cells and prognosis. The cutoff for positive and negative cases is not clearly stated.

Several authors investigated the question of angiogenesis in cervical cancer. In a study of 70 invasive squamous cell carcinomas from Stage IB to Stage IV, biopsy samples of tumor were stained for factor VIII, and capillaries, arterioles, and small venules were counted. Areas of highest density were selected for measurement. An average of the highest three counts under a 400× field was determined to be the vessel count for each tumor. No correlation was found between the vascular density and FIGO stage or disease status, with a mean follow-up of 21 months.[303]

In a study by Schlenger et al.,[311a] two cores of tissue were obtained from Stage IB to Stage IVA cervical cancer greater than 3 cm in size. After staining for factor VIII, a computerized imaging system was used to find the closest vessels and calculated their distances. This preliminary study included 22 women treated by surgery and 17 by radiation, with a mean follow-up of 18 months. Women whose tumor had higher vascularity (mean closest vessels less than 83 microns) had lower disease-free and overall survival rates than those with lower tumor vascularity.

In summary, many of the investigations using new technologies have shown encouraging results to improve routine pathologic examination and to more accurately determine the behavior and outcome of cervical cancers. Because of technical variables and study limitations, additional studies are required to confirm their values and limitations.

REFERENCES

1. Aaro LA, Jacobson LJ, Soule ER. Endocervical polyps. Obstet Gynecol 21:659, 1963.
2. Abdul-Karim FW, Fu YS, Reagan JW, et al. Morphometric study of intraepithelial neoplasia of the uterine cervix. Obstet Gynecol 60:210, 1982.
3. Abdul-Karim FW, Nunez C. Cervical intraepithelial neoplasia after conization: A study of 522 consecutive cervical cones. Obstet Gynecol 65:77, 1985.
4. Abeler VM, Holm R, Nesland JM, Kjorstad KE. Small cell carcinoma of the cervix: A clinicopathologic study of 26 patients. Cancer 73:672, 1994.
5. Abell MR, Gosling JRG. Gland cell carcinoma (adenocarcinoma) of the uterine cervix. Am J Obstet Gynecol 83:729, 1962.
5a. Adam E, Kaufman RH, Melnick JL, et al. Seroepidemiologic studies of herpesvirus type 2 and carcinoma in situ of the cervix. Am J Epidemiol 98:77, 1977.
6. Agnantis NJ, Spandidos DA, Mahera H, et al. Immunohistochemical study of ras oncogene expression in endometrial and cervical human lesions. Eur J Gynaecol Oncol 9:380, 1988.
7. Albores-Saavedra J, Gersell D, Gilks CB, et al. Terminology of endocrine tumors of the uterine cervix: Results of a workshop sponsored by the College of American Pathologists and the National Cancer Institute. Arch Pathol Lab Med 121:34, 1997.
8. Albores-Saavedra J, Larraza O, Poucell S, et al. Carcinoid of the uterine cervix. Cancer 38:2328, 1976.
9. Albores-Saavedra J, Rodriguez-Martinez HR, Larraza-Hernandez O. Carcinoid tumors of the cervix. Pathol Annu 14:273, 1979.
10. Albores-Saavedra J, Young RH. Transitional cell neoplasms (carcinomas and inverted papillomas) of the uterine cervix: A report of five cases. Am J Surg Pathol 19:1138, 1995.
11. Allen HH, Nisker JA, Anderson RJ. Primary surgical treatment in one hundred ninety-five cases of stage IB carcinoma of the cervix. Am J Obstet Gynecol 143:581, 1982.
12. Ambros RA, Park JS, Shah KV, Kurman RJ. Evaluation of histologic, morphometric and immunohistochemical criteria in the differential diagnosis of small cell carcinomas of the cervix with particular reference to human papillomavirus types 16 and 18. Modern Pathol 4:586, 1991.
13. Anders KH, Hall TL, Fu YS. Epidemiologic and histologic studies of female genital warts. In: Fenoglio CM, Wolff MW, Rilke F (eds). Progress in Surgical Pathology. Philadelphia, Field & Wood, 1986, p 33.
14. Andl T, Kahn T, Pfuhl A, et al. Etiological involvement of oncogenic human papillomavirus in tonsillar squamous cell carcinomas lacking retinoblastoma cell cycle control. Cancer Res 58:5, 1998.
15. Anton-Culvar H, Bloss JD, et al. Comparison of adenocarcinoma and squamous cell carcinoma of the uterine cervix: A population-based epidemiologic study. Am J Obstet Gynecol 166:150, 1992.
16. Aurelian L, Manak MM, McKinlay M, et al. "The herpesvirus hypothesis"—Are Koch's postulations satisfied? Gynecol Oncol 12:S56, 1981.
17. Averette HE, Nelson JH, Ng ABP, et al. Diagnosis and management of microinvasive (stage IA) carcinoma of the uterine cervix. Cancer 38:414, 1976.
18. Azodi M, Chambers SK, Rutherford TJ, Kohorn EL, Schwarts PE, Chambers JR. Adenocarcinoma in situ of the cervix: Management and outcome. Gynecol Oncol 73:348, 1999.
19. Babin EA, Davis JR, Hatch KE, Hallum AV. Wilms' tumor of the cervix: A case report and review of the literature. Gynecol Oncol 76:107, 2000.
20. Bachaud JM, Mazabrey D, Berrebi A, et al. Cutaneous metastatic lymphangitis from squamous cell carcinoma of the cervix. Dermatologica 180:163, 1990.
21. Baggish MS, Woodruff JD. Adenoid-basal carcinoma of the cervix. Obstet Gynecol 28:213, 1966.
22. Baltzer J, Koepcke W. Tumor size and lymph node metastases in squamous cell carcinoma of the uterine cervix. Arch Gynecol 227:271, 1979..
23. Baltzer J, Lohe KJ, Koepcke W, et al. Histological criteria for the prognosis in patients with operated squamous cell carcinoma of the cervix. Gynecol Oncol 13:184, 1982.
24. Bamford PN, Ormerod MG, Sloane JP, et al. An immunohistochemical study of the distribution of epithelial antigens in the uterine cervix. Obstet Gynecol 61:603, 1983.
25. Barillot I, Horiot JC, Pigneux J, et al. Carcinoma of the intact uterine cervix treated with radiotherapy alone. A French cooperative study: Update and multivariate analysis of prognostic factors. Int J Rad Oncol Biol Physics 38:969, 1997.
26. Barrett RJ, Davos I, Leuchter RS, et al. Neuroendocrine features in poorly differentiated and undifferentiated carcinomas of the cervix. Cancer 60:2325, 1987.

27. Beecham JB, Halvorsen T, Kolbenstvedt A. Histologic classification, lymph node metastases, and patient survival in stage IB cervical carcinoma: An analysis of 245 uniformly treated cases. Gynecol Oncol 6:95, 1978.

28. Bell DA, Shimm DS, Gang DL. Wilms' tumor of the endocervix. Arch Pathol Lab Med 109:371, 1985.

29. Bemedetto-Panici P, Maneschi F, D'Andrea G, et al. Early cervical carcinoma: The natural history of lymph node involvement redefined on the basis of thorough parametrictomy and giant section study. Cancer 88:2267, 2000.

30. Benda JA, Platz CE, Buchsbaum H, et al. Mucin production in defining mixed carcinoma of the uterine cervix: A clinicopathologic study. Int J Gynecol Pathol 4:314, 1985.

31. Bennett JL, Clement PB. Verrucous carcinoma of the uterine cervix and endometrium. Diagnostic Gynecol Obstet 2:197, 1980.

32. Benson WL, Norris HJ. A critical review of the frequency of lymph node metastasis and death from microinvasive carcinoma of the cervix. Obstet Gynecol 49:632, 1977.

33. Berek JS, Castaldo TW, Hacker NF, et al. Adenocarcinoma of the uterine cervix. Cancer 48:2734, 1981.

34. Berek JS, Hacker NF, Fu YS, et al. Adenocarcinoma of the uterine cervix: Histologic variables associated with lymph node metastasis and survival. Obstet Gynecol 65:46, 1984.

35. Bergeron C, Ferenczy A, Shah KV, et al. Multicentric human papillomavirus infections of the female genital tract: Correlation of viral types with abnormal mitotic figures, colposcopic presentation, and location. Obstet Gynecol 69:736, 1987.

36. Bertrand M, Lickrish GM, Colgan TJ. The anatomic distribution of cervical adenocarcinoma in situ: Implications for the treatment. Am J Obstet Gynecol 157:21, 1987.

37. Bethwaite P, Yeong ML, Holoway L, et al. The prognosis of adenosquamous carcinomas of the uterine cervix. Brit J Obstet Gynecol 99:745, 1992.

38. Biscotti CV, Hart WR. Apoptotic bodies: A consistent morphologic feature of endocervical adenocarcinoma in situ. Am J Surg Pathol 22:434, 1998.

39. Bittencourt AL, Britto JF, Fonseca LE. Wilms' tumor of the cervix: The first report of the literature. Cancer 47:2496, 1981.

40. Bohm JW, Krupp PJ, Lee FY, et al. Lymph node metastasis in microinvasive epidermoid cancer of the cervix. Obstet Gynecol 49:632, 1977.

41. Boon ME, Baak JPA, Kurver PJH, et al. Adenocarcinoma in situ of the cervix: An underdiagnosed lesion. Cancer 48:768, 1981.

42. Boon ME, Kirk RS, Rietveld-Scheffers PEM. The morphogenesis of adenocarcinoma of the cervix—a complex pathological entity. Histopathology 5:565, 1981.

43. Boon ME, Verdonk G. The identification of atypical reserve cells in smears of patients with premalignant and malignant changes in the squamous and glandular epithelium of the uterine cervix. Acta Cytol 22:305, 1978.

44. Borras G, Molina R, Xercavins J, et al. Tumor antigens CA 19.9, CA 125, and CEA in carcinoma of the uterine cervix. Gynecol Oncol 57:205, 1995.

45. Bosch FX, Munoz N, de Sanjose S, et al. Risk factor for cervical cancer in Columbia and Spain. Int J Cancer 53:750, 1992.

46. Bostrom SG, Hart WR. Carcinomas of the cervix with intense stromal eosinophilia. Cancer 47:2887, 1981.

47. Bousfield L, Pacey F, Young Q, et al. Expanded cytologic criteria for the diagnosis of adenocarcinoma in situ of the cervix and related lesions. Acta Cytol 24:283, 1980.

48. Boyce JG, Fruchter RG, Nicastri AD, et al. Vascular invasion in stage I carcinoma of the cervix. Cancer 53:1175, 1984.

49. Brainard JA, Hart WR. Adenoid basal epitheliomas of the uterine cervix. Am J Surg Pathol 22:965, 1998.

50. Brandt B, Lifshitz S. Scalene node biopsy in advanced carcinoma of the cervix uteri. Cancer 47:1920, 1981.

51. Brinton LA, Reeves WC, Brenes MM, et al. Oral contraceptive use and risk of invasive cervical cancer. Int J Epidemiol 19:4, 1990.

52. Brinton LA, Schairer C, Haenszel W, et al. Cigarette smoking and invasive cervical cancer. JAMA 255:3265, 1986.

53. Brinton LA, Tashima KT, Lehman HF, et al. Epidemiology of cervical cancer by cell type. Cancer Res 47:1706, 1987.

54. Brock KE, Berry G, Mock PA, et al. Nutrients in diet and plasma and risk of in situ cervical cancer. J Natl Cancer Inst 80:580, 1998.

55. Broders AC. Carcinoma in situ contrasted with benign penetrating epithelium. JAMA 99:1670, 1932.

56. Burghardt E. Early Histologic Diagnosis of Cervical Cancer. Philadelphia, W.B. Saunders, 1973, p 335.

57. Burghardt E, Girardi F, Lahousen M, et al. Microinvasive carcinoma of the uterine cervix (International Federation of Gynecology and Obstetrics Stage IA) Cancer 67:1037, 1999.

58. Burghardt E, Holzer E. Diagnosis and treatment of microinvasive carcinoma of the cervix uteri. Obstet Gynecol 49:641, 1977.

59. Burghardt E, Pickel H. Local spread and lymph node involvement in cervical cancer. Obstet Gynecol 52:138, 1978.

60. Burk RF. Editorial: Pernicious papillomavirus infection. N Eng J Med 341:1687, 1999.

61. Burke TW, Hoskins WJ, Heller PB, et al. Clinical patterns of tumor recurrence after radical hysterectomy in stage IB cervical carcinoma. Obstet Gynecol 69:382, 1987.

62. Buscema J, Woodruff JD. Significance of neoplastic atypicalities in endocervical epithelium. Gynecol Oncol 17:356, 1984.

63. Buxton EJ, Luesley DM, Wade-Evans T, et al. Residual disease after cone biopsy: Completeness of excision and follow-up cytology as predictive factors. Obstet Gynecol 70:529, 1987.

64. Bychkov V, Rothman M, Bardawil WA. Immunocytochemical localization of carcinoembryonic antigen (CEA), alpha-fetoprotein (AFP), and human chorionic gonadotropin (HCG) in cervical neoplasia. Am J Clin Pathol 79:414, 1983.

65. Cabral GA, Fry D, Marciano-Cabral F, et al. A herpesvirus antigen in human premalignant and malignant cervical biopsies and explants. Am J Obstet Gynecol 145:79, 1983.

66. Cachaza JA, Caballero JJL, Fernandez A, et al. Endocervical polyp with pseudosarcomatous pattern and cytoplasmic inclusions: An electron microscopic study. Am J Clin Pathol 85:633, 1986.

67. Candy J, Abell MR. Progestogen induced adenomatous hyperplasia of the uterine cervix. JAMA 203:323, 1968.

68. Chen RJ, Lin YH, Chen CA, et al. Influence of histologic type and age on survival rates for invasive cervical carcinoma in Taiwan. Gynecol Oncol 73:184, 1999.

69. Cho NH, Ki YT, Kim JW. Correlation between G1 cyclins and HPV in the uterine cervix. Int J Gynecol Pathol 16:339, 1997.

70. Christopherson WM, Nealon N, Gray LA Sr. Noninvasive precursor lesions of adenocarcinoma and mixed adenosquamous carcinoma of the cervix uteri. Cancer 44:975, 1979.

71. Chumas JC, Nelson B, Mann WJ, et al. Microglandular hyperplasia of the uterus cervix. Obstet Gynecol 66:406, 1985.

72. Clement PB. Miscellaneous primary tumors and metastatic tumors of the uterine cervix. Semin Diag Pathol 7:228, 1990.

73. Clement PB, Young RH, Keh P, et al. Malignant mesonephric neoplasms of the uterine cervix: A report of eight cases, including four with a malignant spindle cell component. Am J Surg Pathol 19:1158, 1995.

74. Cohen C, Shulman G, Budgeon LR. Endocervical and endometrial adenocarcinoma: An immunoperoxidase and histochemical study. Am J Surg Pathol 6:151, 1982.

75. Connor JP, Miller DS, Cauer KD, et al. Flow cytometric evaluation of early invasive cervical cancer. Obstet Gynecol 81:367, 1993.

76. Connor JP, Ferreer K, Kane O, Goldberg JM. Evaluation of Langerhans' cells in the cervical epithelium of women with cervical intraepithelial neoplasia. Gynecol Oncol 75:130, 1999.

77. Cooper K, Haffajee Z, Taylor L. Bcl-2 immunoreactivity, human papillomavirus DNA; and cervical intraepithelial neoplasia. Mod Pathol 12:612, 1999.

78. Copeland LJ, Silva EG, Gershenson DM, et al. Superficially invasive squamous cell carcinoma of the cervix. Gynecol Oncol 45:307, 1992.

79. Costa MJ, McIlnay KR, Trelford J. Cervical carcinoma with glandular differentiation: Histological evaluation predicts disease recurrence in clinical stage I or II patients. Hum Pathol 26:829, 1995.

80. Creasman WT. New gynecologic cancer staging. Gynecol Oncol 58:157, 1995.

81. Creasman WT, Fetter BF, Clarke-Pearson DL, et al. Management of stage IA carcinoma of the cervix. Am J Obstet Gynecol 153:164, 1985.

82. Crissman JD, Budhraja M, Aron BS, et al. Histopathologic prognostic factors in stage II and III squamous cell carcinoma of the uterine cervix. Int J Gynecol Pathol 6:97, 1987.

83. Crombach G, Scharl A, Vierbuchen M, et al. Detection of squamous cell carcinoma antigen in normal squamous epithelia and in squamous cell carcinoma of the uterine cervix. Cancer 63:1337, 1989.

84. Crook T, Greenfield I, Howard J, et al. Alterations in growth properties of human papilloma virus type 16 immortalised human cervical keratinocyte cell line correlate with amplification and overexpression of C-myc oncogene. Oncogene 5:619, 1990.

85. Crum CP, Cibas ES, Lee KR. Pathology of Early Cervical Neoplasia. New York, Churchill Livingstone, 1997.

86. Crum CP, Egawa K, Fu YS, et al. Atypical immature metaplasia (AIM): A subset of human papilloma virus infection of the cervix. Cancer 51:2214, 1983.

87. Dabbs DJ, Geisinger KR, Norris HT. Intermediate fil-

88. Daroca PJ, Dhurandhar HN. Basaloid carcinoma of uterine cervix. Am J Surg Pathol 4:235, 1980.

89. Davidson B, Goldberg I, Kopolovic J. Angiogenesis in uterine cervical intraepithelial neoplasia and squamous cell carcinoma: An immunohistochemical study. Int J Gynecol Pathol 16:335, 1997.

90. Daya D, Young RH. Florid deep glands of the uterine cervix. Another mimic of adenoma malignum. Am J Clin Pathol 103:614, 1995.

91. Delgado G, Bundy BN, Fowler WC, et al. A prospective surgical pathological study of stage I squamous carcinoma of the cervix: A Gynecologic Oncologic Group study. Gynecol Oncol 35:314, 1989.

92. Delgado G, Bundy BN, Fowler WC, et al. A prospective surgical pathological study of stage I squamous carcinoma of the cervix: A Gynecological Oncologic Group study. Cancer 69:1750, 1992.

93. Dellas A, Schltheiss E, Holzgreve W, et al. Investigation of the bcl-2 and the C-myc expression in relation to the Ki-67 labeling in cervical intraepithelial neoplasia. Int J Gynecol Pathol 16:212, 1997.

94. Devesa SS. Descriptive epidemiology of cancer of the uterine cervix. Obstet Gynecol 63:605, 1984.

95. Dixit S, Singhal S, Vyas R, et al. Adenoid cystic carcinoma of the cervix. J Postgrad Med 39:211, 1993.

96. Egan AJM, Russell P. Transitional (urothelial) cell metaplasia of the uterine cervix: Morphological assessment of 31 cases. Int J Gynecol Pathol 16:89, 1997.

97. Einhorn N, Patek E, Sjoberg B. Outcome of different treatment modalities in cervix carcinoma stage IB and IIA. Cancer 55:949, 1985.

98. Fawcett KJ, Dockerty MB, Hunt AB. Mesonephric carcinoma of the cervix uteri: A clinical and pathologic study. Am J Obstet Gynecol 95:1068, 1966.

99. Ferenczy A, Richart RM. Female Reproductive System: Dynamics of Scan and Transmission Electron Microscopy. New York, John Wiley & Sons, 1974.

100. Ferguson AW, Svoboda-Newman SM, Frank TS. Analysis of human papillomavirus infection and molecular alterations in adenocarcinoma of the cervix. Mod Pathol 11:11, 1998.

101. Ferry JA, Scully RE. "Adenoid cystic" carcinoma and adenoid basal carcinoma of the uterine cervix: A study of 28 cases. Am J Surg Pathol 12:134, 1988.

102. Ferry JA, Scully RE. Mesonephric remnants, hyperplasia and neoplasia in the uterine cervix: A study of 49 cases. Am J Surg Pathol 14:1100, 1990.

103. Fetissof F, Serres G, Arbeille B, et al. Argyrophilic cells and ectocervical epithelium. Int J Gynecol Pathol 10:177, 1991.

104. Flint A, McCoy JP, Schade WJ, et al. Cervical carcinoma antigen: distribution in neoplastic lesions of the uterine cervix and comparison to other tumor markers. Gynecol Oncol 30:63, 1988.

105. Foushee JHS, Griess FC, Lock FR. Stage IA squamous cell carcinoma of the uterine cervix. Am J Obstet Gynecol 105:46, 1969.

106. Friedell GH, McKay DG. Adenocarcinoma in situ of the endocervix. Cancer 6:887, 1953.

107. Fu YS, Berek JS. Minimal cervical cancer: Definition and histology. In: Grundmann E, Beck L (eds). Minimal Neoplasia—Diagnosis and Therapy. Recent Results in Cancer Research, vol 106. Berlin, Springer-Verlag, 1988, p 47.

108. Fu YS, Berek JS, Hilborne LH. Diagnostic problems

of cervical in situ and invasive adenocarcinoma. Applied Pathol 5:47, 1987.

109. Fu YS, Braun L, Shah KV, et al. Histologic, nuclear DNA, and human papillomavirus studies of cervical condylomas. Cancer 52:1705, 1983.

110. Fu YS, Cheng L, Huang I, et al. DNA ploidy analysis of cervical condyloma and intraepithelial neoplasia obtained by punch biopsy. Analy Quant Cytol Histol 11:187, 1989.

111. Fu YS, Hall TL, Berek JS, et al. Prognostic significance of DNA ploidy and morphometric analyses of adenocarcinoma of the uterine cervix. Anal Quant Cytol Histol 9:17, 1987.

112. Fu YS, Huang I, Beaudenon S, et al. Correlative study of human papillomavirus DNA, histopathology and morphometry in cervical condyloma and intraepithelial neoplasia. Int J Gynecol Pathol 7:297, 1988.

113. Fu YS, Ko JH. Histopathology of preinvasive and invasive squamous neoplasia. In: Rubin SC, Hoskins WJ (eds). Cervical Cancer and Preinvasive Neoplasia. Philadelphia, Lippincott-Raven, 1996, p 77.

114. Fu YS, Reagan JW. Pathology of the Uterine Cervix, Vagina, and Vulva. Philadelphia, W.B. Saunders, 1989.

115. Fu YS, Reagan JW, Fu AS, et al. Adenocarcinoma and mixed carcinoma of the uterine cervix. II: Prognostic value of nuclear DNA analysis. Cancer 49:2571, 1982.

116. Fu YS, Reagan JW, Hsiu JG, et al. Adenocarcinoma and mixed carcinoma of the uterine cervix. I: A clinicopathologic study. Cancer 49:2560, 1982.

117. Fu YS, Reagan JW, Richart RM. Definition of precursors. Gynecol Oncol 12:S220, 1981.

118. Fu YS, Reagan JW, Richart RM, et al. Definition of cervical cancer precursors. In: Grundmann E (ed). Cancer Campaign, vol 8, Cancer of the Uterine Cervix. Stuttgart, Gustav Fischer Verlag, 1985, pp 67–74.

119. Fu YS, Reagan JW, Richart RM, et al. Nuclear DNA and histopathologic studies of genital lesions in DES-exposed progeny. I: Intraepithelial squamous abnormalities. Am J Clin Pathol 72:502, 1979.

120. Fu YS, Temmin L, Olaizola YM, et al. Nuclear DNA characteristics of microinvasive squamous carcinoma of the uterine cervix. In: Fenoglio CM, Wolff MW (eds). Progress in Surgical Pathology, vol I. New York, Masson, 1980, p 398.

121. Fuller AF, Elliot N, Kosloff C, et al. Determinants of increased risk for recurrence in patients undergoing radical hysterectomy for stage IB and IIA carcinoma of the cervix. Gynecol Oncol 33:34, 1989.

122. Gallup DG, Abell MR. Invasive adenocarcinoma of the uterine cervix. Obstet Gynecol 49:596, 1977.

123. Gallup DG, Harper RH, Stock RJ. Poor prognosis in patients with adenosquamous cell carcinoma of the cervix. Obstet Gynecol 65:416, 1985.

124. Geng LI, Conolly DC, Isacson C, et al. Atypical immature metaplasia (AIM) of the cervix: Is it related to high-grade squamous intraepithelial lesion (HSIL)? Human Pathol 30:345, 1999.

125. Gersell DJ, Mazoujian G, Mutch DG, et al. Small-cell undifferentiated carcinoma of the cervix: A clinicopathologic, ultrastructural, and immunocytochemical study of 15 cases. Am J Surg Pathol 12:684, 1988.

126. Giaroli A, Sananes C, Sardi JE, et al. Lymph node metastases in carcinoma of the cervix uteri: Response to neoadjuvant chemotherapy and its impact on survival. Gynecol Oncol 39:34, 1990.

127. Gilks CB, Young RH, Gersell DJ, Clement PB. Large cell carcinoma of the uterine cervix: A clinicopathologic study of 12 cases. Am J Surg Pathol 21:905, 1997.

128. Gloor E, Hurlimann J. Cervical intraepithelial glandular neoplasia (adenocarcinoma in situ and glandular dysplasia). A correlative study of 23 cases with histologic grading, histochemical analysis of mucins, and immunohistochemical determination of the affinity for four lectins. Cancer 58:1272, 1986.

129. Gloor E, Ruzicka J. Morphology of adenocarcinoma in situ of the uterine cervix: A study of 14 cases. Cancer 49:294, 1982.

130. Glucksmann A, Cherry CP. Incidence, histology and response to radiation of mixed carcinomas (adenoacanthomas) of the uterine cervix. Cancer 9:971, 1956.

131. Goldstein NS, Ahman E, Hussian M, et al. Endocervical glandular atypia: Does a preneoplastic lesion of adenocarcinoma in situ exist? Am J Clin Pathol 110:200, 1998.

132. Golijow CD, Mouron SA, Gomez MA, Dulot FN. Differences in K-ras codon 12 mutation frequency between "high-risk" and "low-risk" HPV-infected samples. Gynecol Oncol 75:108, 1999.

133. Graham CE. Cyclic changes in the squamocolumnar junction of the mouse cervix uteri. Anat Rec 155:251, 1966.

134. Grayson W, Taylor LF, Cooper K. Adenoid basal carcinoma of the uterine cervix: Detection of integrated human papillomavirus in a rare tumor of putative "reserve cell" origin. Int J Gynecol Pathol 16:307, 1997.

135. Greer BE, Figge DC, Tamimi HK, et al. Stage IB adenocarcinoma of the cervix treated by radical hysterectomy and pelvic lymph node dissection. Am J Obstet Gynecol 160:1509, 1989.

136. Grenko RT, Abendroth CS, Frauenhoffer EE, et al. Variance in the interpretation of cervical biopsy specimens obtained for atypical squamous cells of undetermined significance. Am J Clin Pathol 114:735, 2000.

137. Groben P, Reddick R, Askin F. The pathologic spectrum of small cell carcinoma of the cervix. Int J Gynecol Pathol 4:42, 1985.

138. Guo Z, Wu F, Asplund A, et al. Analysis of intratumoral heterogeneity of chromosome 3p deletions and genetic evidence of polyclonal origin of cervical squamous cell carcinoma. Hum Pathol 14:54, 2001.

139. Hacker NF, Berek JS, Lagasse LD, et al. Carcinoma of the cervix associated with pregnancy. Obstet Gynecol 59:735, 1982.

140. Halpin TF, Hunter RE, Cohen MB. Lymphoepithelioma of the uterine cervix. Gynecol Oncol 34:101, 1989.

141. Hampton GN, Penny LA, Baergen RN, et al. Loss of heterozygosity in cervical carcinoma; subchromosomal localization of a putative tumor-suppressor gene to chromosome 11q22–24. Proc Natl Acad Sci USA 91:66953, 1994.

142. Hanji D, Gohoa L. Malignant lymphoepithelial lesions of the salivary glands with anaplastic carcinomatous change. Cancer 52:2245, 1983.

143. Hanks GE, Herring DF, Kramer S. Patterns of care outcome studies: Results of the national practice in cancer of the cervix. Cancer 51:959, 1983.

144. Hanselaar A, van Loosbroek M, Schuurbiers O, et al. Clear cell adenocarcinoma of the vagina and cervix:

Update of the central Netherlands registry showing twin age incidence peaks. Cancer 79:2229, 1997.

145. Hanselaar AGJM, Boss EA, Maauger LFAG, Bernheim JL. Cytologic examination to detect clear cell adenocarcinoma of the vagina or cervix. Gynecol Oncol 75: 338, 1999.

146. Harmsel T, Smedts F, Kujiper J, et al. Bcl-2 immunoreactivity increased with severity of CIN: A study of normal cervical epithelia, CIN and cervical carcinoma. J Pathol 179:26, 1996.

147. Harmsel T, Kujipers J, Smedts F, et al. Progressing imbalance between proliferation and apoptosis with increasing severity of cervical intraepithelial neoplasia. Intl J Gynecol Pathol 16:205, 1997.

148. Hasumi K, Ehrmann RL. Clear cell carcinoma of the uterine endocervix with an in situ component. Cancer 42:2435, 1978.

149. Hasumi K, Sakamoto A, Sugano H. Microinvasive carcinoma of the uterine cervix. Cancer 45:928, 1980.

150. Hasumi K, Sugano H, Sakamoto G, et al. Circumscribed carcinoma of the uterine cervix, with marked lymphocytic infiltration. Cancer 39:2503, 1977.

151. Henry RJW, Goodman JDS, Godley M, et al. Immunohistochemical study of cytoplasmic oestradiol receptor in normal, dysplastic and malignant cervical tissue. Br J Obstet Gynaecol 95:927, 1988.

152. Herbst AL, Anderson D. Clear cell adenocarcinoma of the vagina and cervix secondary to intrauterine exposure to diethylstilbestrol. Sem Surg Oncol 6:343, 1990.

153. Herbst AL, Anderson D. Clinical correlations and management of vaginal and cervical clear cell adenocarcinoma. In: Herbst AL, Bern HA (eds). Developmental Effects of Diethylstilbestrol (DES) in Pregnancy. New York, Thieme-Stratton, 1981, p 71.

154. Herrero R, Heldesheim A, Concepcion B, et al. A population based study of human papillomavirus infection and all grades of cervical neoplasia in rural Costa Rica. J Nat Cancer Inst 92:464, 2000.

155. Higgins GE, Phillips GE, Smith LA, et al. High prevalence of human papilloma virus transcripts in all grades of cervical intraepithelial glandular neoplasia. Cancer 70:136, 1992.

156. Hirai U, Takeshima N, Haga A, et al. A clinicopathologic study of adenoma malignum of the uterine cervix. Gynecol Oncol 70:291, 1998.

157. Ho GY, Burk RD, Klein S, et al. Persistent genital human papillomavirus infection as a risk factor for persistent cervical dysplasia. J Nat Cancer Inst 87:1365, 1995.

158. Ho GY, Bierman R, Beardsley L, et al. Natural history of cervicovaginal papillomavirus infection in young women. N Engl J Med 338:423, 1998.

159. Holly EA, Petrakis NL, Friend NF, et al. Mutagenic cervical mucus in women smokers. Am J Epidemiol 122:518, 1985.

160. Hunter RE, Longscope C, Keough P. Steroid hormone receptors in carcinoma of the cervix. Cancer 60:392, 1987.

161. Hurt WG, Silverberg SG, Frable WJ, et al. Adenocarcinoma of the cervix: Histopathologic and clinical features. Am J Obstet Gynecol 129:304, 1977.

162. Inoue T. Prognostic significance of the depth of invasion, and cell types: A study of 628 cases with stage IB, IIA, and IIB cervical carcinoma. Cancer 54:3035, 1984.

163. Ireland D, Cole S, Kelly P, et al. Mucin production in cervical intraepithelial neoplasia and in stage 1b carcinoma of cervix with pelvic lymph node metastases. Br J Obstet Gynecol 94:467, 1987.

164. Ishikawa H, Nakanishi T, Iour T, Kuzuya K. Prognostic factors of adenocarcinoma of the uterine cervix. Gynecol Oncol 73:42, 1999.

165. Jacobs AJ, Marchevsky A, Gordon RE, et al. Oat cell carcinoma of the uterine cervix in a pregnant woman treated with cis-diamine dichloroplatinum. Gynecol Oncol 9:405, 1980.

166. Jensen AB, Rosenthal JR, Olson C, et al. Immunological relatedness of papillomaviruses from different species. J Natl Cancer Inst 64:495, 1980.

167. Johannessen JV, Capella C, Solcia E, et al. Endocrine cell carcinoma of the uterine cervix. Diagn Gynecol Obstet 2:127, 1980.

168. Johnson LD, Easterday CL, Gore H, et al. The histogenesis of carcinoma in situ of the uterine cervix: A preliminary report of the origin of carcinoma in situ in subcylindrical cell anaplasia. Cancer 17:213, 1964.

169. Jonasson JG, Wang HH, Antonioli DA, Ducatman BS. Tubal metaplasia of the uterine cervix: A prevalence study in patients with gynecologic pathologic findings. Int J Gynecol Pathol 11:89, 1982.

170. Jones HW III, Plymate S, Gluck FB, et al. Small cell nonkeratinizing carcinoma of the cervix associated with ACTH production. Cancer 38:1629, 1976.

171. Jones MA, Young RH. Endocervical type A (noncystic) tunnel clusters with cytologic atypia: A report of 14 cases. Am J Surg Pathol 20:1312, 1996.

172. Jones MA, Young RH, Scully RE. Diffuse laminar endocervical glandular hyperplasia: A benign lesion often confused with adenoma malignum (minimal deviation adenocarcinoma). Am J Surg Pathol 15:1123, 1991.

173. Jones MW, Kounelis S, Papadaki H, et al. The origin and molecular characterization of adenoid basal carcinoma of the uterine cervix. Int J Gynecol Pathol 16:307, 1997.

174. Jones MW, Silverberg SG, Kurman RJ. Well-differentiated villoglandular adenocarcinoma of the uterine cervix: A clinicopathologic study of 24 cases. Int J Gynecol Pathol 12:1, 1993.

175. Kaku T, Enjoji M. Extremely well-differentiated adenocarcinoma ("adenoma malignum"). Int J Gynecol Pathol 2:28, 1983.

176. Kaku T. Kanura T, Sakai K, et al. Early adenocarcinoma of the uterine cervix. Gynecol Oncol 65:281, 1997.

177. Kaminski PF, Maier RC. Clear cell adenocarcinoma of the cervix unrelated to diethylstilbestrol exposure. Obstet Gynecol 62:720, 1983.

178. Kaminski PF, Norris HJ. Minimal deviation carcinoma (adenoma malignum) of the cervix. Int J Gynecol Pathol 2:141, 1983.

179. Kamura T, Tsukamoto N, Tsuruchi N, et al. Multivariate analysis of the histopathologic prognostic factors of cervical cancer patients undergoing radical hysterectomy. Cancer 69:181, 1992.

180. Kanbour AI, Stock RJ. Squamous cell carcinoma in situ of the endometrium and fallopian tube as superficial extension of invasive cervical carcinoma. Cancer 42:570, 1978.

181. Kapp DS, LiVolsi VA. Intense eosinophilic stromal infiltration in carcinoma of the uterine cervix: A clinicopathologic study of 14 cases. Gynecol Oncol 16:19, 1983.

182. Kaspar HG, Dinh TV, Doherty MG, et al. Clinical implications of tumor volume measurement in stage I adenocarcinoma of the cervix. Obstet Gynecol 81:296, 1993.

183. Kato H, Torigoe T. Radioimmunoassay for tumor antigen of human cervical squamous cell carcinoma. Cancer 40:1621, 1977.

184. Katz HJ, Davies JNP. Death from cervix uteri carcinoma: The changing pattern. Gynecol Oncol 9:86, 1980.

184a. Keating JT, Cviko A, Riethdorf S, et al. Ki-67, cyclin E, p16^{ink4} are complementary surrogate biomarkers for human papillomavirus-related cervical neoplasia. Am J Surg Pathol 25:884, 2001.

185. Kessler II. Etiological concepts in cervical carcinogenesis. Applied Pathol 5:57, 1987.

186. Kessler II. Etiological concepts in cervical carcinogenesis. Gynecol Oncol 12:S7, 1981.

187. Ketcham AS, Chretien PB, Hoye RC, et al. Occult metastases to the scalene lymph nodes in patients with clinically operable carcinoma of the cervix. Cancer 31:180, 1973.

188. Kiang DT, Bauer GE, Kennedy BJ. Immunoassayable insulin in carcinoma of the cervix associated with hypoglycemia. Cancer 31:801, 1973.

189. Kim PY, Mond BJ, Chabra S, et al. Cervical cancer with paraaortic metastases: Significance of residual paraaortic disease after surgical staging. Gynecol Oncol 69:243, 1998.

190. Kishi Y, Hashimoto Y, Sakamoto Y, et al. Thickness of uninvolved fibromuscular stroma and extrauterine spread of carcinoma of the uterine cervix. Cancer 60:2331, 1987.

190a. Kjorstad KE, Bond B. Stage IB adenocarcinoma of the cervix: Management potential and patterns of dissemination. Am J Obstet Gynecol 150:297, 1984.

191. Koenig C, Turnicky RP, Kankam CF, Tavassoli FA. Papillary squamotransitional cell carcinoma of the cervix: A report of 32 cases. Am J Surg Pathol 21:915, 1997.

192. Kolstad P. Follow-up study of 232 patients with stage Ia1 and 411 patients with stage Ia2 squamous cell carcinoma of the cervix (microinvasive carcinoma). Gynecol Oncol 33:265, 1989.

193. Korhonen MO. Adenocarcinoma of the uterine cervix. Acta Path et Microbiol Scand Sect A. 264(suppl):1, 1978.

194. Korhonen MO. Epidemiological differences between adenocarcinoma and squamous cell carcinoma of the uterine cervix. Gynecol Oncol 10:312, 1980.

195. Koss LG, Durfee GR. Unusual patterns of squamous epithelium of the uterine cervix: Cytologic and pathologic study of koilocytotic atypia. Ann NY Acad Sci 63:1245, 1956.

196. Krebs H, Helmkamp BF, Sevin B, et al. Recurrent cancer of the cervix following radical hysterectomy and pelvic node dissection. Obstet Gynecol 59:422, 1982.

197. Kristensen GB, Kaern J, Abeler VM, et al. No prognostic impact of flow-cytometric measured DNA ploidy and S-phase fraction in cancer of the uterine cervix: A prospective study of 465 patients. Gynecol Oncol 57:79, 1995.

198. Kurman RJ, Jenson AB, Lancaster WD. Papillomavirus infection of the cervix. II: Relationship to intraepithelial neoplasia based on the presence of specific viral structural proteins. Am J Surg Pathol 7:39, 1983.

199. Kurman RJ, Solomon D. The Bethesda System for Reporting Cervical/Vaginal Cytologic Diagnoses. New York, Springer-Verlag, 1994.

200. Kurvinen K, Syrjanen J, Syrjanen S. p53 and bcl-2 proteins as prognostic markers in human papillomavirus-associated cervical lesions. J Clin Oncol 4:2120, 1996.

201. Kyriakos M, Kempson RL, Konikov NF. A clinical and pathological study of endocervical lesions associated with oral contraceptives. Cancer 22:99, 1968.

202. Lagasse LD, Creasman WT, Shingleton HM, et al. Results and complications of operative staging in cervical cancer: Experience of the Gynecologic Oncology Group. Gynecol Oncol 9:90, 1980.

203. Larson DM, Copeland LJ, Stringer CA, et al. Recurrent cervical carcinoma after radical hysterectomy. Gynecol Oncol 30:381, 1988.

204. Larsson G, Alm P, Gullberg B, et al. Prognostic factors in early invasive carcinoma of the uterine cervix: A clinical, histopathologic, and statistical analysis of 343 cases. Am J Obstet Gynecol 146:145, 1983.

205. Lawrence JB, Mazur MT. Adenoid cystic carcinoma: A comparative pathologic study of tumors in salivary gland, breast, lung and cervix. Hum Pathol 13:916, 1982.

206. Lawrence WD, Shingleton GH, Soong S. Ultrastructure and morphometric study of diethylstilbestrol associated lesions diagnosed as cervical intraepithelial neoplasia III. Cancer Res 40:1558, 1980.

207. Lee KR, Sun D, Crum CP. Endocervical intraepithelial glandular atypia (dysplasia): A histopathologic, human papillomavirus and MIB-1 analysis of 25 cases. Hum Pathol 31:656, 2000.

208. Lee KR, Flynn CE. Early invasive adenocarcinoma of the cervix: A histopathologic analysis of 40 cases with observations concerning histogenesis. Cancer 89:1048, 2000.

209. Lee RB, Neglia W, Patk RC. Cervical carcinoma in pregnancy. Obstet Gynecol 58:584, 1981.

210. Leman MH, Benson WL, Kurman RJ, et al. Microinvasive carcinoma of the cervix. Obstet Gynecol 48:571, 1976.

211. Lifshitz S, Buchsbaum HJ. The spread of cervical carcinoma. In: Sciarra JJ (ed). Gynecology and Obstetrics, vol 4. Philadelphia, Harper and Row, 1980.

212. Lindgrin J, Wahlstrom T, Seppala M. Tissue CEA in premalignant epithelial lesions and epidermoid carcinoma of the uterine cervix: Prognostic significance. Int J Cancer 23:448, 1979.

212a. Littman P, Clement PB, Hendricksen B, et al. Glassy cell carcinoma of the cervix. Cancer 37:2238, 1976.

213. Look KY, Rocereto TF. Relapse patterns in FIGO stage IB carcinoma of the cervix. Gynecol Oncol 38:114, 1990.

214. Lorincz AT, Lancaster WD, Temple GF. Detection and characterization of a new human papillomavirus from a woman with dysplasia of the uterine cervix. J Virol 58:225, 1986.

215. Lorincz A, Reid R, Jenson AB, et al. Human papillomavirus infection of the cervix: Relative risk associations of 15 common anogenital types. Obstet Gynecol 79:328, 1992.

216. Lu T, Macasaet MA, Nelson JH Jr. The barrel-shaped cervical carcinoma. Am J Obstet Gynecol 124:596, 1976.

217. Ludwig ME, Lowell DM, LiVolsi VA. Cervical condylomatous atypia and its relationship to cervical neoplasia. Am J Clin Pathol 76:255, 1981.

218. Mackay B, Osborne BM, Wharton JT. Small cell tumor of cervix with neuroepithelial features. Cancer 43:1138, 1979.
219. Magitbay PM, Perrone JF, Stanhope CR, et al. Flow cytometric DNA analysis of early stage adenocarcinoma of the cervix. Gynecol Oncol 75:20, 1999.
220. Majeed GS, Glew S, Bidwell J. An association between LSIL and the high secretory phenotype of IL-BETA. Gynecol Oncol 73:359, 1999.
221. Maier RC, Norris HJ. Coexistence of cervical intraepithelial neoplasia with primary adenocarcinoma of the endocervix. Obstet Gynecol 56:361, 1980.
222. Maier RC, Norris HJ. Glassy cell carcinoma of the cervix. Obstet Gynecol 60:219, 1982.
223. Maiman MA, Fruchter RG, DiMaio TM, Boyce JG. Superficially invasive squamous cell carcinoma of the cervix. Obstet Gynecol 72:399, 1988.
224. Mandai M, Konishi I, Komatsu T, et al. Altered expression of nm 23-HI protein and c-erbB-2 proteins have prognostic significance in adenocarcinoma but not in squamous cell carcinoma of the uterine cervix. Cancer 75:2523, 1995.
225. Martinez I. Relationship of squamous cell carcinoma of the cervix uteri to squamous cell carcinoma of the penis among Puerto Rican women married to men with penile carcinoma. Cancer 24:777, 1969.
226. Masood S, Rhastigan RM, Wilkinson EW, et al. Expression and prognostic significance of estrogen and progesterone receptors in adenocarcinomas of the uterine cervix: An immunocytochemical study. Cancer 72:511, 1993.
227. Matsuyama M, Inoue T, Ariyoshi Y, et al. Argyrophil cell carcinoma of the uterine cervix with ectopic production of ACTH, B-MSH, serotonin, histamine and amylase. Cancer 44:1813, 1979.
228. Matsuyama T, Inoue I, Tsukamoto N, et al. Stage Ib, IIa, and IIb cervix cancer, postsurgical staging, and prognosis. Cancer 54:3072, 1984.
229. Mayer EG, Galindo J, Davis J, et al. Adenocarcinoma of the uterine cervix: Incidence and the role of radiation therapy. Radiology 121:725, 1976.
230. McClugger WG, Maxwell P, Bharucha H. Immunohistochemical detection of metyrothyoneine and MIB-1 in uterine cervical squamous lesions. Int J Gynecol Pathol 17:29, 1998.
231. McGowan L, Young RH, Scully RE. Peutz-Jeghers syndrome with "adenoma malignum" of the cervix: A report of two cases. Gynecol Oncol 10:125, 1980.
232. McIndoe WA, McLean MR, Jones RW, et al. The invasive potential of carcinoma in situ of the cervix. Obstet Gynecol 64:451, 1984.
233. McKelvey JL, Goodlin RR. Adenoma malignum of the cervix: A cancer of deceptively innocent histological pattern. Cancer 16:549, 1963.
234. Meisels A, Fortin R, Roy M. Condylomatous lesions of the cervix. II: Cytologic, colposcopic and histopathologic study. Acta Cytol 21:379, 1977.
235. Meisels A, Morin C. Human papillomavirus and cancer of the uterine cervix. Gynecol Oncol 12:S111, 1981.
236. Mendenhall WM, Thar TL, Bova FJ, et al. Prognostic and treatment factors affecting pelvic control of Stage IB and IIA-B carcinoma of the intact uterine cervix: Treatment with radiation therapy alone. Cancer 53:2649, 1984.
237. Mestwerdt G. Probeexzision and Kolposkopie in der Fruhdiagnose des Portiokarzinoms. Zentralbl Gynaekol 4:326, 1947.
238. Michael H, Grawe L, Kraus FT. Minimal deviation endocervical adenocarcinoma: Clinical and histologic features, immunohistochemical staining for carcinoembryonic antigen, and differentiation from confusing benign lesions. Int J Gynecol Pathol 3:261, 1984.
239. Michael H, Sutton G, Humm MT, et al. Villous adenoma of the uterine cervix associated with invasive adenocarcinoma: A histologic, ultrastructural, and immunohistochemical study. Int J Gynecol Pathol 5:163, 1986.
240. Milde-Langosch K, Schreiber C, Becker G, et al. Human papilloma-virus detection in cervical adenocarcinoma by polymerase chain reaction. Hum Pathol 23:590, 1993.
241. Miller BE, Flax SD, Arherat K, Photopulos G. The presentation of adenocarcinoma of the uterine cervix. Cancer 72:1281, 1993.
242. Mills SE, Austin MB, Randall ME. Lymphoepithelioma-like carcinoma of the uterine cervix. Am J Surg Pathol 9:883, 1985.
243. Mittal KR, Demopoulos RI, Goswami S. Proliferating cell nuclear antigen (cyclin) expression in normal and abnormal cervical squamous epithelia. Am J Surg Pathol 17:117, 1993.
244. Mittal KR, Palazzo J. Cervical condylomas show higher proliferation than do inflamed or metaplastic cervical squamous epithelium. Mod Pathol 11:780, 1998.
245. Mittal KR, Demopoulos RI, Tata M. A comparison of proliferative activity and atypical mitoses in cervical condylomas with various HPV types. Int J Gynecol Pathol 17:24, 1998.
246. Mobius G. Cytological early detection of cervical carcinoma: Possibilities and limitations. Analysis of failures. J Cancer Res Clin Oncol 119:513, 1993.
247. Morice P, Castaigne D, Pautier P, et al. Interest of pelvic and paraaortic lymphadenectomy in patients with stage IB and II cervical carcinoma. Gynecol Oncol 73:106, 1999.
248. Mullins JD, Hilliard GD. Cervical carcinoid ("argyrophil cell" carcinoma) associated with an endocervical adenocarcinoma: A light and ultrastructural study. Cancer 47:785, 1981.
249. Muraoka S, Takahashi T, Ando M, et al. Minute carcinoid tumor of the uterine cervix associated with microinvasive adenocarcinoma, with reference to its histogenesis. Acta Pathol Jpn 37:1183, 1987.
250. Nagao K, Matsuzaki O, Saiga H, et al. A histopathologic study of benign and malignant lymphoepithelial lesions of the parotid gland. Cancer 52:1044, 1983.
251. Naib ZM, Nahmias AJ, Josey WE, et al. Genital herpetic infection: Association with cervical dysplasia and carcinoma. Cancer 23:940, 1969.
252. Naib ZM, Nahmias AJ, Josey WE, et al. Relation of cytohistopathology of genital herpesvirus infection to cervical anaplasia. Cancer Res 33:1452, 1973.
253. Nasu I, Meurer W, Fu YS. Endocervical glandular atypia and adenocarcinoma: A correlation of cytology and histology. Int J Gynecol Pathol 12:208, 1993.
254. Ng ABP, Reagan JW. Microinvasive carcinoma of the uterine cervix. Am J Clin Pathol 52:511, 1969.
255. Ngan HYS, Chan SYW, Wong LC, et al. Serum squamous cell carcinoma antigen in the monitoring of radiotherapy treatment response in carcinoma of the cervix. Gynecol Oncol 37:260, 1990.
256. Nichols TM, Fidler HK. Microglandular hyperplasia

in cervical cone biopsies taken for suspicious and positive cytology. Am J Clin Pathol 56:424, 1971.

257. Nobbenhuis MAE, Walboomers JMM, Helmerhorst TJM, et al. Relation of human papillomavirus status to cervical lesions and consequences for cervical-cancer screening: A prospective study. Lancet 354: 20, 1999.

258. Nucci MR, Clement PB, Young RH. Lobular endocervical glandular hyperplasia, not otherwise specified. Am J Surg Pathol 23:886, 1999.

259. Oka K, Nakano T, Arai T. Adenocarcinoma of the cervix treated with radiation alone: Prognostic significance of S-100 protein and vimentin immunostaining. Obstet Gynecol 79:347, 1992.

260. Oliva E, Clement PB, Young RH. Tubal and tubo-endometrioid metaplasia of the uterine cervix. Unemphasized features that may cause problems in differential diagnosis: A report of 25 cases. Am J Clin Pathol 103:618, 1995.

260a. Orlandi C, Costa S, Terzano P, et al. Presurgical assessment and therapy of microinvasive carcinoma of the cervix. Gynecol Oncol 59:255, 1995.

261. Ostor AG. Natural history of cervical intraepithelial neoplasia: A critical review. Int J Gynecol Pathol 12:186, 1993.

262. Ostor AG. Early invasive adenocarcinoma of the uterine cervix. Int J Gynecol Pathol 19:29, 2000.

263. Ostor A, Rome R, Quinn M. Microinvasive adenocarcinoma of the cervix: A clinicopathologic study of 77 women. Obstet Gynecol 89:88, 1997.

264. Ostor AG, Pagano R, Davoren RAM, et al. Adenocarcinoma in situ of the cervix. Int J Gynecol Pathol 3:179, 1984.

264a. O'Sullivan MJ, Rader JS, Gerhard DS, et al. Loss of heterozygosity at 11q23.3 in vasculoinvasive and metastatic squamous cell carcinoma of the cervix. Hum Pathol 32:475, 2001.

265. Pak HY, Yokota SB, Paladugu RR, et al. Glassy cell carcinoma of the cervix. Cancer 52:307, 1983.

266. Papanicolaou GN. A survey of the actualities and potentialities of exfoliative cytology in cancer diagnosis. Ann Int Med 31:661, 1949.

267. Parente JT, et al. Infrequency of metastasis to ovaries in stage I carcinoma of the cervix. Am J Obstet Gynecol 90:1362, 1964.

268. Park JJ, Genest DR, Sun D, Crum CP. Atypical immature metaplastic-like proliferations of the cervix: Diagnostic reproducibility and viral (HPV) correlates. Human Pathol 30:1161, 1999.

269. Park JJ, Sun D, Quade BJ, et al. Stratified mucin-producing intraepithelial lesions of the cervix: Adenosquamous or columnar cell neoplasia? Am J Surg Pathol 24:1414, 2000.

270. Parker SL, Tong T, Bolden S, Wingo PA. Cancer Statistics, 1997. CA A Cancer Journal for Clinicians 47:5, 1997.

271. Patten SF. Diagnostic Cytology of the Uterine Cervix. Baltimore, Williams & Wilkins, 1978.

272. Paulsen SM, Hansen KC, Nielsen VT. Glassy-cell carcinoma of the cervix: Case report with a light and electron microscopy study. Ultrastruct Pathol 1:377, 1980.

273. Pazdur R, Bonomi P, Slayton R, et al. Neuroendocrine carcinoma of the cervix: Implications for staging and therapy. Gynecol Oncol 12:120, 1981.

274. Peters RK, Chao A, Mack TM, et al. Increased frequency of adenocarcinoma of the uterine cervix in young women in Los Angeles County. J Natl Cancer Inst 76:423, 1986.

275. Pilleron JP, Durand JC, Hamelin JP. Prognostic value of node metastasis in cancer of the uterine cervix. Am J Obstet Gynecol 119:458, 1974.

276. Pins MR, Young RH, Crum CP, et al. Cervical squamous cell carcinoma in situ with intraepithelial extension to the upper genital tract and invasion of tubes and ovaries: Report of a case with human papilloma virus analysis. Int J Gynecol Pathol 16:272, 1997.

277. Piver MS, Chung WS. Prognostic significance of cervical lesion size and pelvic lymph node metastasis in cervical carcinoma. Obstet Gynecol 46:507, 1975.

278. Pratt JH, Jefferies JA. The retained cervical stump. A 25-year experience. Obstet Gynecol 48:711, 1976.

279. Prempree T, Villasanta U, Tang CK. Management of adenoid cystic carcinoma of the uterine cervix (cylindroma). Cancer 46:1631, 1980.

280. Qilzilbash AH. In situ and microinvasive adenocarcinoma of the uterine cervix. Am J Clin Pathol 64:155, 1975.

281. Quade BJ, Park JJ, Crum CP, Sun D, Dutta A. In vivo cyclin E expression as a marker for early cervical neoplasia. Mod Pathol 11:1238, 1998.

282. Rader JS, Gerjard DS, O'Sullivan MJ, et al. Cervical intraepithelial neoplasia III shows frequent allelic loss in 3p and 6p. Journal of Genes, Chromosomes and Cancer, 22:57, 1998.

283. Randall ME, Andersen WA, Mills SE, et al. Papillary squamous cell carcinoma of the uterine cervix: A clinicopathologic study of nine cases. Int J Gynecol Pathol 5:1, 1986.

284. Rawls WE, Lavery C, Marrett LD, et al. Comparison of risk factors for cervical cancer in different populations. Int J Cancer 37:537, 1986.

285. Reagan JW, Fu YS. Histologic types and prognosis of cancers of the uterine cervix. Int J Radiat Oncol Biol Phys 5:1015, 1979.

286. Reagan JW, Ng ABP. The cellular manifestations of uterine carcinogenesis. In: Norris NJ, Hertig AT, Abell MR (eds). The Uterus. Baltimore, Williams & Wilkins, 1973, p 320.

287. Reagan JW, Patten SF Jr. Dysplasia: A basic reaction to injury in the uterine cervix. Ann NY Acad Sci 97:662, 1962.

288. Reagan JW, Seidemann IL, Saracusa Y. Cellular morphology of carcinoma in situ and dysplasia or atypical hyperplasia of uterine cervix. Cancer 6:224, 1953.

289. Reddy EK, Mansfield CM, Hartman GV, et al. Carcinoma of the uterine cervix: Review of experience at University of Kansas Medical Center. Cancer 47:1916, 1981.

290. Reich O, Tamussino K, Lahousen M, et al. Clear cell carcinomas of the uterine cervix: Pathology and prognosis in surgically treated state IB-IIB in women not exposed in utero to diethylstilbestrol. Gynecol Oncol 76:331, 2000.

291. Reid BL, French PW, Singer A, et al. Sperm basic proteins in cervical carcinogenesis: Correlation with socioeconomic class. Lancet 2:60, 1978.

292. Reid R, Greenberg M, Jenson AB, et al. Sexually transmitted papillomaviral infections. I: The anatomic distribution and pathologic grade of neoplastic lesions associated with different viral types. Am J Obstet Gynecol 156:212, 1987.

293. Reid RI, Lorincz AT. New generation of human papillomavirus tests. In: Cervical Cancer and Preinvasive Neoplasia. Rubin SC, Hoskins WJ (eds). Philadelphia, Lippincott-Raven, 1996.

294. Rettenmaier MA, Casanova DM, Micha JP, et al. Radical hysterectomy and tailored postoperative radiation therapy in the management of bulky stage IB cervical cancer. Cancer 63:2220, 1989.

295. Richart RM. Cervical intraepithelial neoplasia: A review. In: Sommers SC (ed). Pathology Annual, vol 8. Norwalk, Conn., Appleton-Century-Crofts, 1973, p 301.

296. Riou G, Barrois M, Le MG, et al. C-myc proto-oncogene expression and prognosis in early carcinoma of the uterine cervix. Lancet 1:761, 1987.

297. Robboy SJ, Welch WR, Young RH. Atypical vaginal adenosis and cervical ectropion: Association with clear cell adenocarcinoma in diethylstilbestrol-exposed offspring. Cancer 54:869, 1984.

298. Roche WD, Norris HJ. Microinvasive carcinoma of the cervix. The significance of lymphatic invasion and confluent patterns of stromal growth. Cancer 36:180, 1975.

299. Ronnett BM, Manos MM, Ransley JE, et al. Atypical glandular cells of undetermined significance (AGUS): Cytologic features, histopathologic results, and human papillomavirus DNA detection. Hum Pathol 30:816, 1999.

300. Rotkin ID. A comparison review of key epidemiological studies in cervical cancer related to current searches for transmissible agents. Cancer Res 33:1353, 1973.

301. Rotkin ID. Adolescent coitus and cervical cancer: Association of related events with increased risk. Cancer Res 27:603, 1967.

302. Rubin SC, Brookland R, Mikuta JJ, et al. Para-aortic nodal metastases in early cervical carcinoma: Long-term survival following extended-field radiotherapy. Gynecol Oncol 18:213, 1984.

303. Rutgers JL, Mattox TF, Vargas MP. Angiogenesis in uterine cervical squamous cell carcinoma. Int J Gynecol Pathol 14:114, 1995.

304. Rutledge FN, Galakatos AE, Wharton JT, et al. Adenocarcinoma of the uterine cervix. Am J Obstet Gynecol 122:236, 1975.

305. Saegusa M, Takano Y, Hasshumura M, et al. The possible role of bcl-2 expression in the progression of tumor of the uterine cervix. Cancer 76:2297, 1995.

306. Saigo PE, Cain JM, Kim WS, et al. Prognostic factors in adenocarcinoma of the uterine cervix. Cancer 57:1584, 1986.

307. Sagae S, Kuzumaki N, Hisada T, et al. Ras oncogene expression and prognosis of invasive squamous cell carcinomas of the uterine cervix. Cancer 63:1577, 1989.

308. Saito K, Saito A, Fu YS, et al. Topographic study of cervical condyloma and intraepithelial neoplasia. Cancer 59:2064, 1987.

309. Sakuragi N, Takeda N, Hareyama H, et al. A multivariate analysis of blood vessel and lymph vessel invasion as predictors of ovarian and lymph node metastases in patients with cervical carcinoma. Cancer 88:2578, 2000.

310. Sasson IM, Haley NJ, Hoffman D, et al. Cigarette smoking and neoplasia of the uterine cervix: Smoke constituents in cervical mucus. N Engl J Med 312:315, 1985.

311. Schiller W, Daro AF, Gollin HA, et al. Small preulcerative invasive carcinoma of the cervix—the spray carcinoma. Am J Obstet Gynecol 65:1088, 1953.

311a. Schlenger K, Hockel M, Mitze M, et al. Tumor vascularity—a novel prognostic factor in advanced cervical carcinoma. Gynecol Oncol 59:57, 1995.

312. Schlesinger C, Silverberg SG. Endocervical adenocarcinoma in situ of tubal type and its relation to atypical tubal metaplasia. Int J Gynecol Pathol 18:1, 1999.

313. Schorge JO, Lee KR, Flynn CD, et al. Stage IA1 cervical adenocarcinoma: Definition and treatment. Obstet Gynecol 93:219, 1999.

314. Schwartz SM, Weiss NS. Increased incidence of adenocarcinoma of the cervix in young women in the United States. Am J Epidemiol 124:1045, 1986.

314a. Scully RE, Bonfiglio TA, Kurman RJ, et al. Histologic Typing of Female Genital Tract Tumors, 2nd ed. Berlin, Springer-Verlag, 1994.

315. Sedlis A, Sol S, Tsukada Y, et al. Microinvasive carcinoma of the uterine cervix: A clinical-pathologic study. Am J Obstet Gynecol 133:64, 1979.

316. Segal GH, Hart WR. Cystic endocervical tunnel clusters. A clinicopathologic study of 29 cases of so-called adenomatous hyperplasia. Am J Surg Pathol 14:895, 1990.

317. Seski JC, Abell MR, Morley GW. Microinvasive squamous carcinoma of the cervix—definition, histologic analysis, late results of treatment. Obstet Gynecol 50:410, 1977.

318. Sevin B, Lu Y, Bloch DA, et al. Surgically defined prognostic parameters in patients with early cervical carcinoma. Cancer 78:1438, 1996.

319. Sevin BU, Nadji M, Averette HE, et al. Microinvasive carcinoma of the cervix. Cancer 70:2121, 1992.

320. Sevin BU, Method MW, Nadji M, et al. Efficacy of radical hysterectomy as treatment for patients with small cell carcinoma of the cervix. Cancer 77:1489, 1996.

321. Shiffman M, Herrero R, Hildesheim A, et al. HPV DNA testing in cervical cancer screening: Results from women in a high-risk province of Costa Rica. JAMA 283:87, 2000.

322. Shingleton HM, Bell MC, Fremgen A, et al. Is there really a difference in survival of women with squamous cell carcinoma, adenocarcinoma, and adenosquamous cell carcinoma of the cervix? Cancer 76:1948, 1995.

323. Shingleton HM, Gore H, Bradley DH, et al. Adenocarcinoma of the cervix. I: Clinical evaluation and pathologic features. Am J Obstet Gynecol 139:799, 1981.

324. Shingleton HM, Lawrence WD, Gore H. Cervical carcinoma with adenoid cystic pattern. Cancer 40:1112, 1977.

325. Sidhu GS, Koss LG, Barber HRK. Relation of histologic factors to the response of stage I epidermoid carcinoma of the cervix to surgical treatment. Obstet Gynecol 35:329, 1970.

326. Silva EG, Brock WA, Gershenson D, et al. Small cell carcinoma of the uterine cervix: Pathology and prognostic factors. Surg Pathol 2:105, 1989.

327. Silva EG, Kott MM, Ordonez NG. Endocrine carcinoma intermediate cell type of the uterine cervix. Cancer 54:1705, 1984.

327a. Silver SA, Devouassoux-Shisheboran M, Mezzetti TP, Tavassoli FA. Mesonephric adenocarcinomas of the uterine cervix: A study of 11 cases with immunohistochemical findings. Am J Surg Pathol 25:379, 2001.

328. Silverberg SG, Hurt WG. Minimal deviation adenocarcinoma ("adenoma malignum") of the cervix. Am J Obstet Gynecol 121:971, 1975.

329. Simon NL, Gore H, Shingleton HM, et al. Study of superficially invasive carcinoma of the cervix. Obstet Gynecol 68:19, 1986.

330. Skyldberg GM, Murry E, Lambkin H, et al. Adenocarcinoma of the uterine cervix in Ireland and Sweden: Human papillomavirus infection and biologic alterations. Mod Pathol 12:675, 1999.

331. Smedts F, Ramaekers F, Troyanovsky S, et al. Keratin expression in cervical cancer. Am J Pathol 141:497, 1992.

332. Smotkin D, Berek JS, Fu YS, et al. Human papillomavirus DNA in adenocarcinoma and adenosquamous carcinoma of the uterine cervix. Obstet Gynecol 68:241, 1986.

333. Solomon D, Schiffman M, Tarone R. Comparison of three management strategies for patients with atypical squamous cells of undetermined significance: Baseline results from a randomized trail. J Natl Cancer Inst 93:293, 2001.

334. Stanhope CR, Smith JP, Wharton JT, et al. Carcinoma of the cervix: The effect of age on survival. Gynecol Oncol 10:188, 1980.

335. Stassart J, Crum CP, Yordan EL, et al. Argyrophilic carcinoma of the cervix: A report of a case with coexisting cervical intraepithelial neoplasia. Gynecol Oncol 13:247, 1982.

336. Steiner G, Friedell GH. Adenosquamous carcinoma in situ of the cervix. Cancer 18:807, 1965.

337. Stendahl U, Willen H, Willen R. Classification and grading of invasive squamous cell carcinoma of the uterine cervix. Acta Radiol Oncol 18:481, 1979.

338. Stendahl U, Willen H, Willen R. Invasive squamous cell carcinoma of the uterine cervix. I: Definition of parameters in a histopathologic malignancy grading system. Acta Radiol Oncol 19:467, 1980.

339. Stewart CJR, Taggart CR, Brett F, Mutch AF. Mesonephric adenocarcinoma of the uterine cervix with focal endocrine cell differentiation. Int J Gynecol Pathol 12:264, 1993.

340. Stock RJ, Zaino R, Bundy BN, et al. Evaluation and comparison of histopathologic grading systems of epithelial carcinoma of the uterine cervix: Gynecologic Oncology Group studies. Int J Gynecol Pathol 13:99, 1994.

341. Stoler MH, Mills SE, Gersell DJ, Walker AN. Small-cell neuroendocrine carcinoma of the cervix: A human papillomavirus type 18-associated cancer. Am J Surg Path 15:28, 1991.

342. Strang P. Cytogenetic and cytometric analyses in squamous cell carcinoma of the uterine cervix. Int J Gynecol Pathol 8:54, 1989.

343. Suh KS, Silverberg SG. Tubal metaplasia of the uterine cervix. Int J Gynecol Pathol 9:122, 1990.

344. Sung HY, Kearney KA, Miller M, et al. Papanicolaou smear history and diagnosis of invasive cervical carcinoma among members of a large prepaid health plan. Cancer 88:2283, 2000.

345. Sutton GP, et al. Ovarian metastases in stage IB carcinoma of the cervix: A Gynecologic Oncology Group study. Am J Obstet Gynecol 166:50, 1992.

346. Tabata M, Ichinoe K, Sakuragi N, et al. Incidence of ovarian metastasis in patients with cancer of the uterine cervix. Gynecol Oncol 28:255, 1987.

347. Tambouret R, Bell DA, Young RH. Microcystic endocervical adenocarcinoma: A report of eight cases. Am J Surg Pathol 24:369, 2000.

348. Tase T, Okagaki T, Clark BA, et al. Human papillomavirus types and localization in adenocarcinoma and adenosquamous carcinoma of the uterine cervix: A study by in situ DNA hybridization. Cancer Res 48:993, 1988.

349. Taylor HB, Irey NS, Norris HJ. Atypical endocervical hyperplasia in women taking oral contraceptives. JAMA 202:637, 1968.

350. Tendler A, Kaufman HL, Kadish AS. Increased carcinoembryonic antigen expression in cervical intraepithelial neoplasia grade 2 and in cervical squamous cell carcinoma. Human Pathol 31:1357, 2000.

351. Teshima S, Shimosato Y, Kishi K, et al. Early stage adenocarcinoma of the uterine cervix. Histopathologic analysis with consideration of histogenesis. Cancer 56:167, 1985.

352. Thelmo WL, Micastri AD, Fruchter R, et al. Mucoepidermoid carcinoma of uterine cervix stage IB: Long-term follow-up, histochemical and immunohistochemical study. Int J Gynecol Pathol 9:316, 1990.

353. Tiltman AJ, Atad J. Verrucous carcinoma of the cervix with endometrial involvement. Int J Gynecol Pathol 1:221, 1982.

354. Timmer PR, Aalders JG, Bouma J. Radical surgery after preoperative intracavitary radiotherapy for stage IB and IIA carcinoma of the uterine cervix. Gynecol Oncol 18:206, 1984.

355. Townsend DE, Richart RM, Marks E, et al. Invasive cancer following outpatient evaluation and therapy for cervical disease. Obstet Gynecol 57:145, 1981.

356. Trivijitsilip R, Mosher R, Sheets EE, et al. Papillary immature metaplasia (immature condyloma) of the cervix: A clinicopathologic analysis and comparison with papillary squamous carcinoma. Human Pathol 29:641, 1998.

357. Tseng CJ, Pao CC, Tseng LH, et al. Lymphoepithelioma-like carcinoma of the uterine cervix: Association with Epstein-Barr virus and human papillomavirus. Cancer 80:91, 1997.

358. Ulbright TM, Gersell DJ. Glassy cell carcinoma of the uterine cervix: A light and electron microscopic study of five cases. Cancer 51:2255, 1983.

359. Ulich TR, Liao SY, Layfield L, et al. Endocrine and tumor differentiation markers in poorly differentiated small-cell carcinoids of the cervix and vagina. Arch Pathol Lab Med 110:1054, 1986.

360. Umezaki K, Sanezumu M, Kanemori H, et al. Immunohistochemical demonstration of aberrant glycosylation and epidermal growth factor receptor in tubal metaplasia of the uterine cervix. Gynecol Oncol 70:40, 1998.

360a. Val-Bernal JF, Pinto J, Garijo MF, Gomez MS. Pagetoid dyskeratosis of the cervix. Am J Surg Pathol 24:1518, 2000.

361. van Nagell JR, Donaldson ES, Gay EC, et al. Carcinoembryonic antigen in carcinoma of the uterine cervix. Cancer 44:944, 1979.

362. van Nagell JR, Donaldson ES, Parker JC, et al. The prognostic significance of cell type and lesion size in patients with cervical cancer treated by radical surgery. Gynecol Oncol 5:152, 1977.

363. van Nagell JR, Donaldson ES, Wood EG, et al. Small cell cancer of the uterine cervix. Cancer 40:2253, 1977.

364. van Nagell JR, Donaldson ES, Wood EG, et al. The clinical significance of carcinoembryonic antigen in the plasma and tumors of patients with gynecologic malignancies. Cancer 42:1527, 1978.

365. van Nagell JR, Greenwell N, Powell DF, et al. Microinvasive carcinoma of the cervix. Am J Obstet Gynecol 145:981, 1983.

366. Vasilev SA, Schlaerth JB. Scalene lymph node sampling in cervical carcinoma: A reappraisal. Gynecol Oncol 37:120, 1990.

367. Vessey MP, Lawless M, McPherson K, et al. Neopla-

sia of the cervix uteri and contraception: A possible adverse effect of the pill. Lancet 2:930, 1983.

368. Wahlstrom T, Lindgren J, Korhonen M, et al. Distinction between endocervical and endometrial adenocarcinoma with immunoperoxidase staining of carcinoembryonic antigen in routine histologic tissue specimens. Lancet 2:1159, 1979.

369. Walker AN, Mills SE, Taylor PT. Cervical neuroendocrine carcinoma: A clinical and light microscopic study of 14 cases. Int J Gynecol Pathol 7:64, 1988.

370. Wallin K-J, Wiklund E, Angstrom T, et al. Type-specific persistence of human papillomavirus DNA before the development of invasive cervical cancer. N End J Med 341:1633, 1999.

370a. Wang T-Y, Chen B-F, Yang Y-C, et al. Histologic and immunophenotypic classification of cervical carcinoma by expression of the p53 homologue p63: A study of 250 cases. Hum Pathol 32:479, 2001.

371. Warner TFCS. Carcinoid tumor of the uterine cervix. J Clin Pathol 31:990, 1978.

372. Watty EI, Johnston LW, Bainborough AR. Polypoid carcinoma of the uterine cervix simulating "pseudosarcoma" and "carcinosarcoma" of esophagus and upper respiratory tract. Diag Gynecol Obstet 3:205, 1981.

372a. Weir MW, Bell DA, Young RH. Transitional cell metaplasia of the uterine cervix and vagina: An underrecognized lesion that may be confused with high-grade dysplasia. Am J Surg Pathol 21:510, 1997.

373. Weiss LK, Kau TY, Sparks BT, Swanson GM. Trends in cervical cancer incidence among young black and white women in metropolitan Detroit. Cancer 73:1849, 1994.

374. Welch WR, Fu YS, Robboy SJ, et al. Nuclear DNA content of clear cell adenocarcinoma of the vagina and cervix and its relationship to prognosis. Gynecol Oncol 15:230, 1983.

375. Wells M, Brown LJR. Glandular lesions of the uterine cervix: The present state of our knowledge. Histopathology 10:777, 1996.

376. Wentz WB, Reagan JW. Survival in cervical cancer with respect to cell type. Cancer 12:384, 1959.

377. White CD, Morley GW, Kumar NB. The prognostic significance of tumor emboli in lymphatic or vascular spaces of the cervical stroma in stage IB squamous cell carcinoma of the cervix. Am J Obstet Gynecol 149:342, 1984.

378. Wielenga G, Old JW, von Haam E. Squamous carcinoma in situ of the uterine cervix. II: Topography and clinical correlations. Cancer 18:1612, 1965.

379. Wilczynski SP, Lin BTY, Xie Y, Paz IB. Detection of human papillomavirus DNA and oncoprotein overexpression are associated with distinct morphological patterns of tonsillar squamous cell carcinoma. Am J Pathol 152:145, 1998.

380. Wilkinson E, Dufour DR. Pathogenesis of micro-

381. Winkler B, Crum CP, Fujii A, et al. Koilocytic lesions of the cervix: The relationship of mitotic abnormalities to the presence of papillomavirus antigens and nuclear DNA content. Cancer 53:1081, 1984.

382. Wisman GBA, DeJong S, Meersma GJ, et al. Telomerase in (pre)neoplastic cervical disease. Human Pathol 31:1304, 2000.

383. Wolf JK, Levenback C, Malpica A, et al. Adenocarcinoma in situ of the cervix: Significance of cone biopsy margins. Obstet Gynecol 88:82, 1996.

384. Wright TC, Denny L, Kuhn L, et al. HPV DNA testing of self-collected vaginal samples compared with cytologic screening to detect cervical cancer. JAMA 283:81, 2000.

385. Wylie-Rosett JA, Romney SL, Slagle NS, et al. Influence of vitamin A on cervical dysplasia and carcinoma in situ. Nutr Cancer 6:49, 1984.

386. Yost NO, Santoso JT, McIntire DD, Iliya FA. Postpartum regression rates of antepartum cervical intraepithelial neoplasia II and III lesions. Obstet Gynecol 93:359, 1999.

387. Young RH, Scully RE. Invasive adenocarcinoma and related tumors of the uterine cervix. Semin Diag Pathol 7:205, 1990.

388. Young RH, Scully RE. Villoglandular papillary adenocarcinoma of the uterine cervix: A clinicopathologic analysis of 13 cases. Cancer 63:1773, 1989.

389. Young RH, Scully RE. Mucinous ovarian tumors associated with mucinous adenocarcinoma of the cervix. Int J Gynecol Pathol 7:99, 1988.

390. Young RH, Scully RE. Atypical forms of microglandular hyperplasia of the cervix simulating carcinoma. Am J Surg Pathol 13:50, 1989.

391. Zaino RJ, Nahhas WA, Mortel R. Glassy cell carcinoma of the uterine cervix. Arch Pathol Lab Med 106:250, 1982.

392. Zaino RJ, Ward S, Delgado G, et al. Histopathologic predictors of the behavior of surgically treated stage IB squamous cell carcinoma of the cervix: A Gynecologic Oncology Group study. Cancer 69:1750, 1992.

393. Zhou C, Gilks CB, Hayes M, Clement PB. Papillary serous carcinoma of the uterine cervix: A clinicopathological study of 17 cases. Am J Surg Pathol 22:113, 1998.

394. Zur Hausen H. Human genital cancer: Synergism between two virus infections or synergism between a virus infection and initiating events? Lancet 2:1370, 1982.

395. Zur Hausen H. Papillomaviruses in human cancer. Appl Pathol 5:19, 1987.

396. Zur Hausen H. Viruses in human cancers. Science 254:1167, 1991.

glandular hyperplasia of the cervix uteri. Obstet Gynecol 47:189, 1976.

9

NONEPITHELIAL AND METASTATIC TUMORS OF THE LOWER GENITAL TRACT

Benign and malignant mesodermal and neurogenic tumors occasionally occur in the female lower genital tract, and especially in the vulva. Specialized mesenchymal tumors of müllerian origin, on the other hand, are more common in the cervix and vagina. Tumor-like conditions, especially those simulating sarcomas, require careful consideration of clinical history and morphologic features to avoid overdiagnosis. Finally, it is important to diagnose metastatic tumors to the lower genital tract correctly for therapeutic and prognostic reasons.

MESODERMAL TUMOR–LIKE CONDITIONS

Nodular Fasciitis

Nodular fasciitis or pseudosarcomatous fasciitis is a benign fibrous proliferation of superficial fascia of subcutaneous tissue or deep fascia overlying muscle, tendon, or bone. It typically has a recent onset, rapid growth, and spontaneous occurrence. The upper extremity is most frequently affected. Only a few cases are reported in the vulva.[63,150]

Vulvar nodular fasciitis presents as a subcutaneous, movable, slightly tender nodule, generally 2 to 3 cm in size and occasionally attached to ischiocavernosus muscle. Histologically, the spindle cells are arranged in interlacing bundles or a storiform pattern. Mitotic figures can be easily found. There is a gradation of collagenous maturation in the stroma ranging from myxomatous early granulation tissue, with hemorrhage, delicate capillaries, and scattered lymphocytes and histiocytes, to mature, hyalinized, keloid-type fibrous tissue (Fig. 9–1). Plasma cells are rare or absent.

Because of the storiform pattern, increased mitotic activity, and poor circumscription, nodular fasciitis may be confused with fibrous histiocytoma, fibrosarcoma, and leiomyosarcoma. A tissue culture–like uniform cell population in varying degrees of collagenization, a small lesion, and a history of recent onset are typical of nodular fasciitis (Fig. 9–2). On the other hand, spindle cell lesions with storiform pattern, nuclear hyperchromasia and atypism, and abundant plasma cells in the stroma are likely to represent neoplasms, such as an inflammatory variant of fibrous histiocytoma.

O'Connell et al.[132] reported on six cases of vulvar nodular fasciitis in females 7 to 51 (mean 34) years of age; all were located on the labia and were 1.5 to 3.5 (mean 2.2) cm in size. Two had cleft-like spaces lined by synovial-like cells, in addition to the typical features. One woman

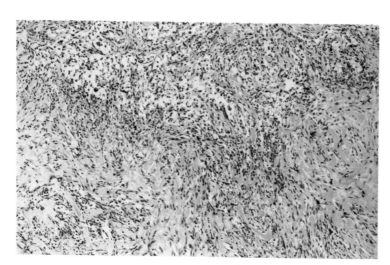

Figure 9–1. Nodular fasciitis. Proliferating spindle cells mix with inflammatory cells. The intercellular matrix varies from edematous, myxomatous to hyalinized, keloid tissue.

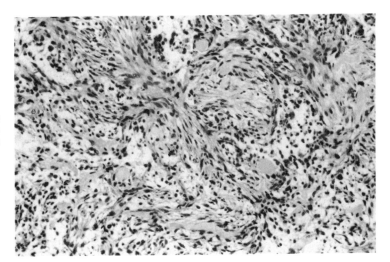

Figure 9–2. Nodular fasciitis. Spindle cells arranged in a storiform pattern mixed with lymphocytes. Plasma cells are rare or absent.

had local recurrence 4 months after excision.[132] Immunohistochemical stains were positive for vimentin in all six lesions, for muscle actin in four of six, and for smooth muscle actin in three of six; none was positive for desmin.

The differential diagnosis includes postoperative spindle cell nodule, which is similar to nodular fasciitis, having high mitotic activity, rapid growth, homogeneous proliferating cells, myxoid cysts, multinucleated giant cells, and keloid component.

Aggressive angiomyxoma is usually larger than 5.0 cm, involves the vulvar, perineal region of reproductive women, and has poorly defined infiltrative borders. Angiomyofibroblastoma is small in size and labial in location. Histologically, it has noninfiltrative smooth borders and mixed hypocellular and hypercellular areas of spindle, plasmacytoid, and epithelioid cells. Myxoid or fibrous stroma has congested blood vessels, has low to absent mitosis, and expresses desmin, estrogen, and progesterone receptor proteins.

Postoperative Spindle Cell Nodule

A fibrous lesion arising at recent surgery sites and closely resembling sarcoma and nodular fasciitis has been designated by Proppe et al.[145] as postoperative spindle cell nodule. They reported eight cases of this entity that occurred in the vagina, urethra, or urinary bladder 5 weeks to 3 months following vaginal hysterectomy, episiotomy, or transurethral resection. All were submucosal and less than 4 cm in size.

The lesion consists of interlacing bundles of plump spindle cells in a background of rich capillary network and scattered chronic inflammatory cells. Stromal edema and hemorrhage are also common. Individual cells have abundant tapering cytoplasm, one to two nucleoli, and high mitotic activity, ranging from one to 25 mitotic figures per 10 high-power fields. Collagen fibrils are generally inconspicuous. Under the electron microscope, spindle cells have the appearance of fibroblasts.

Because of its high degree of cellularity and mitotic activity, this lesion is often considered to be some type of sarcoma, especially leiomyosarcoma, Kaposi's sarcoma, or fibrous histiocytoma. One of the most distinct features is the striking nuclear uniformity and the lack of nuclear hyperchromasia and atypism. Areas of hemorrhage with red blood cells between spindle cells, although mimicking Kaposi's sarcoma, occur sporadically. The storiform pattern commonly found in nodular fasciitis and fibrous histiocytoma is uncommon. With time and further maturation of the reparative tissue, however, different histologic features may emerge. Snover et al.[167] described a 3 cm nodule in the vaginal apex, which was excised 5 months after a hysterectomy and salpingo-oophorectomy. In the nodule, the spindle cells were arranged in a storiform pattern and were low in mitotic activity. Foamy histiocytes and foreign-body giant cells outnumbered sparse lymphocytes.

Despite the alarming histologic features, the benign nature of the spindle cell nodule is supported by the fact that all patients have been well 9 months to 5 years after a limited local excision.

Sclerosing Lipogranuloma

Sclerosing lipogranuloma is a peculiar form of fat necrosis with granulomatous inflammation. Most lesions involve the genitals and buttocks in males. Some of these lesions result from injection of paraffin, mineral oil, and saturated vegetable oil into the skin and subcutaneous areas. Kempson and Sherman[94] described a 55-year-old woman who presented with a 4 × 4 × 8 cm mass on the right vulvar fold. It was rubbery, well delineated, and mobile.

The mass recurred 2 years after local excision. Two additional, similar lesions developed on the abdomen. There was no history of injection of lipid at these sites.

Histologically, fat globules of varying sizes are lined by fat cells, histiocytes, and multinucleated giant cells. Between the fat globules are broad areas of hyalinized fibrous stroma with scattered foci of lymphocytes and plasma cells.

It is important to recognize this benign tumor–like mass because of possible confusion with malignant neoplasm, especially liposarcoma. In sclerosing lipogranuloma, the regional lymph nodes may become enlarged, suggestive of metastasis. Histologically, the lymph nodes have abundant lipid in the cytoplasm of histiocytes. Although this is a peculiar granulomatous form of fat necrosis, it may recur locally or may develop new lesions elsewhere in the body. Complete local excision is recommended.[94]

BENIGN AND MALIGNANT MESODERMAL TUMORS

In a study of 34 benign mesodermal and neurogenic tumors of the vulva, 16 were fibromas, seven were lipomas, five were hemangiomas, two were neurofibromas, two were leiomyomas, one was a ganglioneuroma, and one was a lymphangioma.[110] In the cervix and vagina, benign smooth muscle and vascular tumors are the most common mesenchymal tumors. In most cases, they are asymptomatic until they become large enough to cause pain and a heavy sensation or become ulcerated and cause bleeding, pain, and discharge.

Sarcomas of the vulva, representing 1.8%[39] and 3.0%[47] of all vulvar malignancies, comprise a heterogeneous group of sarcomas. In two series combined, leiomyosarcomas are most common (10 cases, 37%), followed by malignant schwannoma (four cases, 15%), rhabdomyosarcoma (three cases, 11%), fibrosarcoma (two cases, 7%), and malignant fibrous histiocytoma (two cases, 7%).[40,47] Other sarcomas, including dermatofibrosarcoma protuberans, epithelioid sarcoma, malignant hemangiopericytoma, angiosarcoma, endometrial stromal sarcoma, malignant lymphoma, plasmacytoma, malignant mesothelioma, and alveolar soft part sarcoma, have also been reported.[40,48,64,72,142,147] Approximately two thirds of the tumors are located on the labium majus; the other third are located on the labium minus or in the fourchette or Bartholin's gland region. The size of the tumor varies from 2 to 10 cm in greatest dimension. It often appears as a circumscribed mass, which is usually painful. Occasionally, there is associated metastasis to the groin.

Most of the sarcomas involving the cervix and vagina are leiomyosarcoma, rhabdomyosarcoma, and müllerian mixed tumors. Other kinds of sarcomas are much less common. With the exception of rhabdomyosarcoma, most sarcomas affect adult women between 30 and 60 years of age.[47] Prognosis depends on the tumor size, depth of invasion, histologic features, and surgical margins. These findings should be indicated in the pathology reports.

Fibroma

Fibroma of the vulva usually presents as a pediculated, small, firm nodule of so-called fibroma molle (Fig. 9–3). Histologically, the tumor is composed of bundles of mature fibroblasts. The cellularity is mild to moderate. Abundant collagenous stroma sometimes contains myxoid foci. Mitotic figures and nuclear atypia are absent or minimal. Simple excision results in cure.

Lipoma

Lipoma is a soft, round, lobulated mass, which may be pedunculated or sessile. It consists of lobules of mature, well-differentiated fat tissue. Sometimes sclerotic fibrous tissue predominates. Such tumors are referred to as fibrolipomas. Local excision is sufficient for this lesion.

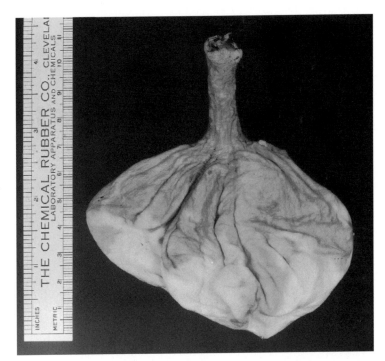

Figure 9–3. A pedunculated fibroma.

Atypical Lipoma and Liposarcoma

Nucci et al.[128] reported six cases of vulvar atypical lipoma in women aged 28 to 69 (median 52) years. Five tumors were located in the labia majora and one was in the clitoral region. Four tumors had the appearance of well-differentiated liposarcoma or atypical lipoma. The other two contained predominantly uniform spindle cells and round epithelioid cells arranged in loose bundles and mixed with lipocytes and lipoblasts. Abundant medium-sized blood vessels occurred in the stroma. Follow-up data were available on five women, including four with no recurrence following excision at 12, 14, 18, and 84 months. One incompletely excised tumor grew slowly over 10 years; this patient was free of disease at 31 months after re-excision.[128]

Hemangiomas may involve any area in the lower genital tract, and especially in the vulva. Several variants have been described.[66] The "strawberry" and cavernous variants are usually found at birth or during early infancy. They appear as raised, lobulated, bright red to purple nodules ranging in size from a few millimeters to several centimeters (Fig. 9–4). Extensive lesions may involve the vaginal wall. Some hemangiomas are known to regress spontaneously over several years.[66]

Hemangioma

The "strawberry" hemangioma consists of lobules of thin-walled, slightly dilated capillaries (Fig. 9–5). Larger feeding vessels are seen in the deep dermis. In young children, the proliferating endothelial cells tend to grow in solid, compact lobules with inconspicuous lumens.

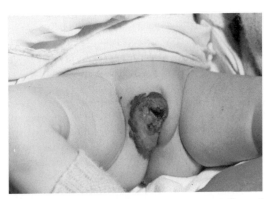

Figure 9–4. Capillary hemangioma presents as an elevated, dark red, well-circumscribed mass.

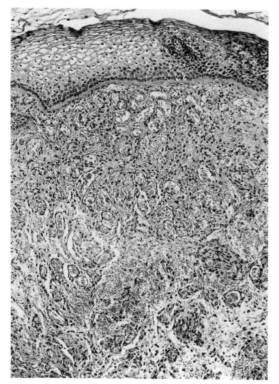

Figure 9–5. Capillary hemangioma consists of dilated capillaries underneath the squamous epithelium.

Occasional mitotic figures may be seen, but nuclear pleomorphism is absent. These hemangiomas are referred to as benign juvenile hemangioendotheliomas.

In cavernous hemangiomas, the vascular spaces are markedly distended. They are separated by septa lined by a layer of flattened endothelial cells and underlying fibrous stroma, which is sometimes hyalinized.

"Senile" hemangiomas are soft, dark, reddish-blue nodules, usually 2 to 3 mm in diameter that usually occur after menopause.[66] Histologically, numerous dilated capillaries are present in the superficial dermis.

Vascular malformations, such as arteriovenous (A-V) fistula, rarely occur in the vulva. An A-V fistula of the right hypogastric artery producing a pulsating swelling of the vagina and a bruit over the same side of the vulva was described by Barnett and Nickerson.[8] Organizing thrombi occur frequently in the hemangioma or vascular malformation. Some have the appearance of Masson's "vegetant intravascular hemangioendothelioma," consisting of villuslike fronds and irregular vascular channels. The plump endothelial cells may reveal mitotic figures. These thrombi should not be misinterpreted as angiosarcoma.

Angiokeratoma

Angiokeratoma of the vulva most often affects women in their reproductive years. In the early stages, it is small and cherry-red in color. Later, with an increase in size, it becomes blue or brown and warty or keratotic in appearance. As a result, it is sometimes mistaken for a nevus, wart, or malignant melanoma. In 50% of cases, the lesions are multiple. The size varies from 2 to 10 mm in diameter but is usually 5 mm. The labium majus is most often involved. The single most important predisposing factor is pregnancy, occurring in 50% of cases.[84] An increase in pelvic venous pressure, resulting from the descent of the fetus into the pelvic inlet is suggested as a possible mechanism. A few women develop angiokeratoma following hysterectomy.[84]

Histologically, the changes are characteristic with markedly dilated capillaries present in the papillary dermis. The overlying epidermis shows hyperkeratosis, parakeratosis, and acanthosis. Characteristically, elongated rete pegs are surrounded by vascular spaces (Fig. 9–6). Organizing thrombi are found in most cases. Local excision often results in cure. In the male, angiokeratoma occurs most often in the scrotum.

Granuloma Pyogenicum

Granuloma pyogenicum of the vulva is usually single, small, and red to brown. It may be sessile or pedunculated.[66] Microscopically, the dermis contains numerous capillaries that are often arranged in a lobular pattern. The endothelial cells are frequently swollen and prominent. Between the capillaries, the stroma is edematous and infiltrated by lymphocytes and plasma cells. The overlying epidermis is attenuated or ulcerated (Fig. 9–7). In the latter, neutrophils are seen in the stroma and the capillaries. There is no agreement as to whether this lesion represents a capillary hemangioma with epidermal ulceration or an exuberant granulation tissue secondary to epidermal ulceration. A similar oral lesion, the granuloma gravidarum, can occur in pregnant women.

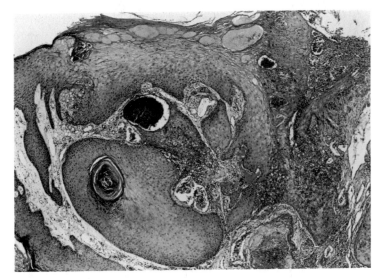

Figure 9–6. Angiokeratoma with surface hyperkeratosis, ulceration, bulky rete pegs, and dilated capillaries.

Lymphangioma and Lymphangiosarcoma

Two types of lymphangioma can occur in the vulvar region.[66] The more common lesion is the so-called lymphangioma simplex, or lymphangioma circumscriptum. Localized groups of small, thin-walled vesicles are present. Microscopically, irregular lymphatic spaces contain lymph or lymphocytes. The vessel wall consists of a layer of endothelium and smooth muscle cells of varying thickness. LaPolla et al.[103] described a patient who developed vulvar lymphangioma circumscriptum and lymphedema of the lower extremity following a radical hysterectomy, pelvic lymphadenectomy, and radiotherapy for cervical squamous carcinoma.

Less frequently, lymphangioma cavernosum causes diffuse swelling of the vulva. The perineum and vagina may be affected. Histologically, lymphatic spaces become cystically dilated. Rarely lymphangiomyomatosis may involve the lung, retroperitoneum, cervix, and pelvic organs. Huey et al.[82] reported a case of lymphangiosarcoma following radiotherapy for vulvar carcinoma.

Other Vascular Tumors

Hemangiopericytoma of the female genital tract usually arises from the uterus and the surrounding soft tissue. Involvement of the cervix,

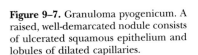

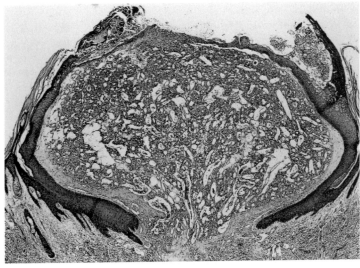

Figure 9–7. Granuloma pyogenicum. A raised, well-demarcated nodule consists of ulcerated squamous epithelium and lobules of dilated capillaries.

vagina, rectovaginal septum, and vulva has been reported.[20,46,80,147] The majority of these tumors are localized and behave in a benign fashion following a complete excision. Hemangiopericytomas associated with high cellularity and mitotic activity, hemorrhage, and necrosis may recur locally and metastasize to distant organs, especially to the lung and bone.[51] Reymond et al.[147] reported on a malignant hemangiopericytoma of the vulva that metastasized to the femur 14 years after the initial diagnosis. Hemangiopericytoma of the genital tract is particularly difficult to distinguish from endometrial stromal tumor. In such cases, analysis by special stains or electron microscopy is necessary.

Glomus tumors of the vulva and vagina associated with local pain and dyspareunia have been reported.[91,95,171] These tumors are firm, well circumscribed, and 1 to 4 cm in size. The uniformly polygonal tumor cells contain abundant eosinophilic cytoplasm. They proliferate around the capillaries and arterioles and sometimes merge with the smooth muscle cells. Perivascular stromal hyalinization may be prominent. Such a tumor may be confused with mixed tumor arising from the sweat gland or vestibular gland.

Angiolymphoid hyperplasia with eosinophilia or Kimura's disease may rarely involve the uterine cervix. Proliferation of medium-sized arteries occurs in the stroma, with marked lymphoid hyperplasia and eosinophilia. The endothelial cells are plump and active in appearance with occasional mitotic figures.

Angiosarcoma involving the vulva has rarely been reported.[40,111] An epithelioid variant of angiosarcoma may occur in the vulva. It is characterized by cords and clusters of cells containing cytoplasmic vacuoles and resembling angioblasts with incomplete luminal formation. It simulates a signet-ring carcinoma.[51] An origin from endothelial cells is supported by the presence of factor VIII by immunohistochemistry and Weibel-Palade bodies by electron microscopy.[51] A low-grade angiosarcoma recently designated as spindle cell hemangioendothelioma shares features of both a cavernous hemangioma and Kaposi's sarcoma.[194]

Aggressive Angiomyxoma

Steeper and Rosai[173] described a series of nine fibromyxomatous tumors that occurred in the vulva, perineum, and pelvis. The patients were young, in their third or fourth decade, and often presented with a labial mass, which was clinically thought to be a Bartholin's cyst. These tumors were usually larger than 10 cm (up to 60 cm) and sometimes extended into the pelvis, ischiorectal fossa, and retroperitoneum.

Fetsch et al.[54] reported on a series of 29 females ranging in age from 16 to 70 (median 34) years. The mass involved pelvis, perineum, vulva, buttock, retroperitoneum, and inguinal regions. The great majority of the tumors were greater than 10 cm in size. The clinical impressions included Bartholin's or vaginal cysts, labial cysts, inguinal or perineal hernia, and lipoma.

The tumors were smooth, lobulated, and partially or completely encapsulated externally and appeared glistening, gelatinous, and homogeneous on the cut surface. This gross appearance corresponded to abundant loose myxoid stroma. The stellate or bipolar-shaped tumor cells had uniform, small nuclei; dense finely granular chromatins; and small nucleoli. Mitotic figures were absent (Figs. 9–8 and 9–9). In a series by Fetsch et al.,[54] the mitotic activity varied from 0 to 4 mitotic figures per 50 high-power fields. In 70% of cases, there was no mitotic activity. No abnormal mitotic figures were found in any of the cases. Parts of the tumors contained randomly distributed blood vessels of varying sizes but lacked the arborizing vascular pattern typically seen in myxoid liposarcomas (see Figs. 9–8 and 9–9). The arteries often exhibited medial hypertrophy. Entrapped fat, small nerve fibers, and mucous glands were sometimes noted.[54]

Although these tumors and intramuscular myxoma share a basic population of bipolar, stellate-shaped cells, Steeper and Rosai[173] believe that these tumors differ from the intramuscular myxoma by having prominent vascular elements. The lack of lipoblasts and plexiform vascular pattern rules out liposarcoma. The absence of nuclear atypism and mitotic activity also rules out other types of sarcoma. Electron microscopic study confirms the presence of fibroblasts, myofibroblasts, capillaries, and pericytes. In a Begin et al. series,[10] the tumor cells have the ultrastructural characteristics of fibroblasts. By immunohistochemistry, the cells react with anti-actin but not with anti–S-100 protein, factor VIII, carcinoembryonic antigen, and keratin.[10] These observations rule out an origin from Schwann cells.

An immunohistochemical study by Fetsch et al.[54] demonstrated the following characteris-

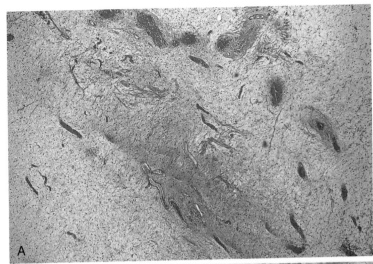

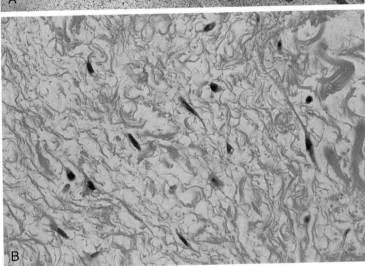

Figure 9–8. Aggressive angiomyxoma. *A,* Broad areas of myxoid stroma containing spindle cells and blood vessels. *B,* Characteristic bipolar spindle cells in a myxoid stroma.

tics: 100% of the tumors tested were positive for desmin and vimentin, 95% were positive for smooth muscle actin, 50% were positive for CD34, 93% were positive for estrogen receptor protein, and 90% were positive for progesterone receptor protein. All tumors were negative for S-100 protein. Ki-67 with antibody MIB1-positive cells were less than 1% in all tumors tested. These authors concluded that the tumor cells have some of the characteristics of fibroblasts and myofibroblasts. These findings help to exclude lipomatous and neurogenic tumors, which are expected to express S-100 protein. The positivity for estrogen and progesterone receptor proteins also raises the possibility of influence by the sex hormones.

Four of the nine women in Steeper and Rosai's[173] series developed local recurrence 21

months to 14 years after the initial excision. After re-excision, all patients were alive and well. The authors designated these tumors as aggressive angiomyxoma to emphasize the prominent vascular components and propensity for local recurrence. In a subsequent report, six of nine women developed recurrent tumor 9 to 84 months following incomplete excision.[10] In the series of Fetsch et al.,[54] 36% of women with follow-up had recurrent tumor from 10 months to 7 years after the initial treatment. None had developed metastasis or died of tumor.

Superficial Angiomyxoma

Fetsch et al.[55] reported on 17 cases of superficial, cutaneous angiomyxoma involving 13 fe-

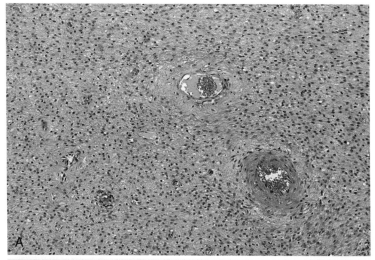

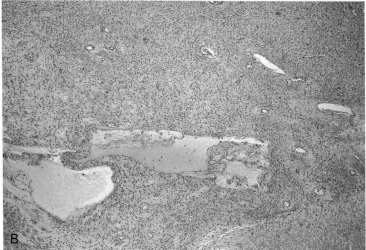

Figure 9–11. Angiomyofibroblastoma. *A,* Sheets of stromal cells and abundant blood vessels of varying thickness. *B,* Hypercellular zone intermixed with hypocellular cystic areas. *C,* Tumor cells have plump to elongated uniform nuclei. *D,* Tumor cells arranged in interlacing bundles with uniform palisaded nuclei and a moderate amount of eosinophilic cytoplasm. (See color section.)

ported by Neilsen et al.[126] An otherwise typical 13 cm angiomyofibroblastoma of the vulva in an 80-year-old woman contained areas of high-grade sarcoma resembling myxoid malignant fibrous histiocytoma. In the benign areas, stains for vimentin, smooth muscle actin, and desmin were positive, but the latter two were absent in the malignant foci. This tumor recurred 2 years following initial excision, and the patient was well 5 months after re-excision. The recurrent tumor was composed entirely of sarcoma with vascular invasion. In the presence of hemorrhage and necrosis, extensive sectioning for histologic examination is recommended to detect malignant foci.

Granter et al.[70] also reported on 13 cases with overlapping features of aggressive angiomyxoma and angiomyofibroblastoma.

Since the initial description of vulvar angiomyofibroblastoma by Fletcher et al.,[57] 52 similar tumors were described in the female vulvo-vaginal, in inguinal and cervical regions, and in the inguinal and scrotal areas of two males.[104]

Laskin et al.[104] reported on 11 tumors in the scrotum or inguinal region of males 39 to 88 (mean 57) years of age, involving superficial soft tissue and 2.5 to 14 cm in size. Vimentin, desmin, and smooth muscle actin were expressed in variable amounts. The authors suggest an origin from perivascular stromal cells.

Cellular Angiofibroma

Angiomyofibroblastoma should be distinguished from cellular angiofibroma of the

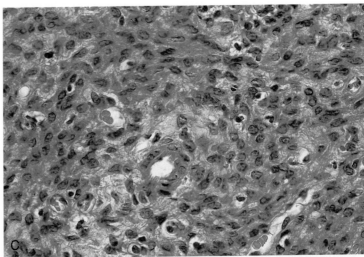

Figure 9–11. *Continued*

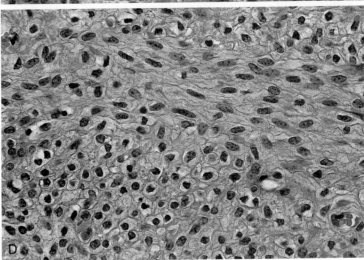

vulva, which was reported by Nucci et al.[127] The four angiofibromas were characterized by a small, well-delineated labial or Bartholin's gland mass of 1.2 to 2.5 cm in size, occurring in women aged 39 to 50 (mean 47) years.

The tumor is highly cellular and consists of two elements: uniform spindle cells and multiple thick-walled blood vessels with hyalinization. Small monotonous tumor cells have uniform nuclei and scant cytoplasm arranged in small bundles. Small aggregates of lipocytes occur in the periphery of the nodule. The stroma has a fibrous or myxoid appearance. There is some resemblance to spindle cell lipoma, but the cellularity is much greater. In addition, mitotic activity in some tumors is high; less than one, five, seven, and 11 mitotic figures per 10 high-power fields, respectively, were noted for

the four reported cases. The borders are usually smooth; however, they did appear irregular and infiltrative in one case. Follow-up data included two women without recurrence at 12 and 19 months, and two patients were lost to follow-up.

Tumor cells in cellular angiofibroma demonstrate vimentin, but not CD34 (positive in spindle cell lipoma), S-100 protein, actin, desmin, keratin, or epithelial membrane antigen (positive in perineurioma). These stains exclude the possibility of neurofibroma, perineurioma, and spindle cell lipoma. Cellular angiofibroma differs from aggressive angiomyxoma and angiomyofibroblastoma in its occurrence in older women, numerous blood vessels with hyalinization, high cellularity and mitotic activity, and negative expression of actin and desmin. For

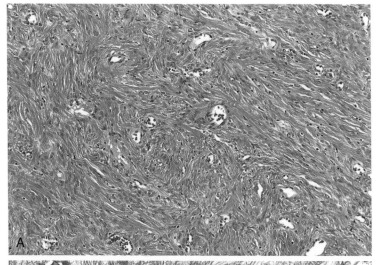

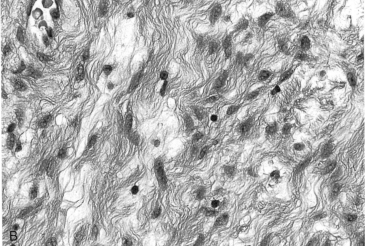

Figure 9–12. Angiomyofibroblastoma. *A*, Tumor with fibrous stroma. *B*, In these areas, the tumor cells have wavy nuclei.

these reasons, the authors recognize the tumor as a distinct entity.

Fibrous Histiocytoma, Dermatofibrosarcoma Protuberans, and Malignant Fibrous Histiocytoma

Included under the term *fibrous histiocytoma* is a spectrum of tumors and tumor-like lesions.[60] Histologically, fibrous and histiocytic elements exist in varying proportions. The fibrous element consists of fibroblasts arranged in a distinct pinwheel, storiform, or spiral nebular pattern, whereas the histiocytes are generally round or polygonal in shape and have finely vacuolated cytoplasm. Xanthomatous cells, multinucleated tumor giant cells, and Touton giant cells appear in varying numbers. Myxoid and inflammatory variants of malignant fibrous histiocytomas need special attention because of their possible confusion with myxoid liposarcoma, nodular fasciitis, and inflammatory pseudotumor.[101,191]

In tissue culture, histiocyte-like cells grow initially from the periphery of the explant, migrate in an ameboid fashion with multiple cell processes and lipid droplets, and subsequently transform into elongated fibroblast-like cells. Fibrohistiocytic tumors were thought to have originated from histiocytes, which act as "facultative fibroblasts."[134] Ultrastructural studies demonstrate that fibroblasts and histiocytes in different stages of differentiation intermingle with undifferentiated mesenchymal cells. In addition, between fibrous and histiocytic cells,

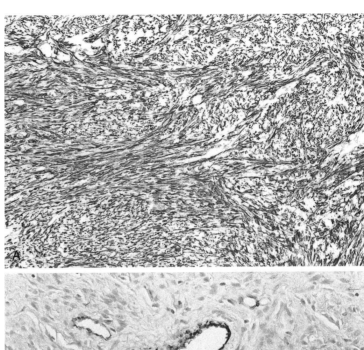

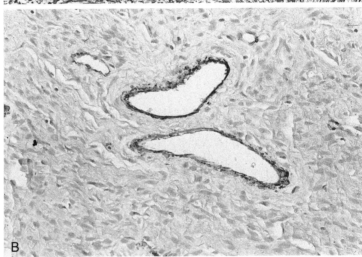

Figure 9–13. Angiomyofibroblastoma. *A,* Immunohistochemical stain for desmin is diffusely positive. *B,* Staining for smooth muscle actin is negative in the tumor cells but positive in the vessel wall. (See color section.)

intermediate cells are also noted. These observations led to the suggestion that undifferentiated stromal cells may differentiate into fibroblastic and histiocytic cells.[60]

Biologically, fibrous histiocytomas encompass the benign group of dermatofibroma, sclerosing hemangioma, and fibroxanthoma; the intermediate group of locally infiltrative but rarely metastatic category of dermatofibrosarcoma protuberans[4,16,170]; and the malignant group, which is capable of local and distant spread.[192]

The histologic appearance of these tumors in the lower genital tract is similar to that of tumors occurring elsewhere. In dermatofibrosarcoma protuberans, proliferating fibroblasts are arranged in a storiform pattern and infiltrate the adjacent fibroadipose by multiple cellular

processes (Fig. 9–14A). The nuclei are uniform in appearance and low in mitotic activity (see Fig. 9–14B). CD34 is uniformly positive (see Fig. 9–14C).

In a report of four cases of dermatofibrosarcoma protuberans of the vulva, one tumor contained areas of fibrosarcoma, which was highly cellular and comprised cells with plump nuclei arranged in a herringbone pattern.[68] Estrogen and progesterone receptor proteins were negative. CD34 was positive in all three tumors studied, including areas of fibrosarcoma.[68]

Ghorbani et al.[68] reviewed 22 cases reported in the literature, including their own four cases. The mean age of the patients was 47 years.[23–83] Tumors were 0.5 to 8.0 cm in size. Three tumors, in addition, had fibrosarcomatous areas in the initial excised specimen. The follow-up

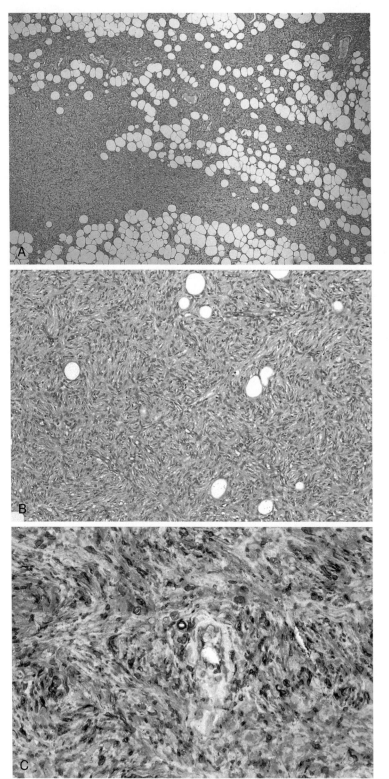

Figure 9–14. Dermatofibrosarcoma protuberans. *A*, Infiltration of adjacent adipose tissue by multiple processes is typical of this tumor. *B*, Tumor cells are arranged in a storiform pattern. *C*, Immunohistochemical stain for CD34 is diffusely positive. (See color section.)

information included that one tumor recurred 2 years later and one woman had no recurrence at 6 months; the third woman was lost to follow-up. Four other women had recurrence. One had positive margins in the initial excision, one had fibrosarcoma in the recurrent tumor, and one had hemivulvectomy with unknown status of excision margin. The fourth woman developed metastases in the lung and abdominal wall.

CD34 was positive in 15 of 33 fibrosarcomas that occurred within the dermatofibrosarcomas.[116] Whether the presence of fibrosarcoma worsened the prognosis remains controversial. A wide resection with clear margins is the treatment of choice.

A deeply seated dermatofibroma can be distinguished from dermatofibrosarcoma by its negative CD34 expression but positivity for factor XIIIa.[2] A positive S-100 protein also helps to exclude dermatofibroma in favor of Schwann cell tumors.

In general, the malignant potential of fibrohistiocytic tumors correlates with increasing depth, tumor size, nuclear pleomorphism, and mitotic activity (Fig. 9–15). Of the four patients with vulvar malignant fibrous histiocytomas, two were alive 5 and 19 months following surgery.[39] The third woman died of widespread disease 11 months after a radical vulvectomy, bilateral groin dissection, and pelvic lymphadenectomy.[76] Metastasis was found in an ipsilateral groin lymph node. The fourth woman was lost to follow-up.[179]

Malignant fibrous histiocytoma of the vagina has been reported.[190] The neoplasm was observed in the posterolateral aspect of the vaginal wall of a 31-year-old woman. Multiple nodules ranging from 0.5 to 2 cm in greatest diameter were present. The submucosal neoplasm was composed of spindle-shaped cells arranged in a poorly defined "cartwheel" pattern. This was associated with abundant collagen. In some areas, the tumor was described as having anaplastic cells associated with mitoses. After radical excision, the patient was free of disease 16 months later.

Pinkston and Sekine[141] reported a case of malignant fibrous histiocytoma that developed after radiotherapy for cervical cancer.

Epithelioid Sarcoma

Epithelioid sarcoma, a malignant tumor of the fascia and tendons, was described by Enzinger[50] in 1970. It typically presents as a slow-growing nodular lesion of the subcutis with multiple satellite nodules. Most of these tumors occur in the extremities of young adults in their third and fourth decades.

Epithelioid sarcoma of the vulva usually involves the labia majora of young adults and appears as a painless mass or Bartholin's cyst.[64,72,142,185] The initial pathologic diagnoses include poorly differentiated metastatic carcinoma, rhabdomyosarcoma, malignant fibrous histiocytoma, and angiosarcoma, attesting to the varied histologic features and the difficulty in determining a diagnosis. An adequate amount of tissue must be obtained for histologic diagnosis.

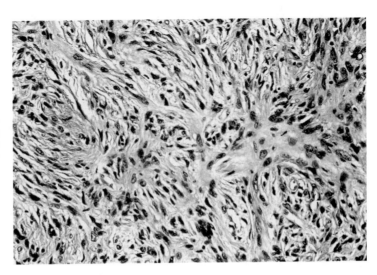

Figure 9–15. Malignant fibrous histiocytoma. The presence of fibroblastic cells arranged in a pinwheel, storiform pattern is a distinct feature of this neoplasm.

On low magnification, the tumor suggests a necrotizing granuloma or infectious process with a nodular or multinodular growth pattern and central necrosis. The predominant cells also resemble epithelioid macrophages in having a polygonal or spindle configuration and abundant eosinophilic cytoplasm (Fig. 9–16). However, the nuclear features are atypical, with prominent nucleoli and mitotic figures. More important, the tumor cells invade the fascia and tendons in a cord-like growth pattern. The overlying skin is sometimes ulcerated.

The histogenesis of this tumor is controversial. Ultrastructural studies have suggested a synovial,[61,136] histiocytic,[50] fibroblastic,[56] or uncertain origin.[14] Both synovial sarcoma and epithelioid sarcoma express cytokeratin, supporting their common origin.[25,51]

Epithelioid sarcoma has a high recurrence rate when inadequately treated. Prat et al.[144] found poor prognosticators to be local recurrence after excision, vascular invasion, and lymph node metastasis. Of their cases, 58% developed metastases, with 42% of these metastasizing to regional lymph nodes and 47% metastasizing to the lungs. The liver and the scalp were also frequent metastatic sites.[144]

Of the five patients with vulvar epithelioid sarcoma, four developed local recurrence and subsequently died of the metastatic disease. The importance of a complete resection was emphasized.[144]

Perrone et al.[138] described four cases of malignant vulvar tumor that share some of the features of epithelioid sarcoma and malignant rhabdoid tumor. One tumor was a typical epithelioid sarcoma. The other three poorly differentiated neoplasms contained tumor cells with eosinophilic cytoplasmic inclusions. All four tumors expressed vimentin, cytokeratin, and epithelial membrane antigen. Stains for desmin, S-100 protein, and gross cystic disease fluid protein-15 were all negative. Electron microscopic study of one tumor demonstrated whorled thick intermediate filaments.

The authors[138] concluded that the three tumors with cytoplasmic inclusions were malignant rhabdoid tumors, although two of them were previously reported as epithelioid sarcoma. Malignant rhabdoid tumor affects infants, adolescents, and young adults and is highly lethal.[118] It contains numerous rhabdoid cells and coagulative necrosis with random distribution. In contrast, epithelioid sarcoma affects young and middle-aged adults. It has nodules of necrotizing granulomas and an indolent clinical course. Rhabdoid cells are few in number.

Malignant Lymphoma

Malignant lymphoma may involve the genital tract, either as a primary tumor or, more frequently, as part of widespread disease.[26,143] The genital tract was involved in 40% of the women who died of malignant lymphoma.[154] Clinical presentation of a genital lymphoma does not differ from that of other, more common primary tumors. Once the diagnosis of lymphoma is established, patients are staged according to both the lymphoma and International Federa-

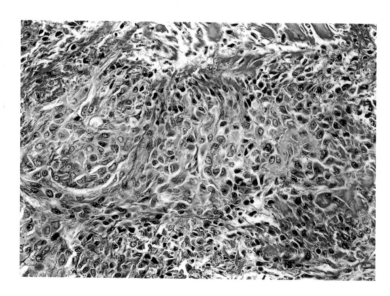

Figure 9–16. Epithelioid sarcoma. Polygonal cells, containing abundant densely eosinophilic cytoplasm, are arranged in solid epithelial sheets or bundles.

tion of Gynecology and Obstetrics (FIGO) criteria.

In 1974, Chorlton et al.[26] identified from the literature 36 cases of localized malignant lymphoma of the female genital tract, excluding the ovary. The most frequently affected site was the cervix (19 cases), followed by the vulva (seven), vagina (five), corpus uteri (four), and broad ligament (one). A similar distribution was also noted in a recent series.[74] Most patients were in their third to sixth decade of life and presented with vaginal bleeding or a palpable mass. The tumors varied in size from 1.7 to 6.0 cm, and some had a sessile or polypoid appearance. The surface was granular, reddened, and sometimes ulcerated.

Malignant lymphoma of the uterus affects women from 20 to 80 years of age, with a median age in the forties.[53] The majority of women are in their fourth or fifth decade of life. The most common symptom is vaginal bleeding. Other symptoms are vaginal discharge, dyspareunia, and pelvic pain. In many women, the cervical smears do not reflect the lymphoma, because the neoplasm is submucosal. Unless there is ulceration, lymphomatous cells are unlikely to appear in the cervical smears. In a literature review, about 10% to 40% of the cervical lymphomas had a positive smear.[53] Cervical lymphomas typically present as diffuse enlargement of the cervix in the form of "barrel-shaped cervix." Less frequently, polypoid nodules or a fungating mass is seen through the external os.[53]

Of the 21 uterine lymphomas described by Harris and Scully,[74] 67% were diffuse large cell type, 28% were follicular lymphomas, and 5% were Burkitt's lymphoma. Rare examples of Hodgkin's lymphomas in the cervix have also been reported. In the cervix, the lymphomatous cells occur beneath an intact cervical mucosa. Stromal fibrosis sometimes is a prominent feature. Lymphomatous cells are sometimes arranged in single file and sometimes are elongated in shape. Small lymphocytes and plasma cells occur in the periphery of the infiltrates.

Microscopic Features

Histologically, 70% to 80% of primary lymphomas of the lower genital tract are diffuse large cell or histiocytic non-Hodgkin's lymphomas. The remaining lesions are nodular or Burkitt's lymphomas.[74] Under low-power magnification, lymphoid infiltrates appear single or multinodular, but the borders are often smooth and pushing rather than infiltrative (Fig. 9–17). The mucosal surface, when included in the biopsy, is intact without ulceration and is separated from the lymphoid infiltration by a thin collagen zone (see Fig. 9–17).

The histologic diagnosis depends on the malignant character of the lymphoid cells and their deep local infiltration. The neoplastic cells are monomorphic, cytologically atypical, and mitotically active (Fig. 9–18). When follicles are present, their borders are ill defined and phagocytosis is absent. Infiltration of the stroma results in prominent fibrosis and Indian file pattern. In the cervix, endocervical glands become widely separated or destroyed.

Differential Diagnosis

A marked lymphoid hyperplasia may be associated with chronic cervicitis. The lymphoid hyperplasia may be nodular (chronic follicular cervicitis) or diffuse. The former contains multiple, discrete germinal centers with active phagocytosis (Fig. 9–19A). The mucosal surface is often ulcerated (Figs. 9–19B and 9–20A). The diffuse form consists of a polymorphic population of plasma cells, mature and immature lymphocytes, histiocytes, and eosinophils. Some of the lymphoid cells are immunoblasts with irregular nuclei and prominent nucleoli (see Fig. 9–20B and C). Clinically, the cervix may appear soft without induration, diffusely enlarged, or involved by tumor. The tissue in this self-limited disease returns to normal after appropriate antibiotic therapy.

Young et al.[194] reported 16 lymphoma-like lesions involving the cervix (10 cases), endometrium (five), and vulva (one). Most patients with a cervical lesion presented with vaginal discharge or bleeding, sometimes postcoital. One had a confirmed infectious mononucleosis. The cervix was described as eroded, ulcerated, nodular, friable, and enlarged. Rarely, the lesions presented as a large, exophytic tumor. The cervix appeared normal in three patients.

The lymphoid infiltrates were diffuse in six samples and mixed diffuse and nodular in three samples. The large lymphoid cells consisted of centroblasts and immunoblasts with active mitosis. More important, the infiltrates were polymorphic, band-like, and superficial, up to 3 mm in depth (see Fig. 9–20A). Mucosal ulceration was common. Stromal sclerosis and perivascular infiltrations were seldom seen. Marker studies by immunoperoxidase stains

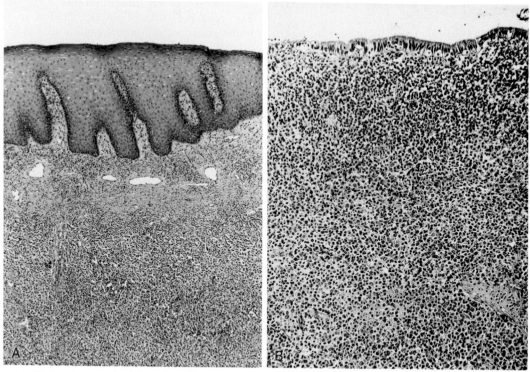

Figure 9–17. Malignant lymphoma. Intact squamous mucosa (*A*) and endocervical epithelium (*B*) are separated from the underlying diffuse lymphoid infiltrates by fibrous tissue. (*A*).

were polyclonal in all samples tested. Available follow-up data suggest a benign process.

Leukemic infiltration, especially granulocytic sarcoma, can be difficult to distinguish from lymphoma. It is important to apply chloracetate esterase stain or immunoperoxidase stain for lysozyme in suspected cases.

In the vulva, inflammatory and infectious diseases may be confused with lymphoma. Infectious mononucleosis has been reported to occur in the vulva, sometimes causing ulcers and sometimes associated with inguinal lymph node enlargement. The diffuse lymphoid infiltrates contain large lymphoid cells, including im-

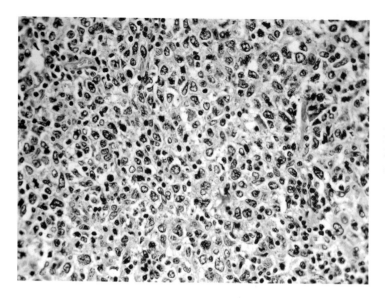

Figure 9–18. Malignant lymphoma. Large lymphoid cells with irregular, convoluted, pleomorphic nuclei mix with smaller, more mature lymphocytes.

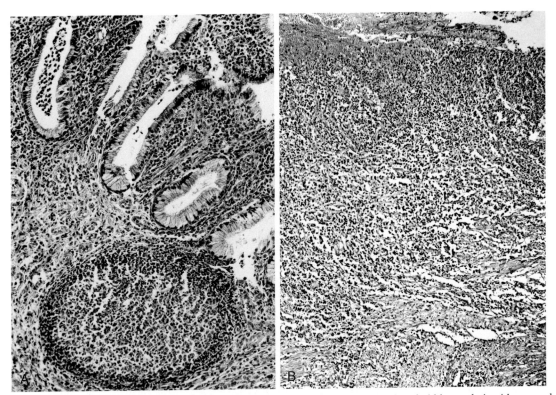

Figure 9–19. *A*, Chronic lymphoid cervicitis with reactive germinal centers. *B*, Benign lymphoid hyperplasia with mucosal ulceration and band-like, superficial infiltrates.

munoblasts with a starry-sky pattern. These immunoblasts are polyclonal by immunohistochemical studies. The lesions heal in 2 to 4 weeks, sometimes with residual scar and discoloration.[53]

Malignant lymphoma may be confused with small cell carcinoma of the cervix. In the latter, the malignant cells demonstrate a smooth nuclear configuration and coarse chromatin aggregates and lack a cleaved appearance. The presence of a nesting pattern and squamous differentiation supports an epithelial origin. With the advent of immunohistochemistry, it is possible to distinguish epithelial and lymphoid cells by using antisera against cytokeratin and common leukocyte antigen. Further study for B and T lymphocyte markers and their clonality is recommended for all possible lymphoid lesions.

Prognosis

Lymphomas of the female genital tract generally respond well to surgery, radiotherapy, and/or chemotherapy, with an overall 5-year survival rate of 73%.[74] When the tumor was localized in the cervix, approximately 90% of the patients survived 5 years or more.[74] When it extended to the lymph node or ovary, the chance of survival decreased to 20%. In general, the prognosis of uterine lymphoma is more favorable than that of ovarian lymphoma. This is attributed to the low clinical stage of the uterine lymphoma at the time of detection.

Granulocytic Sarcoma

Oliva et al.[133] reported on 11 women with granulocytic sarcoma, including ovary in seven, vagina in three, and cervix in one. The patients were ages 13 to 76 (mean 40) years. Diffuse sheets of leukemic cells may appear in cords and pseudoglandular spaces. Although some cells have myeloid differentiation, most cells are primitive. All those tested were positive for chloracetate esterase, lysozyme, and myeloperoxidase, CD68, and CD43.

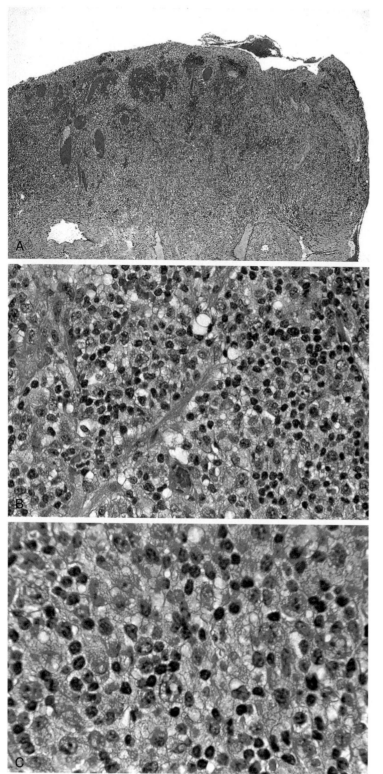

Figure 9–20. Diffuse form of pseudolymphoma of cervix. *A,* Beneath the ulcerated mucosa is a diffuse infiltration of lymphoid cells. The interface with the normal stroma is sharp without irregular infiltrative borders. *B* and *C,* Heterogeneous population of small and large lymphoid cells and histiocytes.

Plasmacytoma

Extramedullary plasma cell tumors are reported to account for 13% of the plasma cell disorders[52,59]; more than three quarters of these tumors occur in the upper airways. Primary plasmacytomas of the vagina are rare.[5,6,48,149] Vaginal tumors are usually isolated and multicentric. They are polypoid and firm and usually have a smooth or nodular surface. Some tumors are elevated above the level of the adjacent normal epithelium. Ulceration of the overlying mucosa may result in bleeding.

On histopathologic examination, there is a localized collection of plasma cells, which displaces the involved tissue. Compared with normal plasma cells, both the cells and their nuclei are enlarged. The "cartwheel" configuration of the nucleus is poorly defined, and multinucleation is common. Whereas multinucleation and macronucleoli are considered to be manifestations of malignant plasmacytomas by some authors,[149] others maintain that the degree of malignancy cannot be assessed by an evaluation of cellular features.[21]

Four of five women with vaginal plasmacytoma were alive and free of disease from 15 months to 4 years after treatment. In one case, cellular evidence provided the first indication of abnormality and also aided in detecting the recurrence. The patient ultimately developed bone involvement, which had not been observed in the previously reported cases of vaginal plasmacytoma within the limited periods of surveillance.[48]

Eosinophilic Granuloma, Langerhans' Histiocytosis

Eosinophilic granuloma, a low-grade histiocytic neoplasm, occurs in the bone, lung, skin, reticuloendothelial system, central nervous system, and other sites. It may be solitary or multifocal. Involvement of the genital tract has been reported. The lesions may involve the endometrium, cervix, vulva, or vagina.[197] Almost all patients presenting with vulvar lesions have disease elsewhere, especially at the base of skull and in bone, lungs, and skin. Diabetes insipidus is also common. The ages of the patients varied from 1.5 to 57 years, with most being between 20 and 50 years of age.[38,117,153]

Grossly, the lesions appeared as nodular, firm, and indurated masses. The vaginal lesions were described as dark brown and papular to ulcerative.[85] Histologically, the cellular infiltrates are polymorphic with a mixture of histiocytes, eosinophils, lymphocytes, plasma cells, and multinucleated giant cells. Histiocytes predominate in most cases and are characterized by eccentrically located, lobulated, irregular nuclei (Fig. 9–21). Nucleoli are prominent. The cytoplasm is abundant and eosinophilic or amphophilic. The cell borders are poorly defined. Eosinophils may be numerous in focal areas.

Ultrastructural studies of histiocytosis X, including eosinophilic granuloma, are helpful for diagnosis. Langerhans' granules are found in the cytoplasm of histiocytes. These are distended vesicles connected to short rods, giving

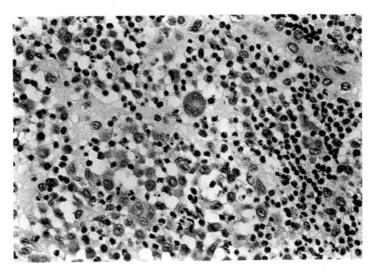

Figure 9–21. Eosinophilic granuloma. Mononuclear and multinucleated histiocytes have abundant cytoplasm and lobulated, irregular nuclei. They are mixed with lymphocytes, plasma cells, and eosinophils.

a tennis racket appearance. Cross bandings of regular periodicity are found within the rods. The presence of Langerhans' granules is one of the distinct features of histiocytosis X.[119]

In immunohistochemical studies, Langerhans' cells react with antisera against S-100 protein, leukocyte antigens, Leu-6 (Langerhans' cell/thymocyte antigen), and Leu-M3 (monocyte, dendritic cell antigen).[9]

Alveolar Soft Part Sarcoma

Alveolar soft part sarcoma was first described by Christopherson et al.[27] It usually originates from the connective tissues of the extremities or from bone. Kasai et al.[90] reported a neoplasm resembling alveolar soft part sarcoma that originated from the lateral vaginal wall near the introitus. The resected tumor measured 7.5 cm in greatest dimension and was circumscribed or encapsulated and firm, white, and covered by an intact vaginal mucosa. The neoplasm was characterized by an organoid pseudoalveolar arrangement of large, oval to polygonal cells with distinct cell boundaries. The cytoplasm contained periodic acid–Schiff (PAS)–positive diastase-resistant material, which, on ultramicroscopic examination, proved to be made up of secretory granules. The authors concluded that the neoplasm resembled an alveolar soft part sarcoma.

Shen et al.[162] described an alveolar soft part sarcoma in the labium majus of a 62-year-old woman. The mass was asymptomatic, mobile, and $4 \times 3 \times 3$ cm in size. At the time of the report, the patient had been free of recurrence 2 years following a radical vulvectomy and bilateral groin node dissection.

Nielsen et al.[124] reported nine cases of alveolar soft part sarcoma, including two in vagina, three in cervix, three in uterine corpus, and one in broad ligament. The patients were 14 to 38 (mean 29) years of age. One woman with vaginal tumor died of lung metastases 25 months after local excision, radiotherapy, and chemotherapy. All other eight women were alive and well from 9 months to 17 years.

Alveolar soft part sarcoma is characterized by loosely cohesive tumor cells, which are arranged in an alveolar, organoid pattern. The cytoplasm is abundant, eosinophilic, and granular. The finding of crystalline, rod-shaped cytoplasmic inclusions by PAS staining or electron microscopy establishes the diagnosis of alveolar soft part sarcoma. The cell of origin of this tumor remains to be determined.

The differential diagnosis of alveolar soft part sarcoma includes epithelioid smooth muscle tumor, rhabdomyosarcoma, granular cell tumor, clear cell adenocarcinoma, paraganglioma, metastatic renal cell carcinoma, and metastatic breast apocrine carcinoma. Immunohistochemical stains are useful and valuable in difficult cases.

When this tumor occurs in the soft tissue, its indolent but slowly aggressive course with a high frequency of lung metastasis through the vascular system is well documented.[162]

Of the 24 cases collected by Nielsen et al,[124] from the literature, one involved vulva, 10 cervix/lower uterine segment, six uterine corpus, and one broad ligament. Patients were aged 8 to 62 (mean 32) years. The tumor was 0.3 to 9.5 (mean 3.5) cm in size. One unique tumor contained melanin pigment.

One of six women with vaginal tumor died of metastasis. All eight women with cervical disease were alive and well from 9 months to 16 years, including one whose disease recurred twice, and one with microscopic metastasis in an obturator lymph node at initial treatment. It appears that the prognosis is better than that of lesions arising from the soft tissue.[124]

BENIGN AND MALIGNANT MÜLLERIAN MESODERMAL TUMORS

Müllerian-related tumors exist in pure or mixed form. The pure form consists of only one type of mesenchymal tissue, which may be homologous (endometrial stroma, smooth muscle) or heterologous (skeletal muscle, bone, cartilage). The mixed form contains more than one type of mesoderm or both epithelial and sarcomatous elements. These neoplasms are believed to arise from the multipotential cells of the müllerian duct.[187] They may be completely benign, highly malignant, or locally aggressive with low metastatic potential.

Leiomyoma and Leiomyosarcoma

Vulva

Smooth muscle tumors of the vulva may arise from the arrector pili muscle, the erectile tissue, or the insertions of the round ligament. Tavassoli and Norris[177] reported on a series of 32 benign and malignant smooth muscle tumors of the vulva. The ages of the patients varied from 18 to 66 years, with a median of 35 years. All the patients presented with a palpable mass, which was located in the labium majus in 14 patients, the area of Bartholin's gland in 11 patients, the clitoris in four patients, and the labium minus in three patients. The size of the tumors ranged from 1.4 to 7 cm. Only five tumors were greater than 5 cm in size. All the pregnant women experienced an increase in size of the tumor with progression of the pregnancy.[177]

Histologically, all but one of the tumors were composed of spindle-shaped cells arranged in interlacing bundles and whorls. The exception was an epithelioid variant.[177] A smooth muscle origin was recognized by the longitudinal fibrils demonstrable by trichrome stain, nuclear palisading, and clear halos around the cross-sectioned nuclei (Fig. 9–22).

Some degree of cellular atypia was found in 14 tumors (44%) (Fig. 9–23). The presence or absence of nuclear atypism did not correlate with mitotic activity or recurrence. The margins of the tumor were well circumscribed in 25 tumors, irregularly infiltrative in three tumors, and indeterminate in four tumors.

The size, margins, and mitotic activity were related to local recurrence.[177] Only two of 27 tumors less than 5 cm in size recurred, compared with two of five tumors greater than 5 cm. Of the tumors with less than five mitotic figures per 10 high-power fields, 8% recurred, in contrast to one of six tumors with greater than five mitotic figures per 10 high-power fields. Only two of 25 tumors with well-circumscribed borders recurred, compared

with two of three tumors with infiltrative borders. However, the authors concluded that no single morphologic criterion is completely reliable in the prediction of recurrence.[177] In the absence of local infiltration or distant metastasis, smooth muscle tumors that are greater than 5 cm in size or that have more than five mitotic figures per 10 high-power fields are likely to recur locally.[177]

Of the 25 cases of vulvar smooth muscle tumors reported by Nielsen et al.,[125] 19 had follow-up of more than a month (mean 58 months). Tumors that meet at least three of the following four criteria are classified as leiomyosarcoma: 5 cm or more in dimension, five or more mitotic figures per 10 high-power fields, infiltrative borders, and moderate or severe nuclear atypia. Tumors having one of the above features are designated as leiomyoma, and those having any of the two criteria are diagnosed as atypical leiomyoma.[125]

Of the four women with leiomyosarcoma, two recurred at 3 months and 4 months, and both were free of disease at 3 years following modified radical vulvectomy and wide excision. The third woman died of tumor at 7 months, with metastatic disease in the lung and bone. The fourth woman was free of disease 2.5 years following modified radical vulvectomy and radiotherapy.[125]

Only one of 15 atypical leiomyomas and benign leiomyomas recurred. It recurred 10 years after initial excision, and the patient was free of disease for 2.5 years following re-excision.[125]

Other reported leiomyosarcomas of the vulva all had more than 10 mitotic figures per 10

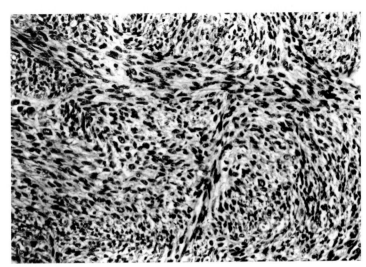

Figure 9–22. Leiomyoma. High-power view showing bundles of smooth muscle cells cut at varying planes. Longitudinal cuts along the nuclear long axis often reveal nuclear palisading, whereas perinuclear halo is apparent in cross sections.

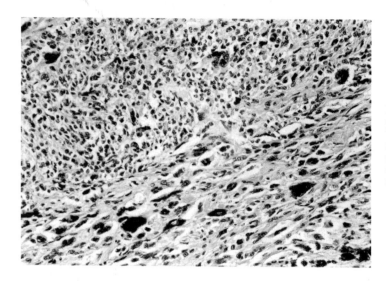

Figure 9–23. A moderate degree of nuclear atypia occurs in this leiomyoma. The affected nuclei are hyperchromatic, irregular, and multinucleated. Nucleoli are inconspicuous, and mitotic figures are less than one per 10 high-power fields.

high-power fields, including abnormal forms.[40] They are relatively slow growing and tend to recur locally (five of 10 cases). Metastases to distant organs developed in five of 10 cases (two to the lung, one to the liver, and two widely disseminated).[40,47]

Nielsen et al.[125] reviewed 36 vulvar leiomyosarcomas reported in the literature. Of these, 11 metastasized. Those that metastasized ranged from 3 to 15 (mean 9) cm in size, as compared with 4 to 15 (mean 6) cm for nonmetastatic tumors. Characteristically, distant metastasis was preceded by one more local recurrence, lung being the most common site. None metastasized to the regional lymph nodes.

Vagina

Smooth muscle tumors are reported to be the most common mesenchymal tumors identified in the vagina of adult women.[92] Their gross appearance is variable depending on the extent of hyalinization, the degree of cellularity, and the presence of necrosis or edema. Most neoplasms are isolated and well circumscribed, and only a few appear as irregular nodules or have an adjacent smaller satellite nodule.

Of the 60 vaginal smooth muscle tumors reported by Tavassoli and Norris,[176] 35 had no evidence of mitosis, whereas mitoses were identified in the remaining 25 tumors. In only seven neoplasms, the number of mitotic figures was greater than five per 10 high-power fields. Degenerative changes were common. Hyalinization was observed in almost half the neoplasms. Edema, hemorrhage, and focal necrosis were

less frequent. A myxoid change was observed in six tumors.

Five tumors recurred following local excision, and all of these had more than five mitoses per 10 high-power fields. Four of the five cases had moderate to marked atypia. All neoplasms were greater than 3 cm in greatest dimension.[176] Four women with recurrent tumors were alive without disease after re-excision.[176] One neoplasm recurred during pregnancy on three occasions within a 3-year period. This tumor enlarged during pregnancy and became smaller after parturition. Other tumors were also observed to grow during pregnancy.[176] The fifth woman with tumor recurrence died of pulmonary metastasis 10 months after the initial diagnosis. This neoplasm was ulcerated, infiltrative, and mitotically active (16 mitoses in 10 high-power fields).

Other authors have also reported vaginal leiomyosarcomas.[39,113,160,182] There is no predilection as to the site of origin. The neoplasms may present as a small or bulky, firm mass with circumscribed or infiltrative borders. The neoplasms are not encapsulated. There is considerable variation in their gross appearance.[39,113,182] Histopathologic examination demonstrates that the tumors are composed of interlacing bundles of cells with elongated, round-ended nuclei. The cytoplasm is acidophilic and contains myofibrils.

Mitotic activity and nuclear abnormalities are more common in recurrent tumors (Figs. 9–24 and 9–25). It is proposed that vaginal smooth muscle tumors having more than five mitoses per 10 high-power fields and moderate or

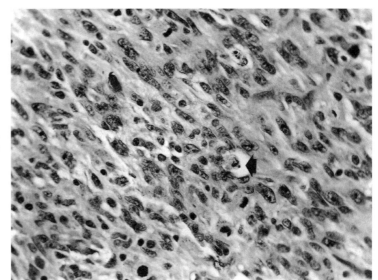

Figure 9–24. Vaginal leiomyosarcoma with bizarre cells and atypical mitoses (*arrow*).

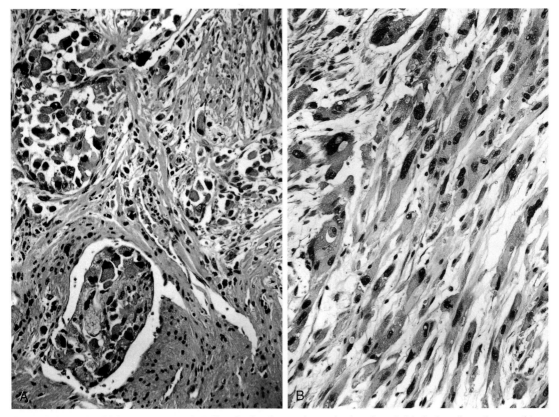

Figure 9–25. Vaginal leiomyosarcoma. *A,* Infiltrative borders and vascular invasion. *B,* Marked nuclear pleomorphism.

marked cellular atypia be designated as leiomyosarcoma.[182]

In dealing with smooth muscle neoplasms, adequate sampling is essential. A minimum of one block is recommended for each 2 cm of tumor diameter; some authors prefer one block per centimeter of tumor.[176]

Cervix

Leiomyoma of the cervix may be submucosal, pedunculated, or intramural, causing diffuse enlargement of the cervix. Its histologic appearance is similar to that of leiomyoma of the vagina and vulva.

Among 661 consecutive total hysterectomy specimens, 427 (64.6%) leiomyomas were found in the uterine wall and only four (0.6%) involved the cervix. In only two cases was this finding considered to be of clinical significance; both had multiple leiomyomas of the uterus. In other cases, the tumor size was less than 10 mm.[180]

Leiomyosarcoma of the cervix affects women in their fifth to seventh decade of life. They present with vaginal bleeding and large polypoid masses replacing the cervix. Histologically, the neoplastic cells demonstrate varying degrees of nuclear atypism. Of the eight cases reported by Abell and Ramirez,[1] all had more than 10 mitotic figures per 10 high-power fields. Rarely, the tumor cells contained abundant lipid in the cytoplasm, simulating xanthomatous cells.[71]

After surgery or radiotherapy, six of the eight patients were dead of their disease. The remaining two were free of disease 6 and 10 years following surgery.[1]

Rhabdomyoma

Rhabdomyomas are divided into adult type and fetal type. In the female genital tract, rhabdomyomas occur mainly in the vagina in the form of fetal type.[42,45,54,62,69,108,124] The mean age at detection was 45.3 years, the youngest patient being 34 years and the oldest being 56 years. The tumors may arise from the anterior or posterior vaginal wall and have a polypoid appearance or may present as nodular growths ranging from 1 to 11 cm in greatest dimension.

The stratified squamous epithelium overlying the neoplasm is usually intact. Beneath the epithelium is a loose connective tissue stroma composed of plump stellate or spindle-shaped cells with oval nuclei (Fig. 9–26A and B). Scattered in the stroma are bundles of large strap-shaped or aggregates of racket-shaped cells with abundant acidophilic cytoplasm. The nuclei are centrally or eccentrically located and may have prominent nucleoli (Fig. 9–27A and B). Mitoses are not identified. Within the acidophilic cytoplasm, there are often discernible fibers with evidence of cross striations. The tumor cells are separated one from another by loose collagenous connective tissue and thin-walled vascular spaces. The tumors are circumscribed but not encapsulated.

Under electron microscopic study, the tumor cells closely resemble mature striated muscle. Myofilaments join several Z bands together in succession, forming repeated sarcometric units with transverse rows of Z bands accounting for the cross striations. I bands are identified as light areas surrounding the Z bands. Between successive I bands are electron-dense areas corresponding to A bands. H bands are not readily identified.[69,108]

Rhabdomyosarcoma

Rhabdomyosarcoma is the most common malignant tumor involving the urogenital tract of infants and children. In females, it occurs more frequently in the vagina and cervix and less often in the vulva and urinary bladder.[34,35] The majority of rhabdomyosarcomas of the female genital tract, like those occurring in the mucosa-lined cavitary organs, appear as multiple grape-like growths of so-called sarcoma botryoides (see Fig. 9–19). This is believed to be a variant of embryonal rhabdomyosarcoma with a distinct gross and microscopic appearance and location. The alveolar variants typically occur in the vulva and perineum of patients between 13 and 20 years of age.[35]

Clinical Features

Rhabdomyosarcoma of the vulva presents as a mass or cyst in the labium majus, the fourchette, or the perineum. Most patients are younger than 20 years of age.[34,35,47,130,174] Rhabdomyosarcoma of the vagina is similarly a disease of infants and young children.[78] Among 58 reported cases,[78] 85% to 90% occurred in females younger than 5 years, and two thirds were detected during the first 2 years of life. In

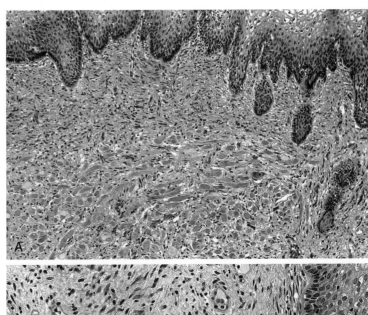

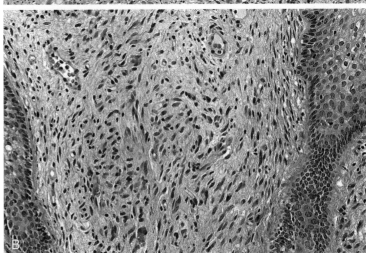

Figure 9–26. Vaginal rhabdomyoma. *A,* Beneath the intact squamous mucosa is a cellular fibrous stroma and mature skeletal muscle cells. *B,* Higher magnification of uniform fibroblasts.

some cases, the tumor was found at birth.[129,131] Only four cases appeared after the onset of puberty. The mean patient age in the reported cases was 38.3 months. The oldest patient, aged 41 years, previously had enucleation of both eyes for retinoblastoma in early life.[109]

The presenting symptoms are vaginal mass and/or vaginal bleeding in 83% of the reported cases. A vaginal mass without bleeding is the most common and main complaint.[78] Symptoms related to the urinary tract and lower bowel were caused by extravaginal spread and advanced tumor.

In sarcoma botryoides, the tumor appears as 2 to 3 mm papillae or small nodules arising from a hypertrophic vaginal mucosa. With time, the tumor becomes pedunculated or produces sessile polyp-like masses up to 3 to 4 cm in diameter (Figs. 9–28 and 9–29). The individual polypoid mass has a shiny, white, translucent, edematous, or myxomatous appearance. Less frequently, it is large, solitary, smooth-surfaced, and sometimes cystic.

Initially, the tumor grows in an expansile fashion, filling the vagina. Later, the tumor may protrude from the vagina or involve the labia minora, cervix, bladder, and pelvic organs.

Most rhabdomyosarcomas of the vagina arise from the anterior wall. The site of origin is related to the mode of spread and future course. With involvement of the anterior wall, the lesion is likely to extend to the vesicovaginal septum and posterior bladder wall. A posterior wall tumor generally spreads to the rectovaginal septum and, rarely, into the rectum. Extension into the pelvic organs often leads to ascites and abdominal enlargement. Enlargement of inguinal lymph nodes

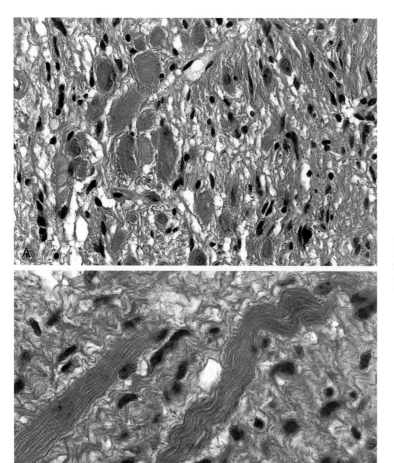

Figure 9–27. Vaginal rhabdomyoma. *A,* Racket-shaped rhabdomyocytes with abundant eosinophilic cytoplasm. *B,* Elongated mature rhabdomyocytes with cross striations.

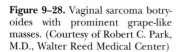

Figure 9–28. Vaginal sarcoma botryoides with prominent grape-like masses. (Courtesy of Robert C. Park, M.D., Walter Reed Medical Center)

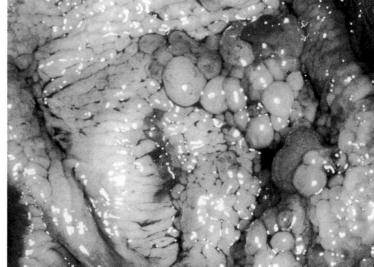

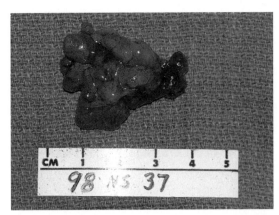

Figure 9–29. Locally excised cervical sarcoma botryoides consisting of multiple polypoid nodules, some of which have a grayish edematous appearance.

secondary to metastasis occurs with some frequency.

Embryonal rhabdomyosarcoma of the cervix, in most cases, has a multinodular, polypoid, glistening, and gelatinous appearance (Fig. 9–30).

Microscopic Features

Sarcoma botryoides demonstrates three zones, each made up of distinct cellular elements (Figs. 9–31A and 9–32). Immediately beneath the squamous mucosa is a highly cellular layer of undifferentiated spindle or round cells and rhabdomyoblasts. This is the so-called cambium layer. When present, it is helpful in making the diagnosis. Cross striations are often found in the rhabdomyoblasts of the cambium layer.

Beneath the cambium layer is a central, relatively acellular myxoid stroma made up of spindle and stellate-shaped cells whose nuclei may not appear anaplastic (Fig. 9–31B). Myxoid degeneration and microcystic formation of the stroma sometimes predominate in the biopsy specimen.

In the third zone, the tumor cells are similar to those of ordinary embryonal rhabdomyosarcomas (Fig. 9–31C). Islands of mature hyaline cartilage occur in some embryonal rhabdomyosarcomas (Fig. 9–31D).[75,109] Of the 13 cases of cervical sarcoma botryoides, 45% of the tumors contained mature cartilage.[41]

Embryonal rhabdomyosarcoma consists of primitive mesenchymal cells and rhabdomyoblasts. Rhabdomyoblasts have abundant, dense, eosinophilic cytoplasm and are round or racket- or strap-shaped. Immunohistochemical stains for actin, desmin, and myoglobin readily identify these cells (Figs. 9–32 and 9–33). The undifferentiated cells are round or spindle-

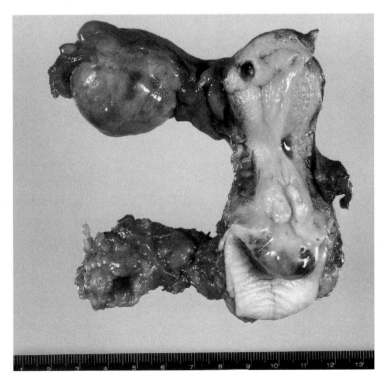

Figure 9–30. Radical hysterectomy for embryonal rhabdomyosarcoma of the cervix presenting as a bulging mass with a smooth, glistening, hemorrhagic surface.

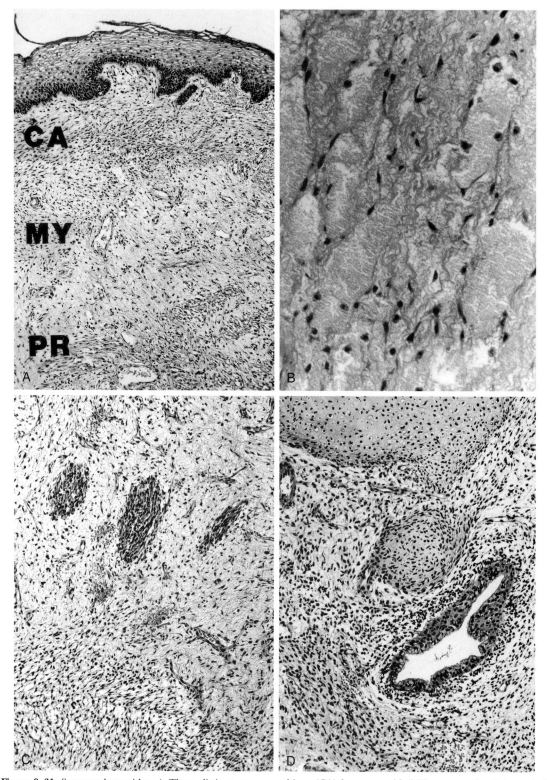

Figure 9–31. Sarcoma botryoides. *A,* Three distinct zones: cambium (CA) layer, myxoid (MY) zone, and cellular, primitive (PR) tissue. *B,* The myxoid zone may simulate a benign tissue because of the hypocellularity, microcystic spaces, and lack of nuclear atypism. *C,* In the third zone, the cellular elements resemble ordinary embryonal rhabdomyosarcoma consisting of primitive spindle cells and rhabdomyoblasts. *D,* Islands of mature hyaline cartilage.

Figure 9–11. Angiomyofibroblastoma. *A,* Sheets of stromal cells and abundant blood vessels of varying thickness. *B,* Hypercellular zone intermixed with hypocellular cystic areas. *C,* Tumor cells have plump to elongated uniform nuclei. *D,* Tumor cells arranged in interlacing bundles with uniform palisaded nuclei and a moderate amount of eosinophilic cytoplasm. *Illustration continued on following page*

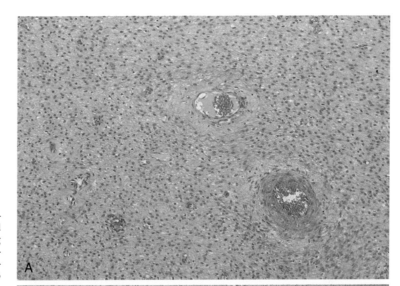

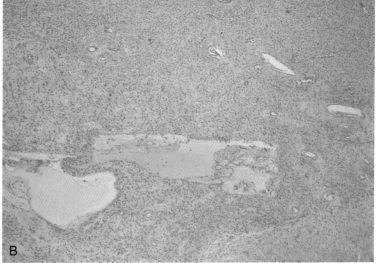

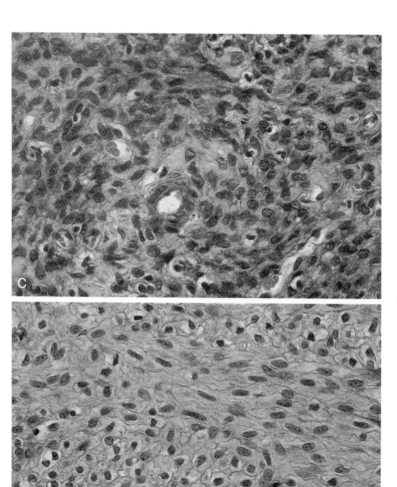

Figure 9–11. *Continued*

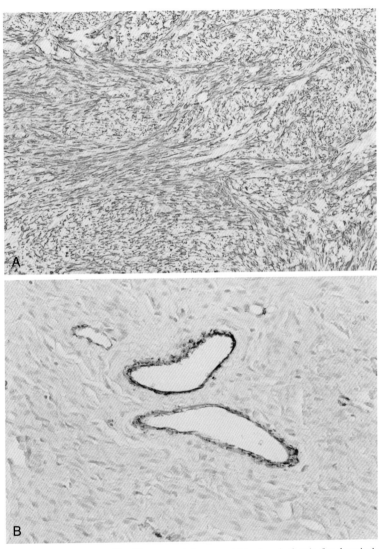

Figure 9–13. Angiomyofibroblastoma. *A*, Immunohistochemical stain for desmin is diffusely positive. *B*, Staining for smooth muscle actin is negative in the tumor cells but positive in the vessel wall.

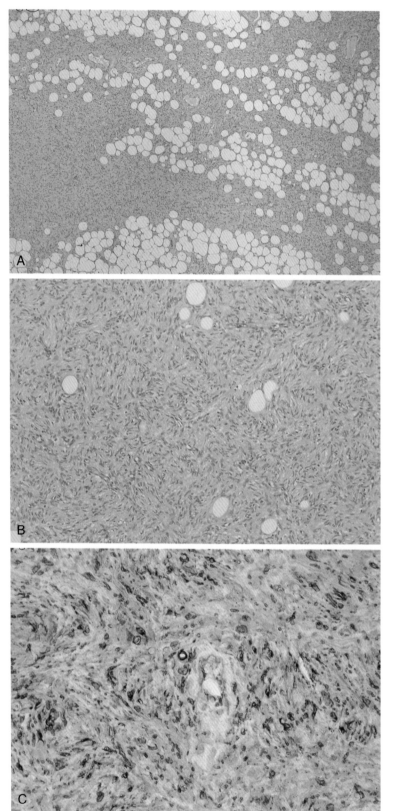

Figure 9–14. Dermatofibrosarcoma protuberans. *A,* Infiltration of adjacent adipose tissue by multiple processes is typical of this tumor. *B,* Tumor cells are arranged in a storiform pattern. *C,* Immunohistochemical stain for CD34 is diffusely positive.

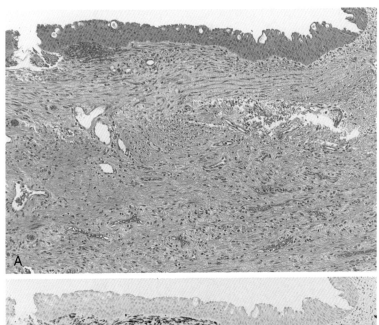

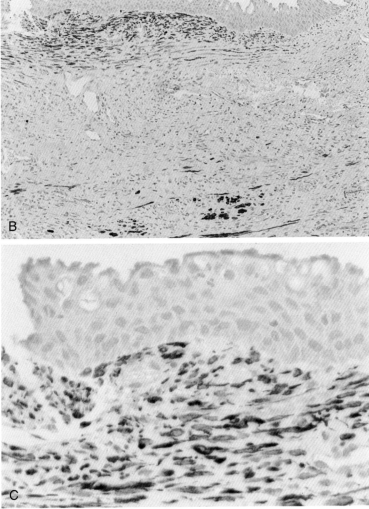

Figure 9–32. Sarcoma botryoides. *A,* Low-power view with three distinct zones: hypercellular cambium layer beneath the squamous mucosa, hypocellular zone in the middle, followed by cellular embryonal tissue. *B,* Immunohistochemical stain for myoglobin demonstrates rhabdomyoblasts in the cambium layer and deeper embryonal tissue. *C,* Higher magnification of rhabdomyoblasts in the cambium layer.

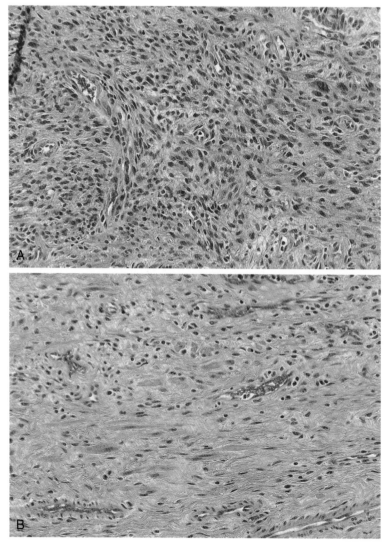

Figure 9–33. Embryonal rhabdomyosarcoma. *A,* Highly cellular primitive tissue with atypical cells in the right field. *B,* Round to oval to elongated cells suggestive of muscle differentiation. *C,* Immunohistochemical stain of myoglobin in area comparable to *B* confirms rhabdomyoblastic differentiation.

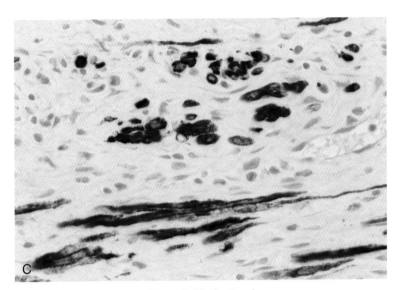

Figure 9–33. *Continued*

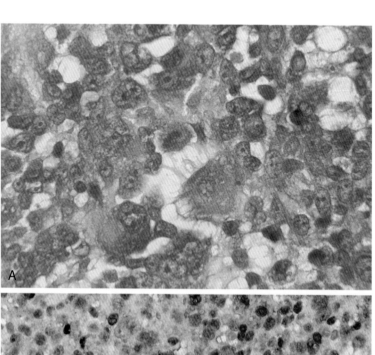
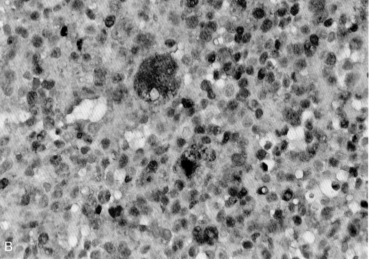

Figure 9–52. Malignant melanoma of vagina. *A*, Highly pleomorphic cells with some resemblance to rhabdomyoblasts. *B*, Immunohistochemical stain for S-100 protein is strongly positive and supports malignant melanoma.

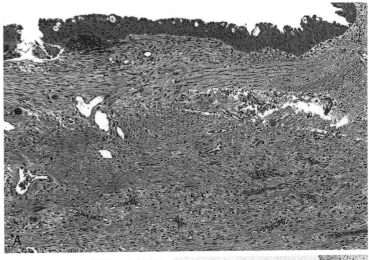

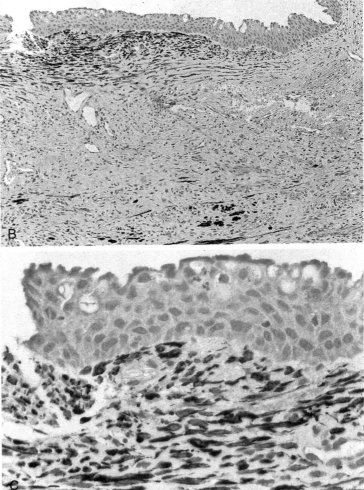

Figure 9–32. Sarcoma botryoides. *A,* Low-power view with three distinct zones: hypercellular cambium layer beneath the squamous mucosa, hypocellular zone in the middle, followed by cellular embryonal tissue. *B,* Immunohistochemical stain for myoglobin demonstrates rhabdomyoblasts in the cambium layer and deeper embryonal tissue. *C,* Higher magnification of rhabdomyoblasts in the cambium layer. (See color section.)

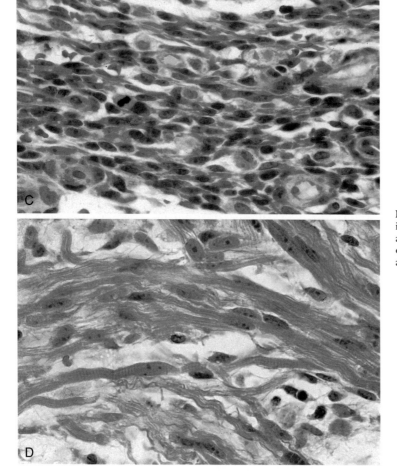

Figure 9–34. *Continued C,* Elongated immature cells with increased mitotic activity. *D,* Elongated rhabdomyoblasts with eosinophilic cytoplasm and cross striations.

aments, which are found in a variety of mesenchymal cells and therefore are not specific for rhabdomyoblasts. In better-differentiated cells, myofibrils consisting of thin (60 to 80 Å, actin) and thick (120 to 250 Å, myosin) filaments are present. With further polymerization of myofibrils, Z, I, H, and M bands in the order of development are found. The presence of actin and myosin filaments as an organized unit of myofibrils is the earliest identifiable rhabdomyoblastic differentiation.

In a review of 44 rhabdomyosarcomas studied with electron microscopy, six had cross striations visible by light microscopy, and 18 (41%) had demonstrable thin and thick filaments by electron microscopy. The remaining rhabdomyosarcomas demonstrated only thin actin filaments.[120] The lack of rhabdomyoblastic differentiation by electron microscopy can be at-

tributed to a sampling error or an inherent lack of differentiation of the tumor cells. Although ultrastructural studies confirm only 41% (18 of 44) of rhabdomyosarcomas, the ultrastructural features nonetheless help to rule out neoplasms such as undifferentiated carcinoma, malignant lymphoma, and Ewing's sarcoma.

Immunoperoxidase stain for intracellular myoglobin is useful for demonstrating immature rhabdomyoblasts, which lack cross striations or are few in number in the hematoxylin-eosin–stained sections.[123] In a series of 17 rhabdomyosarcomas, 13 (76%) were positive for myoglobin, including five of five embryonal type, five of seven alveolar type, and three of five pleomorphic type.[36] The presence of myoglobin is diagnostic for skeletal muscle differentiation. Actin and desmin are also useful in the confirmation of smooth or skeletal muscle origin.

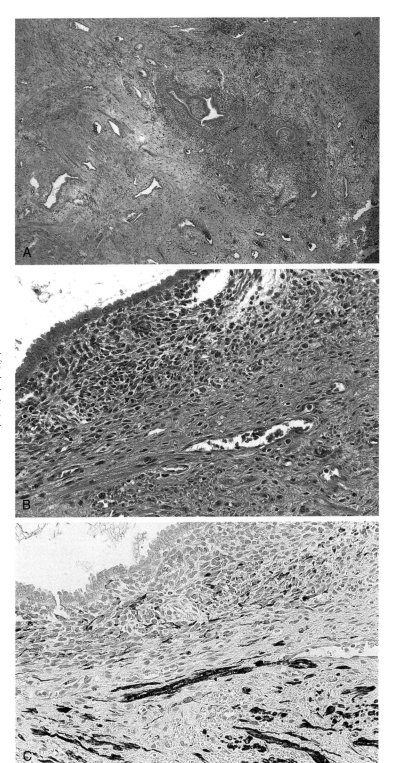

Figure 9–35. Cervical embryonal rhabdomyosarcoma. *A,* Low-power view of hypercellular zone around the endocervical glands. *B,* Higher magnification of *A* illustrates cellular primitive cells and adjacent rhabdomyoblasts. *C,* Immunohistochemical stain for myoglobin highlights rhabdomyoblasts.

Differential Diagnosis

In dealing with a polypoid lesion of the genital tract in infants, children, and young adults, the possibility of rhabdomyosarcoma should always be kept in mind. Benign polyps and neurogenic tumors usually enter into consideration because of the polypoid configuration and myxoid stroma. The stromal cells of these benign changes, although they may exhibit nuclear atypism, lack a hypercellular zone beneath the mucosa, the cambium layer.

Prognosis

The prognosis of rhabdomyosarcoma is generally poor owing to frequent pelvic recurrence or metastases. Metastases are most likely to occur in the inguinal lymph nodes and lungs, and they occur less frequently in bone. Surgical resection and additional chemotherapy seem to provide some hope for long-term survival in early cases. With combined therapy, the 5-year survival rate is 25% or better.[34,35]

In a literature review of the cases of 13 women with cervical sarcoma botyroides,[41] one patient died of the tumor 1 year after total abdominal hysterectomy and chemotherapy. The other 12 women were alive and well for 1 to 8 (mean 3.5) years.[41] Most of the patients had total abdominal hysterectomy, pelvic nodal dissection, and chemotherapy. However, a few patients had only polypectomy and were free of disease for 5 years. In correlating various pathologic parameters with the prognosis, only deep myometrial invasion of the cervical wall was associated with fatal outcome. The tumor size, presence or absence of a stalk, level of mitotic activity, degree of nuclear atypia, and presence or absence of cartilage were not associated with prognosis in this group. The authors pointed out that vaginal sarcoma botryoides, in contrast, has a poor prognosis.[41]

Stromal Sarcoma

Vagina

Endometrial stromal sarcoma was reported in the vagina to be associated with endometriosis of the vagina.[12,39] In a case reported by Ulbright and Kraus,[184] the vaginal tumor had a dense, fibrous stroma containing islands of endometrial stroma–like cells. The endometrial stroma–like cells involved vascular spaces. Mitotic activity was low at less than one mitotic figure per 10 high-

power fields. There was focal cellular pleomorphism. Otherwise, the lesion resembled well-differentiated endometrial stromal sarcoma.

Cervix

Cervical stromal sarcoma is a homologous sarcoma derived from the substantia propria of the cervix. Abell and Ramirez[1] reported on 12 cases, all but one of which occurred in perimenopausal or postmenopausal women. All of these women presented with abnormal vaginal bleeding. Under examination, all but one had space-occupying masses, most of which were polypoid. The other women presented with an indurated ulcer. The sarcomatous cells were predominantly stellate and, less frequently, spindle-shaped. The cytoplasm had an angular, reticular appearance. The nuclei were hyperchromatic, large, and relatively uniform. The number of mitotic figures exceeded 10 per 10 high-power fields in all cases. Stromal edema was marked in focal areas, resulting in compact, hypercellular islands surrounded by less cellular myxoid tissue. The endocervical glands were compressed by rather than destroyed by neoplastic cells.

Prognosis is closely related to the degree of differentiation. Neoplasms that were well differentiated and superficially located had a better prognosis. All patients with poorly differentiated tumors died 2 to 24 months following diagnosis. Well-differentiated neoplasm should be distinguished from cervical polyps and papillary adenofibroma. Appropriate immunohistochemical stains should be used to distinguish poorly differentiated neoplasm from large cell and anaplastic lymphomas, rhabdomyosarcoma, and small cell carcinoma.

Mixed Mesodermal Tumors

Most mixed mesodermal tumors occur in the uterine corpus and rarely in the cervix, fallopian tube, ovary, or pelvis. Based on a spectrum of morphology and clinical behavior, four categories have been recognized: (1) müllerian adenofibroma, (2) adenomyoma and atypical polypoid adenomyoma, (3) müllerian adenosarcoma, and (4) malignant mixed mesodermal sarcoma.

Müllerian Adenofibroma

The adenofibroma consists of benign epithelium and stroma in a papillary pattern. It is well demarcated from the adjacent tissue, without evidence of invasion (Figs. 9–36 and 9–37). The lining epithelium is usually of the endometrial or endocervical type. The stroma, depending on the site of origin, may contain fibroblasts, endometrial stromal cells, smooth muscle, or a mixture of any of these. The cellularity is generally mild to moderate, with a tendency to become more cellular adjacent to the gland or the surface epithelium. The mitotic activity of the stromal cells is low, at usually less than three mitotic figures per 10 high-power fields (see Fig. 9–37).[196]

Adenomyoma and Atypical Polypoid Adenomyoma

Adenomyoma of the lower genital tract is rare. Both the endocervical type and the usual type of adenomyoma have been reported in the cervix. Gilks et al.[68a,68b] reported 10 cases of endocervical type and three examples of the usual type of adenomyoma in the cervix. In the endocervical type, eight lesions appeared as a polypoid mass projecting into the cervical canal and varied from 1.3 to 8.0 cm in size. The other two tumors originated from the deep cervical stroma and extended into the pelvis; they measured 11 and 23 cm in size.

Most of the glands were lined by a layer of endocervical mucinous cells and occasionally by tubal cells. These glands proliferated to form buddings but maintained a lobulated pattern.

Some of the glands were cystic. The surrounding stromal tissue was made up of benign smooth muscle cells without notable nuclear atypia or increased mitotic activity (Fig. 9–38A and B).[68b] Carcinoembryonic antigen was present in the cytoplasm of endocervical cells in two of five cases studied.

Of the 30 usual type of uterine adenomyomas reported, three tumors originated from the cervix and the remaining 27 from the uterus. The age of patients ranged from 26 to 64 (mean 47) years. Most patients presented with vaginal bleeding. All three women with cervical adenomyoma had a polypoid nodule visualized near the cervical os. Gross appearance varied from solid to cystic.[68b]

Histologically, endometrial glands are closely associated with endometrial stromal cells and smooth muscle cells (Fig. 9–39A and B). Occasional glands are lined by tubal, endocervical, and/or squamous cells. No mitotic activity was seen in 67% of adenomyomas. However, in the remaining 33% up to five mitotic figures per 10 high-power fields were counted. In adenomyomas, the glandular cells do not demonstrate nuclear atypia.

In contrast, atypical polypoid adenomyoma (APA) contains overcrowded, complex endometrial glands with frequent squamous metaplasia (Fig. 9–40A and B). In addition, moderate to severe nuclear atypia occurs in the glandular cells (see Fig. 9–40C). The second elements are cellular fibrous stroma and

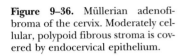

Figure 9–36. Müllerian adenofibroma of the cervix. Moderately cellular, polypoid fibrous stroma is covered by endocervical epithelium.

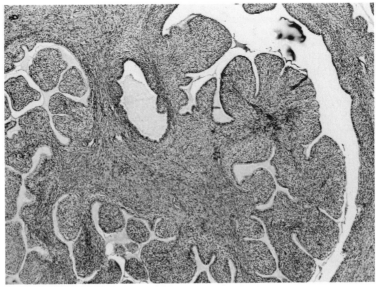

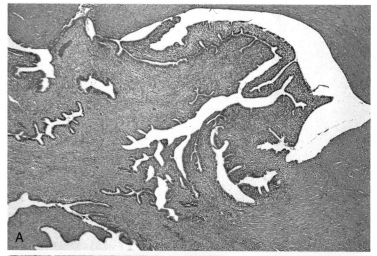

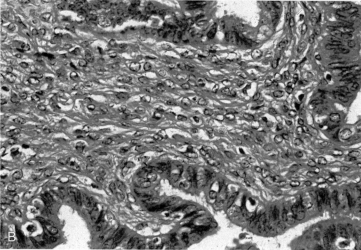

Figure 9–37. Müllerian adenofibroma of the cervix. *A,* Branching papillary glands and moderately cellular fibrous stroma. *B,* Ciliated tubal cells line the glandular space. Fibroblasts reveal mild nuclear atypia but no increase in mitotic activity.

smooth muscle cells (see Fig. 9–40D). The mitotic activity in most cases is low at less than two mitotic figures per 10 high-power fields. In rare cases, this number may increase to five.[109a]

Of the 33 women who underwent hysteroscopic examination, 28 had atypical polypoid adenomyomas described as polypoid lesions, including 16 lesions in the fundus, 11 in the lower uterine segment, and one in the endocervical canal. Three lesions were described as multiple polyps (one case) or a prolapsed polyp from the cervical os (two cases).[109a] Thus, a significant number of atypical polypoid adenomyomas involve the lower uterine segment or cervical canal. The abnormal tissue is often seen in the endometrial curettage specimen

and, less frequently, in endocervical curettage and polypectomy specimens.

Atypical polypoid adenomyoma is a disease of young and premenopausal women with a mean age of 39.9 years.[109a] Some women initially presented with infertility problems and were able to conceive following removal of the tumor, and therefore, it is important not to overdiagnose this tumor as adenocarcinoma; thus, close attention should be paid to the character of the stroma. In the presence of fibromuscular stroma, the possibility of adenomyoma and atypical polypoid adenomyoma should be considered and confirmed by immunohistochemical stains, such as for smooth muscle actin and desmin.

In atypical polypoid adenomyomas contain-

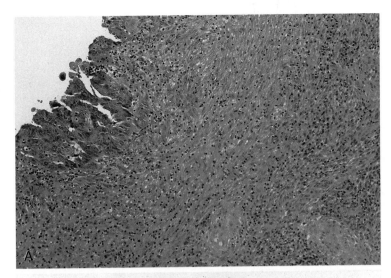

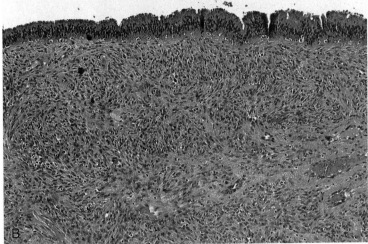

Figure 9–38. Adenomyoma of endocervical type. *A,* Hyperplastic endocervical glands and underlying fibromuscular stroma with chronic inflammation. *B,* Endocervical lining cells and whorls of smooth muscle cells.

ing areas of highly complex glands the term *APA with low malignant potential* is suggested by Longacre et al. to emphasize possible myometrial invasion.[109a] Local excision of atypical polypoid adenomyomas and close follow-up of patients are recommended.[109a]

Müllerian Adenosarcoma

The second group of tumors was initially described and designated by Clement and Scully[31] as müllerian adenosarcoma characterized by benign epithelium but with malignant homologous or heterologous stroma. The atypical stromal cells have a tendency to infiltrate, and usually more than three mitoses per 10 high-power fields are evident.[196]

Adenosarcomas are generally well circumscribed, sessile, polypoid, and sometimes papillary. Of the 24 patients with adenosarcomas of the uterus discussed by Zaloudek and Norris,[196] six (24%) had tumor recurrence locally and four (16%) had metastasis outside the pelvis. Only two adenosarcomas involved the cervix.[196] Both patients were 15 years old and had localized, superficial tumors. No recurrence was noted 4 and 6 years after local excision and trachelectomy, respectively.[196] Several additional cervical adenosarcomas have been reported.[79,155,175]

The growth pattern under low magnification mimics that of cystosarcoma phyllodes of the breast. Papillary and glandular spaces are surrounded and compressed by cellular stroma

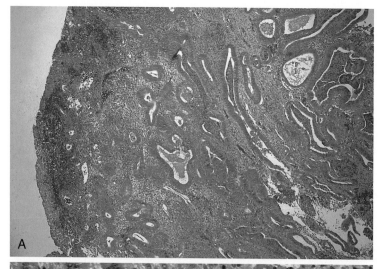

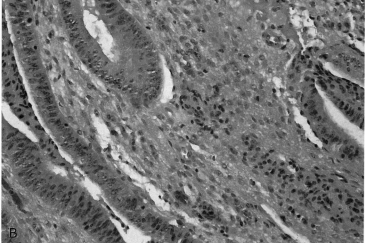

Figure 9–39. Adenomyoma of usual type in the cervix. *A,* Polypoid nodule consists of hyperplastic endometrial glands and fibromuscular stroma. *B,* Higher magnification reveals proliferative endometrial glands and fibromuscular stroma without nuclear atypia.

(Fig. 9–41A and B). Papillary fronds frequently project into cystic spaces or the mucosal surface. The stroma is particularly cellular around the glands (see Fig. 9–41A and B). When the tumor arises from the cervix, the glands are usually lined by endocervical type cells and sometimes undergo squamous metaplasia. The stromal cells usually have the appearance of endometrial stromal cells with moderate or severe nuclear atypia. Heterologous elements may occur. Mitotic activity is increased but is variable from area to area and from tumor to tumor (see Fig. 9–41C).

Morphologic distinction between müllerian adenofibroma and adenosarcoma is sometimes difficult because of the overlap in stromal cellularity and nuclear atypia. Zaloudek and Norris[196] recommend classification as adenosar-coma if the tumor manifests one or more of the following features: (1) four or more mitotic figures per 10 high-power fields, (2) a marked atypia of stromal cells, (3) the presence of malignant heterologous elements, and (4) myometrial invasion. Among these criteria, mitotic activity is most useful.

Jones and Lefkowitz[87] reported on 12 cases of cervical adenosarcoma. Patient age varied from 13 to 67 (mean 37) years. The soft papillary, polypoid mass ranged from 1.5 to 4.5 cm in size. The diagnostic features included a distinct hypercellular zone beneath the mucosal surface and around the glands and increased mitotic activity, with 4 to 28 (mean 7) mitotic figures per 10 high-power fields. One tumor also contained cartilage, and another had rhabdomyosarcoma.

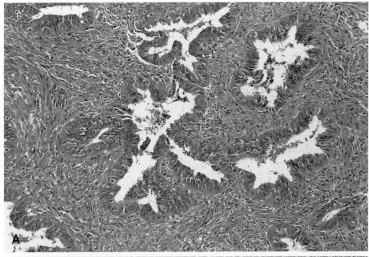

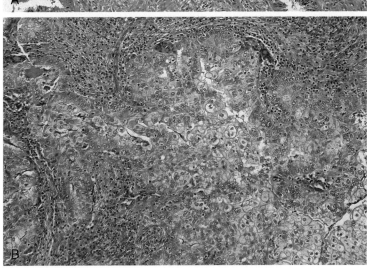

Figure 9–40. Atypical polypoid adenomyoma of cervix. *A,* Branching papillary hyperplastic endometrial glands are surrounded by fibromuscular stroma. *B,* Complex endometrial glands undergo morlues of squamous metaplasia.

At the time of report, nine patients were alive and well, and one died of abdominal metastasis a year after diagnosis. One developed vaginal recurrence 9 months after hysterectomy, which was excised, and the patient was well for 10.8 years. The last woman was lost to follow-up. Overall, the prognosis is favorable, influenced mostly by the depth of myometrial invasion. The treatment options include complete local excision in young women, and hysterectomy and bilateral salpingo-oophorectomy for older patients.[87]

Malignant Mixed Mesodermal Sarcoma

The third group, malignant mixed mesodermal sarcoma, is also the most common and the most malignant. The tumor is composed of both ma-

lignant epithelium and stroma. In addition to cellular anaplasia, the stromal cells have more than 10 mitotic figures per 10 high-power fields. Abell and Ramirez[1] reported on six cases of primary malignant mixed mesodermal sarcoma of the cervix. All the patients died of recurrence or metastasis within 15 months of diagnosis.

Müllerian mixed mesodermal sarcoma involving the cervix is usually secondary to that of the endometrium and presents as a polypoid mass. In biopsy specimens, the tumor may consist largely of rhabdomyosarcoma. This finding in perimenopausal or postmenopausal women should raise the possibility of malignant mixed mesodermal sarcoma of the uterine corpus.

Clement et al.[32] reported on cervical malignant mixed mesodermal sarcoma in nine

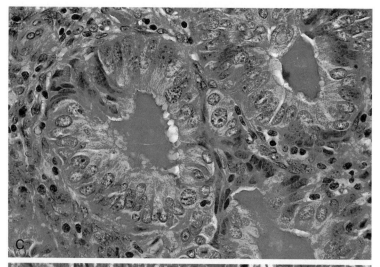

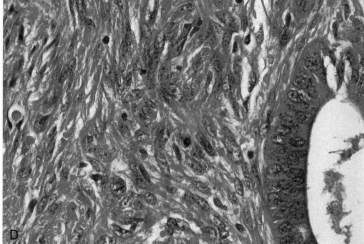

Figure 9–40. *Continued C,* Moderate nuclear atypia of endometrial cells with disorderly nuclear arrangement, uneven distribution of chromatin particles, and small nucleoli. *D,* Smooth muscle cells have plump nuclei and fibrillar cytoplasm.

women 23 to 87 (mean 65) years of age. All presented with visible cervical mass associated with abnormal bleeding or abnormal cervical smear. FIGO stage was IB in seven women and II in one woman. Available follow-up data included that four women were alive and well without disease, and three died of tumor or had tumor recurrence. A review of reported cases also found dismal outcomes, especially following treatment by local excision and radiotherapy.

Unusual features included a wide range of carcinomas, from basaloid carcinoma, squamous cell carcinoma, and adenoid cystic carcinoma to endometrioid and endocervical adenocarcinomas.[32,114] Endometrial stromal sarcoma, fibrosarcoma, and myxoid sarcoma were predominant mesodermal elements. Chon-

drosarcoma and rhabdomyosarcoma occurred in two tumors.[32]

BENIGN AND MALIGNANT NEUROGENIC TUMORS

Neurofibroma and Schwannoma

Benign Schwann cell tumor of the genital tract most often involves the vulva. Neurofibroma is usually superficial, solitary, polypoid, and small, often less than 3 cm. However, giant neurofibromas larger than 20 cm have been reported.[188] Nearly 50% of patients with vulvar neurofibroma have manifestations of von Recklinghausen's disease. In a series of 53 women

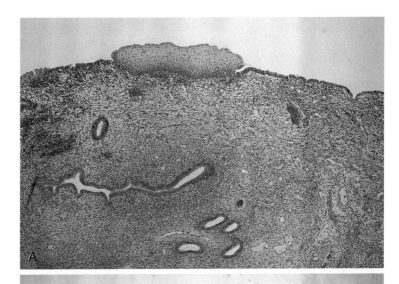

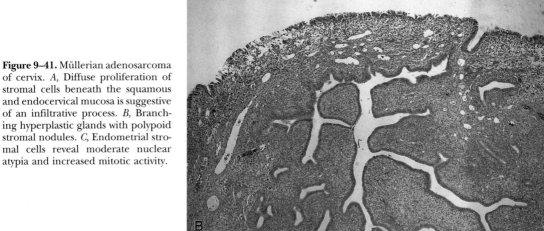

Figure 9–41. Müllerian adenosarcoma of cervix. *A,* Diffuse proliferation of stromal cells beneath the squamous and endocervical mucosa is suggestive of an infiltrative process. *B,* Branching hyperplastic glands with polypoid stromal nodules. *C,* Endometrial stromal cells reveal moderate nuclear atypia and increased mitotic activity.

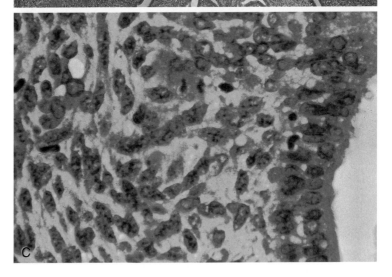

with von Recklinghausen's disease, 18% had vulvar lesions.[161] Schwannoma is encapsulated and situated deep in the soft tissue.[81] Clitoral involvement by neurofibroma or schwannoma may simulate hermaphroditism or adrenogenital syndrome.

Microscopically, neurofibroma has a myxoid stroma and comma-shaped, wavy cells arranged in loose aggregates or bundles. Mast cells are sometimes present. Schwannoma, on the other hand, contains alternating areas of cellular Antoni A and hypocellular, myxoid, sometimes cystic Antoni B. In the former, bundles of Schwann cells demonstrate nuclear palisading. Perivascular hyalinization, accumulation of foamy cells, and hemorrhage are common. Cells with hyperchromatic, pyknotic, irregular nuclei can occur in both neurofibroma and schwannoma. Mitotic activity is rare or absent.

The differential diagnosis includes traumatic neuroma, occurring in the area of trauma or previous surgery. It consists of scar tissue and proliferating nerve fibers, which retain the regular bundle pattern and myelinated nerve sheath. Smooth muscle tumors can be distinguished from Schwann cell tumors by their positive immunoreactivity with desmin and actin but negative response with S-100 protein. Fibrous tumors and fibrous histiocytomas are nonreactive with desmin or S-100 protein. Schwann cells react only with the antibody of S-100 protein and not with desmin.

Granular Cell Tumor (Myoblastoma)

Granular cell tumors have been found in almost every part of the body. Approximately 35% of the tumors involve the head and neck region, 30% occur in the skin and soft parts, and the remaining affect various internal organs.[13] About 7% of all granular cell tumors involve the vulva.[13]

Clinical Features

The majority of vulvar granular cell tumors involve the labium majus and present as a discrete, firm, raised, and usually superficial mass. Involvement of the clitoris may cause priapism.[43,165] The size varies from 1 to 4 cm. The overlying skin tends to be depigmented and sometimes ulcerated. Grossly, the tumor is pale yellow to gray, nonencapsulated, firm, and gritty.

Only rarely are cases of granular cell myoblastomas involving the vagina reported.

Geschicter[67] reported the first myoblastoma of the vagina in 1934, and Koskela[96] reported an additional case in 1964. In the case described by Koskela,[96] a pear-sized mass was identified 2 cm from the urethral meatus in the anterior vaginal wall. This was clinically believed to be a vaginal cyst. The excised well-circumscribed mass primarily consisted of large cells with abundant granular cytoplasm. The nuclei were relatively small. The author concluded that the cyst formation within the tumor was a secondary phenomenon. There was no evidence of recurrence when the patient was examined 3.5 years later.

Microscopic Features

Microscopically, the tumor cells are arranged in bundles, fascicles, cords, or diffuse sheets. The individual cells are polygonal or spindle-shaped. The nuclei are uniformly round or oval and sometimes hyperchromatic (Fig. 9–42). The most distinctive feature is the abundant, granular, eosinophilic cytoplasm that stains bright red with trichrome stain and is reactive with PAS stain. The cell borders are indistinct, and mitotic figures are rare. In two thirds of cases, there is pseudoepitheliomatous hyperplasia of the overlying skin and the rete pegs extend into the underlying tumor (Fig. 9–43). In some cases, the branching and irregularly sized and shaped rete pegs extend as deep as 2.5 mm into the dermis.[13] A superficial biopsy of such lesions may lead to an erroneous diagnosis of squamous cell carcinoma, especially when the skin surface is absent or ulcerated. It is a good practice to look for granular cells in the stroma of a suspected squamous cell carcinoma. The presence of granular cells strongly suggests the possibility of pseudoepitheliomatous hyperplasia coexisting with granular cell tumor.

Histogenesis

Under the electron microscope, the granular cytoplasm corresponds to numerous intracytoplasmic, membrane-bound lysosomes that are electron dense and irregular in shape. The lysosomes frequently become coalescent and form a larger granular mass. Mitochondria are irregular in shape and sometimes degenerated. Myelin figures and whorls of membranes indistinguishable from those found in Schwann cells are present. These ultrastructural features, the presence of basal lamina and long-spacing

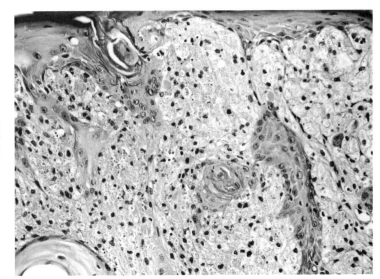

Figure 9–42. Granular cell tumor. The tumor cells contain coarsely granular and eosinophilic cytoplasm. The nuclei are uniform in size and shape.

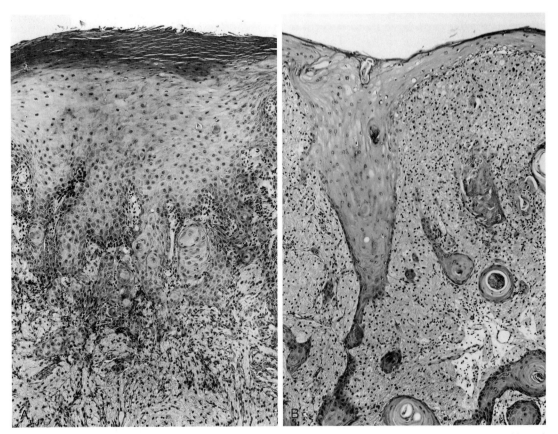

Figure 9–43. Granular cell tumor with pseudoepitheliomatous hyperplasia. Long and irregular rete pegs extend into the dermis as isolated nests and squamous pearls. Note the absence of nuclear atypia in the overlying squamous epithelium.

collagen fibers (Luse bodies), and expression of S-100 protein by immunohistochemistry support a Schwann cell origin.[7,65,168,169]

Prognosis

Most granular cell tumors are benign and do not recur after complete excision. Rarely, the tumor may infiltrate locally.[165] It should be emphasized that about 3% of all granular cell tumors are multicentric in origin[13] and should not be confused with malignant variants.

Malignant Granular Cell Tumor

A review of the literature reveals 26 cases reported as malignant granular cell tumor.[151] Because both benign and malignant granular cell tumors express carcinoembryonic antigen (CEA) by immunohistochemistry, this tumor marker is not useful in separating the two.[151,164] The only reliable criterion is the presence of local invasion or metastasis. Nuclear atypia alone is not a reliable indicator of malignancy.

Three malignant granular cell tumors of the vulva have been reported.[112,151,157] The case reported by Sadler and Dockerty[157] is mostly likely a pleomorphic sarcoma rather than a malignant granular cell tumor. Magori and Szegvari[112] described a 49-year-old woman with metastasis to the regional lymph nodes. The patient was alive 35 months after surgery. Robertson et al.[151] described a 33-year-old patient who had a 3 cm smooth, hard, mobile mass of the right labium majus for 18 years. This was removed by local excision. Four and one-half years later, two of three right inguinal lymph nodes were involved by tumor. In the original tumor, only occasional mitoses were present. There was, however, infiltration of a vein. In the lymph node metastases, numerous mitoses were present.

This author examined a case of malignant granular cell tumor of the vulva with multiple satellite nodules and metastasis to the right inguinal lymph nodes (Fig. 9–44). Although the nucleoli were prominent, no significant nuclear atypia or increase in mitotic activity was noted (see Fig. 9–44). The prognosis of malignant granular cell tumor is poor, with 60% of the patients in reported cases dying from recurrence within a few years of initial treatment.[151]

Paraganglioma

This is a rare tumor of the vagina. In one reported case, the neoplasm measured 3 cm in greatest dimension and occurred in the anterior vaginal wall close to the introitus.[139] The tumor was "shelled out" and found to be composed of cells having a granular cytoplasm. The nuclei were relatively small and somewhat varied in size. Nucleoli were prominent in a few cells. Mitoses were not identified. Argentaffin granules were observed with special stain. Neurosecretory granules were demonstrated by electron microscopy.

Malignant Schwannoma

Five cases of malignant schwannoma have been reported in the vulvar region, including two on the labium majus, one on the labium minus, one in the perianal area, and one in the ischiorectal fossa.[40,47,106] At diagnosis, the ages of the patients were 25, 29, 40, 44, and 45 years, respectively.

The histologic appearance of malignant schwannoma is highly variable, contributing to the difficulty in establishing the diagnosis. In the majority of cases, the tumor cells are arranged in interlacing bundles resembling fibrosarcoma or in a storiform pattern simulating fibrous histiocytoma. The presence of nuclear palisading is a helpful feature for the diagnosis. The tumor is highly cellular, and mitoses are abundant. Rhabdomyoblasts, cartilage, and even glandular epithelium may occur within the malignant schwannoma. Rarely, many of the malignant cells assume the appearance of granular cells, resembling those in granular cell tumor.[153]

Unless there is associated benign neurofibromatous tissue, attachment to major nerves, or clinically known von Recklinghausen's disease, the diagnosis of malignant schwannoma is difficult to establish without immunohistochemical stains. Of the five cases of vulvar malignant schwannomas reported, two had benign neurofibromatous tissue identified histologically, and one had the clinical features of von Recklinghausen's disease. Because of the lack of major nerves in the vulvar region, it may not be possible to demonstrate an origin from peripheral nerves.

Lawrence and Shingleton[106] studied a vulvar malignant schwannoma with the electron mi-

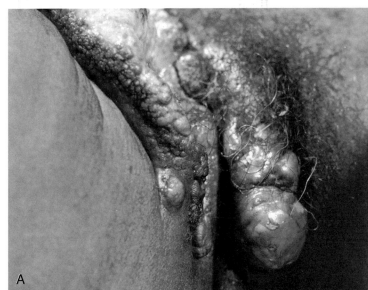

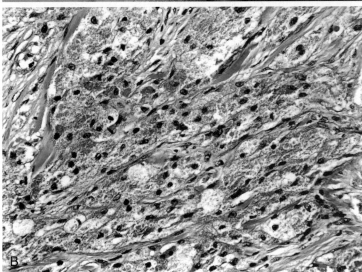

Figure 9–44. Malignant granular cell tumor of the right labium majus. *A,* In addition to the main mass, there are multiple satellite nodules and metastasis to the inguinal lymph nodes. *B,* Bundles of tumor cells contain characteristic granular, eosinophilic cytoplasm. The uniform nuclei have slightly enlarged nuclei and small nucleoli.

croscope. The cells contained abundant mitochondria and rough endoplasmic reticulum and were sometimes arranged in concentric whorls. The cytoplasmic processes were attenuated. Basal lamina was present in focal areas. However, neurofilaments and long-spacing collagen fibrils of so-called Luse bodies, frequently found in benign Schwann cell tumors, were not identified. Similar findings were reported by Taxy et al.[178] In their opinion, ultrastructural findings in malignant schwannoma provided supportive evidence for, rather than constituting specific morphologic features of, a Schwann cell origin. Important ultrastructural findings included basal lamina formation and slender, interdigitating, overlapping cytoplasmic processes occasionally connected with poorly formed tight junctions. The cytoplasmic microfilaments were scant or absent. Electron microscopic study was helpful in confirming the diagnosis of malignant schwannoma in eight of 14 cases.[178] Using the immunoperoxidase technique, only about 50% of malignant schwannomas were positive for S-100 protein.[193]

At the time of the report, four of five women with malignant schwannoma were free of tumor 1, 1.5, 2, and 9 years after radical surgery.

The fifth patient died of multiple pulmonary metastases.[40,47,106]

Keel et al.[93] reported on three cases of malignant schwannoma of the cervix, in women aged 25, 65, and 73 years. The tumors measured 1.3 cm, 4 cm, and 5 cm in size, respectively, and the mass was polypoid and necrotic. Whorls of highly cellular interlacing bundles of spindle cells resembled features of fibrosarcoma with alternating areas of hypocellular myxoid tissue. There were also benign fibromatous areas with spindle cells in a hypocellular, hyalinized stroma. One tumor contained epithelioid cells with round nuclei, prominent nucleoli, and abundant eosinophilic cytoplasm. All three tumors were positive for S-100 protein and vimentin. Stains for cytokeratin, desmin, and melanoma antigen with HMB-45 were all negative. All patients underwent hysterectomy; one developed abdominal and pelvic masses 20 months later. Two recent cases had no follow-up information.[93]

Junge et al.[88] reported a 1.2 cm malignant schwannoma in a 45-year-old woman. The tumor cells were mitotically active, necrotic, and S-100 positive. Sloan[166] reported a case of pigmented malignant schwannoma in a 47-year-old woman, who presented with vaginal bleeding and a 4 cm mass at the os. Tumor cells were mitotically active and locally infiltrative and contained melanin in the cytoplasm.

MELANOCYTIC LESIONS

Hypopigmentation

A decrease in or an absence of pigmentation on the vulvar skin may be the result of inherited disorders, such as vitiligo and albinism, or postinflammatory depigmentation of so-called leukoderma.[58] In vitiligo and partial albinism, the depigmented areas are smooth and well defined. In vitiligo, the melanocytes are decreased in number or completely absent. In albinism, the melanocytes, although normal in appearance and number, fail to produce melanin because of a lack of tyrosinase activity.

Leukoderma involves a temporary loss of pigmentation that is usually secondary to infection, trauma, or ulceration. Candidal and herpetic infections and syphilitic ulcers are common underlying causes.[58] The affected skin is thinner than normal and lacks the normal number of melanocytes.

Pigmented Nevi

Hyperpigmentation of the vulvar skin is most often due to pigmented nevi of various forms. Lentigo simplex is the most common pigmented lesion of the vulva. It is a smooth, dark brown spot measuring 1 to 5 mm in diameter. The epidermis shows elongation of the rete pegs in which melanin pigment and melanocytes are increased in the basal layer. Clinically, the lesion may simulate junctional nevus, but the lack of junctional activity helps to distinguish it from the latter.

Juvenile, junctional, intradermal, and compound nevi occasional occur on the vulva.[23] Most vulvar nevi are of the junctional type.[58] Their histologic appearance is similar to that of nevi found elsewhere in the body. The development of ulceration, change in size or color, or an inflammatory reaction with a collar of erythema should raise the possibility of malignant transformation and justifies excision.[58] During pregnancy, pigmented nevi may become darker and more prominent. Microscopically, active junctional nests, large nucleoli, and increased mitotic activity may occur (Fig. 9–45). Knowledge of pregnancy status is important to avoid overdiagnosis. In irritated or inflamed nevus, a heavy lymphocytic infiltration is present in the dermis. Dysplastic nevus may occur in the vulva (Fig. 9–46A and B) With multiple levels of sectioning, evidence of epidermal or dermal invasion usually becomes apparent in the case of malignant melanoma.

Blue Nevus

Benign pigmented lesions are rarely reported in the vagina. Tobon and Murphy[181] described a blue nevus located in the apex of the vagina. Beneath an intact, stratified, squamous epithelium were irregular groupings of elongated, thin melanocytes with delicate dendritic processes arranged parallel to the basal cell layer. Many of the cells were obscured by melanin pigment. The pigmented cells were separated from the overlying epithelium by a thin band of collagenous connective tissue. Cellular blue nevus has been reported to involve the hymeneal ring, vagina, and cervix.[115]

Blue nevus of the cervix is typically found incidentally in the endocervix of hysterectomy specimens (Fig. 9–47).[137] Rare cases of vulvar blue nevus have been reported to undergo malignant change.[30]

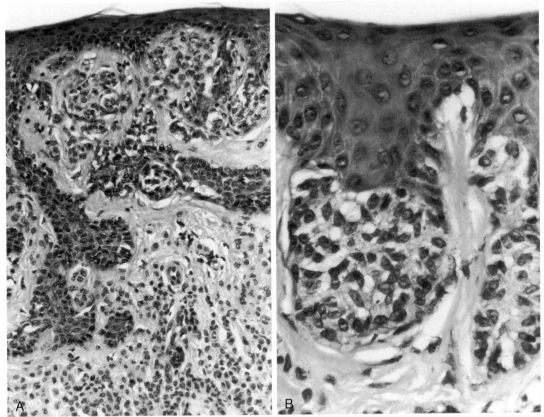

Figure 9–45. *A,* Compound nevus of the vulva in a pregnant woman. The junctional nests of nevus cells appear active and are associated with mild nuclear atypia. *B,* Higher magnification reveals nuclear irregularity and micronucleoli.

Malignant Melanoma

Vulva

Clinical Features

Malignant melanoma of the vulva, constituting 9.8% to 9.9% of all vulvar malignancies and 3.4% of all melanomas in females, is the second most common malignant tumor of the vulva.[30,121,122] It predominantly affects postmenopausal women, with a peak incidence in the sixth to eighth decades of life. Of affected women, 30% are younger than 50 years, including a few in their twenties.[122]

The most common complaints include a mass in the vulvar or inguinal region, bleeding, and pruritus. A few patients note recent changes in pre-existing moles. At the time of detection, the lesions vary from 0.5 to 10 cm in size, with a mean diameter of 2.5 cm.[30] Two thirds of the lesions are pigmented and variously described as black, blue, brown, or gray.[89]

The configuration may be flat, polypoid, nodular, or ulcerated (Fig. 9–48). Melanoma may simulate a urethral caruncle, labial furuncle, Bartholin's gland abscess, hemangioma, or pigmented nevus.[156] The sites of involvement in one series included labia majora (41%), labia minora (34%), clitoris (11%), and more than one site in the remaining 14% of cases.[30] Overall, 55% originated from the squamous mucosa, and 43% originated from hair-bearing skin. The labia minora and clitoris are more commonly involved in other series.[89,122]

Microscopic Features

The majority of the melanomas exhibit atypical melanocytes migrating through the squamous epithelium, as is characteristic of superficial spreading melanoma (Fig. 9–49).[30] Nodular melanoma is less common.[30] Extensive involvement of peripheral nerve fibers, although rare, has been reported.[189]

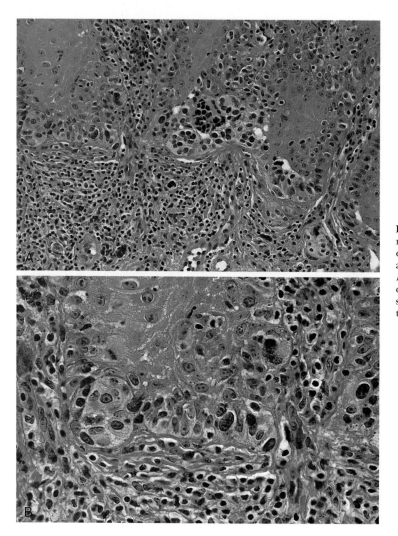

Figure 9–46. Dysplastic junctional nevus. *A,* Nests of atypical nevus cells at junctional location. There is also moderate chronic inflammation. *B,* Higher magnification illustrates nuclear enlargement, irregularity, and small nucleoli. No epidermal migration of atypical cells is seen.

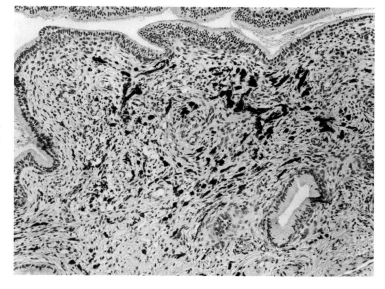

Figure 9–47. Blue nevus of the endocervix. Pigmented, dendritic cells mix with nonpigmented cells.

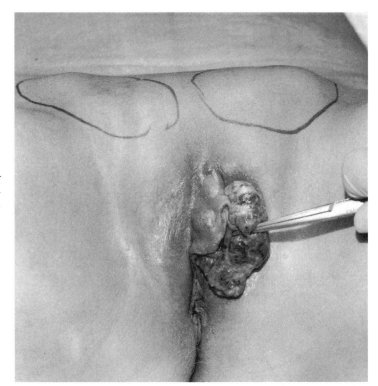

Figure 9–48. Malignant melanoma of the left vulva with metastasis to both inguinal lymph nodes. It is nodular and pigmented in appearance.

In the presence of characteristic epidermal and dermal invasion, the diagnosis of malignant melanoma usually poses no difficulty. The loose cellular aggregates, nuclear pleomorphism, prominent nucleoli, mitoses, and fine melanin pigment further support the diagnosis. Melanoma cells have divergent appearances and may resemble nevoid, epithelioid, small, and spindle cells. Some cells are pleomorphic and bizarre in appearance (Figs. 9–50, 9–51, and 9–52A). Numerous mitoses occur in a majority of cases. Vascular invasion is uncommon. In dealing with an ulcerating and amelanotic melanoma, the differential diagnosis includes squamous cell carcinoma, undifferentiated carcinoma, and some types of sarcoma. A definitive

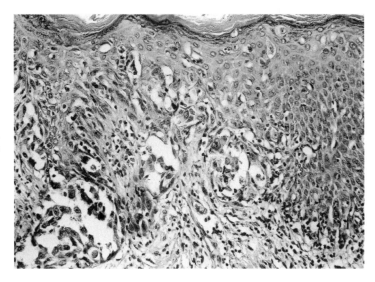

Figure 9–49. Malignant melanoma. Markedly atypical melanocytes proliferate at the junctional positions and migrate through the epidermis.

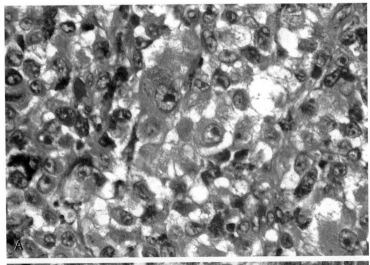

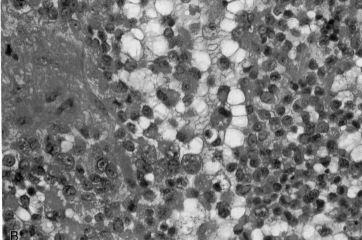

Figure 9–50. Malignant melanoma. *A,* Large round to oval epithelioid cells with abundant melanin pigment. *B,* Loosely cohesive small melanoma cells.

Figure 9–51. Malignant melanoma, spindle cell type. Some cells have vacuolated cytoplasm resembling "balloon" cells.

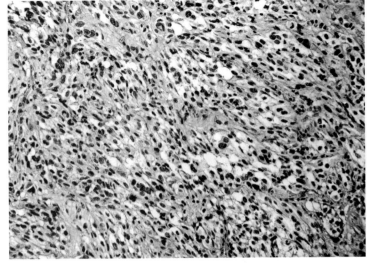

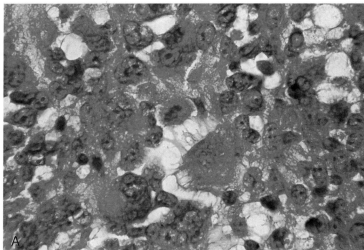

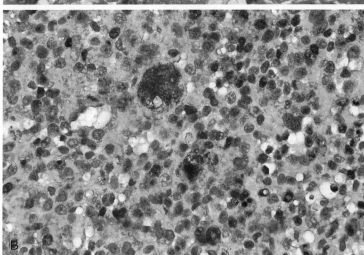

Figure 9–52. Malignant melanoma of vagina. *A,* Highly pleomorphic cells with some resemblance to rhabdomyoblasts. *B,* Immunohistochemical stain for S-100 protein is strongly positive and supports malignant melanoma. (See color section.)

diagnosis is readily made by a positive reaction with S-100 protein and melanoma antigen by immunoperoxidase stains (Fig. 9–52B).

Prognosis

The prognosis for patients with vulvar melanoma strongly correlates with Clark's level and Breslow's tumor thickness.[19] In a series reported by Phillips et al.,[140] 100%, 50%, and 25% of patients with Clark's level II, III, and IV to V invasion, respectively, were free of disease after treatment. All patients with a melanoma less than 0.76 mm in depth had no recurrence of disease, compared with only 33% (four of 12) of patients with a melanoma greater than 1.25 mm in depth.[140]

Because of the lack of a well-defined papillary dermis in the vulvar area, Chung et al.[30] modified the original Clark's classification as follows:

Level II. Tumor thickness of 1 mm or less, as measured from the granular layer or epithelial surface.

Level III. Tumor thickness between 1 mm and 2 mm.

Level IV. Tumor thickness greater than 2 mm but not extending to the fat.

Level V. Extension into the fat.

Using this modified scheme, the mortality rate for vulvar melanoma confined to level II is 0%; for levels III and IV, it is 60%; and for level V, it is 80%.

The size of the lesion is also important. The 5-year survival rate for patients with melanomas less than 2 cm in diameter is 71%, compared with 0% for those with lesions greater than 2 cm in diameter.[89] These findings, however, are based on a relatively small number of cases.

In a detailed analysis of 75 women with vulvar malignant melanoma, the independent prognostic factors include FIGO stage, tumor localization, groin metastasis, tumor thickness, angioinvasion, and DNA ploidy pattern. Scheistroen et al.[159] reported that the 5-year survival rate for women with Stage I disease was 63% and with Stage II was 44%; for patients with Stage III and Stage IV disease, there were no survivals. Women with tumor in the clitoris or multifocal disease have no survivals. In the absence of groin metastasis, the 5-year survival rate was 56% as compared with no survival when the groin lymph node was positive. The 5-year survival rate for tumor thickness up to 1.5 mm was 89%; 1.6 to 5 mm, 55%; and greater than 5 mm, 27%. In the absence of angio-invasion, the 5-year survival rate was 71% as compared with 20% with angio-invasion. The DNA ploidy pattern was closely related to 5-year survival rates, which are 61%, 44%, and 33%, respectively, for women with diploid, tetraploid, and aneuploid tumors.[159]

In a study by Bradgate et al.[18] of 50 women with vulvar melanoma, the significant prognostic factors include clinical stage, patient age, tumor ulceration, cell type, and mitotic rate. Tumor thickness was not of prognostic significance, because the majority of patients in this study had deep melanomas. Women over 65 years of age had a worse prognosis than younger women. The 5-year survival rates were 58% for Stage I disease, 55% for Stage II, and 0% for Stage III and Stage IV disease. Of the 18 women with lymph node metastasis, 17 died in 2 years, and none survived more than 5 years. The 5- and 10-year survival rates without groin or lymph node metastasis were 55% and 35%, respectively. Epithelioid cell melanomas had a worse prognosis than that for spindle cell melanoma and mixed type. When the mitotic activity was low at zero to four mitotic figures per 10 high-power fields, the 5-year survival rate was 57%, as compared with 24% when the mitotic activity was higher.[18]

Of patients undergoing inguinal lymphadenectomy, approximately 50% had histologically confirmed metastasis. In the absence of lymph node metastasis, the 5-year survival rate was 38%, compared with 13% for women with nodal involvement.[30] One of the major problems was the development of recurrent tumor in the local site or regional lymph node in as many as 40% of the cases following definitive surgery.[122] Because of this, most authors propose radical vulvectomy with bilateral inguinal-femoral lymph node dissection as the minimal surgical treatment.

In a review of 157 cases of vulvar melanoma reported in the literature, the absolute 5-year survival rates following radical surgery varied from 14% to 50%, with a mean of 30%.[30] This is comparable to the 5-year survival rate of 34% for patients with cutaneous melanoma of the nongenital region[120] but significantly lower than the 59% survival rate reported for patients with squamous cell carcinoma of the vulva.

Vagina

Melanoma is rare in the vagina.[28,105] In 1980, Chung et al.[29] cited 81 published cases. The neoplasm was observed in women ranging from 37 to 72 years of age. The presenting complaints included vaginal bleeding, vaginal discharge, pelvic pain, or a pelvic mass. The lesions varied in size. The smallest reported by Chung et al.[29] was 0.5 cm in diameter, whereas the largest involved the entire anterior vaginal wall. The lower vagina was the most common site of origin.

Most melanomas are raised above the vaginal surface. The overlying mucosa is denuded or ulcerated. In most cases, lateral spread of melanoma cells is extensive and often beyond the tumor borders. The junctional melanocytes may be lentiginous, or an admixture of pagetoid and lentiginous cells may be present.

Vaginal melanomas have a poor prognosis. The crude 5-year survival rate was 21% in the series reported by Chung et al.[29] Compared with melanomas arising in other sites, vaginal melanoma is less likely to be limited in extent at the time of detection.

Borazjani et al.[17] reported on 10 vaginal melanomas ranging from 1.5 to 5 cm in size. The mean depth was 7.5 mm. The mean survival time was 15 months and the mean period to recurrence was 8 months. Melanomas with a mitotic count of less than six mitotic figures per 10 high-power fields had a better prognosis than those with higher rates.[17]

The preferred treatment is radical surgery. Local recurrence is closely related to the lateral spread of melanoma cells to involve the resection margins (Fig. 9–53A and B).

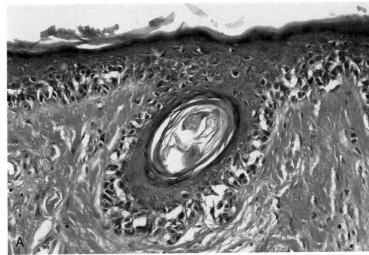

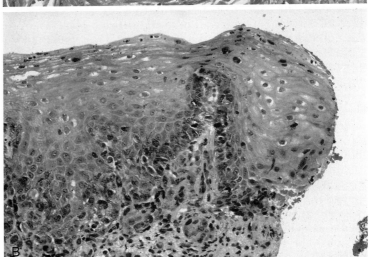

Figure 9–53. Malignant melanoma. *A,* Extensive lateral spread of melanoma cells along the basal cell layer. *B,* Lateral extension of melanoma cells involves the excision margin.

Cervix

In the female genital tract, about 300 primary vulvar, 80 vaginal, and only 12 cervical melanomas have been reported.[73,121] At the time of diagnosis, most patients had an exophytic, polypoid mass that was gray, blue, or black in color. Histologically, the tumor cells resemble poorly differentiated carcinoma. Melanin pigment may be scanty or absent. Junctional activity is present in only 50% of the cases.[86] In the reported cases with adequate follow-up, most patients died 6 months to 14 years following diagnosis. In a literature review by Kristiansen et al.,[98] most patients were found to die of their disease within 3 years of the diagnosis.

OTHER PRIMARY TUMORS

Endodermal Sinus Tumor (Yolk Sac Tumor)

Endodermal sinus tumor occurs primarily in the gonads. In females, about 20 cases of extranodal endodermal sinus tumor have been reported, mostly in the vagina but occasionally in the pelvis, broad ligament, retroperitoneum, maxillary sinus, cervix, and pineal gland. Four tumors involved the vulvar region.[22,49,186]

Ungerleider et al.[186] reported the case of a 14-year-old female who presented with a 4 × 1 cm nodular, indurated mass in the right labium majus. An exploratory laparotomy revealed multicystic ovaries without evidence of malignant tumor on wedge resection. Fallopian tubes, uterus, round ligaments, retroperitoneum, and visceral organs appeared to be normal. The patient underwent radical vulvectomy with unilateral inguinal lymphadenectomy and subsequent whole-pelvis irradiation and chemotherapy with vincristine, actinomycin, and cyclophosphamide. The patient died of widespread metastases 23 months after surgery. Serum alpha-fetoprotein consistently was not detectable.

Castaldo et al.[22] reported on a 2-year-old girl with a 1.2 × 1.5 × 1.0 cm firm, tan nodule involving the entire clitoris. A complete wide local excision was performed. At laparotomy, biopsies of ovaries and pelvic lymph nodes were free of tumor. Serum alpha-fetoprotein was not detectable. The patient was free of disease for 42 months following surgery without adjunctive chemotherapy.

Krisnamurthy and Sampat[97] reported a 7 × 6 cm mass in the left labium majus of a 26-year-old pregnant woman. After local excision, the tumor recurred in the vulva and left inguinal lymph nodes. Despite re-excision, left inguinal node dissection, and adjuvant chemotherapy, the patient died of pleural involvement 11 months later. Dudley et al.[49] described a 6 cm tumor in the right labium majus and ipsilateral femoral lymph node of a 22-month-old girl. She underwent local and pelvic radiotherapy and chemotherapy and subsequently a radical vulvectomy and bilateral groin and pelvic node dissections. The patient died 6 months later with metastasis in the vertebrae. In a case described by Rezaizadeh and Woodruff[148] the neoplasm

filled the upper vagina and was adherent to the lateral vaginal wall. The infant, aged 22 months, died 3 months after therapy.

The histologic appearance of the tumor is similar to that occurring in the gonads. The primitive embryonal cells are arranged in microcystic, tubular, papillary, or reticular pattern (Fig. 9–54). The stroma is sometimes myxomatous. Schiller-Duval bodies, consisting of clusters of cells with a central capillary projection into a microcystic space, are present (Fig. 9–55). Eosinophilic, spherical, hyaline droplets can be found in the cytoplasm and extracellular spaces of most tumors. These hyaline globules are PAS positive and are made up of alpha-fetoprotein and basement membrane material as demonstrated by immunohistochemical stains.[100] Serum alpha-fetoprotein level is a useful marker for the diagnosis and follow-up of patients with germ cell tumors.

The prognosis of endodermal sinus tumor is poor. Less than 10% of patients with ovarian endodermal sinus tumors have lived beyond 24 months following surgery.[186] Three of four patients with vulvar endodermal sinus tumor died of metastatic disease. The only survivor at the time of the report had a small, 1 cm tumor.

Choriocarcinoma

Most choriocarcinomas seen in the cervix represent a direct extension, recurrence, or metastasis from the uterine primary tumor. About 40 primary cervical choriocarcinomas have been reported in Japan.[158,183] The age of the patients

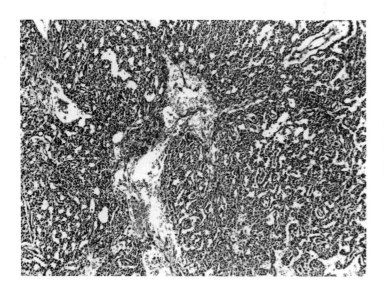

Figure 9–54. Endodermal sinus tumor of the vagina. Tumor cells are arranged in tubular and papillary patterns. (Courtesy of J.D. Woodruff, M.D., Baltimore, Maryland)

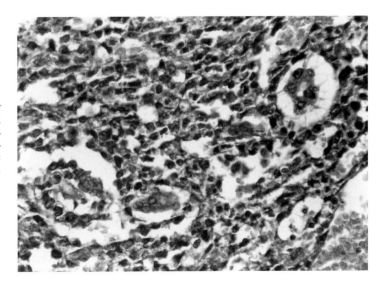

Figure 9–55. Endocervical sinus tumor of the vagina. Primitive embryonal cells form Schiller-Duval bodies, which consist of a cluster of cells with a central capillary core projecting into a microcystic space. (Courtesy of J.D. Woodruff, M.D., Baltimore, Maryland)

varied from 23 to 52 years, with the majority being in their fourth decade of life.[158] Approximately 60% of the patients had a preceding hydatidiform mole, and the remaining patients had term delivery or spontaneous abortion.[158] The suggested mechanisms for the development of primary cervical choriocarcinoma include metastasis from a regressed uterine choriocarcinoma and malignant transformation of cervical pregnancy or misplaced trophoblasts from uterine pregnancy.[3,146]

Most patients with cervical choriocarcinoma present with vaginal bleeding, which is sometimes profuse. The tumor is characterized by soft, nodular, hemorrhagic, necrotic tissue with bizarre blood vessels visible by colposcopy.

Histologically, sheets of pleomorphic cytotrophoblasts and syncytiotrophoblasts without villus formation are present (Fig. 9–56). Necrosis and hemorrhage are prominent. With hysterectomy and chemotherapy, the prognosis is favorable in the absence of disseminated disease.[183]

Ewing's Sarcoma/Primitive Neuroectodermal Tumor (PNET) and Other Tumors

Cenacchi et al.[23] reported on a case of Ewing's sarcoma/PNET in the cervix of a 36-year-old woman. The 7.0 cm cystic, hemorrhagic, necrotic, and well-circumscribed mass ex-

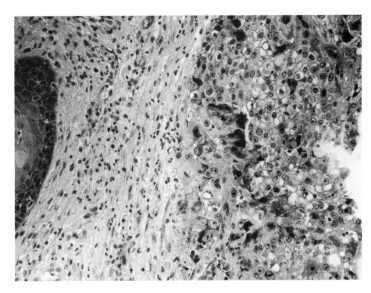

Figure 9–56. Metastatic choriocarcinoma of the cervix. Sheets of cytotrophoblasts and syncytiotrophoblasts without placental villi. (Courtesy of Frank Vellios, M.D., Atlanta, Georgia)

panded the cervix. Sheets of small, round tumor cells contained PAS-positive glycogen and were weakly positive for neuron-specific enolase and surface glycoprotein antigen p30/32 MIC2, supporting the diagnosis of Ewing's sarcoma/PNET.

Benatar et al.[11] reported on a 10 cm polyp protruding from the cervix of an 11-year-old female. The tumor turned out to be an external Wilms' tumor originating from the uterus, nephrogenic blastema tissue, and rhabdomyoblastoma. Extensive recurrence developed in the abdomen 7 months following polypectomy. The authors also reviewed three similar cases reported in the literature. All were teenagers or young adults who had no evidence of disease 2 to 9.6 years following hysterectomy.

Vang et al.[186a] reported on two cases of Ewing's sarcoma/PNET from the vaginal wall of a 35-year-old woman and the vulvar dermis of a 28-year-old female. The diagnosis was further confirmed by the presence of *MIC2* gene, EWS/FL-1 chimeric transcript, and positive immunostain for CD99. Following local excision and chemotherapy/radiotherapy, both patients were free of disease 18 months and 19 months after diagnosis.[186a]

Osteosarcoma of the cervix and uterus most commonly occurs as part of malignant mixed mesodermal sarcoma and adenosarcoma. Rarely, primary osteosarcoma involves the cervix. Bloch et al.[15] reported on such a case associated with hyperplastic and atypical mesonephric rests. The 65-year-old woman presented with vaginal bleeding and was found to have a 3×2 cm necrotic mass attached to the endocervix by a stalk. She was free of disease 23 months following radical hysterectomy and bilateral salpingo-oophorectomy and radiotherapy to the pelvis.

METASTATIC AND SECONDARY TUMORS

Secondary neoplasms of the female genital tract occur by direct extension of the adjacent genital neoplasm, by metastasis from an extragenital site through lymphatic and hematogenous channels, or as peritoneal implants. The first mode of spread most commonly involves the vagina (109 cases, 62%), followed by ovary (30 cases, 17%), and vulva (14 cases, 8%).[115] In contrast, extragenital neoplasms are more likely to involve ovary

(113 cases, 76%), followed by vagina (20 cases, 13%), endometrium (seven cases, 5%), and cervix (five cases, 3%).[115] A more detailed discussion of the individual sites is given in the following sections.

Vulva

In one study, metastatic and secondary tumors of the vulva, constituting 8% of all vulvar malignancies, were the third most frequent group of neoplasms, preceded by invasive squamous carcinoma (51%) and squamous carcinoma in situ (25%).[37] Cervical cancers were the single most frequent primary tumors, followed by cancers of the endometrium, urethra, and kidney.[37] The remaining tumors included malignant lymphoma and cancers of the vagina, ovary, and breast. Overall, 73% were primary tumors of the genital tract and 18% were of the urinary tract. Other authors have reported rare cases of malignant melanoma, choriocarcinoma, neuroblastoma, and carcinomas of the lung, rectum, breast, and stomach that metastasized to the vulva.[37,44]

In a study by Dehner,[44] 46% of the secondary tumors were detected within a year, and 27% were detected more than a year after the diagnosis of the primary tumor. The remaining 27% of the secondary neoplasms were detected concurrently with the primary tumor. The majority of the secondary tumors were solitary (73%), and others were multiple (23%) or diffuse (4%). They occurred most frequently on the labia majora (64%), followed by the clitoris (23%) and labia minora (13%).

Histologically, most metastatic tumors have the same degree of differentiation as that in the primary tumor. Characteristically, metastatic squamous carcinomas are localized to the dermis and subcutis. The intact overlying skin may be helpful in differentiating the neoplasms from primary vulvar squamous carcinoma. Metastatic adenocarcinomas of the endometrium, cervix, kidney, and breast usually involve the epidermis (Figs. 9–57 and 9–58). The most consistent finding is the presence of vascular invasion in all biopsies, regardless of the primary site, suggesting that most vulvar metastases are the result of hematogenous and lymphatic spread.[44] Vulvar metastasis is usually associated with advanced disease and a poor prognosis, with 91% of patients dying of the disease within a year of detection.[44]

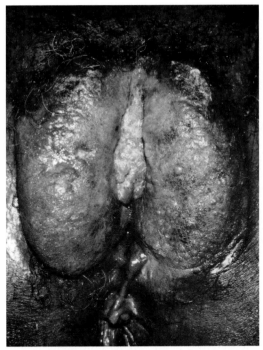

Figure 9–57. Bilateral, diffuse vulvar tumor secondary to adenocarcinoma of the cervix.

Vagina

In a review of 355 invasive carcinomas involving the vagina, only 58 (16%) neoplasms represented primary neoplasia; the remaining 84% were secondary.[77] The most common primary site was the cervix (32%), followed in order of frequency by the endometrium (18%), colon and rectum (9%), ovary (5%), vulva (6%), and urinary bladder and urethra (4%). These tumors reached the vagina by direct extension, local recurrence, or lymphatic spread.[77]

Of the 164 squamous cell carcinomas, 44 (27%) were primary and the remaining 120 (73%) were secondary. Among the latter, 95 (79%) originated from the cervix, 17 (14%), from the vulva, and eight (7%) from both the cervix and the vulva. There were 152 adenocarcinomas, including 12 primary clear cell carcinomas of the vagina. The remaining 140 (92%) were secondary. Of these, 45 (32%) arose from the endometrium, 37 (26%) from the rectum and colon (Fig. 9–59), and 24 (17%) from the ovary.[77] Other, less common tumors included transitional cell carcinoma of the urinary bladder and urethra, malignant mixed mesodermal sarcoma, malignant melanoma, choriocarcinoma, and cloacogenic carcinoma of the anus.

Cervix

Secondary tumors of the uterine cervix most commonly originate from endometrial neoplasms by direct extension. Poorly differentiated adenocarcinoma and adenosquamous carcinoma of the endometrium were prone to involve the cervix, presenting as Stage II cancer. Ovarian and tubal carcinomas may occasionally spread to the cervix.[32] Metastasis to the

Figure 9–58. Same case as in Figure 9–57. Adenocarcinoma beneath the intact squamous epithelium invades the fibrous stroma and vascular lymphatic spaces.

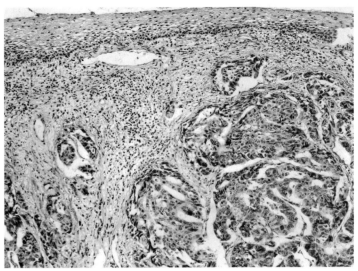

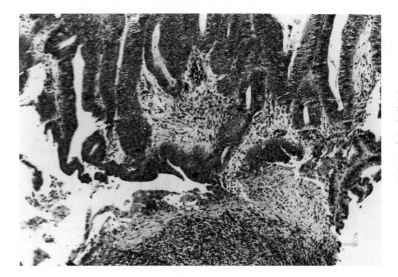

Figure 9–59. This vaginal tumor consists of tall, columnar cells with pseudostratified, picket-fence nuclear arrangement. Some of the cells have vacuolated cytoplasm, suggestive of mucus secretion. The tumor represents local recurrence of colonic carcinoma.

cervix by embolic phenomena is relatively uncommon owing to the low vascularity of the cervical fibromuscular stroma and its centrifugal drainage through lymphatic channels.[107]

Lemoine and Hall[107] reviewed the literature and added 33 new cases to those reported. They accepted 25 gastric, 23 ovarian, 21 colonic, and 14 breast carcinomas as well-documented metastatic tumors to the cervix. Other, less common primary tumors include renal cell carcinoma, transitional cell carcinoma of the renal pelvis and urinary bladder, pancreatic carcinoma, and melanoma of the skin.[107] About 25% of the uterine metastases have no known primary tumors; such occult primary lesions are most likely to be found in the stomach, pancreas, or kidney.[99]

Several cellular and histologic features may aid in localizing the primary tumor. Cellular arrangements in single file and in cords strongly suggest a breast carcinoma (Figs. 9–60A and B and 9–61A). Tumor cells derived from infiltrating lobular carcinoma of the breast often contain intracytoplasmic lumens (Fig. 9–61B). Abundant, clear cytoplasm raises the question of renal cell carcinoma and clear cell adenocarcinoma. Signet-ring cells may derive from the gastrointestinal tract and breast. Columnar-shaped malignant cells with parallel nuclear arrangement favor colonic carcinoma. In dealing with poorly differentiated tumors, immunostains are useful.

In a review of the literature of metastatic breast carcinoma to the cervix, 80% of women had treatment for breast cancer, and of the remaining cases, cervical and breast carcinomas were detected at about the same time.[32,195]

The median interval between the cervical and breast tumors was 1 year, and the longest interval was 9 years. Of women with cervical disease, 90% also had metastasis in the endometrium or myometrium, or both. The metastatic tumor cells frequently had a signet-ring appearance or single-file arrangement. The median survival from the time of detection of cervical metastasis was 12 months.[32,195]

Of the approximately 30 metastatic gastric carcinomas to the cervix, most had the appearance of poorly differentiated signet-ring adenocarcinoma.[32] Of the 22 cases of colonic carcinoma metastatic to the cervix, most were associated with recurrent tumor in the pelvis. The cervical metastasis occurred 3 to 60 months following colectomy.[32]

Immunohistochemical stains for cytokeratin 7 and cytokeratin 20 using monoclonal antibodies are particularly useful in identifying primary tumors.[28] Cytokeratin 7 is expressed by most carcinomas, with the exception of those from the colon, prostate, kidney, and thymus as well as carcinoid tumor and Merkel cell tumor. Most of the squamous cell carcinomas of various sites are negative for cytokeratin 7. An exception is cervical squamous cell carcinoma, which is positive for cytokeratin 7 in 87% of cases. Almost all colorectal carcinomas and Merkel cell tumors express cytokeratin 20. This antigen is also likely to be

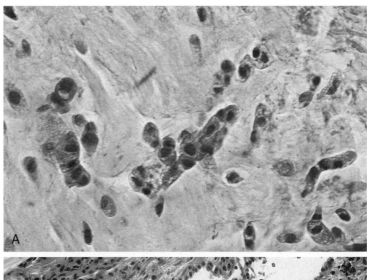

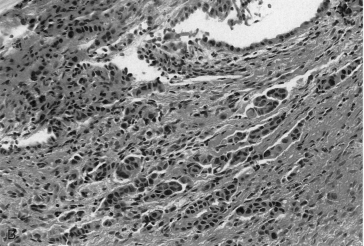

Figure 9–60. Metastatic infiltrating ductal carcinoma of the breast to cervix. *A,* In this endocervical curettage, atypical cells appear in isolated form and cords. These cells have abundant eosino-philic cytoplasm and slightly irregular nuclei without enlargement. In the absence of breast cancer history, these cells can be easily interpreted as reactive endocervical cells. *B,* Cervical biopsy reveals cords and nests of tumor cells invading the endocervix and consistent with breast primary tumor.

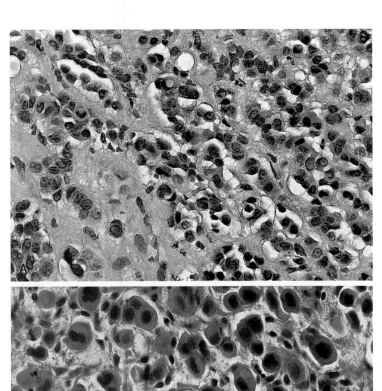

Figure 9–61. Metastatic infiltrating lobular carcinoma of the breast to cervix. *A,* The majority of tumor cells are arranged in single files. *B,* Some tumor cells contain intracytoplasmic lumens.

positive in pancreatic carcinoma, gastric carcinoma, and transitional cell carcinomas of the urinary tract.[28]

REFERENCES

1. Abell MR, Ramirez JAG. Sarcomas and carcinosarcomas of the uterine cervix. Cancer 31:1176, 1973.
2. Abenoza P, Lillemoe T. CD34 and factor VIIIa in the differential diagnosis of dermatofibroma and dermatofibrosarcoma protuberans. Am J Dermatopathol 15:429, 1993.
3. Acosta-Sison H. Apparent metastatic chorioepithelioma without demonstrable primary chorionic malignancy in the uterus. Report of three cases: A new possible explanation of its occurrence. Obstet Gynecol 10:165, 1957.
4. Agress R, Figge DC, Tamimi H, et al. Dermatofibrosarcoma protuberans of the vulva. Gynecol Oncol 16:288, 1983.
5. Andersen P. Extramedullary plasmacytomas. Acta Radiol 32:365, 1949.
6. Appleberg G. Plasmacytoma of the vagina. Acta Radiol 39:83, 1953.
7. Armin A, Connelly E, Rowden G. An immunoperoxidase investigation of S100 protein in granular cell myoblastoma: Evidence of Schwann cell derivation. Am J Clin Pathol 79:37, 1983.
8. Barnett JM, Nickerson CW. Vaginal arterio-venous fistula. Am J Obstet Gynecol 120:197, 1974.
9. Beckstead JH, Wood GS, Turner RR. Histiocytosis X cells and Langerhans' cells: Enzyme histochemical and immunologic similarities. Hum Pathol 15:826, 1984.
10. Begin LR, Clement PB, Kirk ME, et al. Aggressive angiomyxoma of pelvic soft parts: A clinicopathologic study of nine cases. Hum Pathol 16:621, 1985.
11. Benatar B, Wright C, Freinkel AL, Cooper K. Primary extrarenal Wilms' tumor of the uterus presenting as a cervical polyp. Int J Gynecol Pathol 17:277, 1998.
12. Berkowitz RS, Ehrmann RL, Knapp RC. Endometrial stromal sarcoma arising from vaginal endometriosis. Obstet Gynecol 51:348, 1978.
13. Birch HW, Sondag DR. Granular cell myoblastoma of the vulva. Obstet Gynecol 18:443, 1961.
14. Bloustein PA, Silverberg SG, Waddell WR. Epithelioid sarcoma: Case report with ultrastructural review, histogenetic discussion, and chemotherapeutic data. Cancer 38:2390, 1976.
15. Bloch T, Roth LM, Stehman FB, et al. Osteosarcoma of the uterine cervix associated with hyperplastic and atypical mesonephric rests. Cancer 62:1594, 1988.
16. Bock JE, Andreasson B, Thorn A, et al. Dermatofibrosarcoma protuberans of the vulva. Gynecol Oncol 20:129, 1985.
17. Borazjani G, Prem KA, Okagaki T, et al. Primary malignant melanoma of the vagina: A clinicopathologic analysis of 10 cases. Gynecol Oncol 37:264, 1990.
18. Bradgate MG, Rollason TP, McConkey CC, Powell JL. Malignant melanoma of the vulva: A clinicopathologic study of 50 women. Br J Obstet Gynecol 97:124, 1990.
19. Breslow A. Tumor thickness, level of invasion and node dissection in stage I cutaneous melanoma. Am Surg 182:571, 1975.
20. Buscema J, Rosenshein NB, Taqi F, et al. Vaginal hemangiopericytoma: A histopathologic and ultrastructural evaluation. Obstet Gynecol 66:828, 1985.
21. Castaldo E, Meyer I. Solitary and multiple plasma-cell tumors of the jaws and oral cavity. Oral Surg Oral Med Oral Pathol 22:628, 1966.
22. Castaldo TS, Petrilli ES, Ballon SC, et al. Endodermal sinus of the clitoris. Gynecol Oncol 9:376, 1980.
23. Cenacchi G, Pasquinelli G, Montanaro L, et al. Primary endocervical extraosseous Ewing's sarcoma/PNET. Int J Gynecol Pathol 17:83, 1998.
24. Ceremsak RJ. Benign rhabdomyoma of the vagina. Am J Clin Pathol 52:604, 1969.
25. Chase DR, Weiss SW, Enzinger FM, et al. Keratin in epithelioid sarcoma. Am J Surg Pathol 8:435, 1984.
26. Chorlton I, Karnei RF, King FM, et al. Primary malignant reticuloendothelial disease involving the vagina, cervix and corpus uteri. Obstet Gynecol 44:735, 1974.
27. Christopherson, WM, Foote FW Jr, Stewart F. Alveolar soft part sarcomas: Structurally characteristic tumors of uncertain histogenesis. Cancer 5:100, 1952.
28. Chu P, Wu E, Weiss LM. Cytokeratin 7 and cytokeratin 20 expression in epithelial neoplasms: A survey of 435 cases. Mod Pathol 13:962, 2000.
29. Chung AF, Casey MJ, Flannery JT, et al. Malignant melanoma of the vagina: Report of 19 cases. Obstet Gynecol 55:720, 1980.
30. Chung AF, Woodrugg JM, Lewis JL Jr. Malignant melanoma of the vulva: A report of 44 cases. Obstet Gynecol 45:638, 1975.
31. Clement PB, Scully RE. Müllerian adenosarcoma of the uterus: A clinicopathologic analysis of ten cases of a distinct type of müllerian mixed tumor. Cancer 34:1138, 1974.
32. Clement PB. Miscellaneous primary tumors and metastatic tumors of the uterine cervix. Semin Diagn Pathol 7:228, 1990.
33. Clement PB, Zubovits JT, Young RH, Schully RE. Malignant mullerian mixed tumor of the uterine cervix: A report of nine cases of a neoplasm with morphology often different from its counterpart in the corpus. Int J Gynecol Pathol 17:211, 1998.
34. Copeland LJ, Gershenson DM, Saul PB, et al. Sarcoma botryoides of the female genital tract. Obstet Gynecol 66:262, 1985.
35. Copeland LJ, Sneige N, Strainger CA, et al. Alveolar rhabdomyosarcoma of the female genitalia. Cancer 56:849, 1985.
36. Corson JM, Pinkus GS. Intracellular myoglobin—a specific marker for skeletal muscle differentiation in soft tissue sarcomas: An immunoperoxidase study. Am J Pathol 103:384, 1981.
37. Covington EE, Brendle WK. Breast carcinoma with vulvar metastasis. Obstet Gynecol 23:910, 1964.
38. Craig JM, Castleman B. Case records of MGH: Eosinophilic granuloma of the vulva. N Engl J Med 282:862, 1970.
39. Davis, I, Abell MR. Sarcomas of the vagina. Obstet Gynecol 47:342, 1976.
40. Davis I, Abell MR. Soft tissue sarcoma of the vulva. Gynecol Oncol 4:70, 1976.
41. Daya DA, Scully RE. Sarcoma botryoides of the uterine cervix in young women: A clinicopathological study of 13 cases. Gynecol Oncol 29:290, 1988.

42. De MN, Tribede BP. Skeletal muscle tissue tumor. Br J Surg 28:17, 1940.

43. Degefu S, Dhurandhar N, O'Quinn AG, et al. Granular cell tumor of the clitoris in pregnancy. Gynecol Oncol 19:246, 1984.

44. Dehner LP. Metastatic and secondary tumors of the vulva. Obstet Gynecol 42:47, 1973.

45. Delaini G. Considerazion: Anatomo-cliniche su di un eccezionale reperto di rabdomioma della vagina. Ateneo Parmense (Acta Biomed) 2–7:341, 1956.

46. DeSousa LM, Lash AF. Hemangiopericytoma of the vulva. Am J Obstet Gynecol 78:295, 1959.

47. DiSaia PJ, Rutledge F, Smith JP. Sarcoma of the vulva: Report of 12 patients. Obstet Gynecol 38:1802, 1971.

48. Doss LL. Simultaneous extramedullary plasmacytomas of the vagina and vulva: A case report and review of the literature. Cancer 41:2468, 1978.

49. Dudley AG, Young RH, Lawrence WD, et al. Endodermal sinus tumor of the vulva in an infant. Obstet Gynecol 61:768, 1983.

50. Enzinger FM. Epithelioid sarcoma, a sarcoma simulating a granuloma or carcinoma. Cancer 26:1029, 1970.

51. Enzinger FM, Weiss SW. Soft Tissue Tumors. St. Louis, C.V. Mosby, 1983.

52. Ewing MR, Foote FW Jr. Plasma cell tumors of the mouth and upper air passages. Cancer 5:499, 1952.

53. Ferry JA, Young RH. Malignant lymphoma, pseudolymphoma, and hematopoietic disorders of the female genital tract. Pathol Ann 26(part I):227, 1991.

54. Fetsch JF, Laskin WB, Lefkowitz M, et al. Aggressive angiomyxoma: A clinicopathologic study of 29 female patients. Cancer 78:79, 1996.

55. Fetsch JF, Laskin WB, Tavassoli FA. Superficial angiomyxoma (cutaneous myxoma): A clinicopathologic study of 17 cases arising in the genital region. Int J Gynecol Pathol 16:325, 1997.

56. Fisher ER, Horvat B. The fibrocystic origin of so-called epithelioid sarcoma. Cancer 30:1074, 1972.

57. Fletcher CDM, Tsang WYW, Fisher C, et al. Angiomyofibroblastoma of the vulva: A benign neoplasm distinct from aggressive angiomyxoma. Am J Surg Pathol 16:373, 1992.

58. Friedrich EG Jr. Vulvar Disease. Philadelphia, W.B. Saunders, 1976.

59. Fruhling L, Chadli A. Le sarcome plasmacytaire extrasquelettique. Ann Anat Pathol (Paris) 8:317, 1963.

60. Fu YS, Gabbiani G, Kaye GI, et al. Malignant soft tissue tumors of probable histiocytic origin (malignant fibrous histiocytoma), general consideration and electron microscopic and tissue culture studies. Cancer 35:176, 1975.

61. Gabbiani G, Fu YS, Kaye GI, et al. Epithelioid sarcoma: A light and electron microscopic study suggesting a synovial origin. Cancer 30:486, 1972.

62. Gad A, Eusebi V. Rhabdomyoma of the vagina. J Pathol 115:179. 1975.

63. Gaffney EF, Majmudar B, Bryan JA. Nodular fasciitis (pseudosarcomatous fasciitis) of the vulva. Int J Gynecol Pathol 1:307, 1982.

64. Gallup DG, Abell MR, Morley G. Epithelioid sarcoma of the vulva. Obstet Gynecol 48:14S, 1976.

65. Garancis JC, Komorowski RA, Kuzma JF. Granular cell myoblastoma. Cancer 25:542, 1970.

66. Gardner HL, Kaufman RJ. Benign Diseases of the Vulva and Vagina, 2nd ed. Boston, G.K. Hall, 1981.

67. Geschicter CF. Tumors of muscle. Am J Cancer 22:378, 1934.

68. Ghorbani RP, Malpica A, Ayala AG. Dermatofibrosarcoma protuberans of the vulva: Clinicopathologic and immunohistochemical analysis of four cases, one with fibrosarcomatous change, and review of literature. Int J Gynecol Pathol 18:366, 1999.

68a. Gilks CB, Clement PB, Hart WR, Young RH. Uterine adenomyomas excluding atypical polypoid adenomyomas and adenomyomas of endocervical type. Int J Gynecol Pathol 19:195, 2000.

68b. Gilks CB, Young RH, Clement PB, et al. Adenomyomas of the uterine cervix of endocervical type. Mod Pathol 9:220, 1996.

69. Gold JH, Bossen EH. Benign vaginal rhabdomyoma: A light and electron microscopy study. Cancer 27:2283, 1976.

70. Granter SR, Nucci MR, Fletcher CDM. Aggressive angiomyxoma: Reappraisal of its relationship to angiomyofibroblastoma in a series of 13 cases. Histopathology 30:3, 1997.

71. Grayson W, Fourie J, Tiltman AJ. Xanthomatous leiomyosarcoma of the uterine cervix. Int J Gynecol Pathol 17:89, 1998.

72. Hall D, Grimes MM, Goplerud DR. Epithelioid sarcoma of the vulva. Gynecol Oncol 9:237, 1980.

73. Hall DJ, Schneider V, Goplerud DR. Primary malignant melanoma of the uterine cervix. Obstet Gynecol 56:525, 1980.

74. Harris NL, Scully RE. Malignant lymphoma and granulocytic sarcoma of the uterus and vagina. Cancer 53:2530, 1984.

75. Hart WR, Craig JR. Rhabdomyosarcoma of the uterus. Am J Clin Pathol 70:217, 1978.

76. Hensley FT, Friedrich EG. Malignant fibroxanthoma: A sarcoma of the vulva. Am J Obstet Gynecol 116:289, 1973.

77. Hilborne LH, Fu YS. Intraepithelial, invasive and metastatic neoplasms of the vagina. In: Wilkinson EJ (ed). Pathology of the Vulva and Vagina. New York, Churchill Livingstone, 1987, pp 181–207.

78. Hilgers RD, Malkasian FD, Jr, Soule EH. Embryonal rhabdomyosarcoma (botryoid type) of the vagina. Am J Obstet Gynecol 107:484, 1970.

79. Hirschfield L, Kahn LB, Chen S, et al. Müllerian adenosarcoma with ovarian sex cord-like differentiation: A light- and electron-microscopic study. Cancer 57:1197, 1986.

80. Hiura M, Nagai N. Vaginal hemangiopericytoma: A light microscopic and ultrastructural study. Gynecol Oncol 21:376, 1985.

81. Huang HJ, Yamabe T, Tagawa H. A solitary neurilemmoma of the clitoris. Gynecol Oncol 15:103, 1983.

82. Huey GR, Stehman FB, Roth LM, et al. Lymphangiosarcoma of the edematous thigh after radiation therapy for carcinoma of the vulva. Gynecol Oncol 20:394, 1985.

83. Hulagu C, Erez S. Juvenile melanoma of clitoris. J Obstet Gynecol Br Comm 80:89, 1973.

84. Imperial R, Helwig EB. Angiokeratoma of the vulva. Obstet Gynecol 29:307, 1967.

85. Issa PY, Salem PA, Brihi E, et al. Eosinophilic granuloma with involvement of the female genitalia. Am J Obstet Gynecol 137:608, 1980.

86. Jones HW, Droegemuller W, Makowski EL. A primary melanocarcinoma of the cervix. Am J Obstet Gynecol 111:959, 1971.

87. Jones MW, Lefkowitz M. Adenosarcoma of the uterine cervix: A clinicopathological study of 12 cases. Int J Gynecol Pathol 14:223, 1995.

88. Junge J, Horn T, Bock J. Primary malignant schwannoma of the uterine cervix. Br J Obstet Gynecol 96:111, 1989.

89. Karlen JR, Piver MS, Barlow JJ. Melanoma of the vulva. Obstet Gynecol 45:181, 1975.

90. Kasai K, Yoshida Y, Okmura M. Alveolar soft part sarcoma in the vagina; clinical features and morphology. Gynecol Oncol 9:227, 1980.

91. Katz VI, Askin FB, Bosch BD. Glomus tumor of the vulva: A case report. Obstet Gynecol 67:435S, 1986.

92. Kaufman RH, Gardner HL. Tumors of vulva and vagina: Benign mesodermal tumors. Clin Obstet Gynecol 8:953, 1965.

93. Keel SB, Clement PB, Prat J, Young RH. Malignant schwannoma of the uterine cervix: A study of three cases. Int J Gynecol Pathol 17:223, 1998.

94. Kempson RL, Sherman A. Sclerosing lipogranuloma of the vulva. Am J Obstet Gynecol 101:854, 1968.

95. Kohorn EI, Merino MJ, Goldenhersh M. Vulvar pain and dyspareunia due to glomus tumor. Obstet Gynecol 67:41S, 1986.

96. Koskela O. Granular cell myoblastoma of the vagina. Ann Chir Gynaec Fenn 53:270, 1964.

97. Krishnamurthy SC, Sampat MB. Endodermal sinus (yolk sac) tumor of the vulva in a pregnant female. Gynecol Oncol 11:379, 1981.

98. Kristiansen SB, Anderson R, Cohen DM. Primary malignant melanoma of the cervix and review of the literature. Gynecol Oncol 47:398, 1992.

99. Kumar NB, Hart WR. Metastases to the uterine corpus from extragenital cancers: A clinicopathologic study of 63 cases. Cancer 50:2163, 1982.

100. Kurman RJ, Scardino PT, McIntire KR, et al. Cellular localization of alpha-fetoprotein and human chorionic gonadotropin in germ cell tumors of the testis using an indirect immunoperoxidase technique. Cancer 40:2136, 1977.

101. Kyriakos M, Kempson RL. Inflammatory fibrous histiocytoma, an aggressive and lethal lesion. Cancer 37:1584, 1976.

102. Lane N, Lattes R, Malm J. Clinicopathological correlation in a series of 117 malignant melanomas of the skin of adults. Cancer 11:1025, 1958.

103. LaPolla J, Foucar E, Leshin B, et al. Vulvar lymphangioma circumscriptum: A rare complication of therapy for squamous cell carcinoma of the cervix. Gynecol Oncol 22:363, 1985.

104. Laskin WB, Fetsch JF, Mostofi FK. Angiomyofibroblastoma-like tumor of the male genital tract. Am J Surg Pathol 22:6, 1998.

105. Laufe LE, Bernstein ED. Primary malignant melanoma of the vagina. Obstet Gynecol 37:148, 1971.

106. Lawrence WD, Shingleton HM. Malignant schwannoma of the vulva: A light and electron microscopic study. Gynecol Oncol 6:527, 1978.

107. Lemoine NR, Hall PA. Epithelial tumors metastatic to the uterine cervix. Cancer 57:2002, 1986.

108. Leone PB, Taylor HB. Ultrastructure of a benign polypoid rhabdomyoma of the vagina. Cancer 31:1414, 1973.

109. Levene M. Congenital retinoblastoma and sarcoma botryoides of the vagina. Cancer 13:532, 1960.

109a. Longacre TA, Chung MH, Rouse RV, Hendrickson MR. Atypical polypoid adenofibroma (atypical polypoid adenomyoma) of the uterus: A clinicopathologic study of 55 cases. Am J Surg Pathol 20:1, 1996.

110. Lovelady SB, McDonald JR, Waugh JM. Benign tumors of the vulva. Am J Obstet Gynecol 42:309, 1941.

111. Maddox JC, Evans HL. Angiosarcoma of skin and soft tissue. Cancer 48:1907, 1981.

112. Magori Von A, Szegvari M. Rezidivierender und metastasierender Abrikossoff-Tumor der Vulva. Zeutbl Pathol Pathol Anat 117:265, 1973.

113. Malkasian GD, Welch JS, Soule EM. Primary leiomyosarcoma of the vagina. Am J Obstet Gynecol 86:730, 1963.

114. Mathoulin-Portier M, Penault-Llorca F, Labit-Bouvier C, et al. Malignant mullerian mixed tumor of the uterine cervix with adenoid cystic component. Int J Gynecol Pathol 17:91, 1998.

115. Mazur MT, Hsueh W, Gersell DJ. Metastases to the female genital tract: Analysis of 325 cases. Cancer 53:1978, 1984.

116. Mentzel T, Beham A, Katenkamp D, et al. Fibrosarcomatous (high grade) dermato-fibrosarcoma protuberans: Clinicopathologic and immunohistochemical study of a series of 41 cases with emphasis on prognostic significance. Am J Surg Pathol 22:576, 1998.

117. Miodovnik M, Adatto R, Adoni A, et al. Vulvar eosinophilic granuloma. Acta Obstet Gynecol Scand 58:565, 1979.

118. Molenaar WM, DeJong B, Dam-Meiring A, et al. Epithelioid sarcoma or malignant rhabdoid tumor of soft tissue? Epithelioid immunophenotype and rhabdoid karyotype. Hum Pathol 20:347, 1989.

119. Morales AR, Fine G, Horn RJ Jr. Langerhans' granules in a localized lesion of the eosinophilic granuloma type. Lab Invest 20:412, 1969.

120. Morales AR, Fine G, Horn RC Jr. Rhabdomyosarcoma: An ultrastructural appraisal. In: Sommers SC (ed). Pathology Annual, vol 7, Norwalk, Conn., Appleton-Century-Crofts, 1972, p 81.

121. Morrow CP, DiSaia PJ. Malignant melanoma of the female genitalia: A clinical analysis. Obstet Gynecol Surg 31:233, 1976.

122. Morrow CP, Rutledge F. Melanoma of the vulva. Obstet Gynecol 39:745, 1972.

123. Mukai K, Varela-Duran J, Nomchovitz E. The rhabdomyoblast in mixed mullerian tumors of the uterus and ovary: An immunohistochemical study of myoglobin in 25 cases. Am J Clin Pathol 74:101, 1980.

124. Nielsen GP, Oliva E, Young RH, et al. Alveolar soft part sarcoma of the female genital tract: A report of nine cases and review of the literature. Int J Gynecol Pathol 14:283, 1995.

125. Nielsen GP, Rosenberg AE, Koerner FC, et al. Smooth-muscle tumors of the vulva: A clinicopathologic study of 25 cases and review of the literature. Am J Surg Pathol 20:779, 1996.

126. Nielsen GP, Young RH, Dickersin FR, Rosenberg AE. Angiomyofibroblastoma of the vulva with sarcomatous transformation ("angiomyofibrosarcoma"). Am J Surg Pathol 21:1104, 1997.

127. Nucci MR, Granter SR, Fletcher CDM. Cellular angiofibroma: A benign neoplasm distinct from angiomyo-fibroblastoma and spindle cell lipoma. Am J Surg Pathol 21:636, 1997.

128. Nucci MR, Fletcher CDM. Liposarcoma (atypical lipomatous tumors) of the vulva. Int J Gynecol Pathol 17:17, 1998.

129. Ober WB, Edgecomb JH. Sarcoma botryoides in female genital tract. Cancer 7:75, 1954.
130. Ober WB, Palmer RE, Glassy FJ. Rhabdomyosarcoma of the vulva and vagina. Arch Pathol 56:364, 1953.
131. Ober WB, Smith JA, Rouillard FC. Congenital sarcoma botryoides of vagina: Report of 2 cases. Cancer 11:620, 1958.
132. O'Connell JX, Young RH, Nielsen GP, et al. Nodular fasciitis of the vulva: A study of six cases and literature review. Int J Gynecol Pathol 16:117, 1997.
133. Oliva E, Ferry JA, Young RH, et al. Granulocytic sarcoma of the female genital tract: A clinicopathologic study of 11 cases. Am J Surg Pathol 21:1156, 1997.
134. Ozzello L, Stout AP, Murray MR. Cultural characteristics of malignant histiocytomas and fibrous xanthomas. Cancer 16:331, 1963.
135. Pack GT, Oropeza R. A comparative study of melanoma and epidermoid carcinoma of the vulva: A review of 44 melanomas and 58 epidermoid carcinomas (1920–1965). Rev Surg 24:305, 1968.
136. Patchefsky A, Soriano R, Kostianovsky M. Epithelioid sarcoma: Ultrastructural similarity to nodular synovitis. Cancer 39:143, 1977.
137. Patel DS, Shagavan BS. Blue nevus of the uterine cervix. Human Pathol 16:79, 1985.
138. Perrone T, Swanson PE, Twigg L, et al. Malignant rhabdoid tumor of the vulva: Is distinction from epithelioid sarcoma possible? Am J Surg Pathol 13:848, 1989.
139. Pezeshkpour G. Solitary paraganglioma of the vagina—report of a case. Am J Obstet Gynecol 14:80, 1982.
140. Phillips GL, Twiggs LB, Okagaki T. Vulvar melanoma: A microstaging study. Gynecol Oncol 14:80, 1982.
141. Pinkston JA, Sekine I. Postirradiation sarcoma (malignant fibrous histiocytoma) following cervical cancer. Cancer 49:434, 1982.
142. Piver MS, Tsukada GY, Barlow J. Epithelioid sarcoma of the vulva. Obstet Gynecol 40:839, 1972.
143. Popoff NA, Malinin TI. Cytoplasmic tubular arrays in cells of American Burkitt's lymphoma. Cancer 37:275, 1976.
144. Prat J, Woodruff JM, Marcove RL. Epithelioid sarcoma: An analysis of 22 cases indicating the prognostic significance of vascular invasion and regional lymph node metastases. Cancer 41:1472, 1978.
145. Proppe KH, Scully RE, Rosai J. Postoperative spindle cell nodules of genitourinary tract resembling sarcomas: A report of eight cases. Am J Surg Pathol 8:101, 1984.
146. Rashbaum M, Daub WW, Lisa JR. Primary cervical choriocarcinoma. Am J Obstet Gynecol 64:451, 1952.
147. Reymond RD, Hazra TA, Edlow DW, et al. Haemangiopericytoma of the vulva with metastasis to bone 14 years later. Br J Radiol 45:765, 1972.
148. Rezaizadeh MM, Woodruff JD. Endodermal sinus tumor of the vagina. Gynecol Oncol 6:459, 1978.
149. Rio F. Considerazioni su un raro caso di plasmocitoma della vagina. Arch Ital Pathol Clin Tumori 1:321, 1957.
150. Roberts W, Daly JW. Pseudosarcomatous fasciitis of the vulva. Gynecol Oncol 11:383, 1981.
151. Robertson AJ, McIntosh W, Lamont P, et al. Malignant granular cell tumor (myoblastoma) of the vulva: Report of a case and review of the literature. Histopathology 5:69, 1981.
152. Rodriguez HA, Ackerman LV. Cellular blue nevus: Clinicopathologic study of 45 cases. Cancer 21:393, 1968.
153. Rose PG, Johnston GC, O'Toole RV. Pure cutaneous histiocytosis X of the vulva. Obstet Gynecol 64:587, 1984.
154. Rosenberg SA, Diamond HD, Craver LF. Lymphosarcoma: The effects of therapy and survival in 1,269 patients in a review of 30 years experience. Ann Intern Med 53:877, 1960.
155. Roth LM, Pride GL, Sharma HM. Müllerian adenosarcoma of the uterine cervix with heterologous elements. Cancer 37:1725, 1976.
156. Rutledge FN. Malignant melanoma of the vulva. In: Neoplasms of the Skin and Malignant Melanoma. Chicago, Year Book Medical Publishers, 1976, p 401.
157. Sadler WP, Dockerty MG. Malignant myoblastoma vulvae. Am J Obstet Gynecol 6:1047, 1951.
158. Saito M. Axuma T, Nakamura K, et al. On ectopic choriocarcinoma. World Obstet Gynecol 17:459, 1965.
159. Scheistroen M, Trope C, Koern J, et al. Malignant melanoma of the vulva: Evaluation of prognostic factors with emphasis on DNA ploidy in 75 patients. Cancer 75:72, 1995.
160. Schram M. Leiomyosarcoma of vagina: Report of a case and review of the literature. Obstet Gynecol 17:459, 1965.
161. Schreiber MM. Vulvar von Recklinghausen's disease. Arch Dermatol 88:3202, 1963.
162. Shen JT, D'Áblaing G, Morrow CP. Alveolar soft part sarcoma of the vulva: Report of a case and review of literature. Gynecol Oncol 13:120, 1982.
163. Shimamura K, Osmura Y, Ueyama Y, et al. Malignant granular cell tumor of right sciatic nerve. Cancer 53:524, 1984.
164. Shousha S, Lyssiotis T. Granular cell myoblastoma: Positive staining for carcino-embryonic antigen. J Clin Pathol 32:219, 1979.
165. Slavin RE, Christie JD, Swedo J, et al. Locally aggressive granular cell tumor causing priapism of the crus of the clitoris. Am J Surg Pathol 10:497, 1986.
166. Sloan D. Diagnosis of a tumor with an unusual presentation in the pelvis. Am J Obstet Gynecol 159:826, 1988.
167. Snover DC, Phillips G, Dehner LP. Reactive fibrohistiocytic proliferation simulating fibrous histiocytoma. Am J Clin Pathol 76:232, 1981.
168. Sobel HJ, Marquet E. Granular cells and granular cell lesions. In: Sommers SC (ed). Pathology Annual, vol 9. Norwalk, Conn., Appleton-Century-Crofts, 1974, p 43.
169. Sobel HJ, Marquet E, Schwarz R. Is schwannoma related to granular cell myoblastoma? Arch Pathol 95:396, 1973.
170. Soltan MH. Dermatofibrosarcoma protuberans of the vulva: Case report. Br J Obstet Gynecol 88:203, 1981.
171. Spitzer M, Molho L, Seltzer VI, et al. Vaginal glomus tumor: Case presentation and ultrastructural findings. Obstet Gynecol 66:86S, 1985.
172. Steeper TA, Piscioli F, Rosai J. Squamous cell carcinoma with sarcoma-like stroma of the female genital tract: Clinicopathologic study of four cases. Cancer 52:890, 1983.
173. Steeper TA, Rosai J. Aggressive angiomyxoma of the female pelvis and perineum. Am J Surg Pathol 7:463, 1983.

174. Talerman A. Sarcoma botryoides presenting as a polyp on the labium majus. Cancer 32:994, 1973.

175. Tang C-K, Toker C, Harriman B. Müllerian adenosarcoma of the uterine cervix. Human Pathol 12:579, 1981.

176. Tavassoli FA, Norris HJ. Smooth muscle tumors of the vagina. Obstet Gynecol 53:689, 1979.

177. Tavassoli FA, Norris HJ. Smooth muscle tumor of the vulva. Obstet Gynecol 53:213, 1979.

178. Taxy JB, Battifora H, Trujillo Y, et al. Electron microscopy in the diagnosis of malignant schwannoma. Cancer 48:1381, 1981.

179. Taylor RN, Bottles K, Miller TR, et al. Malignant fibrous histiocytoma of the vulva. Obstet Gynecol 66:145, 1985.

180. Tiltman AJ. Leiomyomas of the uterine cervix: A study of frequency. Int J Gynecol Pathol 17:231, 1998.

181. Tobon H, Murphy AI. Benign blue nevus of the vagina. Cancer 40:3174, 1977.

182. Tobon H, Murphy AI, Salazar H. Primary leiomyosarcoma of the vagina: Light and electron microscopic observations. Cancer 32:450, 1973.

183. Tsukamoto N, Nakamura M, Kashimura M, et al. Primary cervical choriocarcinoma. Gynecol Oncol 9:99, 1980.

184. Ulbright TM, Kraus FT. Endometrial stromal tumors of extra-uterine tissue. Am J Clin Pathol 76:371, 1981.

185. Ulbright TM, Brokaw SA, Stehman FB, et al. Epithelioid sarcoma of the vulva: Evidence suggesting a more aggressive behavior than extra-genital epithelioid sarcoma. Cancer 52:1462, 1983.

186. Ungerleider RS, Donaldson SS, Warnke RA, et al. Endodermal sinus tumor: The Stanford experience and the first reported case arising in the vulva. Cancer 41:1627, 1978.

186a. Vang R, Taubenberger JK, Mannion CM, et al. Primary vulvar and vaginal extraosseous Ewing's sarcoma/primitive neuroectodermal tumor: Diagnostic confirmation with CD99 immunostaining and reverse transcriptase–polymerase chain reaction. Int J Gynecol Pathol 19:103, 2000.

187. Vellios F, Ng ABP, Reagan JW. Papillary adenofibroma of the uterus: A benign mesodermal mixed tumor of müllerian origin. Am J Clin Pathol 60:543, 1973.

188. Venter PF, Rohm GF, Slabber CF. Giant neurofibromas of the labia. Obstet Gynecol 57:128, 1981.

189. Warner TF, Hafez GR, Buchler DA. Neurotropic melanoma of the vulva. Cancer 49:000, 1982.

190. Webb, MJ, Symmonds RE, Weiland LH. Malignant fibrous histiocytoma of vagina. Am J Obstet Gynecol 119:190, 1974.

191. Weiss SW, Enzinger FM. Myxoid variant of malignant fibrous histiocytoma. Cancer 39:1672, 1977.

192. Weiss SW, Enzinger FM. Malignant fibrous histiocytoma, an analysis of 200 cases. Cancer 41:2250, 1978.

193. Weiss SW, Enzinger FM. Spindle cell hemangioendothelioma: A low-grade angiosarcoma resembling a cavernous hemangioma and Kaposi's sarcoma. Am J Surg Pathol 11:521, 1986.

194. Young RH, Harris NL, Scully RE. Lymphoma-like lesions of the lower female genital tract: A report of 16 cases. Int J Gynecol Pathol 4:289, 1985.

195. Yzogi R, Sandstad J, Munoz AK. Breast cancer metastasizing to the uterine cervix. Cancer 61:2558, 1988.

196. Zaloudek CJ, Norris HJ. Adenofibroma and adenosarcoma of the uterus: A clinicopathologic study of 35 cases. Cancer 48:354, 1981.

197. Zinkham WH. Multifocal eosinophilic granuloma: Natural history, etiology and management. Am J Med 60:457, 1976.

INDEX

Note: Page numbers followed by the letter f refer to figures; those followed by the letter t refer to tables.